CLINICAL LABORATORY MEDICINE

CLINICAL
LABORATORY MEDICINE

Clinical Application of Laboratory Data

RICHARD RAVEL, M.D.

Director of Laboratories, St. Mary Hospital, Quincy, Illinois

THIRD EDITION

YEAR BOOK MEDICAL PUBLISHERS, INC.

Chicago • London

Reprinted, November 1969
Reprinted, September 1970
Reprinted, February 1972
Second Edition, 1973
Reprinted, April 1974
Reprinted, December 1974
Reprinted, January 1976
Third Edition, 1978

Library of Congress Catalog Card Number: 77-77386

International Standard Book Number: 0-8151-7096-3

Preface to Third Edition

CONTINUED CHANGE in the repertoire of the clinical laboratory necessitates a new edition. As in previous editions, the aim is to provide as much useful information as possible which may assist the understanding, selection and interpretation of laboratory tests. A new chapter has been added for serum level monitoring of therapeutic drugs. The chapters covering endocrine tests have been rewritten. Many other areas had to be revised. New tests have been added: for example, aminoglycoside serum level, amylase clearance/creatinine clearance ratio in pancreatitis, beta-subunit of hCG in tumor diagnosis, CPK isoenzymes, DNA antibody in rheumatoid-collagen disorders, estrogen receptor assay, ferritin assay, parathyroid hormone assay, prolactin assay, thyrotropin-releasing factor test, tumor-seeking radiopharmaceuticals, urine myoglobin and uroporphyrinogen-I-synthetase assay in acute intermittent porphyria. As far as possible, everything has been brought up to date. As in previous editions, information on nuclear medicine procedures has been incorporated; and now some data on ultrasound and on computerized axial tomography are included.

A major problem has been the fact that while new tests continue to be announced and new information about standard procedures must be recorded, out-of-date tests refuse to disappear from clinical use. Data on these tests have been retained in this edition, although frequently relocated. In the future it may be necessary simply to list the test and provide one or two references.

RICHARD RAVEL

Preface to First Edition

THE CLINICAL LABORATORY has a major role in modern medicine. A bewildering array of laboratory procedures is available, each of which has its special usefulness and its intrinsic problems, its advantages and its drawbacks. Advances in biochemistry and radioisotopes, to name only two conspicuous examples, are continually adding new tests or modifying older methods toward·new usefulness. It seems strange, therefore, that medical education has too often failed to grant laboratory medicine the same prominence and concern that are allotted to other subjects. If ever a comprehensive, systematic and critical teaching system were needed, it is for this complex and heterogeneous topic. It would seem that if one were to consider ordering any laboratory procedure, several things should be known about that test, including:

1. In what situations is the test diagnostic, and in what situations does the test provide information without being diagnostic?

2. What commonly available tests give similar information, and when should one be used in preference to the others?

3. What are the disadvantages of the test and possibilities of error or false results?

The fact that this type of information is not adequately disseminated is quickly brought home to a clinical pathologist, who supervises the clinical laboratory and at the same time acts as liaison to clinicians on laboratory problems. It becomes quickly evident in two ways—the continually rising number of laboratory procedure requests and even a casual inspection of patients' hospital charts. Unnecessary tests represent severe financial and personal inconvenience to the patient; inappropriate tests or tests done under improper conditions mean wasted or misleading information, and often a loss of precious time.

In laboratory medicine, textbooks are available, as in all areas of general medicine considered detailed enough to warrant a specialty status. These fall into two groups: those mainly for the technician and those designed for clinicians. Technician-oriented books necessarily stress the technical aspects of individual tests, with emphasis on cookbook methodology. Textbooks for the clinician vary considerably in approach. Some excellent works concentrate almost exclusively on one subject or subspecialty, such as hematology. Many others combine technician methodology with discussion to varying degrees of the clinical aspects of tests. The latter aspect often suffers due to inevitable limitations imposed by mere length. Some texts which emphasize the clinical approach may be criticized on the grounds that they neglect either adequate attention to possible limitations

vii

and sources of error in each particular laboratory procedure, or fail to delineate the background or the technical aspects of the tests enough to provide a clear picture as to just what information the test actually can provide.

This volume attempts to meet these criticisms. Its aim is to provide enough technical and clinical information about each laboratory procedure included so as to allow adequate understanding, selection and interpretation of these procedures. Many of the laboratory tests require varying amounts of individual discussion. Others are noted in the context of the diseases in which they may be useful. In addition, most of the common diseases in which laboratory tests render significant assistance are briefly outlined, and the role of the laboratory in each is explained. Also included are a considerable number of diseases or conditions which are uncommon or even rare, but which may be considered important from various points of view — either as well-known entities, diagnostic problems or cases which may benefit from early diagnosis and therapy.

There is a great temptation for a work of this type to become encyclopedic. Brevity and succinctness are preserved, therefore, at some cost, hopefully with more gain than loss. Probably the most striking examples are the chapters on infectious diseases and parasitology. In most cases, description of clinical syndromes and specific organisms has been eliminated or markedly reduced, because this book is not intended to be a treatise on internal medicine. Emphasis is on material which seems more directly concerned with selection and interpretation of laboratory tests. Nevertheless, a few diseases (such as leptospirosis) are important from the standpoint of laboratory diagnosis because their signs and symptoms mimic other conditions, so the clinical findings are included in some detail. On the other hand, syphilis serology has a chapter to itself due to confusion which surrounds the multiplicity of available tests. Likewise, certain subjects are discussed at unusual length. These are topics which, in my experience, seem to be common problem areas. The aim is to provide a reasonably thorough, yet compact, survey of laboratory medicine. This book is meant to provide some area of assistance to anyone who is engaged in clinical medicine, and to provide, in a sense, a reasonably comprehensive course in clinical pathology.

It is anticipated that the style and format of this book may be criticized; either because the uninitiated reader might gain an impression that laboratory medicine can be reduced to a relatively few rules or protocols, or that one approach to diagnosis is presented as though all others were invalid. Such inferences are not intended.

It should be obvious that no person could write a book covering clinical pathology entirely from his own experience. On the other hand, adequate citation of references would be a tremendous undertaking in itself. A compromise is therefore offered. At the ends of the chapters there are lists of suggested readings, composed of selected references which include textbooks with general or specific coverage, papers on certain specific subjects and occasionally an article selected because of an unusually inclusive bibliography. Due to spare considerations, those references with more than two authors have been listed in the first author's name only. This book is only a beginning; the reader is urged to consult these papers and others on individual subjects in order to broaden the information presented here, and to evaluate contrasting points of view.

An Appendix is provided, in order to include certain information which is useful but which seemed better presented separately from the regular text. Much of this is in tabular form.

I wish to express my deep appreciation to the following members of the University of Miami Medical School faculty, and to several others, who critically reviewed portions of the manuscript and made many valuable suggestions:

J. Walter Beck, Ph.D., Associate Professor of Pathology, Department of Parasitology.

George W. Douglas, Jr., M.D., Chief, Microbiology Section, Communicable Disease Center, U.S. Public Health Service.

N. Joel Ehrenkranz, M.D., Professor of Medicine, Division of Infectious Diseases.

Mary J. Harbour, M.D., Instructor, Department of Radiology.

Martin H. Kalser, M.D., Ph.D., Professor of Medicine, Division of Gastroenterology.

Robert B. Katims, M.D., Assistant Professor of Medicine, Department of Endocrinology.

Howard E. Lessner, M.D., Associate Professor of Medicine, Division of Hematology.

Joel B. Mann, M.D., Assistant Professor of Medicine, Division of Renal Disease and Endocrinology.

Leslie C. Norins, M.D., Chief, Venereal Disease Research Laboratory, Communicable Disease Center, U.S. Public Health Service.

William L. Nyhan, M.D., Ph.D., Professor of Pediatrics.

John A. Stewart, M.D., Assistant Chief, Virology Section, Communicable Disease Center, U.S. Public Health Service.

Thomas B. Turner, M.D., Director, John Elliot Blood Bank, Miami, Fla.

Table of Contents

1 / Basic Hematologic Tests and Classification of Anemia

HEMATOLOGY is the study of the blood, the cellular elements of the blood and the metabolic processes by which the blood components are formed. The major emphasis in hematology is given to the three cellular elements of the blood—red cells, white cells and platelets—the plasma proteins, electrolytes, fluid and other constituents being covered elsewhere in this book. Each of the three cellular elements will be discussed separately for reasons of convenience.

MAJOR HEMATOLOGIC TESTS

There are several tests that form the backbone of laboratory diagnosis in hematology.

Hemoglobin (Hb)

This is the oxygen-carrying compound contained in red cells. Hemoglobin can be measured chemically, and the amount of Hb/100 ml of blood can be used as an index of the oxygen-carrying capacity of the blood. Total blood Hb depends mostly on the number of RBC (the Hb carriers) but also (to a much lesser extent) on the amount of Hb in each RBC. A low hemoglobin level thus indicates anemia. Depending on the method used and the care with which the laboratory checks its spectrophotometers, hemoglobin values are accurate to 2–3%. Older methods (Sahli) used a chemical technique in which the final compound was compared visually against a colored glass standard; at best, this gives 2–3 times the average error of methods using a good spectrophotometer.

Normal values are most frequently quoted as 14–18 gm/100 ml for males and 12–16 gm/100 ml for females (grams/100 ml is often abbreviated gm% or gm/dl). Some reports indicate lower values, expecially in women, so that it is probably better not to consider a patient anemic until Hb is less than 13 gm in males and 11 gm in females. Infants have different normal limits (p. 477). In addition, several investigators found a significant decrease in Hb (up to 1.0 gm) when one sample was obtained after some time in the upright position followed by another specimen after overnight bed rest. Finally, there is some evidence that heavy smokers have slightly increased Hb concentration (0.5 gm or more) compared to nonsmokers.

RBC Count

The number of RBC per cu mm gives an indirect estimate of the hemoglobin content of the blood. Blood cell counting chamber (hemocytometer) methods give average errors of 4–8%, or even more – depending on the experience of the technician. Automatic counting machines reduce this error to about 2–4%. However, many smaller laboratories do not have these machines. Normal values are 4.5–6.0 million/cu mm for males and 4.0–5.5 million/cu mm for females.

Hematocrit (HCT)

After centrifugation, the height of the red cell column is measured and compared with the height of the original whole blood. The percentage of red cell mass to original blood volume is the hematocrit. Anticoagulated whole blood is centrifuged in a special tube. Since whole blood is made up essentially of RBC and plasma, after centrifugation the percentage of packed red cells gives an indirect estimate of the number of RBC/100 ml of whole blood (and thus, in turn, is an indirect estimate of the amount of hemoglobin). Hematocrit thus depends mostly on the number of RBC, but there is some effect (to a much lesser extent) from the average size of the RBC. Normal values are 40–54% for males and 37–47% for females. The HCT is usually about three times the hemoglobin value (assuming no marked hypochromia). The average error in HCT procedures is about 1–2%. Microhematocrits are generally as accurate as the older standard Wintrobe (macrohematocrit) technique. The HCT may be changed by position and heavy smoking in the same manner as Hb is changed.

Indices (Wintrobe Indices)

Wintrobe introduced a very useful method to demonstrate certain characteristics of red cells.

MEAN CORPUSCULAR VOLUME (MCV). – This concept utilizes the effect that the average size of the RBC has on the HCT. If the average RBC size is increased, the same number of RBC will have a slightly larger cell mass and thus a slightly increased HCT reading; the opposite happens if the average RBC size is smaller than normal. The MCV is therefore calculated from the HCT and RBC count as follows:

$$\frac{HCT \times 10}{^*RBC\ count} = MCV \quad \text{(HCT in \%; RBC in millions/cu mm*; MCV in cubic microns [cu } \mu\text{])}$$

Normal values are 87 ± 5 cu μ (manual) and 90 ± 10 cu μ (Coulter Counter). Heavy smoking may increase MCV as much as 3 cu μ.

MEAN CORPUSCULAR HEMOGLOBIN (MCH). – This concept gives an estimate of the amount of hemoglobin in the average red cell; this is done by comparing the blood Hb level to the RBC count as follows:

$$\frac{Hb \times 10}{^*RBC\ count} = MCH \quad \text{(Hb in gm/100 ml; RBC in millions/cu mm*; MCH in micromicrograms [} \mu\ \mu\text{g])}$$

Normal values are $29 \pm 2\mu\ \mu$ (manual) and $30 \pm 4\mu\ \mu$ (Coulter Counter).

MEAN CORPUSCULAR HEMOGLOBIN CONCENTRATION (MCHC). – This

---

*Use the number of millions rather than the actual count; e.g., 4,560,000 = 4.56 million.

concept estimates the average concentration of hemoglobin in the average RBC. It differs from MCH in that the average RBC concentration of Hb depends on RBC size as well as on the actual amount of Hb contained in the RBC. MCHC is calculated as follows:

$$\frac{Hb \times 100}{HCT} = MCHC \qquad \text{(Hb in gm/100 ml; HCT in \%; MCHC in \%)}$$

Normal values are 34 ± 2% (manual) and 34 ± 3% (Coulter Counter).

Several factors should be mentioned.

1. As an index of red cell hemoglobin, the MCHC is often more reliable than the MCH, since the MCHC does not incorporate the relatively inaccurate RBC count procedures. It is true that macrocytic or microcytic (larger or smaller than normal) RBC will alter the MCHC independently of the hemoglobin values. However, in those diseases where there is significant overall macrocytosis or microcytosis, the RBC counts of the blood are changed (decreased) in addition to the changes in average RBC size. Since HCT depends on the number of RBC more than on average RBC size, the decrease in RBC number more than compensates for the relatively small effect that RBC size has on the HCT. Therefore, in most clinical situations, alterations in average RBC size alone do not affect the MCHC significantly.

2. The various indices are affected only by *average* cell measurements, either of size or of quantity of hemoglobin. This is especially noticeable in the indices dependent on average RBC size (MCV and, to some extent, MCHC). There may be considerable variation in size between individual red cells (anisocytosis), but the indices do not show this, since they take into account only the average size.

3. Examination of a well-made peripheral blood smear will give most of the same information as the indices. Indices are not a substitute for examination of the peripheral blood smear, but they may be helpful in confirming equivocal cases. Indices are only as accurate as the various counts and procedures (plus calculation) that went into their preparation.

Examination of Wright-Stained Peripheral Blood Smear

This procedure gives a vast amount of information. It allows visual estimation of the amount of hemoglobin in RBC and the overall size of RBC. In addition, alterations in size, shape and structure of individual red cells (p. 37) or white cells are visible, which may have diagnostic significance in certain diseases. Pathologic early forms of the blood cells are also visible. Finally, a good estimate of the platelet count can be made in most cases from the peripheral smear alone.

The peripheral smear is the most useful laboratory procedure in hematology. There obviously are many limitations; for example, a peripheral smear cannot demonstrate the presence of anemia per se, which must be detected by means of either the Hb, HCT or RBC count. Also, many etiologies of anemia show peripheral blood changes that are nonspecific. In some cases in which the peripheral smear is highly suggestive, it may not be so in early stages of the disease. Even if characteristic cell changes are present, there may be different underlying causes for the same morphologic type of anemia, different causes that call for different treatment. Finally, there are some conditions that produce anemia without any demonstrable morphologic changes in the RBC of the peripheral smear. The same comments about RBC may, in general, also be applied to the white cells of the peripheral smear. However, it is often possible to predict leukocytosis by comparing the overall visual ratio of WBC to RBC. A differential count of the various WBC forms is done from the peripheral smear.

Reticulocyte Count

Reticulocytes occupy an intermediate position between nucleated RBC in the bone marrow and mature (nonnucleated fully hemoglobinated) RBC. After the normoblast (metarubricyte) nucleus is extruded from the cell, some remnants of nuclear material remain for a short time. It is possible to stain this material using vital staining techniques and dyes such as methylene blue or cresyl blue. The material then is seen microscopically in the form of dark blue dots arranged in loose aggregates or reticulum. The reticulocyte count is an index of the production of mature red cells by the blood-forming organs, mostly the bone marrow. Increased reticulocyte counts mean an increased number of RBC being put into the peripheral blood in response to some stimulus. In exceptionally great reticulocyte responses, there may even be nucleated RBC pushed out into the peripheral blood due to massive red cell production activity of the bone marrow. Except in a very few diseases, such as erythroblastosis, peripheral blood nucleated RBC are usually few in number and of later maturity stage when they do appear. Reticulocytes are not completely mature RBC; therefore, when reticulocytes appear in the peripheral blood they may be slightly larger than normal RBC. This may give a slightly macrocytic MCV and show macrocytes on peripheral smear. Also, reticulocytes may sometimes have a slightly bluish (basophilic) tinge with Wright's stain (although this often does not occur); this phenomenon is called polychromatophilia, and results because the reticulocyte is not yet a mature RBC, and therefore does not have a full complement of (reddish-staining) hemoglobin.

Some authorities advocate correcting the reticulocyte count by the number of RBC to differentiate a true increase in reticulocyte production from a situation in which reticulocyte quantity is unchanged but RBC number is decreased. This may be done by multiplying the reticulocyte (%) count by the quotient of patient HCT divided by average normal HCT (47 for men and 42 for women). Alternatively, one can obtain the absolute number of reticulocytes by multiplying the reticulocyte count (%) by the RBC count.

WBC Count

This may be done using either a hemocytometer or machine (such as the Coulter Counter). The error produced by hemocytometer counts is about 4–8%, but may be higher with inexperienced personnel. Coulter counts have approximately 2–4% error. The machine has the disadvantage that WBC counts over 100,000/cu mm become increasingly inaccurate unless a dilution is used. In addition, some of the abnormal lymphocytes of lymphocytic leukemia are unusually fragile and may be destroyed when the specimen is prepared for a machine count, thus giving a false low value. With either hemocytometer or machine, nucleated RBC are counted as WBC, so a correction has to be made on the basis of the percentage of nucleated RBC (to 100 WBC) found on the peripheral smear.

Normal values are most often quoted as 5,000–10,000/cu mm. Several studies suggest that 4,500–11,000 would be more correct. However, there is a significant overlap of normal and abnormal between 4,500–5,000 and 10,000–11,000, especially the latter area. There is some evidence that normal range for blacks may be at least 500/cu mm lower than normal range for whites. Alterations in WBC levels are discussed in Chapter 5.

Platelet Count

The usual procedure that employs a hemocytometer counting chamber and a standard microscope has approximately a 10–20% error. A somewhat similar method that makes use of a phase contrast microscope has a reported error of about 8%. Platelet counting machines can reduce the error even further. Normal values are 150,000–300,000/cu mm for direct counts.

Bone Marrow Aspiration

Bone marrow aspiration is of help in several situations: (1) to demonstrate the diagnosis of megaloblastic anemia; (2) to establish the diagnosis of leukemia or multiple myeloma; (3) to show whether deficiency of one or more of the peripheral blood cellular elements is due to a deficiency in the bone marrow precursors (bone marrow hypoplasia); (4) to document a deficiency in body iron stores in certain cases of suspected iron-deficiency anemia; (5) in certain selected cases, to demonstrate metastatic neoplasm or some types of infectious disease (culture or histologic sections may be preferred to routine Wright-stained smears).

These nine procedures are the basic tests of hematology. Intelligent selection and interpretation of these procedures usually can go far toward solving the vast majority of hematologic problems. Other tests may be ordered to confirm or rule out a diagnosis suggested by the results of preliminary study. These other tests will be discussed in association with the diseases in which they are useful.

However, once again, certain points should be made. Laboratory tests in hematology are no different from any other laboratory tests. Two or more tests that give essentially the same information in any particular situation should not be ordered. For example, it is rarely necessary to order Hb, HCT and RBC count all together unless indices are needed. As a matter of fact, either the Hb or the HCT is usually sufficient, although, initially, the two are often ordered together as a check on each other. (As it is the least accurate, the RBC count is rarely helpful.) Both the WBC count and differential are usually done initially. If both are normal, there usually is no need to repeat the differential count if the (total) WBC count remains normal and there are no morphologic abnormalities of the RBC and WBC.

Another point to be stressed is the proper collection of specimens. The timing of collection is sometimes extremely important. Transfusion therapy may cause a megaloblastic bone marrow to lose its diagnostic megaloblastic features, sometimes in as little as 12 hours. On the other hand, transfusion will not affect a bone marrow that has no iron. Capillary blood (finger puncture) is best for making peripheral blood smears, because oxalate anticoagulant causes marked artifacts in WBC morphology and even will slightly alter the RBC. EDTA anticoagulant will cause a false decrease in HCT (Hb is not affected) if the amount of blood collected is less than half the proper volume (for the amount of EDTA in the tube). When capillary (fingerstick) blood is used to make HCT, Hb or cell counts, too much squeezing of the finger or other poor technique may result in dilution of the blood by tissue juice and give falsely low values. On the other hand, dehydration may result in hemoconcentration and produce falsely high values. This may mask an anemia actually present, or, when the patient is properly hydrated, a repeat determination may give the false impression of a sudden drop in values, such as might otherwise come from an acute bleeding episode. If very severe, hemoconcentration may simulate polycythemia.

ANEMIA – CLASSIFICATION

Although anemia may be defined as a decrease in hemoglobin concentration, it may result from a pathologic decrease in the red cell count. Since mature RBC are fully saturated with hemoglobin, such a decrease means that total blood hemoglobin will also be affected. Anemia is a symptom of some underlying disease, and is not a diagnosis. There always is a cause, and most of the causes may be discovered by a relatively few simple procedures. The greatest help in finding the underlying disease responsible comes from knowing the common causes of anemia, getting a good history, doing a thorough physical examination, and ordering a logical sequence of laboratory tests based on what the situation and other findings suggest.

Classification of anemia is helpful because it provides a handy reference for differential diagnosis. There are several possible classifications; each is helpful in some respects.

Anemia may be classified according to pathogenesis. Using this concept, three mechanisms may be responsible.

1. *Deficiency of vital hematopoietic raw material – "factor deficiency anemia."* – The most common causes of deficiency anemia are iron deficiency and deficiency of vitamin B_{12} and/or folic acid.

2. *Failure of the blood-forming organs to produce or to deliver mature RBC to the peripheral blood – "production-defect anemia."* – This may be due to (a) replacement of marrow by fibrosis or by neoplasm (primary or metastatic); (b) hypoplasia of the bone marrow, most commonly produced by certain chemicals; or (c) toxic suppression of marrow production or delivery without actual marrow hypoplasia, found to variable extent in some patients with certain systemic diseases. The most common of these are severe infection, chronic renal disease, widespread malignancy (without extensive marrow replacement), rheumatoid-collagen diseases and hypothyroidism. (These conditions may sometimes be associated with an element of hemolytic anemia.)

3. *RBC loss from the peripheral blood – "depletion anemia."* – This is commonly due to (a) hemorrhage, acute or chronic (causing escape of RBC from the vascular system); (b) hemolytic anemia (RBC destroyed or RBC survival shortened within the vascular system), or (c) hypersplenism (splenic sequestration).

A second classification is based on a morphologic approach. Depending on the appearance of the RBC on a peripheral blood smear and/or Wintrobe indices, anemias may be characterized as microcytic, normocytic or macrocytic. They may be further subdivided according to the average amount of RBC hemoglobin, resulting in hypochromia or normochromia. (Macrocytic RBC may appear hyperchromic on peripheral smear, but this is an artifact due to an enlarged and, therefore, thicker cell that, being thicker, does not transmit light through the central portion as it would normally.)

I. Microcytic
  A. Hypochromic
    1. Chronic iron deficiency (most frequent cause)
    2. Thalassemia
    3. Occasionally in certain chronic systemic diseases
  B. Normochromic
    Very uncommon; may be simulated by spherocytosis; present to mild degree in some cases of infection

II. Normocytic
  A. Hypochromic
    1. Some cases of anemia due to systemic diseases
    2. Many cases of lead poisoning
  B. Normochromic
    1. Acute blood loss
    2. Hemolytic anemia
    3. Bone marrow replacement or hypoplasia
    4. Hypersplenism
    5. Many cases of anemia due to systemic diseases
    6. Some cases of lead poisoning

III. Macrocytic
  A. Hypochromic
    Some cases of macrocytic anemia with superimposed iron deficiency
  B. Normochromic
    1. Pernicious anemia
    2. Malabsorption (vitamin B_{12} and/or folic acid)
    3. Folic acid deficiency
    4. Reticulocytosis
    5. Some cases of chronic liver disease and hypothyroidism
    6. Some cases of aplastic anemia

The more common causes of anemia will be discussed in greater detail in the following chapters. Only the more common hematologic diseases will be covered. No attempt will be made to list every known entity or every disease that either produces or is associated with anemia. For a more complete coverage, several excellent textbooks on hematology are available.

REFERENCES

Diggs, L. W., et al.: *The Morphology of Blood Cells* (North Chicago, Il: Abbott Laboratories, 1954).

Dutcher, T. F.: Erythrocyte indices and corpuscular constants revisited, Lab. Med. 2:32, 1971.

Friedman, G. D., et al.: Smoking habits and the leukocyte count, Arch. Environ. Health 26:137, 1973.

Furlong, M. B.: Interpreting the reticulocyte count, Postgrad. Med. 54:207, 1973.

Gilmer, P. R., Jr., and Koepke, J. A.: The reticulocyte: an approach to definition, Am. J. Clin. Pathol. 66:262, 1976.

Harris, J. W., and Kellermeyer, R. W.: *The Red Cell* (2d ed.; Cambridge, MA: Harvard University Press, 1970).

Helman, N., and Rubenstein, L. S.: The effects of age, sex and smoking on erythrocytes and leukocytes, Am. J. Clin. Pathol. 63:35, 1975.

Mayer, G. A.: Diurnal, postural and postprandial variations in hematocrit, Can. Med. Assn. J. 93:1006, 1965.

Miale, J. B.: *Laboratory Medicine — Hematology* (4th ed.; St. Louis: The C. V. Mosby Company, 1972).

Perrotta, A. L., et al.: The polychromatophilic erythrocyte, Am. J. Clin. Pathol. 57: 471, 1972.

Pollycove, M., and Tono, M.: Studies of the erythron, Semin. Nucl. Med. 5:11, 1975.

Sandoz Atlas of Haematology (2d ed.; Basel, Switzerland: Sandoz Ltd., 1952).

Smith, C. H.: *Blood Diseases of Infancy and Childhood* (2d ed.; St. Louis: The C. V. Mosby Company, 1966).

Wheby, M. S.: Using a clinical laboratory in the diagnosis of anemia, Med. Clin. North Am. 50:1689, 1966.

Whitfield, C. L.: The patient with anemia: Diagnosis, The New Physician 16:184, 1967.

Williams, W. J., et al.: *Hematology* (New York: McGraw-Hill Book Co. Inc., 1972).

Wintrobe, M. M.: *Clinical Hematology* (7th ed.: Philadelphia: Lea & Febiger, 1974).

2 / Factor Deficiency Anemia

IRON

IRON is utilized from the diet in the ferrous form, absorbed mostly in the upper and middle small intestine, and coupled to a protein known as transferrin after a series of complicated physiologic reactions. The bone marrow RBC precursors utilize part of the iron; some of the excess is stored by bone marrow reticulum cells in the form of hemosiderin. This creates a storehouse of iron available in cases of deficiency. Deficiency may be created in two ways: (1) a chronic deficiency in dietary or available iron or (2) a loss of blood hemoglobin of such magnitude that normal amounts of dietary iron are not sufficient for replacement.

Acute blood loss can usually be handled without difficulty if the bleeding episode is not too prolonged and if tissue iron stores are adequate. The anemia that develops from acute bleeding is normocytic and normochromic and is not the type characteristic of chronic iron deficiency. Changes in hematocrit (HCT) are discussed elsewhere (p. 104). Chronic bleeding, however, is often sufficient to exhaust body iron stores from continued attempts by the bone marrow to restore the blood hemoglobin level. If this occurs, a hypochromic-microcytic type of anemia eventually develops. Chronic bleeding may be in the form of slow tiny daily loss; intermittent losses of small to moderate size not evident clinically; or repeated, more widely spaced, larger bleeding episodes. Chronic iron deficiency may develop with normal diet but naturally is hastened if the diet is itself borderline or deficient in iron.

In adults anemia due to pure dietary iron deficiency is extremely uncommon. Most of these cases arise from such malabsorption diseases as sprue, which, strictly speaking, is not a dietary problem. A more common etiology is iron deficiency of pregnancy, brought on by a combination of iron utilization by the fetus superimposed on previous iron deficiency due to excessive menstrual bleeding or multiple pregnancies.

By far the most common cause of chronic iron deficiency in adolescents or adults is excessive blood loss. In males, this is usually from the gastrointestinal tract. In females, it may be either GI or vaginal bleeding. Therefore, in females a careful inquiry about the frequency, duration and quantity of menstrual bleeding is essential. An estimate of quantity may be made from the number of menstrual pads used. In males and females below age 40 peptic ulcer is probably the most frequent GI etiology. After age 40 GI carcinoma is more common and should always be ruled out. Hemorrhoids are sometimes the cause of chronic iron deficiency anemia; but since hem-

9

orrhoids are very common it should never be assumed, without further investigation, that the anemia is due only to hemorrhoids.

If excessive vaginal bleeding is suspected, a careful vaginal examination with a Papanicolaou (Pap) smear should be done. If necessary, a gynecologist should be consulted. For possible GI bleeding an occult blood test on a stool sample should be ordered on at least three separate days. However, one or more negative stool guaiacs do not rule out GI cancer or peptic ulcer since these lesions may bleed intermittently. If a patient is over age 40 and stool guaiacs are negative, it would probably be best to do a sigmoidoscopy and a barium enema. If the barium enema result is negative and no other cause for the iron deficiency anemia can be demonstrated, it would be wise to repeat the barium enema in 3–4 months, in case a lesion was missed. The lower GI tract studies are particularly stressed as important for detection of carcinoma because colon carcinoma has an excellent cure rate if discovered in the early stages. Gastric carcinoma, on the other hand, has a very poor cure rate by the time it becomes demonstrable. The detection of peptic ulcer and the differential diagnosis of gastrointestinal lesions by selection of appropriate laboratory tests are discussed in more detail in Chapter 26. In addition to peptic ulcer, gastric hiatus hernia is sometimes associated with iron deficiency anemia.

In infants there is a different situation. The infant grows rapidly and must make hemoglobin to keep up with expanding blood volume. The demands of rapid growth may lead to iron depletion at age 6 months to 2 years because most of the infant's iron comes from the hemoglobin possessed at birth. Premature infants are therefore more likely to develop iron deficiency because their hemoglobin volume at birth is less. Since milk contains relatively small amounts of iron, infants on prolonged milk diets are more apt to have iron deficiency.

Under the experimental situation of a normal adult on a normal diet made iron deficient by repeated phlebotomy, it takes about 3 months before significant anemia (Hb more than 2 gm/100 ml below normal) appears. The first laboratory indication of iron deficiency is a bone marrow that shows absent marrow iron. The next test to show abnormal results is the serum iron level. When anemia becomes manifest, it is moderately hypochromic but only slightly microcytic; marked hypochromia and microcytosis are relatively late manifestations of iron lack. When the anemia is treated, these tests return to normal in the reverse order. Even with adequate therapy it takes several months before bone marrow iron appears again.

The reticulocyte count is normal in uncomplicated chronic iron deficiency anemia. Superimposed acute blood loss or other factors, such as adequate iron in the hospital diet, may cause reticulocytosis. For a short time following recent (acute) hemorrhage, the Wintrobe MCV may be normal or even increased due to the reticulocytosis. The reticulocyte response to iron therapy (3–7%) is somewhat less than that seen with treatment of megaloblastic anemia.

Serum iron (SI) levels are decreased in iron deficiency anemia. Normal values vary according to the method used, but less than 50 μg/100 ml is usually considered low. The plasma total iron-binding capacity (TIBC) is increased in 75% of cases. Since both the serum iron and the plasma iron-binding capacity have fairly wide normal ranges, a simultaneous plasma iron and TIBC is more helpful than the S1 alone. Normally, the TIBC is about one-third saturated. It will be much less saturated in chronic iron deficiency anemia (p. 479).

The peripheral blood smear in severe cases shows marked hypochromia and microcytosis and, in addition, considerable anisocytosis and poikilocytosis. This means that not all the RBC are microcytes. The microcytes of iron deficiency have to be differentiated from spherocytes; this is usually not difficult, since in chronic iron deficiency, even the microcytes have hypochromia. Bone marrow aspiration shows mild erythroid hyperplasia and absent marrow iron.

VITAMIN B_{12}

Vitamin B_{12} is absorbed in the ileum with the aid of "intrinsic factor" produced by the gastric glands of the stomach. Vitamin B_{12} deficiency may have three causes: (1) dietary lack, which is rarely sufficient by itself to cause anemia; (2) deficiency of intrinsic factor, leading to pernicious anemia, and (3) malabsorption syndromes involving the ileum mucosa or B_{12} handling by the ileum.

Besides direct damage to ileal mucosa, various causes of B_{12} malabsorption include bacterial overgrowth in the intestine (blind loop syndrome), infestation by the fish tapeworm, severe pancreatic disease and interference by certain medications (p. 473). Achlorhydria is reported to produce decreased release or utilization of B_{12} from food, although intestinal absorption of B_{12} is not affected. Vitamin B_{12} deficit may be accompanied by folic acid deficiency in some conditions.

Vitamin B_{12} deficiency can usually be proved by serum B_{12} assay. Therefore, a "therapeutic trial" of oral B_{12} (p. 436) is seldom needed. In patients with severe anemia of unknown etiology it is often useful to freeze a serum specimen before blood transfusion therapy begins since B_{12} and folic acid measurements (or other tests) may be desired later. Severe liver disease or myeloproliferative disorders (with high WBC counts) produce elevated B_{12} binding protein levels and falsely raise total serum B_{12} values.

Deficiency of either vitamin B_{12} or folic acid eventually leads to development of megaloblastic anemia. The RBC precursors in the marrow become slightly enlarged and develop a peculiar sievelike appearance of the nuclear chromatin, called megaloblastic change. This affects all stages of the precursors. The bone marrow typically shows considerable erythroid hyperplasia as well as megaloblastic change. Not only are the red cells affected but also the white cells and platelets. In far-advanced megaloblastic anemia there is a peripheral blood leukopenia and thrombocytopenia in addition to anemia; in early cases there may be anemia only. The bone marrow shows abnormally large metamyelocytes and band neutrophils. Macrocytosis is usually present in the peripheral blood, along with considerable anisocytosis and poikilocytosis. Hypersegmented polymorphonuclear neutrophils are characteristically found in the peripheral blood, although their number may be few or the degree of hypersegmentation may be difficult to separate from normal variation.

The diagnosis of megaloblastic anemia is made from bone marrow aspiration. This should be done as soon as possible and definitely before transfusion, since the characteristic megaloblastic changes can quickly disappear, even though the anemia is not affected by such a small amount of B_{12} or folic acid. The diagnosis of pernicious anemia is made by gastric aspiration and the Schilling test with and without intrinsic factor, as described in Chapter 25 (p. 298). The classic Schilling test response in pernicious anemia is low absorption ("positive test") without intrinsic factor and normal absorption with added intrinsic factor, while primary small bowel disease produces impaired B_{12} absorption both with and without intrinsic factor. However, some cases of pernicious anemia are reported to display a Schilling test response typical of primary small bowel malabsorption; after treatment with parenteral B_{12}, the Schilling test results became typical of pernicious anemia. A bone marrow should be the first procedure done in cases of macrocytic anemia because not all cases of megaloblastic anemia have positive Schilling test results (without intrinsic factor), and because the Schilling test will eliminate megaloblastic changes.

Treatment with oral B_{12} plus intrinsic factor evokes a reticulocyte response of 5–15%. The same thing will occur after a Schilling test, due to the nonisotopic B_{12} given parenterally.

A megaloblastic bone marrow is not diagnostic of folic acid or B_{12} deficiency. Some features of megaloblastic change may appear whenever intense marrow erythroid hyperplasia takes place, such as occurs in severe hemolytic anemia. Similar changes may also be found in chronic myelofibrosis; insideroblastic anemias; in "preleukemia" and DiGuglielmo's syndrome; in some patients with neoplasia, cirrhosis and uremia; and associated with certain drugs, such as diphenyhydantoin (Dilantin).

FOLIC ACID

The main causes of folic acid deficiency are: (1) dietary deficiency (most common cause, especially common in chronic alcoholism), (2) primary small intestine malabsorption syndrome, (3) pregnancy and (4) anticonvulsant drugs.

Folic acid deficiency causes a megaloblastic anemia that may be indistinguishable from pernicious anemia in every laboratory respect (except the behavior of the Schilling test with and without intrinsic factor). It may also be indistinguishable clinically, except that neurologic symptoms do not occur from folic acid deficiency. Folic acid therapy will improve most hematologic abnormalities of pernicious anemia, even though the pernicious anemia defect is vitamin B_{12} and not folic acid, but folic acid therapy alone can make pernicious anemia neurologic damage worse. Therefore, it is necessary to differentiate B_{12} and folic acid problems.

Folic acid deficiency can be proved by serum folic acid measurement. If the test is being done by the original microbiologic assay system, any antibiotic therapy must cease for a full week before patient serum can be drawn. Radioimmunoassay (RIA) is less complicated than bacterial methods and is not affected by antibiotics; therefore, RIA has made folate measurement more practical. Unfortunately, because serum folate measurement is not ordered frequently, smaller laboratories will probably not do the test for economic reasons. Serum folic acid levels fall below normal limits 3–4 weeks after dietary or absorption-induced deficiency begins. Tissue folate (measured by RBC folate assay) becomes abnormal some time after serum levels fall, with a corresponding lag in the return to normal later. Therefore, RBC folate assays may be helpful if serum folate is normal following a few meals containing folic acid. On the other hand, B_{12} deficiency will interfere with incorporation of folate into RBC and lead to RBC folate deficiency while serum folate levels may be normal. In addition, RIA methods may produce falsely decreased serum folate values in severe liver or kidney disease.

The "therapeutic trial" and certain other tests are discussed in Chapter 35.

Malabsorption syndromes associated with folic acid deficiency are most often due to primary small bowel disease. These are discussed in Chapter 25. A small but significant percentage of pregnant women have folic acid deficiency, although by far the most common cause of deficiency anemia in pregnancy is iron deficiency. Folic acid deficiency in pregnancy may be due to dietary defect plus fetal demands; sometimes no good explanation is possible. One clue may be a report that oral contraceptive pills can be associated with folic acid and vitamin B_6 deficiency. Dietary defect occasionally causes megaloblastic anemia in nonpregnant adult females or in adult males. This is most common in chronic alcoholics with liver disease. Certain anticonvulsant drugs, especially Dilantin and Mysoline, can on occasion produce a macrocytic megaloblastic anemia that responds best to folic acid. A considerable number of patients taking these drugs have macrocytosis without anemia. The actual percentage of those in whom anemia develops is extremely small. It should be noted that megaloblastic anemia due to pregnancy, diet or anticonvulsant drugs shows normal Schilling test results.

PYRIDOXINE

Pyridoxine (vitamin B_6) is necessary for synthesis of delta-aminolevulinic acid, a precursor of heme. Pyridoxine-deficient patients develop microcytic-hypochromic anemia. Both idiopathic and secondary forms exist; the most frequently mentioned secondary type is due to therapy with isoniazid (INH). Pyridoxine anemia is included in the sideroblastic anemias, a group whose characteristics are hypochromic RBC, elevated serum iron with increased saturation of iron-binding capacity, bone marrow erythroid hyperplasia and presence of bone marrow "ring" sideroblasts. Ring sideroblasts are normoblasts with abnormal numbers of iron-stainable cytoplasmic granules, sufficient to form a ring around the nucleus. Sideroblastic anemias may be hereditary, idiopathic, acquired or secondary; the secondary types are most frequently associated with severe alcoholism, antituberculosis drugs (such as INH) and lead poisoning. Bone marrow may be normoblastic or, less frequently, may exhibit some degree of megaloblastic change.

REFERENCES

Beutler, E., et al.: A comparison of the plasma iron, iron-binding capacity, sternal marrow iron and other methods in the clinical evaluation of iron stores, Ann. Intern. Med. 48:60, 1958.

Briggs, M., and Staniford, M.: Oral contraceptives and blood-iron, Lancet 2:742, 1969.

Brown, E. B.: Clinical aspects of iron metabolism, Semin. Hematol. 3:314, 1966.

Comitta, B. M., and Nathan, D. G.: Anemia in adolescence: Disturbances of iron balance, Postgraduate Med. 57:143, 1975.

Conrad, M. E., and Crosby, W. H.: The natural history of iron deficiency induced by phlebotomy, Blood 20:173, 1962

Crosby, W. H.: Mucosal block: An evaluation of concepts relating to control of iron absorption, Semin. Hematol. 3:299, 1966.

DeLeeuw, N. K. M., et al.: Iron deficiency and hydremia in normal pregnancy, Medicine 45:291, 1966.

Doscherholmen, A.: Plasma absorption of cyanocobalamin Co^{57}: Diagnostic value in vitamin B_{12} malabsorption states. Arch. Intern. Med. 134:1019, 1974.

Editorial: Pyridoxine-responsive anemia, J.A.M.A. 180:684, 1962.

Editorial: Achlorhydria and anaemia, Lancet 2:27, 1960.

Eichner, E. R., and Hillman, R. S.: The evolution of anemia in alcoholic patients, Am. J. Med. 50:218, 1971.

Emerson, P. M., and Wilkinson, J. H.: Lactate dehydrogenase in the diagnosis and assessment of response to treatment of megaloblastic anemia, Br. J. Haematol. 12:678, 1966.

Erlandson, M. E.: Iron metabolism and iron deficiency anemia, Pediatr. Clin. North Am. 9:673, 1962.

Fudenberg, H., and Estren, S.: Non-addisonian megaloblastic anemia, Am. J. Med. 25:198, 1958.

Herbert, V.: B_{12} and Folate Deficiency, in Rothfeld, B. (ed.): *Nuclear Medicine in Vitro* (Philadelphia; J. B. Lippincott Co., 1974), p. 69.

Herbert, V.: Detection of malabsorption of vitamin B_{12} due to gastric or intestinal dysfunction, Semin. Nucl. Med. 2:220, 1972.

Hines, J. D., and Grasso, J. A.: The sideroblastic anemias, Semin. Hematol. 7:86, 1970.

Jacobs, A.: Iron overload—clinical and pathologic aspects, Semin. Hematol. 14:89, 1977.

Kahn, S. B.: Recent advances in the nutritional anemias, Med. Clin. North Am. 54:631, 1970.

Lindenbaum, J.: Folic acid deficiency in sickle cell anemia, N. Engl. J. Med. 269:875, 1963.

McIntire, P. A.: Use of radioisotope techniques in the clinical evaluation of patients with megaloblastic anemia, Semin. Nucl. Med. 5:79, 1975.

Paine, C. J., et al.: Oral contraceptives, serum folate and hematologic status, J.A.M.A. 231:731, 1975.

Pollycove, M.: Iron metabolism and kinetics, Semin. Hematol. 3:235, 1966.

Pritchard, J. A.: Hemoglobin regeneration in severe iron-deficiency anemia, J.A.M.A. 195:717, 1966.

Spector, I., and Hutter, A. M., Jr.: Folic acid deficiency in neoplastic disease, Am. J. Med. Sci. 252:419, 1966.

Spurling, C. L., et al.: Juvenile pernicious anemia, New England J. Med. 271:995, 1964.

Streiff, R. R.: Folic acid deficiency anemia, Semin. Hematol. 7:23, 1970.

Sullivan, A. L., and Weintraub, L. R.: Sideroblastic anemias: An approach to diagnosis and management, Med. Clin. North Am. 57:335, 1973.

Waxman, S., et al.: Drugs, toxins and dietary amino acids affecting vitamin B_{12} or folic acid absorption or utilization, Am. J. Med. 48:599, 1970.
Weir, D. R., et al.: Serum proteins and blood vitamins in anemia of the chronically ill – Possible role of protein undernutrition, J. Chronic Dis. 22:407, 1969.
Wenk, R. E.: Significance of iron measurements, Postgrad. Med. 45:59, 1969.
Worwood, M.: Clinical biochemistry of iron, Semin. Hematol. 14:3, 1977.

3 / Production-Defect Anemia

ANEMIA due to inadequate erythropoiesis without factor deficiency may be classified in several ways. One system is based on the mechanism involved; either marrow failure to incorporate adequate supplies of hematopoietic raw materials (such as iron) into red cell precursors, failure to release mature red cells from the marrow or destruction of red cell precursors in the marrow. From a clinical point of view, it is easier to divide production-defect anemias into two categories—those due to a hypoplastic bone marrow and those with normally cellular marrow that are associated with certain systemic diseases.

HYPOPLASTIC MARROW

Conditions which produce a hypoplastic marrow affect the bone marrow directly, either by actual replacement or by toxic depression of red cell precursors. Bone marrow examination is the main diagnostic or confirmatory test.

REPLACEMENT OF MARROW BY FIBROSIS.—This condition is commonly termed myelofibrosis, is usually idiopathic and leads to a clinical syndrome called myeloid metaplasia. The peripheral blood picture is similar in many ways to that of chronic myelogenous leukemia. Many include this condition in the group of "myeloproliferative syndromes," and a more complete discussion is given in Chapter 6.

REPLACEMENT OF MARROW BY NEOPLASM.—The types of tumors most commonly metastatic to bone marrow, the laboratory abnormalities produced and the main hematologic findings are covered in Chapter 32. The anemia of neoplasia is usually normocytic and normochromic. Iron-deficiency anemia secondary to hemorrhage may be present if the tumor has invaded or originated from the GI tract. Besides extensive marrow replacement ("myelophthisic anemia"), neoplasia may produce anemia with minimal bone involvement or even without any marrow metastases; in these patients, there seems to be some sort of toxic influence on the marrow production and release mechanism. In occasional cases of widespread neoplasm, a hemolytic component (shortened RBC life span) has been demonstrated.

Multiple myeloma is a neoplasm of plasma cells which is difficult to separate from the group of leukemias on one hand and the category of malignant lymphomas on the other. Myeloma initially or eventually involves the bone marrow and produces a moderate normocytic-normochromic anemia.

16

The diagnosis of multiple myeloma is covered in Chapter 21. Despite pro-liferation of plasma cells in the bone marrow, appearance of more than an occasional plasma cell in the peripheral blood is very uncommon. Periph-eral blood RBC often display the phenomenon of rouleau formation, a pil-ing up of red cells like a stack of coins. This is not specific for myeloma, and is most often associated with hyperglobulinemia.

APLASTIC ANEMIA. — Patients with this disease have severe anemia, often progressive and fatal, and bone marrow aspiration reveals hypoplasia or aplasia of red cell precursors. In addition, WBC and/or platelets may be involved. In 50% or more of the patients, the reason for bone marrow changes is unknown. In the remainder, the most common known etiologies are destruction by toxins and idiosyncratic reactions. Of course, the two terms are related, but in one group the disease is caused by exposure to chemicals or toxins that affect everyone, whereas in the other group mar-row aplasia develops as an idiosyncratic reaction to a drug or chemical that does not have this effect on most other people. The exact cause of aplastic anemia cannot be found in at least 50% of cases.

The most common known causes in the general toxin group are chemi-cals, such as benzene, and excessive x-ray and radioactive compound expo-sure. This group causes pancytopenia (anemia, leukopenia and thrombocy-topenia) and is most often fatal, although occasionally persons do recover. Leukemia is an occasional late development if the patient survives long enough.

A great variety of drugs and chemicals have been reported to cause idio-syncratic reactions. The effects range from pancytopenia to any combina-tion of single or multiple blood element defect. Bone marrow aspiration usually shows a deficiency in the particular cell precursor involved, al-though, especially with megakaryocytes, this is not always true. These pa-tients most often recover if they can be supported long enough, although a considerable number die from superimposed infection.

The drugs most often implicated are:

Pancytopenia — Chloramphenicol (Chloromycetin), Phenylbutazone (Bu-tazolidin), Mesantoin, gold preparations, nitrogen mustard compounds, Myleran and other antileukemic drugs. In addition, chloramphenicol therapy may produce the "gray syndrome" in premature infants and new-borns.

Leukopenia — Chlorpromazine (Thorazine), promazine (Sparine), phenyl-butazone, thiouracil, antileukemic drugs, sulfonamides.

Thrombocytopenia — Quinidine, Furadantin, sulfonylureas, chlorthia-zide.

The anemia produced is of the normocytic-normochromic type. Reticulo-cyte counts are usually low (although they sometimes might be slightly elevated if the patient is in a recovery phase). About one third of aplastic anemia patients have a macrocytic peripheral blood smear.

As noted, bone marrow aspiration is usually essential for diagnosis, and can be used to follow any response to therapy. However, there are prob-lems not always taken into account. A false impression of marrow hypocel-lularity may be produced by hemodilution of the marrow specimen, by aspiration at a place which has unusually large amounts of fatty tissue, and by poor slide preparation technique. Occasional completely "dry" puncture is not uncommon in normal persons, due to considerable variability in the bone marrow distribution. Therefore, the diagnosis should never be made on the basis of a single failure to obtain marrow. Also, a bone marrow biopsy—or at least a clot section (clotted marrow aspirate processed like an ordinary histologic specimen)—is more reliable than a smear for estimating cellularity. This is especially true for megakaryocytes. On the other hand, a smear is definitely more valuable for demonstrating abnormal morphology. Both can usually be done at the same time.

SYSTEMIC DISEASE

RENAL DISEASE.—Anemia of moderate degree is frequently found in association with uremia. Some investigators claim it is almost always present when the BUN is persistently over twice normal, and often appears before this level. Patients with prolonged but potentially reversible azotemia (such as acute renal failure) often develop anemia until the kidneys recover. Transient types of azotemia usually do not produce anemia unless azotemia is prolonged or due to the underlying cause itself. The anemia of actual renal insufficiency develops regardless of the cause of the uremia.

The peripheral blood RBC are usually normocytic and normochromic; there is often mild-to-moderate anisocytosis. There sometimes may be mild hypochromia, and occasionally some degree of microcytosis. In some cases "burr" cells are found; these are triangular shrunken RBC with irregular pointed projections from the surface.

Bone marrow usually shows normal cellularity, although some cases have mild RBC hypoplasia. Marrow iron is adequate. Serum iron is usually normal, but about 20–30% of patients have low serum iron, even though they do not have iron deficiency. Reticulocyte counts are usually normal; occasionally, they may be slightly elevated.

The pathophysiology involved is not well understood. The primary known abnormality is a lack of incorporation of iron into RBC within the bone marrow. There is depression both of hemoglobin synthesis and of formation and release of mature RBC into the peripheral blood. In 10–15% of patients there is also decreased RBC survival in the peripheral blood, although the hemolytic aspect is usually not severe. In the late stages of uremia there may be a bleeding tendency due to coagulation defects, most commonly thrombocytopenia. Platelet function may be abnormal even with normal numbers of platelets. The effect of hemorrhage, if it occurs, is separate and additional to the anemia of chronic renal disease.

ANEMIA OF NEOPLASIA.—This anemia is usually normocytic-normochromic with normal reticulocyte counts, unless there is hemorrhage or chronic blood loss. A hemolytic component is present in a considerable minority of patients, but hemolysis is generally mild and is not detectable except with radioisotope red cell survival procedures. Occasionally, hemolysis may be severe, especially with chronic lymphocytic leukemia and malignant lymphomas. Thrombocytopenia may be found in certain types of leukemia and in myelophthisic anemias. Fibrinolysins may appear in occasional cases of widespread malignancy, most often prostate carcinoma.

ANEMIA OF INFECTION. — Mild-to-moderate anemia is frequently seen in association with subacute or chronic infection. The mechanism of this anemia is not well understood, but there seems to be a decreased rate of erythropoiesis, coupled in some patients with slightly shortened RBC survival and failure to utilize iron normally. The anemia of infection does not usually develop unless the infection lasts a month or more, although occasionally anemia may develop rapidly in severe acute infection, such as septicemia. Also, chronic infection generally is of at least moderate severity. Such situations include bronchiectasis, salpingitis, abscess of visceral organs or body cavities, or severe pyelonephritis. Anemia is a common finding in subacute bacterial endocarditis and in the granulomatous diseases such as tuberculosis or sarcoidosis. The anemia is usually normocytic and normochromic, but sometimes is hypochromic. Reticulocyte counts are usually normal, although occasionally they may be slightly increased. Bone marrow aspiration shows either normal marrow or hyperplasia of the granulocytes. Serum iron is usually low or low normal, and plasma total iron-binding capacity is reduced (in iron deficiency anemia the TIBC is elevated).

RHEUMATOID-COLLAGEN DISEASE GROUP. — This frequently is associated with mild-to-moderate normocytic-normochromic anemia. Again, reticulocytes are usually normal and the bone marrow is unremarkable. Apparently there is decreased erythropoiesis with a slightly shortened RBC survival, but there is disagreement about the factor of RBC survival.

CHRONIC LIVER DISEASE. — The type and frequency of anemia in liver disease vary with the type and severity of hepatic dysfunction, but anemia has been reported in up to 75% of patients. It is most frequently seen in far-advanced cirrhosis. Extensive metastatic carcinoma of the liver may produce the same effect, although it is difficult to say whether the liver involvement or the neoplasm itself is the real cause. About one third to one half of those with anemia have a macrocytosis; about one-third are normocytic. Some have a hypochromia because of gastrointestinal blood loss. Target cells in varying numbers are a fairly frequent finding on peripheral blood smear.

Macrocytic anemia in liver disease is most often found in severe chronic liver damage; such anemia is not usually caused by acute liver disease, even when severe, or by chronic disease of only slight or mild extent. A small but significant percentage of hepatic macrocytic anemias are megaloblastic, usually secondary to folic acid dietary deficiency, although most are not megaloblastic and will not be corrected by folic acid treatment. A macrocytic peripheral blood smear may be present even when there is a normal Hb or HCT, and sometimes even with a normal MCV.

Gastrointestinal bleeding occurs in a considerable number of cirrhotic patients; often it is very slight and intermittent. Esophageal varices are present in some; other lesions may be demonstrated in other patients. In a considerable proportion of cases the source of the bleeding cannot be located.

Anemia and other cytopenias, especially thrombocytopenia, may be occasionally produced by the effects of liver disease on the spleen. Hypersplenism occurs in some of the patients with portal vein hypertension and its resulting splenic congestion (see p. 36). In severe chronic (or massive acute) liver disease, coagulation problems may result from insufficient hepatic synthesis of several blood coagulation factors.

Some liver-diseased patients have shortened RBC survival demonstrated only by using radioactive isotope studies and show no evidence of GI bleeding. There is no clinical or laboratory evidence of hemolysis otherwise. Zieve's syndrome is a rare combination of hyperlipemia, cirrhosis and hemolytic anemia. This hemolytic anemia has reticulocytosis and the other classic findings of hemolysis.

Unless blood loss is a factor, and excluding those cases of megaloblastic anemia, the bone marrow is unremarkable in liver disease, and reticulocytes are usually close to normal. Not all cases of anemia in liver disease can be explained.

HYPOTHYROIDISM. — Anemia is found in 30–60% of cases. About one third of the anemic patients have a macrocytic type, most of the remainder being either normocytic-normochromic or normocytic-hypochromic. A small percentage are hypochromic-microcytic.

The hypochromic type responds to a combination of iron and thyroid hormone preparation. The iron deficiency component is frequently produced by excessive menstrual bleeding; in patients without demonstrable blood loss there is speculation that decreased intestinal iron absorption may occur, since thyroid hormone is known to increase intestinal carbohydrate absorption. Most of the macrocytic cases respond only to thyroid hormone. The bone marrow is not megaloblastic and is sometimes slightly hypocellular. Reticulocytes are usually normal. Isotope studies reportedly show normal survival time in most cases. Lack of thyroid hormone seems to have a direct effect on erythropoiesis, since thyroid extract therapy cures both the myxedema and the anemia (unless there is superimposed iron deficiency). A minority of the macrocytic cases have folic acid or B_{12} deficiency, presumably secondary to decreased intestinal absorption. Thyroid hormone is required in addition to folic acid or B_{12}. About 5% have actual pernicious anemia, with megaloblastic bone marrow.

To conclude this discussion, it should be noted that the normocytic-normochromic anemia of systemic diseases has often been called "simple chronic anemia," although the pathophysiology is apparently far from simple. The disease categories listed are only the most common. In many cases, the diagnosis is one of exclusion; the patient has anemia for which no definite etiology can be found, so whatever systemic disease he has is blamed for the anemia. In these patients, it is important to rule out treatable serious diseases; this especially is true for hypochromic anemias (where blood loss might be occurring) and macrocytic anemias (which may be due to B_{12} or folic acid deficiency). A normocytic-normochromic picture may be due to an occult underlying disease, such as malignant lymphoma or multiple myeloma.

REFERENCES

Burns, S. L.: Anemia in rheumatoid arthritis, Med. Clin. North Am. 52:527, 1968.
Cartwright, G. E.: The anemia of chronic disorders, Semin. Hematol. 3:351, 1966.
Clement, D. H.: Aplastic anemia, Pediatr. Clin. North Am. 9:703, 1962.

Corr, W. P., et al.: Hematologic changes in tuberculosis, Am. J. Med. Sci. 248:709, 1964.

Dawson, R. B., Jr.: Drug-induced blood dyscrasias—prevention and diagnosis, Med. Times 96:671, 1968.

Ellis, L. D., and Westerman, M. P.: Autoimmune-hemolytic anemia and cancer, J.A.M.A. 193:962, 1965.

Fein, H. G., and Rivlin, R. S.: Anemia in thyroid disease, Med. Clin. North Am. 59: 1133, 1975.

Friedman, I. A., and Schwartz, S. O.: The Relation Between the Liver and the Hematopoietic System, in Popper, H., and Schaffner, F. (eds.): *Progress in Liver Diseases* (New York: Grune & Stratton, Inc., 1961), vol. 1, p. 134.

Harris, J. W., and Kellermeyer, R. W.: *The Red Cell* (2d ed.; Cambridge, MA: Harvard University Press, 1970).

Hattersley, P. G.: Macrocytosis of the erythrocytes: A preliminary report, J.A.M.A. 189:997, 1964.

Higgins, M. R., et al. Anemia in hemodialysis patients, Arch. Intern. Med. 137:172, 1977.

Hines, J. D., and Grasso, J. A.: The sideroblastic anemias, Semin. Hematol. 7:86, 1970.

Huguley, C. M.: Hematological reactions, J.A.M.A. 196:122, 1966.

Leikin, S. L.: Hematologic aspects of renal disease, Pediatr. Clin. North Am. 11:667, 1964.

Maldonado, J. E., et al.: The thymus gland and its relationship to the hematopoietic and immunologic systems: A review, Mayo Clin. Proc. 39:60, 1964.

Marks, P. A., et al.: Hemolytic anemia associated with liver disease, Med. Clin. North Am. 47:711, 1963.

Martin, E. W., et al.: *Hazards of Medication* (Philadelphia: J. B. Lippincott, Co., 1971).

Movitt, E. R., et al.: Idiopathic true bone marrow failure, Am. J. Med. 34:500, 1963.

Pisciotta, A. V.: Drug-induced leukopenia and aplastic anemia, Clin. Pharmacol. Ther. 12:13, 1971.

Pisciotta, A. V.: Idiosyncratic hematologic reactions to drugs, Postgrad. Med. 55:105, 1974.

Sullivan, A. L., and Weintraub, L. R.: Sideroblastic anemias: an approach to diagnosis and management, Med. Clin. North Am. 57:335, 1973.

Waldon, H. A.: Anemia of lead poisoning: A review, Br. J. Ind. Med. 23:83, 1966.

Weiss, A. J.: Hematologic complications of renal disease, Med. Clin. North Am. 47: 1001, 1963.

4 / Depletion Anemia

TWO TYPES OF DEPLETION ANEMIA are possible: abnormal loss of red cells from the circulation and abnormal destruction of red cells within the circulation. Red cell loss due to hemorrhage has been covered elsewhere (blood volume, p. 103; iron-deficiency anemia, p. 9). Intravascular RBC destruction is called hemolytic anemia. In general, there are two major types of hemolytic anemia. In one category, destruction is relatively slow, and, although RBC survival is shortened, the only laboratory test that demonstrates this fact is radioisotope study using tagged RBC. In the other category, hemolysis or shortened RBC life span is sufficient to cause abnormality in one or more standard laboratory tests.

Two etiologic groups comprise most of the hemolytic anemias: those primarily due to intracorpuscular RBC defects and those primarily due to extracorpuscular agents acting on the RBC. This provides a rational basis for classification.

I. Due primarily to intracorpuscular defects
   A. Hemoglobinopathies
   B. Congenital nonspherocytic hemolytic anemias
   C. Congenital spherocytosis
   D. Paroxysmal nocturnal hemoglobinuria
II. Due primarily to extracorpuscular agents
   A. Isoimmune antibodies
   B. Autoimmune antibodies
   C. Toxins (lead, bacterial toxins)
   D. Parasites (malaria)
   E. Systemic diseases
   F. Hypersplenism

LABORATORY TESTS IN HEMOLYTIC ANEMIAS

Certain laboratory tests are extremely helpful in suggesting or demonstrating the presence of hemolytic anemia. Which tests give abnormal results, and to what degree, depends of course on the severity of the hemolytic process and possibly also on its duration.

RETICULOCYTE COUNT.—This is significantly elevated in nearly all active hemolytic anemias, and the degree of reticulocytosis corresponds to some extent with the degree of anemia. The highest counts appear after acute hemolytic episodes. The reticulocyte count is a valuable screening test for active hemolytic anemia, and reticulocyte counts of more than 5%

22

should suggest this diagnosis. Other conditions that give a similar reticulocyte response are acute bleeding and deficiency anemias after initial treatment (note that sometimes the treatment may be dietary only). It usually takes 2–3 days after acute hemolysis to obtain the characteristic reticulocyte response.

SERUM HAPTOGLOBIN. — Haptoglobins are alpha$_2$ globulins that bind any free hemoglobin (Hb) liberated by intravascular RBC destruction. Haptoglobin can be estimated as haptoglobin-binding capacity or measured directly (p. 92). Decreased serum or plasma haptoglobins usually mean that hemolysis has occurred, and that some of the haptoglobins have been made unavailable because of binding to free hemoglobin. Haptoglobins also are decreased in situations with considerable extravascular RBC destruction, such as congenital spherocytosis or Rh incompatibility reactions (p. 92). Haptoglobins are fairly sensitive indicators of hemolytic anemia; however, congenital absence of haptoglobin occurs in about 3% of blacks and rarely in whites.

PLASMA METHEMALBUMIN. — After the binding capacity of haptoglobin is exhausted, free hemoglobin combines with albumin to form a compound known as methemalbumin. This can be demonstrated with a spectroscope. The presence of methemalbumin means that intravascular hemolysis has occurred to a considerable extent. It also suggests that the episode was either continuing or relatively recent, because otherwise the haptoglobins would be replenished and once again take over the hemoglobin removal duty from albumin.

FREE HEMOGLOBIN IN PLASMA OR URINE. — This occurs when all the plasma protein-binding capacity for free hemoglobin is exhausted, including albumin. There normally is a small amount of free hemoglobin in the plasma, probably because some artifactual hemolysis is unavoidable in drawing blood and processing the specimen. This is less when plasma is used instead of serum. If increased amounts of free hemoglobin are found in plasma, and artifactual hemolysis due to poor blood-drawing technique (very frequent, unfortunately) can be ruled out, then a relatively severe degree of intravascular hemolysis is probable. If the degree of hemolysis is marked, this is often accompanied by free hemoglobin in the urine (hemoglobinuria). In chronic hemolysis, the urine may contain hemosiderin, located in urothelial cells or casts.

DIRECT COOMBS TEST. — This test is helpful when a hemolytic process is suspected or demonstrated. It detects a wide variety of both isoantibodies and autoantibodies which have attached to the patient's red cells. This is discussed in Chapter 9. The indirect Coombs test is often wrongly ordered in such situations. The indirect Coombs test forms a part of certain special techniques for antibody identification and by itself is usually not helpful in most clinical situations. If an antibody is demonstrated by the direct Coombs test, an antibody identification test should be requested. The laboratory will decide what techniques to use, depending on the situation.

SERUM UNCONJUGATED ("INDIRECT-ACTING") BILIRUBIN. — This is often elevated in hemolysis of at least moderate degree. Slight or mild degrees of hemolysis will often show no elevation. The direct-acting (conjugated) fraction is usually not elevated significantly in jaundice due to purely hemolytic cause. Except in blood bank problems, serum bilirubin is not as helpful in diagnosis of hemolytic anemias as most of the other tests and often shows equivocal results.

RBC SURVIVAL STUDIES. – Red cell survival can be estimated in vivo by tagging some of the patient's red cells with a radioactive isotope, such as ^{51}Cr, drawing daily blood samples for isotope counting and determining in this way how long it takes for the tagged cells to disappear from the circulation. Survival studies are most useful to demonstrate low-grade hemolytic anemias, situations in which bone marrow production is able to keep pace with red cell destruction but is not able to keep the red cell count at normal levels. Low-grade hemolysis often presents as anemia whose etiology cannot be demonstrated by the usual methods. There are, however, certain drawbacks to this procedure. If anemia is actually due to chronic occult extravascular blood loss, tagged red cells will disappear from the circulation by this route and simulate decreased intravascular survival. A minor difficulty is the fact that survival data are only approximate, because certain technical aspects of isotope red cell tagging limit the accuracy of measurement.

THE HEMOGLOBINOPATHIES

At birth, approximately 80% of the infant's hemoglobin is fetal-type hemoglobin (Hb F), which has a greater affinity for oxygen than the adult type. By age 6 months, all except 1–2% is replaced by adult hemoglobin (Hb A). Persistence of large amounts of Hb F is abnormal. There are a considerable number of abnormal hemoglobins, which differ structurally and biochemically to varying degrees from normal Hb A. The clinical syndromes produced in persons having certain of these abnormal types are called the hemoglobinopathies. The most important of these abnormal hemoglobins in the Western Hemisphere are thalassemia, sickle cell and hemoglobin C. Hemoglobin E is comparably important in Southeast Asia. All the abnormal hemoglobins are genetically transmitted, just as normal Hb A is. Therefore, since each person has two genes for each trait (such as hemoglobin type), one gene on one chromosome received from the mother and one gene on one chromosome received from the father, a person can be either homozygous (two genes with the trait) or heterozygous (only one of the two genes with the trait). When present in double dose (homozygous), the syndrome produced by the abnormal hemoglobin is usually much more severe than if the abnormality were present only in a single dose (heterozygous, only one of the two genes carrying the trait). This also allows genes for two different abnormal hemoglobins to be present in the same person (double heterozygosity).

Sickle Cell Hemoglobin

Several disease states may be due to the abnormal hemoglobin gene called sickle hemoglobin (Hb S). When Hb S is present on both genes (SS), the disease produced is called sickle cell anemia. When Hb S is present on one gene and the other gene has normal Hb A, it is called sickle trait. Sickle hemoglobin is found mostly in blacks, although it may occur in populations along the northeastern Mediterranean and in a few other areas. The incidence of sickle trait in blacks in the United States is about 8%, and of sickle cell anemia, less than 1%. The S gene may also be found in combination with a gene for another abnormal hemoglobin, such as hemoglobin C (Hb C).

SICKLE CELL ANEMIA. — Sickle cell (SS) anemia symptoms are not usually manifest until age 6 months or later. On the other hand, survival over age 40 is not frequent. Anemia is of moderate or severe degree, and the patient often has slight jaundice (manifested by scleral icterus). The patients seem to adapt surprisingly well to their anemic state, and apart from easy fatigability, or perhaps weakness, have few symptoms until a so-called crisis develops. The crisis of sickle cell disease is often due to small infarcts in various organs, but in some cases the reason is unknown. Abdominal pain or bone pain are the two most common symptoms, and the pain may be extremely severe. There usually is an accompanying leukocytosis, which, if associated with abdominal pain, may suggest acute intra-abdominal surgical disease. The crisis ordinarily lasts 5–7 days. In most cases, there is no change in hemoglobin levels during the crisis.

Other commonly found abnormalities in sickle cell disease are chronic leg ulcers (usually over the ankles), hematuria and a loss of urine-concentrating ability. Characteristic bone abnormalities are frequently seen on x-ray films, especially of the skull. Gallstones are increased in frequency. There may be various neurologic signs and symptoms. The spleen may be palpable in a few early cases, but eventually it becomes smaller than normal, due to repeated infarcts. The liver is palpable in occasional cases.

As mentioned, the anemia is moderate to severe. There is moderate anisocytosis. Target cells are characteristically present, but are fewer than 30% of the RBC. Sickled cells are found in the peripheral blood smear in many, although not all, of the patients. Sometimes they are very few and take a careful search. There are usually nucleated RBC of the orthochromic or polychromatophilic normoblast stages, most often ranging from 1 to 10 per 100 WBC. Polychromatophilic RBC are usually present. Howell-Jolly bodies appear in a moderate number of patients. The WBC count may be normal or there may be a mild leukocytosis, which sometimes may become moderate in degree. There is often a "shift to the left" (when in crisis, this becomes more pronounced), and sometimes even a few myelocytes are found. Platelets may be normal or even moderately increased.

The laboratory features of active hemolytic anemia are present, including moderate or even marked reticulocytosis.

Diagnosis rests on first demonstrating the characteristic sickling phenomenon, and then doing hemoglobin electrophoresis to find out if the abnormality is SS disease or some combination of another hemoglobin with the S gene. Bone marrow shows marked erythroid hyperplasia, but a bone marrow is not helpful and is therefore not indicated for diagnosis of suspected sickle cell disease. Screening tests for sickle hemoglobin are discussed in Chapter 35.

Sickle hemoglobin is less soluble than normal adult hemoglobin when oxygen tension is lowered, and the sickle hemoglobin forms crystalline aggregates under these circumstances that distort the RBC shape into a sickle shape. A sickle preparation ("sickle cell prep") may be done in two ways. A drop of blood from a finger puncture is placed on a slide, coverslipped, and the edges sealed with petrolatum. The characteristic sickled forms may be seen after 6 hours (or earlier), but may not appear for nearly 24 hours. A more widely used procedure is to add a reducing substance, 2% sodium metabisulfite, to the blood before coverslipping. This speeds the reaction markedly, with the preparation becoming readable in 15–60 minutes. Many laboratories have experienced difficulty with sodium metabisulfite, since it may deteriorate during storage, so that other chemical methods, such as dithionate (p. 438), under a variety of trade names are becoming standard screening procedures. The sickle preparation may be negative early in life, presumably because most of the hemoglobin is still fetal hemoglobin (Hb F). Finally, these tests are not specific for Hb S, because several rare non-S hemoglobins will produce a "sickle reaction" with metabisulfite or with dithionate.

Hemoglobin electrophoresis allows good separation of Hb S from Hb A and C. In SS disease, 75–95% is Hb S and the remainder is Hb F.

The sickle cell preparation is almost always positive in homozygous (SS) disease, except in young infants, if the test is properly done. On peripheral smear, certain other abnormal RBC shapes may be confused with sickle cells. The most common of these are ovalocytes and schistocytes (burr cells). Ovalocytes are somewhat rod-shaped RBC that, on occasion, may be found normally in small numbers but that may also appear due to another genetically inherited abnormality, hereditary ovalocytosis. Compared to sickle cells, the ovalocytes are not usually curved and are fairly well rounded at each end, lacking the sharply pointed ends of the classic sickle cell. Schistocytes may be found in certain severe hemolytic anemias, usually of a toxic or an antigen-antibody type. They are red cells in the process of destruction. They are smaller than normal RBC, misshapen and have one or more spinous processes on the surface. Overall form may be triangular, star-shaped or a stubby short crescent; none of these closely resembles the more slender, smooth and regular sickle cell.

SICKLE CELL TRAIT.—This is the heterozygous combination of one gene for sickle (S) hemoglobin with one gene for normal adult (A) hemoglobin. There is no anemia, and no clinical evidence of any disease except for two situations: some persons with S trait develop splenic infarcts under hypoxic conditions, such as flying at high altitudes in nonpressurized airplanes, and some persons develop hematuria. On paper electrophoresis, 20–45% of the hemoglobin is sickle type, with the remainder being normal adult type. The metabisulfite sickle preparation is usually positive; although a few patients have been reported negative, some believe that every person with sickle hemoglobin will have a positive sickle preparation if it is properly done.

SICKLE-CELL HEMOGLOBIN C (SC) DISEASE.—This combines one gene for sickle (S) hemoglobin with one for Hb C. About 20% of patients do not have anemia and are asymptomatic. In the others a disease is produced that may be much like that of SS disease but is usually milder. Compared to sickle cell (SS) disease, the anemia is usually only of mild or moderate degree, although sometimes it may be severe. Crises are less frequent; abdominal pain has been reported in 30%. Bone pain is almost as common as in SS disease, but is usually much milder. Idiopathic hematuria is found in a substantial minority of cases. Chronic leg ulcers occur but are not frequent. Skull x-ray abnormalities are not frequent, but may be present.

There are some differences from SS disease. In SC disease, aseptic necrosis in the head of the femur is common; this can occur in SS disease but is not frequent. Splenomegaly is common in SC disease, with a palpable spleen in 65–80% of the patients. Finally, target cells are more frequent on the average than in SS disease (due to the Hb C gene), although the number present varies considerably from patient to patient and cannot be used as a differentiating point unless over 30% of the RBC are involved. Nucleated RBC are not common in the peripheral blood. Sickle cells may or may not be present in the peripheral smear; if present, they are usually few in number. White cell counts are usually normal, except in crises or with superimposed infection.

Sickle preparations are usually positive. Hemoglobin electrophoresis establishes a definitive diagnosis.

Hemoglobin C

HEMOGLOBIN C DISEASE. — This is the double dose homozygous state (CC) for the Hb C gene. The C gene is said to be present in only about 3% of blacks in the United States, so that homozygous Hb C (CC) disease is not common. The C gene may be homozygous (CC), in combination with normal hemoglobin (AC), or in combination with any of the other abnormal hemoglobins (such as SC disease). Episodes of abdominal and bone pain may occur, but usually are not severe. Splenomegaly is generally present. The most striking feature of the peripheral blood smear is the large number of target cells, always over 30% and often close to 90%.

Diagnosis is by means of hemoglobin electrophoresis.

HEMOGLOBIN C TRAIT. — This is the combination of the C gene and the normal hemoglobin (A) gene. There is no anemia nor any symptoms. The only abnormality is the presence of variable numbers of target cells in the peripheral blood smear.

Thalassemia

Strictly speaking, there is no thalassemia hemoglobin. Thalassemia is a complex group of genetically inherited abnormalities in hemoglobin synthesis. There are three main clinical types: thalassemia major, which has over 50% fetal (F) hemoglobin; thalassemia minor, which has normal amounts of fetal hemoglobin but usually has increased amounts of a variant of normal hemoglobin called Hb A_2, and combinations of the thalassemia gene with other abnormal hemoglobins. The thalassemia gene is found most commonly in persons of Greek or southern Italian origin and is also rather frequent in other countries which border the Mediterranean.

Actually, the situation is much more complicated than this description implies. The globin portion of normal hemoglobin (Hb A_1) is composed of two pairs of polypeptide (amino acid) chains, one pair called alpha and the other beta. All normal hemoglobins have two alpha chains, but certain hemoglobins have amino acid chains different from beta that make up the second chain pair. Thus, Hb A_2 has two delta chains, and Hb F has two gamma chains in addition to the two alphas. All three of these hemoglobins (A_1, A_2 and F) are normally present in adult RBC, but A_2 and F normally are only in trace amounts. One polypeptide chain from each pair is inherited from each parent, so that one alpha chain and one beta chain are derived from the mother, and the other alpha and beta chain from the father. The thalassemia gene may involve either the alpha or the beta chain. In the great majority of cases, the beta is affected; genetically speaking, it would be more correct to call such a situation a beta thalassemia. If the condition is heterozygous, only one of the two beta chains is affected; this supposedly leaves only one beta chain (instead of two) available for Hb A_1 synthesis, thus resulting in a partial decrease of normal hemoglobin (A_1) synthesis and a relative increase in A_2 hemoglobin. This produces the clinical picture of thalassemia minor. In a homozygous beta thalassemia, both of the beta chains are affected; this apparently results in marked suppression of normal hemoglobin A_1 synthesis and leads to a compensatory increase in gamma chains; the combination of increased gamma chains with the non-affected alpha chains produces marked elevation of Hb F. This gives the clinical syndrome of thalassemia major. It is also possible for the thalassemia gene to affect the alpha chains; in heterozygous alpha thalassemia, Hb A_1 production is mildly curtailed, but no Hb A_2 or F increase occurs because they also need alpha chains. If the alpha thalassemia is homozygous, hemoglobin production, in most cases, apparently is curtailed enough to be lethal in utero or in neonatal life. Hemoglobin Bart's, in which all four chains are gamma, and Hb H, in which all four chains are beta, are extreme forms of alpha chain disorders.

THALASSEMIA MAJOR (COOLEY'S ANEMIA). — This disease produces a severe anemia, which is accompanied by a considerable number of normoblasts in the peripheral blood. The nucleated RBC are most often about one-third or one-half the number of WBC, but may even exceed them. There are often Howell-Jolly bodies and considerable numbers of polychromatophilic RBC. The mature red cells are usually very hypochromic, with considerable anisocytosis and poikilocytosis, and there are moderate numbers of target cells. The mean corpuscular volume (MCV) is microcytic. White cell counts are often mildly increased, and there may be mild granulocytic immaturity, sometimes even with myelocytes present. Platelets are normal. Skull x-ray films show abnormal patterns similar to those in sickle cell anemia, but even more pronounced. Death most often occurs in childhood or adolescence.

Diagnosis is suggested by a severe anemia with very hypochromic RBC, moderate numbers of target cells, many nucleated RBC and a family history of Mediterranean origin. The sickle preparation is negative. Definitive diagnosis depends on the fact that in thalassemia major, fetal hemoglobin (Hb F) is elevated (10–90% of the total hemoglobin, usually over 50%). Hb F has approximately the same migration rate as Hb A_1 on paper electrophoresis, so the two cannot easily be separated by this technique. However, Hb F is much more resistant to denaturation by alkali than is Hb A_1. This fact is utilized in the alkali denaturation test. The hemoglobin solution is added to a certain concentration of NaOH and, after filtration, the amount of hemoglobin in the filtrate (the undenatured Hb) is measured and compared to the original total quantity of hemoglobin. One report cautions that if the red cells are not washed sufficiently before preparing the hemoglobin solution, reagents of some manufacturers may produce false apparent increase in Hb F.

THALASSEMIA MINOR. — This variation of thalassemia produces a mild (or sometimes moderate) anemia, which is most often asymptomatic. It is characterized by mildly or moderately hypochromic and microcytic RBC with moderate poikilocytosis and a varying (usually not great) number of target cells. Nucleated RBC are not found in the peripheral smear. Splenomegaly may be present.

The main laboratory abnormality in thalassemia minor is an increased amount of A_2 hemoglobin. (This is true for heterozygous beta thalassemia; A_2 is not elevated in the less common heterozygous alpha thalassemia.) As noted previously, A_2 is a variant of adult Hb A_1, and is normally present in quantities up to 2.5% or 3.0%. In (beta) thalassemia minor, A_2 is elevated, ranging from 3.5 to 10%. Fetal (F) Hb is normal. A_2 Hb cannot be demonstrated on paper electrophoresis; cellulose acetate or the more complicated and time-consuming starch-block electrophoresis is required for diagnosis. These methods, especially starch techniques, are not available in many laboratories.

Thalassemia minor must sometimes be differentiated from iron deficiency anemia because of the hypochromic-microcytic status of the red cells. The serum or plasma iron is high-normal or elevated and the plasma total iron-binding capacity is considerably decreased (i.e., the TIBC is much more saturated than normal). Bone marrow iron is increased.

SICKLE-THALASSEMIA. — This produces a condition analogous to S-C disease — clinically similar in many respects to SS anemia but considerably milder. Sickle cell preparations are positive. There is often a considerable number of target cells. In these patients, 60 – 80% of the hemoglobin is Hb S, with 0 – 2% being Hb F and the remainder, if any, composed of Hb A. This means that paper electrophoresis may give either an SS or an SA pattern. When the hemoglobin is SA type (rather than the SF combination that may be found in some cases of homozygous sickle cell disease) and there is over 50% sickle hemoglobin, this suggests S-thalassemia. Also, sickle trait does not usually have the clinical picture of S-thalassemia. When the pattern is SS, the diagnosis is difficult. Clues are a syndrome much milder than one would expect with SS disease and the presence of more target cells and hypochromia than one would expect. Family studies are often necessary to look for thalassemia minor in one of the parents.

To conclude the hemoglobinopathies, certain observations should be made. First, a sickle preparation should be done on all black patients who have anemia, hematuria, abdominal pain or arthralgias. This should be followed up with hemoglobin electrophoresis if the sickle preparation is positive or if peripheral blood smears show significant numbers of target cells. However, if the patient has had these studies done previously, there is no need to repeat them. Second, these patients may have other diseases superimposed on their hemoglobinopathies. For example, unexplained hematuria in a person with sickle hemoglobin may be due to carcinoma and should not be blamed on the hemoglobinopathy without investigation. Likewise, when there is hypochromia and microcytosis, one should rule out chronic iron deficiency (e.g., chronic bleeding). This is especially true when the patient has sickle trait only, since this does not usually produce anemia. The leukocytosis found as part of SS disease (and to a lesser degree in S-C and S-thalassemia) may mask the leukocytosis of infection. As mentioned, finding significant numbers of target cells suggests one of the hemoglobinopathies. However, target cells are often found in chronic liver disease; they may be seen in any severe anemia in relatively small numbers, and may sometimes be produced artifactually at the thin edge of a blood smear.

Several reports indicate that decreased MCV (p. 2) detected by automated hematology cell counters is a useful screening method for thalassemia as well as for chronic iron deficiency anemia. Occasional patients with other hemoglobinopathies may also be found.

Electrophoresis has been mentioned repeatedly as a means of detecting and differentiating various abnormal hemoglobins. Different electrophoresis methods produce different results, and there may be variance between manufacturers who supply the same basic methods. For example, filter paper separates Hb A, S and C; F migrates with A, and A_2 with C. Cellulose acetate has considerable diversity, but many techniques can detect A, F and S, with C and A_2 migrating together. Citrate agar has the same general pattern as cellulose acetate, but Hb D, E and G migrate with A on citrate agar, while on cellulose acetate they travel with S. Citrate agar gives a little better separation of F from A in newborn cord blood.

CONGENITAL NONSPHEROCYTIC HEMOLYTIC ANEMIAS

The red cell contains many enzymes involved in various metabolic activities. Theoretically any of these may be affected by congenital or possibly by acquired dysfunction. The most frequent congenital abnormalities are associated with enzymes that participate in metabolism of glucose. After glucose is phosphorylated to glucose-6-phosphate by hexokinase, about 10% of the original molecules follow the oxidative hexose monophosphate (pentose) pathway, and about 90% traverse the anaerobic Embden-Meyerhof route. The only common defect associated with clinical disease is produced by glucose-6-phosphate dehydrogenase (G-6-PD) deficiency, which is a part of the hexose monophosphate shunt. The primary importance of this sequence is its involvement with metabolism of reduced glutathione (GSH), which is important in protecting the red cell from damage by oxidizing agents. The next most frequent abnormality, pyruvate kinase defect, a part of the Embden-Meyerhof pathway, is very uncommon, and other enzyme defects are rare. The various RBC enzyme defects (plus the unstable hemoglobins) are sometimes collectively referred to as the congenital nonspherocytic anemias.

Those RBC enzyme defects of the hexose monophosphate shunt and others involved in glutathione metabolism are sometimes called Heinz-body anemias. The term also includes many of the unstable hemoglobins and a few idiopathic cases. Heinz bodies are small, round, dark-staining, intraerythrocytic inclusions of varying size, which are only visualized when stained by supravital stains (not ordinary Wright's or Giemsa). In most cases, the Heinz bodies must be induced by oxidizing agents before staining.

Glucose-6-Phosphate Dehydrogenase (G-6-PD) Defect

This is a sex-linked genetic defect carried on the female (X) chromosome. To obtain full expression of its bad effects, the gene must not be opposed by a normal X chromosome. Therefore, the defect is most severe in males (XY) and in the much smaller number of females in whom both X chromosomes have the abnormal gene. Those females with only one abnormal gene ("carrier" females) have varying expressions of bad effect, ranging from completely asymptomatic to only moderate abnormality even under stimulation, which is greater than that needed to bring out the defect clinically in affected males or homozygous females.

The G-6-PD defect is found mainly in blacks and to a lesser extent in persons whose ancestors came from Mediterranean countries such as Italy or Greece. The defect centers in the key role of G-6-PD in the pentose phosphate glucose metabolic cycle of RBC. When RBC get older, they normally have less ability to utilize the pentose phosphate (oxidative) cycle, which is an important pathway for utilization of glucose, although secondary to the Embden-Meyerhof (nonoxidative) glycolysis cycle. When the defective G-6-PD status is superimposed on the older erythrocyte, utilization of the pentose phosphate shunt is lost. This cycle is apparently necessary to protect the integrity of the RBC against certain chemicals. Currently it is thought that these chemicals act as oxidants and that reduced nicotinamide-adenine dinucleotide phosphate (NADPH) from the pentose cycle is the reducing agent needed to counteract their effects. At any rate, exposure to certain chemicals in sufficient dosage results in destruction of erythrocytes with a sufficiently severe G-6-PD defect. About 11% of American black males are affected. Their defect is relatively mild, since their younger RBC contain about 10% of normal enzyme activity, enough to resist drug-induced hemolysis. When the RBC become older, they lose nearly all G-6-PD activity and will be destroyed. In affected persons of Mediterranean origin, all RBC regardless of age contain less than 1% G-6-PD activity.

As noted, before drug exposure the susceptible patients do not have anemia. After a hemolytic drug is given, acute hemolysis is usually seen on the second day, but sometimes not until the third or fourth day. All the classic laboratory signs of nonspecific acute hemolysis are present. The degree of anemia produced in blacks is only moderate, because only the older cell population is destroyed. If the drug is discontinued, hemolysis stops in 48–72 hours. If the drug is continued, anemia continues at a plateau level, with only a small degree of active hemolysis taking place as the RBC advance to the susceptible cell age. Whites have a more severe defect and, therefore, more intense hemolysis, which continues unabated as long as the drug is administered.

Many drugs have been reported to cause this reaction in G-6-PD defective persons. The most common ones are the following: antimalarials, sulfas, nitrofurantoin (Furadantin) family, and aspirin and similar analgesics, such as phenacetin. Hemolysis induced by various infections has been frequently reported and may also occur in uremia and diabetic acidosis.

Several screening tests for G-6-PD deficiency are available, among which are methemoglobin reduction (Brewer's test), glutathione stability, dye reduction, ascorbate test and fluorescent spot tests. Assay procedures can also be done. During hemolytic episodes in blacks, dye reduction and glutathione stability tend to give false normal results. Blood transfusions may temporarily invalidate all tests for G-6-PD deficiency in blacks and whites.

Once again, the same caution applies to G-6-PD that was necessary with the hemoglobinopathies. Hemolytic anemia in those groups known to have a high incidence of this defect should always raise the suspicion of its presence. However, even if the patient has the defect, this does not exclude the possibility that the actual cause of hemolysis was something else.

Unstable Hemoglobins

This is a group of rare hemoglobins with the common laboratory feature of increased susceptibility to heat denaturation. Autohemolysis (demonstrated by an autohemolysis test) is increased in many patients, but not all. Although unstable hemoglobins are usually categorized as Heinz body anemias, Heinz bodies may not be present except after splenectomy or during an acute hemolytic episode. The degree of anemia and splenic size are variable among the different hemoglobins. Since many rare hemoglobins migrate with more common varieties, electrophoretic detection is not reliable and depends on the system used as well as on the particular hemoglobin involved.

HEREDITARY (CONGENITAL) SPHEROCYTOSIS

This is another genetically transmitted red cell defect. Most of the patients are English or northern Europeans. A dominant gene is involved, whose incidence apparently is not frequent but also not rare. The defect is manifest as spherocytosis of varying numbers of the red cells; in some patients relatively few, in other patients many.

Most patients are asymptomatic unless a crisis develops. The development of symptoms most often begins in childhood. There may be no anemia at all, or any variation from mild to moderate. The crisis of congenital spherocytosis is intermittent and varies in frequency. It is due to sudden hypoplasia of the bone marrow of unknown cause that usually lasts 6–10 days. During the crisis, anemia may become severe. Between crises, patients may be completely asymptomatic or may have very mild jaundice (scleral icterus). If anemia is present, there may be a slight or mild reticulocytosis and slightly to mildly elevated serum indirect bilirubin. There is a considerably increased incidence of gallstones.

The spherocytes are not destroyed in the blood stream but are sequestered, removed and destroyed in the spleen. Splenomegaly usually is present. Therefore, splenectomy satisfactorily cures the patient's symptoms because marrow RBC production can then keep up with the presence of spherocytes, which have a shorter life span than normal RBC.

The most useful diagnostic test in congenital spherocytosis is the osmotic fragility test. RBC are placed in bottles containing decreasing concentrations of NaCl. When the concentration becomes too dilute, normal RBC begin to hemolyze. Spherocytes are more susceptible to hemolysis in hypotonic saline than normal RBC, so that spherocytes begin hemolyzing at concentrations above the normal range. This will be true when there are significant degrees of spherocytosis from any cause, not just congenital spherocytosis. Incidentally, target cells are resistant to hemolysis in hypotonic saline and begin to hemolyze at concentrations below those of normal RBC. Osmotic fragility is not reliable in the newborn unless the blood is incubated at 37° C for 24 hours prior to testing. This may be necessary in a minority of adults.

Spherocytes are often confused with nonspherocytic small RBC (microcytic RBC). A classic spherocyte is smaller than normal RBC size, is round and does not demonstrate the usual central clear area. (The relatively thin center associated with normal biconcave disk shape is lost as the red cell becomes a sphere.)

PAROXYSMAL NOCTURNAL HEMOGLOBINURIA

This is a rare but famous etiology for hemolytic anemia. The disease consists of a chronic hemolytic anemia with crisis episodes of hemoglobinuria, which most often occur at night. It usually affects young or middle-aged adults. The anemia is usually of moderate degree except during crisis, when it may be severe. A crisis is reflected by all the usual laboratory parameters of severe hemolysis, including elevated plasma hemoglobin. No spherocytosis or demonstrable antibodies are present. The disease gets its name because hemoglobinuric episodes change urine collected during or just after sleep to a red or brown color due to large amounts of hemoglobin. Urine formed during the day is clear. Various stimuli are known to precipitate attacks in some cases; these include infections, surgery and blood transfusion.

In addition to severe anemia leukopenia is extremely common, and thrombocytopenia is fairly common. This is in contrast to most other hemolytic anemias, where hemolysis usually provokes leukocytosis.

A good screening test is a urine hemosiderin examination. However, a positive urine hemosiderin may be otained in many cases of chronic hemolytic anemia of various types and also may be produced by frequent blood transfusions, especially if given over periods of weeks or months. A much more specific test is the acid hemolysis (Ham) test. The RBC of paroxysmal nocturnal hemoglobinuria (PNH) are more susceptible to hemolysis in acid pH. Therefore, serum is acidified to a certain point that does not affect normal RBC but will hemolyze the RBC of PNH.

A more recently reported test, claimed to be as good or better than the Ham procedure, is called the sugar-water test.

HEMOLYTIC ANEMIAS DUE TO EXTRACORPUSCULAR AGENTS

Isoagglutinins (Isoantibodies)

As explained in Chapter 10 these anemias are hemolytic reactions caused by antibodies within the various blood group systems. The classification, symptomatology and diagnostic procedures necessary for detection of such reactions and identification of the etiology are discussed in that chapter.

Autoagglutinins (Autoantibodies)

These are antibodies produced by an individual against certain of his own body cells. In this discussion those produced against his own red blood cells are the ones in question. This disease has been called "autoimmune hemolytic anemia" or "acquired hemolytic anemia."

Autoantibodies of the autoimmune hemolytic anemias form two general categories: those which react best in vitro above room temperature (37° C, warm autoantibodies) and those which react best in vitro at cold temperatures (cold autoantibodies or cold agglutinins). For each type there are two general etiologies, idiopathic and secondary to some known disease.

Warm autoantibodies are the most frequent type, and the idiopathic variety is twice as frequent as that secondary to known disease. Clinically, in the warm type the anemia appears at any age and may be either chronic or acute. When chronic, it is more often relatively low grade. When acute, it is often severe and fatal. The laboratory signs are those of any hemolytic anemia and depend on the degree of anemia. Thus, there are varying degrees of reticulocyte elevation. The direct Coombs test (p. 81) is usually, although not always, positive. Most of the patients have spherocytes in the peripheral blood, especially if the anemia is acute. There is often splenomegaly.

Cold agglutinins (cold autoantibodies) are much less frequent. They are seen mostly in adults and more often in the elderly. The idiopathic and secondary forms have a nearly equal incidence. Clinically, the disease is often worse in cold weather. Raynaud's phenomenon is common. Splenomegaly is not common. Laboratory abnormalities are not as marked as in the warm autoantibody type, except for a usually positive direct Coombs test. The anemia tends to be less severe. The reticulocyte count is usually increased, but often only slightly. Spherocytes are more often absent than present. WBC and platelets are usually normal unless altered by underlying disease. However, exceptions to the above statements may occur, with severe hemolytic anemia present in all its manifestations. As noted in the discussion of primary atypical pneumonia (p. 187), cold agglutinins may occur in many normal persons, but only in titers up to 1:64. In symptomatic anemia due to cold agglutinins the cold agglutinin titer is almost always over 1:1000.

The causes of acquired hemolytic anemia of the secondary type, either warm or cold variety, can be divided into three main groups. The most frequent occurrence is with chronic lymphocytic leukemia, to a lesser extent in lymphocytic lymphoma, and occasionally with Hodgkin's disease. The second group in order of frequency is the collagen diseases, notably lupus.

The third is a miscellaneous category, including systemic diseases in which the development of overtly hemolytic anemia is relatively rare, but does happen from time to time. These diseases include viral infections, severe liver disease, ovarian tumors, and carcinomatosis. It should be emphasized that in all of the groups of diseases mentioned above, anemia is a common or even frequent finding, but that the anemia is usually not due to hemolytic anemia—at least not of the overt or symptomatic type. Anemias of systemic disease were discussed earlier (p. 18).

Toxins

CHEMICAL.—Lead poisoning is the most frequent in this group. Ingestion of paint containing lead used to be frequent in children and still happens occasionally. Auto battery lead, gasoline fumes and homemade whiskey are the most common causes in adults. It takes several weeks of chronic exposure to develop symptoms, unless a large dose is ingested. The anemia produced is most often mild to moderate, and the usual reason for seeing the patient is development of other systemic symptoms, such as convulsions from lead encephalopathy, abdominal pain or paresthesias of hands and feet. The anemia is more often hypochromic, but may be normochromic; it is usually normocytic. Basophilic stippling of red cells is often very pronounced, and forms a classic diagnostic clue to this condition. Basophilic stippling may occur in any severe anemia, especially the hemolytic anemias, but when present in unusual quantity should suggest lead poisoning unless the cause is already obvious. The stippled cells are reticulocytes, which, for some unknown reason, appear in this form in these patients. However, in some patients, basophilic stippling is minimal or absent. In lead poisoning there is usually increased urinary excretion of coproporphyrin type III, and this fact provides a very useful screening test (p. 432, however, in a few cases there may be normal results).

Other chemicals were mentioned in the discussion on glucose-6-phosphate dehydrogenase deficiency anemia (p. 31). Benzene toxicity was discussed in the hypoplastic bone marrow anemias (p. 17). Other chemicals that often produce a hemolytic anemia if taken in sufficient dose include naphthalene, toluene, phenacetin and distilled water given intravenously. Severe extensive burns often produce acute hemolysis to varying degree.

BACTERIAL.—*Clostridium welchii* septicemia often produces a severe hemolytic anemia with spherocytes. Hemolytic anemia is rarely seen with tuberculosis. The anemia of infection is usually not overtly hemolytic, although there may be a minor hemolytic component (not demonstrable by the usual laboratory tests).

Parasites

Among hemolytic anemias due to parasites, malaria is by far the most frequent. It has to be considered in persons who have visited endemic areas and who have suggestive symptoms or no other etiology for their anemia. The diagnosis is made from peripheral blood, best obtained morning and afternoon for 3 days. Organisms within parasitized RBC may be few, and often will be missed unless the laboratory is notified that malaria is suspected. A thick-drop special preparation is the method of choice for diagnosis. With heavy infection, the parasites may be identified in an ordinary (thin) peripheral blood smear. A hemolytic anemia is produced with the usual reticulocytosis and other laboratory abnormalities of hemolysis. Most patients have splenomegaly. *Bartonella* infection occurs in South America, most often in Peru. This is actually a bacterium rather than a parasite, but in many textbooks is usually retained in the parasite category. The organisms infect RBC and cause hemolytic anemia similar clinically to malaria.

Systemic Diseases

Hemolytic anemia is most often seen with certain types of reticuloendothelial malignancy (chronic lymphocytic leukemia and lymphocytic lymphoma), but may occur in collagen diseases and rarely in systemic illnesses or severe acute infections (p. 19). In most diseases where it occurs the actual incidence is very low or rare. Even in the higher-incidence groups, such as certain reticuloendothelial malignancies and, to a lesser extent, the collagen diseases, it is not very common. Further discussion is located in the section on hemolytic anemias due to autoimmune antibodies (p. 82).

Hypersplenism

This is a poorly understood entity whose main feature is an enlarged spleen associated with a deficiency in one or more blood cell elements. The most common is thrombocytopenia, but there may be a pancytopenia or any combination of anemia, leukopenia, and thrombocytopenia. Hypersplenism may be primary or, more commonly, secondary to any disease that causes splenic enlargement. However, it should be noted that splenic enlargement in many cases does not produce hypersplenism effects. Portal hypertension with secondary splenic congestion is the most common etiology; the usual cause of this is cirrhosis. If anemia is produced in hypersplenism, it is normocytic and normochromic without reticulocytosis. Bone marrow examination in hypersplenism shows either mild hyperplasia of the deficient peripheral blood element precursors or normal marrow.

Several mechanisms have been proposed to explain the various effects of hypersplenism. To date, the weight of evidence favors sequestration in the spleen. In some cases, the spleen may destroy blood cells already damaged by immunologic or congenital agents; in some cases, the action of the spleen cannot be completely explained.

INVESTIGATION OF A PATIENT WITH ANEMIA

To conclude the presentation of anemia, the thing most needed is a rational and systematic approach to diagnosis. Anemia is a symptom, not a disease. Most of the causes can be localized by utilizing available information plus a relatively few laboratory tests. When anemia is discovered (usually by the appearance of a low hemoglobin or hematocrit value), the first thing is to determine whether anemia really exists. The abnormal result should be confirmed by redrawing the specimen. Then, if the patient is not receiving intravenous fluids that might produce hemodilution, the next step is to get a WBC count, differential, red cell indices, reticulocyte count and a description of RBC morphology from the peripheral smear. It is wise to personally look at the peripheral smear in addition, because many technicians do not routinely pay much attention to the RBC of a peripheral smear (this is the main reason for getting indices). A careful history and physical examination must be performed. To some extent, the findings on the peripheral smear and indices help suggest areas to emphasize particularly (p. 478).

1. If the RBC are hypochromic and microcytic, chronic blood loss must always be ruled out carefully.

2. If the RBC show macrocytosis, the possibility of megaloblastic anemia must always be investigated.

3. If the RBC are not markedly hypochromic and microcytic, if macrocytosis due to megaloblastic anemia is ruled out and if the reticulocyte count is significantly elevated, two main possibilities should be considered: acute blood loss and hemolytic anemia. The reticulocyte count is usually 5% or over in these cases. However, the possibility of a deficiency anemia responding to therapy should not be forgotten, and also the possibility that macrocytosis may be due to a reticulocytosis.

4. In a basically normocytic-normochromic anemia where there is no significant reticulocytosis and either leukopenia or thrombocytopenia (or both) is present, hypersplenism, bone marrow depression or a few systemic diseases (such as lupus) are the main possibilities. Presence of rouleaux would raise the question of myeloma.

5. Appearance of certain RBC abnormalities in the peripheral blood suggests certain diseases. Considerable numbers of target cells suggest one of the hemoglobinopathies or chronic liver disease. Marked basophilic stippling points toward lead poisoning. Sickle cells mean sickle cell anemia. Nucleated RBC indicate either bone marrow replacement or unusually marked bone marrow erythropoiesis, most commonly seen in hemolytic anemias. Significant rouleau formation suggests monoclonal gammopathy or hyperglobulinemia. Spherocytes usually indicate an antigen-antibody type of hemolytic anemia, but may mean congenital spherocytosis or a few other kinds of hemolytic anemia. Schistocytes (burr cells) are usually associated with certain types of hemolytic anemia or with uremia. They have also been reported in various other conditions, such as hypothyroidism and alcoholism. Macrocytes are frequently produced by reticulocytosis, but are also associated with megaloblastic anemias, cirrhosis, chronic alcoholism, hypothyroidism and aplastic anemia.

Once the basic underlying process is identified, the etiology can usually be isolated by selective laboratory tests plus the help of physical examination and careful history.

In general, it is best to perform diagnostic studies before giving blood transfusions, although in many cases the diagnosis can be made despite transfusion. Usually, appropriate blood specimens for the appropriate tests can be obtained before transfusion of blood is actually begun, since blood for type and crossmatching must first be drawn anyway. A peripheral blood smear is often helpful to indicate what tests will be needed.

REFERENCES

Amorosi, E. L.: Hypersplenism, Semin. Hemat. 2:249, 1965.
Beutler, E.: Genetic disorders of red cell metabolism, Med. Clin. North Am. 53:813, 1969.

Cooper, H. A., and Hoagland, H. C.: Fetal hemoglobin, Mayo Clin. Proc. 47:402, 1972.

Costea, N., and Eipe, J.: Erythrocyte antibodies in autoimmune hemolytic anemia, Postgrad. Med. 55:63, 1974.

Crosby, W. H.: Hypersplenism, in DeGraff, A. C., and Creger, W. P. (eds.): *Annual Review of Medicine* (Palo Alto, CA: Annual Reviews, Inc., 1962), vol. 13, p. 127.

Fairbanks, V. F., and Fernandez, M. N.: The identification of metabolic errors associated with hemolytic anemia, J.A.M.A. 208:316, 1969.

Furlong, M. B.: Drug-induced immune hemolytic anemia, Postgrad. Med. 56:193, 1974.

Hartmann, R. C., and Krantz, S. B.: Paroxysmal nocturnal hemoglobinuria and pure red cell aplasia, Postgrad. Med. 55:141, 1974.

Hoffman, G. C.: Thalassemia minor – a common disorder, Lab. Med. 6:13, 1975.

Honig, G. R.: Hemoglobinopathies and thalassemia: abnormalities of hemoglobin structure, function, and synthesis, Postgrad. Med. 55:77, 1974.

Kruger, H. C., and Burgert, E. O.: Hereditary spherocytosis in 100 children, Mayo Clin. Proc. 41:821, 1966.

McCurdy, P. R.: Abnormal hemoglobins and pregnancy, Am. J. Obstet. Gynecol. 90: 891, 1964.

McElfresh, A. E.: Congenital microspherocytosis, Pediatr. Clin. North Am. 9:665, 1962.

Mengel, C. E., et al.: Anemia during acute infections: role of glucose-6-phosphate dehydrogenase deficiency in Negroes, Arch. Intern. Med. 119:287, 1967.

Motolsky, A. G., and Stamatoyannopoulos, G.: Clinical implications of glucose-6-phosphate dehydrogenase deficiency, Ann. Intern. Med. 65:1329, 1966.

Necheles, T. F., and Allen, D. M.: Heinz-body anemias, N. Engl. J. Med. 280:203, 1969.

Newman, D. R., et al.: Studies on the diagnostic significance of hemoglobin F levels, Mayo Clin. Proc. 48:199, 1973.

Okuno, T., and Chou, A.: The significance of small erythrocytes, Am. J. Clin. Pathol. 64:48, 1975.

Orkin, S. H., and Nathan, D. G.: The thalassemias, N. Engl. J. Med. 295:710, 1976.

Prankard, T. A. J., and Bellingham, A. J. (ed.): Haemolytic anaemias, Clinics in Haematol. 4, Feb. 1975.

Van Eys, J.: Recent progress in genetic hemolytic disorders: a practical approach, Pediatr. Clin. North Am. 17:449, 1970.

Weatherall, D. J. (ed.): Abnormal haemoglobins, Clinics in Haematol. 3, June 1974.

Woods, W. E., and O'Neill, B.: Sucrose haemolysis: A simple screening test for paroxysmal nocturnal haemoglobinuria, Med. J. Aust. 56:21, 1969.

5 / White Blood Cells and Leukocytosis

WHITE BLOOD CELLS (leukocytes) form the first line of defense of the body against invading microorganisms. Neutrophils and monocytes respond by phagocytosis; lymphocytes and plasma cells apparently produce antibodies. Besides nonspecific response to infection by either bacteria or virus, alterations in the normal leukocyte blood picture may provide a diagnostic clue in certain specific diseases, both benign and malignant. Nonneoplastic leukocyte alterations may be quantitative, qualitative or both, the qualitative aspects demonstrating an increased degree of immaturity, morphologic alteration in cellular structure, or increased quantity of certain less commonly found types of WBC.

Normal white cell maturation sequence begins with the blast form, presumably itself derived from fixed tissue reticulum cells. In the myelocytic (granulocytic or neutrophilic) series (Table 5–1) the blast is characterized by a large nucleus with delicate interlacing chromatin, one or more nucleoli and a relatively scanty basophilic cytoplasm without granules. Next in sequence is the progranulocyte (promyelocyte), which is essentially similar to the blast except for the appearance of cytoplasmic granules. This gives rise to the myelocyte. The myelocyte nuclear chromatin is more condensed, no nucleolus is present, and the nucleus itself is round or oval, sometimes with a slight flattening along one side. The cytoplasm is mildly basophilic and has granules to varying degrees, although sometimes granules are absent. There often is a small localized pale or clear area next to the flattened portion (if present) of the nucleus, the so-called myeloid spot. Next, the nucleus begins to indent; when it does, the cell is called a metamyelocyte (juvenile). As the metamyelocyte continues to mature, the nucleus becomes more and more indented; the nuclear chromatin becomes more and more condensed, clumped and dark-stained; and the cytoplasm becomes less and less basophilic. The entire cell size becomes somewhat smaller, with the nucleus taking up less and less space. Finally, the band (stab) neutrophil stage is reached. There is some disagreement over just what constitutes a band as opposed to a metamyelocyte on the one hand and a mature polymorphonuclear on the other. Basically, a band is distinguished from a late metamyelocyte when the nucleus has indented over half its diameter, and the nucleus has formed a curved rod structure which is roughly the same thickness throughout. The final stage is the polymorphonuclear neutrophil. The nucleus has segmented into two or more lobes, at least one of which is connected only by a threadlike filament to the next.

39

TABLE 5-1.—TERMINOLOGY OF BLOOD CELLS

SERIES	CLASSIC TERMINOLOGY	SYNONYMS
Granulocytic	Myeloblast	
	Promyelocyte	Progranulocyte
	Myelocyte	
	Metamyelocyte	Juvenile cells
	Band granulocyte	Stab cells
	Segmented granulocyte	Polymorphonuclear cells
	Hypersegmented granulocyte	
Erythroid	Pronormoblast	Rubriblast
	Basophilic normoblast	Prorubricyte
	Polychromatophilic normoblast	Rubricyte
	Orthochromic normoblast	Metarubricyte
	Reticulocyte	
	Erythrocyte	
Lymphocytic	Lymphoblast	
	Prolymphocyte	
	Lymphocyte	
Plasmocytic	Plasmablast	
	Proplasmocyte	
	Plasmocyte	Plasma cell
Monocytic	Monoblast	
	Promonocyte	
	Monocyte	

The nuclear chromatin is dense and clumped. The cytoplasm is a very slightly eosinophilic color, or at least there is no basophilia. There usually are small irregular granules, which often are indistinct. The separation point of the polymorphonuclear from the band is the presence of the filament connection between lobes. Beginning lobe formation occurs in late band forms. When the constriction becomes a thin wire the cell is a segmented granulocyte ("poly"). In some cases a bandlike nucleus is folded in such a way as to hide the possibility of a thin constricted area; the cell is then classified as a segmented form. When multiple nuclear segmentation occurs and the clearly segmented portions number more than five, the cell is termed hypersegmented. Naturally, there are transition forms between any of the maturation stages just enumerated (Fig 5-1).

Monocytes are often confused with metamyelocytes or bands. The monocyte tends to be a larger cell. Its nuclear chromatin is a little less dense than the myeloid cell, and instead of being clumpy it is a little more strandlike. The nucleus typically has several pseudopods, which sometimes are obscured by being superimposed on the remainder of the nucleus and have to be looked for carefully. Sometimes, however, a monocyte nuclear shape is found that resembles a metamyelocyte. The monocyte cytoplasm is light blue or light gray, is rather abundant and frequently has a cytoplasm border that appears frayed or has small irregular tags or protrusions. The granules of a monocyte, when present, usually are very tiny or pinpoint in size, a little smaller than those of a neutrophil. In some cases, the

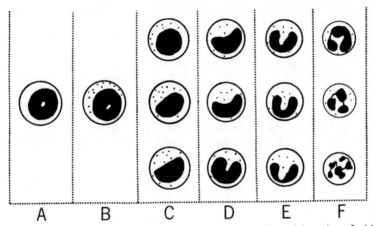

Fig 5–1.—Maturation sequence of granulocytic (myelocytic) series. **A,** blast; **B,** promyelocyte; **C,** myelocyte (*top,* early stage; *bottom,* late stage); **D,** meta-myelocyte (*top,* early stage; *bottom,* late stage); **F,** segmented granulocyte (*top,* early stage; *bottom,* hypersegmented late stage).

best differentiation is to find undisputed bands and compare their nucleus and cytoplasm with that of the cell in question.

The normal range for peripheral blood WBC is 4,500–11,000/cu mm. Most persons fall into the area of 5,000–10,000/ cu mm, but there is significant overlap between normal and abnormal in the wider range, especially between 10,000 and 11,000/cu mm.

Total neutrophils	50–70%
Segmented neutrophils (polys)	50–70%
Bands (stabs)	3– 5%
Metamyelocytes (juveniles)	0– 1%
Lymphocytes	20–40%
Monocytes	0– 7%
Eosinophils	0– 5%
Basophils	0– 1%

Neutrophilic Leukocytosis

Infection and inflammation.—This is the most frequent cause. Besides an increase in total neutrophil count, there often is some degree of immaturity ("shift to the left"—the maturation sequence of Schilling used to be diagrammed with the more mature forms going toward the right and the immature forms progressing toward the left). Usually a shift to the left centers in the early segmented and band neutrophil stages. Leukocytosis is most often seen with bacterial infection; viral infections, in general, tend to have normal counts or even leukopenia. The granulomatous infections (tuberculosis, sarcoid) most often have normal WBC counts, but tuberculosis occasionally demonstrates a leukocytosis. Typhoid fever is a bacterial infection that usually does not have a WBC increase; on the other hand, a neutrophilic leukocytosis may be present in 30% or more persons with severe ECHO virus infection. Overwhelming infection, particularly in debilitated persons or the elderly, may fail to show leukocytosis.

Certain neutrophil cytoplasmic inclusions are associated with infection (although also seen in tissue destruction, burns and similar toxic states); these include toxic granulation and Döhle bodies. Toxic granulation is accentuation of normal neutrophilic cytoplasm granules, which become enlarged or appear as short, rod-shaped structures of irregular width, either dark blue-black or the same color as the nucleus. Döhle bodies are moderate-sized, light blue structures most frequently located next to the cytoplasmic border.

Tissue Destruction. — This may be due to burns, abscess, trauma, hemorrhage, infarction, carcinomatosis, active alcoholic cirrhosis or surgery, and is often accompanied by varying degrees of leukocytosis. The leukocytosis varies in severity and frequency according to the etiology and the amount of tissue destruction.

Metabolic Toxic States. — The most frequent of these include uremia, diabetic acidosis, acute gout attacks and convulsions. A similar situation prevails to some extent during the last phase of pregnancy.

Certain Drugs and Chemicals. — Adrenal cortical steroids, lithium or asthma therapy with epinephrine, have been reported frequently to produce significant leukocytosis. Poisoning by various chemicals, especially lead, is another cause. (Certain drugs may, on the other hand, sometimes cause leukopenia due to idiosyncratic bone marrow depression.)

Other causes are: *Acute hemorrhage* or *severe hemolytic anemia,* acute or chronic.

Heavy cigarette smoking.

Myelogenous leukemia and myeloproliferative syndromes, including some cases of polycythemia vera.

Monocytosis

Monocytosis may occur in the absence of leukocytosis. It is most frequently found in typhoid fever, tuberculosis, subacute bacterial endocarditis and during the recovery phase of some cases of acute infection. Malaria and leishmaniasis (kala-azar) are frequent causes outside the United States. Monocytic leukemia and "preleukemia" (p. 53) also enter the differential diagnosis.

Eosinophilia

Parasites. — Eosinophilia is most often associated with roundworms and infestation by various flukes. In the United States, roundworms predominate, such as *Ascaris, Strongyloides,* and *Trichinella (Trichina).* The condition known as visceral larva migrans, caused by the nematode *Toxocara canis* (common in dogs) is sometimes seen in man. In *Trichinella* infection an almost diagnostic triad is bilateral upper eyelid edema, severe muscle pain and eosinophilia (eosinophilia, however, may be absent in overwhelming infection).

Acute Allergic Attacks. — Asthma, hay fever and other allergic reactions may be associated with eosinophilia.

Certain Extensive Chronic Skin Diseases. — Eosinophilia is often found in pemphigus; it also may appear in psoriasis and several other cutaneous disorders.

Certain Bacterial Infections. — Eosinophilia may occur in scarlet fever and brucellosis.

Miscellaneous Conditions. — Eosinophilia is reported in 20% of periarteritis nodosa cases and 25% of sarcoidosis. It also has been reported in up to 20% of Hodgkin's disease, but is usually not impressive. Many diseases, including metastatic carcinoma, have been reported to produce eosinophilia, but these are either unusual diseases or unusual findings in more common diseases, and the fact is mentioned only as a reminder of this possibility.

Basophilia
The most frequent cause is chronic myelogenous leukemia. Basophils may be increased in the other "myeloproliferative" diseases, and occasionally in certain nonmalignant conditions.

Lymphocytosis
Usually this accompanies a normal or decreased total white count. Viral infection is the most common etiology. Sometimes a neutropenia (such as occurs with agranulocytosis) will produce a "relative" type of lymphocytosis (actually a pseudolymphocytosis), since the total lymphocytes remain the same but the neutrophils are greatly decreased. A real lymphocytosis with leukocytosis occurs in pertussis, infectious lymphocytosis, infectious mononucleosis and some infants with adenovirus infection.

Neonatal Leukocytosis
At birth, there is a leukocytosis of 18,000 – 22,000 for the first 1 – 3 days. This drops sharply at 3–4 days to levels between 8,000 and 16,000. At roughly 6 months, approximate adult levels are reached, although the upper limit of normal is more flexible. Although the postnatal period is associated with neutrophilia, lymphocytes slightly predominate thereafter until about age 4 – 5 years, when adult values for total WBC count and differential become established (p. 477).

REFERENCES

Branam, G. E., and Paff, J. R.: Plasma cells and plasmacytoid lymphocytes in the peripheral blood, Lab. Med. 6:24, 1975.
Conrad, M. E.: Hematologic manifestations of parasitic infections, Semin. Hemat. 8: 267, 1971.
Donohugh, D. L.: Eosinophils and eosinophilia, Calif. Med. 104:421, 1966.
Dutcher, T. F.: Bands, polys, and atypical lymphs — one more time! Lab. Med. 6:19, 1975.
Ferenzi, G. W.: The significance of neutropenia, Med. Clin. North Am. 46:245, 1962.
Gilliland, B. C., and Evans, R. S.: The immune cytopenias, Postgrad. Med. 54:195, 1973.

Hildebrand, F. L., et al.: Eosinophilia of unknown cause, Arch. Intern. Med. 113:129, 1964.

John, T. J.: Leukocytosis during steroid therapy, Am. J. Dis. Child. 111:68, 1966.

Kuvin, S. F., and Brecher, G.: Differential neutrophil counts in pregnancy, N. Engl. J. Med. 266:877, 1962.

Maldonado, J. E.: Monocytosis: A current appraisal, Mayo Clin. Proc. 40:248, 1965.

Miller, F. F.: Eosinophilia in the allergic population, Ann. Allergy 23:177, 1965.

Twomey, J. J., and Leavell, B. S.: Leukemoid reactions to tuberculosis, Arch. Intern. Med. 116:21, 1965.

Vaisrub, S.: On the fringes of smoke rings, J.A.M.A. 234:520, 1975.

Weitzman, M.: Diagnostic utility of white blood cell and differential cell counts, Am. J. Dis. Child. 129:1183, 1975.

Welsh, J. D., et al.: The incidence and significance of the leukemoid reaction in patients hospitalized with pertussis, South. Med. J. 52:643, 1959.

Wood, T. A., and Frenkel, E. P.: The atypical lymphocyte, Am. J. Med. 42:923, 1967.

Zacharski, L. R., and Linman, J. W.: Lymphocytopenia: Its causes and significance, Mayo Clin. Proc. 46:168, 1971.

Zacharski, L. R., et al.: The lymphocyte, Mayo Clin. Proc. 42:431, 1967.

6 / Leukemia, Lymphomas and Myeloproliferative Syndromes

A CONSIDERATION of the origin and maturation sequence of white blood cells is helpful in understanding the classification and behavior of the leukemias and their close relatives, the malignant lymphomas. Most authorities agree that the basic cell of origin is the fixed tissue reticulum cell. Figure 6-1 shows the normal WBC development sequence. The corresponding malignancy is included in parentheses at each stage.

Note that malignancy may be centered at each major stage in the development sequence of the blood cells. In general, the earlier the stage at which malignancy is centered, the worse the patient's prognosis. Thus, a leukemia whose predominant cell is the myeloblast has a much worse prognosis than one whose predominant cell is the myelocyte.

Acute leukemia is a term originally defined as a leukemia which, if untreated, would be expected to allow an average life span of less than 6 months. The predominant cell is usually the blast (or closely related cells such as the promyelocyte). In most cases, there are over 25% blasts in the peripheral blood, and this criterion is the usual basis for establishing the diagnosis of acute leukemia. The one major exception to this is monocytic leukemia, which behaves like acute leukemia, even though the number of monoblasts may be very low.

Chronic leukemia is one which, if untreated, would on the average be expected to permit a life span of more than 1 year. The predominant cell forms are more mature; generally, the prognosis is best for those with the most mature forms. Thus, chronic lymphocytic leukemia has a better prognosis than chronic granulocytic (myelocytic) leukemia.

Subacute leukemia falls between the acute and chronic types.

Leukemia itself is a term which implies malignancy of one of the white cell types, ordinarily implying a situation in which the total number of white cells in the peripheral blood is increased (above the normal range).

Subleukemic leukemia is sometimes used to characterize a leukemia in which the total peripheral blood WBC count is within normal range but a significant number of immature cells (usually blasts) are present. *Aleukemic leukemia* is used when the peripheral blood count is normal (or, more often, decreased) and no abnormal cells are found in the peripheral blood. The diagnosis of subleukemic or aleukemic leukemia is made by bone marrow examination. Over 20% blasts in the bone marrow usually means leukemia, and 10-20% is suspicious.

Stem cell leukemia or acute blastic leukemia are terms often applied

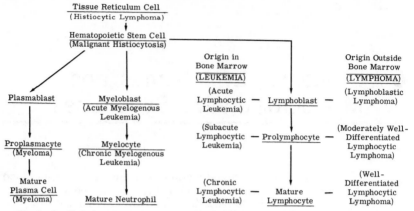

Fig 6–1.—Relationship of leukemia and malignant lymphoma to normal WBC maturation sequence.

when nearly all the white cells are blasts and no definite differentiating features are present. Myeloblasts and lymphoblasts are morphologically almost identical. In some cases, it is possible to distinguish between blast types, but for practical purposes it should not be considered reliable. In most cases, the differentiation is made on other information, such as the age of the patient and the types of cells accompanying the blasts. Cytochemical stains are sometimes helpful (p. 439). *Auer rods* are small rod-shaped structures that sometimes are present in the cytoplasm of blasts. When present, these are diagnostic of myeloid cells. They may also be found in the myelomonocytic form of monocytic leukemia.

The malignant lymphomas are basically similar to the lymphocytic leukemias; both derive from the lymphocyte series, but the leukemias originate in the bone marrow, whereas the lymphomas start outside the marrow, usually in lymph nodes. The lymphomas and their close relative, Hodgkin's disease, will be discussed later (see p. 53).

ACUTE LEUKEMIA

As noted before, this disease is rapidly fatal. It is most common in children, but a second peak in frequency is found after age 60. Acute lymphocytic leukemia is the usual childhood type, with acute myelogenous being most frequent thereafter. Monocytic leukemia is less frequent than lymphocytic or myelogenous; it tends to behave in an acute fashion, and occurs mainly in adults, including those of middle age.

Acute leukemia usually has over 25% blasts in the peripheral blood and over 50% blasts in the bone marrow. Sometimes the peripheral blood has fewer than 25%, especially if there is a leukopenia. The total peripheral WBC count is most often mildly to moderately elevated (15,000–50,000), but a sizable minority of patients have either counts in the normal range or leukopenia. Anemia is present and is generally of moderate to severe degree. If not present initially, it develops later. Thrombocytopenia is also found in most cases.

Lymph nodes often are not palpable, although lymphadenopathy of mild degree may be present—especially late in the disease. The spleen is either normal or only slightly enlarged in most cases. Generally speaking, enlargement of visceral organs is related to the duration of leukemia, so that the chronic leukemias are usually the ones with marked organomegaly or adenopathy. A fair number of acute leukemia cases develop ulcerative lesions in the oral mucous membranes or gums—occasionally elsewhere, as in the gastrointestinal tract. Hemorrhagic phenomena are frequent, due to the thrombocytopenia. Superimposed infection is common, and is probably the most frequent cause of death.

Several diseases can simulate the clinical and sometimes part of the laboratory picture of acute leukemia.

Infectious mononucleosis is frequently a problem because of the leukocytosis (or initial leukopenia) plus the atypical lymphocytes. However, infectious mononucleosis almost never has anemia and only rarely has thrombocytopenia. The bone marrow of infectious mononucleosis is normal, and is not infiltrated by significant numbers of the atypical lymphocytes. The Paul-Bunnell test (p. 184) is negative in leukemia.

Aplastic anemia may simulate acute leukemia because of peripheral blood pancytopenia. The bone marrow, however, is usually hypoplastic. Agranulocytosis often has mouth lesions and has leukopenia, but there is no anemia or thrombocytopenia.

Certain viral diseases, such as mumps, measles and whooping cough, are occasionally associated with considerably elevated WBC counts. There may be occasional atypical lymphocytes. There is no anemia or thrombocytopenia. A disease called infectious lymphocytosis occurs in children, but is uncommon. WBC counts may be 40,000–90,000—all mature lymphocytes. This condition lasts only a few days. There are no abnormal cells, no anemia or thrombocytopenia, and there is a normal bone marrow.

Overwhelming infection may cause immature cells and even a few blasts to appear in the peripheral blood of infants and young children, and sometimes other toxic bone marrow stimulation has the same effect. There is often anemia and sometimes thrombocytopenia. Bone marrow aspiration may be hypercellular and show marked myeloid hyperplasia but does not usually show the number of blasts found in leukemia. The peripheral blood blasts are usually less than 5%. They decrease in number and disappear when the underlying disease is treated.

MONOCYTIC LEUKEMIA

As noted, this entity has the clinical and laboratory aspects of acute leukemia. In monocytic leukemia, however, the number of actual blasts may be low in both the peripheral blood and bone marrow. Instead of blasts there are cells resembling monocytes.

Monocytic leukemia has been subdivided into two types: (1) the so-called pure type (monocytic leukemia of Schilling) and (2) the myelomonocytic type (monocytic leukemia of Naegeli).

Myelomonocytic leukemia is by far the most frequent variety. It actually is a form of myelogenous leukemia, in which the leukemic cells have features both of the more differentiated myeloid line and of the more primitive histiocytic precursors of the myeloid cells. The nucleus is histiocytic; the cytoplasm tends to be myelocytic. There may be accompanying myeloid cells that are nonmonocytic, less-immature forms; if so, this helps make the diagnosis. Sometimes the cells are indistinguishable from those of "pure" monocytic leukemia (Schilling type), but eventually some of them develop myeloid features. If Auer rods are found, this establishes the myeloid derivation of the cells.

Diseases accompanied by a monocytosis are sometimes confused with monocytic leukemia. Bone marrow aspiration provides the differentiation. The most common of these diseases are tuberculosis, subacute bacterial endocarditis and typhoid fever.

CHRONIC LYMPHOCYTIC LEUKEMIA

This disease is usually found after the age of 50. It is more common in males. Average survival is 3–7 years, with an appreciable number of patients alive even at 8–10 years. White cell counts usually range from 50,000 to 200,000. Most of the white cells are lymphocytic; of these lymphocytes, most (often nearly all) are mature types. In some cases there may be a considerable number of prolymphocytes and even some blasts, but this is not common. There is mild-to-moderate normocytic-normochromic anemia, usually without reticulocytosis. Platelets are often decreased, but this may not occur until late in the disease. The bone marrow contains at least 20% lymphocytes and usually over 50%. There is splenomegaly, usually to at least moderate degree, and often moderate adenopathy. Occasionally, the splenomegaly and adenopathy are marked. There is a considerable tendency to infection, and this is often the cause of death. A Coombs-positive autoimmune hemolytic anemia is reported in 5–10% of cases; a Coombs-negative hemolytic anemia, often without a reticulocytosis, eventually develops in 15–25% of cases.

CHRONIC MYELOGENOUS (GRANULOCYTIC) LEUKEMIA (CML)

This entity is most common between the ages of 20 and 50 and is rare in childhood. There usually is an increased (total) peripheral white blood cell count, most often in the 50,000–200,000 range. There is usually a predominance of myeloid cells having intermediate degrees of maturity, such as the myelocyte and early metamyelocyte. As a matter of fact, the peripheral blood often looks like a bone marrow. Anemia is usually present, although initially it is often slight. Later, anemia becomes moderate. There may be mild reticulocytosis with polychromatophilia and there occasionally are a few nucleated RBC in the peripheral blood. Platelets are either normal or increased. Average patient survival is 2–4 years. Terminally, a picture of acute leukemia often develops, the so-called blast crisis, associated with severe anemia, thrombocytopenia, and the myeloblastic type of peripheral blood and bone marrow.

Bone marrow aspiration in CML shows a markedly hypercellular marrow due to the granulocytes, with intermediate degrees of immaturity. In this respect, it resembles the peripheral blood picture.

On physical examination, there are varying degrees of adenopathy and organomegaly. The spleen is often greatly enlarged, and the liver may be moderately enlarged. Lymph nodes are often easily palpable, but generally are only slightly to moderately increased in size.

One characteristic of CML is the finding of increased numbers of basophils in the peripheral blood. The reason for the basophilia is not known.

One interesting nonhematologic aspect of CML is the presence in most, but not in all, cases of a specific chromosome abnormality in the leukemic cells. No other neoplasm thus far has such a consistent finding. The chromosome involved is number 22 (formerly thought to be number 21) of the 21–22 group in the Denver classification (G-group by letter classification); this contains a characteristic deformity and is called the Philadelphia chromosome. The Philadelphia chromosome is found in approximately 85% of patients (reported range, 75–92%). Those not having it seem as a group to have a worse prognosis. The significance of this genetic abnormality is not clear, since most cases of CML have no apparent inheritance. Also, acute myelogenous leukemia or the cells of the acute (blastic) terminal crisis of CML do not possess the Philadelphia chromosome.

When CML has the typical picture of a WBC count over 100,000 with myelocytic predominance, increased platelets, and a basophilia, the diagnosis is reasonably safe. Two conditions that otherwise may be hard to differentiate are myeloid metaplasia and leukemoid reaction. Leukemoid reaction is an abnormally marked granulocytic response to some bone marrow stimulus, most commonly infection. Leukemoid reaction is basically the same process as an ordinary leukocytosis, except in the degree of response. The expected peripheral blood WBC count elevation is even more marked than usual, and may reach the 50,000–100,000 range in some cases. Instead of the mild degree of immaturity expected, which would center in the band neutrophil (stab neutrophil) stage, the immature tendency ("shift to the left") may be extended to earlier cells, such as the myelocyte. The bone marrow may show considerable myeloid hyperplasia with unusual immaturity. However, the number of early forms in either the peripheral blood or bone marrow is not usually as great as the classic case of granulocytic leukemia. There is no basophilia, although the increased granulation often seen in neutrophils during severe infection ("toxic granulation") is sometimes mistaken for basophilia. The bone marrow in leukemoid reaction is moderately hyperplastic and may show mild immaturity, but again is not quite as immature as in CML. Splenomegaly and lymphadenopathy may be present in a leukemoid reaction due to the underlying infection, but the spleen is usually not as large as the spleen found in classic CML.

A disease that is often very difficult to separate from CML is agnogenic (idiopathic) myeloid metaplasia (AMM). This is most common in the age group 50–60. The syndrome results from bone marrow failure and subsequent extra-medullary hematopoiesis on a large scale in the spleen and sometimes in the liver and lymph nodes. Actually, the extramedullary hematopoiesis is compensatory and therefore is not idiopathic (agnogenic), but the bone marrow failure is. The bone marrow is most commonly replaced by fibrous tissue (myelofibrosis), but sometimes the syndrome of AMM may occur with normally cellular or even hypercellular marrow, at least in the early stages. The average life span is 5–7 years. There is a normochromic anemia of mild-to-moderate degree. There usually is a moderate degree of reticulocytosis and polychromatophilia, more so than with CML. There tends to be a moderate degree of anisocytosis and poikilocytosis, somewhat more than with CML. Abnormal RBC shapes are fairly frequent in AMM, and teardrop forms are very characteristic, although sometimes similar shapes may be found in CML. Nucleated RBC are more frequent in AMM than in CML.

The WBC counts in AMM are most often in the 20,000–50,000 range and very seldom reach 100,000; however, WBC counts within normal range are not uncommon. Peripheral blood differential counts are similar to CML. There may be basophilia, although this is not as common as in CML. Splenomegaly is usually marked, just as in CML, even when the WBC count is relatively low. Platelets are normal or increased, and giant platelets are often found. Giant platelets may be found in CML, but they are not common.

Bone marrow examination is the most valuable differentiating test between CML and AMM; CML has a hypercellular marrow with moderate immaturity, AMM most often has a hypocellular or fibrotic marrow. Often no marrow can be obtained, and sometimes a bone biopsy is necessary to make sure the difficulty was not due to poor technique rather than to actual absence of marrow. Sometimes x-ray films will show bone sclerosis, but this is not always true.

Although it would seem by the preceding discussion that differentiation between CML and AMM should be easy, the differences outlined may be slight and may at times appear in either disease. In fact, CML and AMM have been classified together under the term "myeloproliferative syndrome."

A useful test to differentiate leukemoid reaction, CML and AMM is the *leukocyte alkaline phosphatase (LAP) stain*. A fresh peripheral blood smear is stained with a reagent that colors the alkaline phosphatase granules normally found in the cytoplasm of mature and moderately immature neutrophils. One hundred neutrophils are counted; each neutrophil is graded 0 to 4 plus, depending on the amount of alkaline phosphatase it possesses, and the total count (score) for the 100 cells is added up. In most patients with leukemoid reaction, simple leukocytosis and leukocytosis of pregnancy or estrogen therapy (birth control pills), and in 80–90% of polycythemia vera patients, the score is higher than normal range. In AMM, about two thirds of patients have elevated values; about 25% fall within normal limits; and about 10% are low. In CML, about 90% are below normal, but 5–10% reportedly have normal values. Values may be normal in CML during remission, blast crisis or superimposed infection. In acute leukemia, values may be low, normal or high; the percentage in each category differs with cell type but not enough to provide adequate cell type diagnosis. Overlap and borderline cases occur to limit the usefulness of the test in establishing a definitive diagnosis; however, when values are obtained that are well out of normal range, the result can be very helpful in problem cases. However, an experienced technician is needed to make the test reliable, because the test reagents often give trouble, and the reading of the results is often not easy. Therefore, diagnosis should not be based on this test alone. In obvious cases, there is no need to do this test.

In many patients with "active" Hodgkin's disease, LAP is elevated. Infectious mononucleosis in early stages is associated with low or normal values in 95% of cases. In sickle cell anemia, LAP is decreased even though WBC are increased; however, if infection is superimposed, there may be an LAP increase (although a normal LAP does not rule out infection). Low values are found in paroxysmal nocturnal hemoglobinuria.

One other source of confusion with CML is the so-called leukoerythroblastic marrow response seen occasionally with certain diseases, such as septicemia, and widespread carcinomatous replacement of bone marrow. Anemia is present, and both immature white cells and also nucleated RBC may sometimes appear in the peripheral blood. A bone marrow usually is diagnostic in widespread marrow neoplasia; blood cultures and neutrophil alkaline phosphatase are helpful in septicemia. A Philadelphia chromosome study may be necessary in a few diagnostic problems.

POLYCYTHEMIA

Polycythemia is an increase in the total blood red cells over normal range. This usually entails a concurrent increase in hemoglobin and hematocrit. Since various studies disagree somewhat on the values which should be considered the upper limits of normal, partially arbitrary criteria are used to define polycythemia. A hemoglobin of over 18 gm/100 ml for men and 16 gm/100 ml for women with a hematocrit of over 55% for men and 50% for women are generally considered polycythemic levels.

Polycythemia may be divided into three groups: primary (polycythemia vera), secondary and relative.

Polycythemia vera has sometimes been included with chronic myelogenous leukemia and agnogenic myeloid metaplasia as myeloproliferative diseases. Polycythemia vera is most frequent between the ages of 40 and 70. In classic cases, peripheral blood WBC and platelets are also increased along with the RBC; however, this is not always found. The peripheral blood WBC count is over 10,000/cu mm in 50-70% of the cases. About 20-30% have a leukocytosis over 15,000/cu mm of relatively mature forms; about 10% have a leukocytosis over 15,000/cu mm with a moderate degree of neutrophil immaturity (myelocytes and metamyelocytes present). Platelets are elevated in about 25% of cases. There may be small numbers of polychromatophilic RBC in the peripheral blood, but these are not usually prominent. Splenomegaly occurs in 60-90% of patients, and is more common in those with a leukocytosis. Hepatomegaly is less frequent, but still common (40-50%). Bone marrow aspiration usually shows marrow hyperplasia, with classically an increase in all three blood element precursors—WBC, RBC and megakaryocytes. A marrow section is much more valuable than marrow smears to demonstrate this. Serum uric acid is elevated in up to 40% of cases, due to the increased red cell turnover.

Clinically, there is an increased incidence of peptic ulcer and gout, and a definite tendency toward the development of venous thrombosis.

The classic triad of greatly increased red cell mass (Hb and HCT), leukocytosis with thrombocytosis and splenomegaly, make the diagnosis obvious. However, the hemoglobin and hematocrit are often only moderately elevated, and some or all of the other features may be lacking. The problem then is to differentiate between polycythemia vera and the other causes of polycythemia.

True polycythemia refers to an increase in the total red cell mass (quantity). Relative polycythemia is a term used to describe a normal total red cell mass which falsely appears increased, due to decrease in plasma volume. Dehydration is the most common etiology for relative polycythemia; in most cases, the hematocrit is high normal or only mildly increased, but occasionally it may be substantially elevated. In simple dehydration, other blood constituents, such as the WBC, electrolytes, and urea nitrogen (BUN), also tend to be elevated (falsely). The most definitive test is a blood volume study (p. 103), which will demonstrate that the red cell mass is normal. Stress polycythemia (Gaisböck's syndrome) also is a relative polycythemia due to diminished plasma volume. Most persons affected are middle-aged males; there is a strong tendency toward mild degrees of hypertension, arteriosclerosis and obesity.

Secondary polycythemia is a true polycythemia, but, as the name implies, it has some specific underlying etiology for the increase in red cell mass. The most common cause is hypoxia. This usually is due to chronic lung disease or to congenital heart disease (although it is also seen in those who live at high altitudes). Cushing's syndrome is rather frequently associated with mild, sometimes moderate, polycythemia. A much less common etiology is certain tumors, most frequently renal carcinoma (hypernephroma) and hepatic carcinoma (hepatoma). There are several other causes, such as marked obesity (Pickwickian syndrome), but these are rare.

Laboratory tests allow differentiation of these conditions from polycythemia vera.

1. Blood volume measurements (red cell mass plus total blood volume, p. 104) can rule out relative polycythemia. Relative polycythemia has a decreased total blood volume (or plasma volume) and a normal red cell mass.

2. Arterial blood oxygen saturation studies frequently help to rule out hypoxic (secondary) polycythemia. Arterial oxygen saturation should be normal in polycythemia vera and decreased in hypoxic (secondary) polycythemia. Caution is indicated, however, since patients with polycythemia vera may have some degree of lowered PO_2 or oxygen saturation from a variety of conditions superimposed on their hematologic disease.

3. Bone marrow aspiration or biopsy is often useful, as stated earlier. If aspiration is performed, a marrow section (from clotted marrow left in the syringe and fixed in formalin, then processed like a tissue biopsy) is much better than marrow smears for this purpose. However, even bone marrow sections are not always diagnostic. In one study, about 5% of patients displayed normal or slightly increased overall marrow cellularity in conjunction with normal or only slightly increased numbers of megakaryocytes.

4. Serum uric acid levels may be useful in some cases. If the uric acid is elevated, this would be a point in favor of polycythemia vera, since secondary polycythemia has normal uric acid values. However, since uric

acid is normal in many cases of polycythemia vera, a normal value is not helpful.

5. Leukocyte alkaline phosphatase is elevated in approximately 90% of patients; the elevation occurs regardless of the WBC count.

DI GUGLIELMO'S SYNDROME

Two categories are usually included. In one, often termed erythremic myelosis, the peripheral blood contains many nucleated RBC and varying numbers of immature granulocytes. Anemia is present, and the disease behaves like acute leukemia. In the second and more frequent category the disease begins as some combination of anemia, leukopenia or thrombocytopenia, with anemia most often present. The peripheral blood RBC are usually normochromic and often display anisocytosis and poikilocytosis with varying numbers of oval macrocytes. Small numbers of immature granulocytes are present in a considerable number of patients. Some have monocytosis. The bone marrow is most often hypercellular, although it may be hypocellular. There is increase in both nucleated RBC and immature WBC and frequently in megakaryocytes also. The most typical feature is early RBC precursors with some megaloblastic-like features ("megaloblastoid"). Sideroblasts may be numerous. This entire pattern is often called erythroleukemia.

Some have noted that the form of Di Guglielmo's syndrome without marked peripheral blood erythroblastosis often procedes to myelomonocytic leukemia (less frequently, acute granulocytic leukemia); and therefore do not consider this phase as Di Guglielmo's but as "preleukemia."

MALIGNANT LYMPHOMAS

Histologic Classification

The malignant lymphomas are derived from lymphoid tissue, such as lymph nodes. Lymph nodes are composed of two parts, germinal centers and lymphoreticular tissue. The germinal centers contain lymphoblasts and reticulum cells; these produce the mature lymphocytes and reticulum cells that form the remainder of the lymphoid tissue. Therefore, three main types of cells exist in lymph nodes (and other lymphoid tissue): reticulum cells, lymphoblasts and lymphocytes. Malignancy may arise from any of these three cell types, as noted before in the discussion on leukemia. According to the classification of Rappaport, the malignant lymphomas are divided into three types based on whatever cell of origin is suggested by microscopic appearance: lymphocytic lymphoma, histiocytic lymphoma (formerly called reticulum cell sarcoma) and Hodgkin's disease. Lymphocytic lymphoma (formerly called lymphosarcoma) may, in turn, be subdivided into well-differentiated and poorly differentiated (lymphoblastic), depending, of course, on the predominant degree of differentiation of the lymphoid cells (Table 6–1). Besides the degree of differentiation, malignant lymphomas may exist in two architectural patterns—nodular and diffuse. In the nodular type, the lymphomatous tissue is distributed in focal aggregates or nodules. In the diffuse type, the lymphomatous cells diffusely and completely replace the entire lymph node or the nonlymphoid area

TABLE 6-1.—HISTOLOGIC CLASSIFICATION
OF NON-HODGKIN'S MALIGNANT LYMPHOMAS
(RAPPAPORT)

CELL TYPE	HISTOLOGIC TISSUE PATTERN	
Lymphocytic lymphoma		
Well differentiated	Nodular (rare)	Diffuse
Poorly differentiated	Nodular	Diffuse
Histiocytic lymphoma	Nodular	Diffuse
Mixed cell (lymphocytic-histiocytic)	Nodular	Diffuse
Undifferentiated	Nodular	Diffuse

invaded. Hodgkin's disease, which will be discussed later, also exists in a nodular or diffuse form, although the nodular variety is rare. In the malignant lymphomas as a whole, the diffuse pattern is more frequent than the nodular one.

In general, the nodular pattern carries a better prognosis than the corresponding diffuse pattern. The better the cell differentiation, the better the prognosis, just as in the leukemias. The most frequent histologic types of non-Hodgkin's lymphoma are poorly differentiated lymphocytic and mixed types.

Histiocytic lymphoma may be found with different nuclear types, but the various possible subclassifications all have roughly the same prognosis. Untreated histiocytic lymphoma has a prognosis comparable to that of acute leukemia. The same is true for the poorly differentiated lymphocytic lymphomas. Treatment is somewhat more effective against these neoplasms than it is for acute leukemia.

The nodular form of lymphoma has been called Brill-Symmer's disease, or giant follicular lymphoma. This was originally thought to have a relatively good prognosis. However, many feel that this terminology should be abandoned, since evidence exists that prognosis depends as much on the cell type as the architectural pattern. This would suggest that the poorly differentiated or more primitive cell types do not have a good prognosis even when they appear in a nodular ("follicular") form.

Rappaport's classification has been criticized by various investigators. Some wish to include more subclassification and others feel that the terminology does not reflect cell origin correctly. Many cases which would be classified as histiocytic by Rappaport's criteria have been shown to display reactions to special stains that are more typical of lymphoid cells than histiocytes. Nevertheless, Rappaport's classification is the one most frequently used in the United States and seems to provide a fairly reliable index of prognosis.

Most classifications of hematopoietic malignancies are based on cell morphology and tissue pattern (often including interpretation of cell origin or even cell function as estimated from morphology). Work has been presented that characterizes malignancies involving lymphocytes according to phylogenetic origin of the cells. Lymphocytes have two origins; thymus-derived (T), which functionally are responsible for delayed hypersensitivity cell-mediated immune reactions, and bursa- or bone marrow-derived

(B), which are involved with immune reactions characterized by immuno-globulin (antibody) production. Both B and T cells are derived from pre-cursors in bone marrow, which early in life produce cells that are differen-tiated into T-cells by the thymus and into B-cells within bone marrow or certain areas elsewhere. T-cells in lymph nodes are located in the deep layers of the cortex and in a thin zone surrounding germinal centers. These cells (or their derivatives) directly attack antigens and are responsible for delayed hypersensitivity reactions (as exemplified by the tuberculosis skin test reaction), immune response against certain types of infection and neo-plasms, graft-host reactions and various autoimmune disorders. The classic procedure for measuring T-cell function is the migration inhibition factor (MIF) assay. B-cells are located in the outer cortex of lymph nodes and within germinal centers. They are precursors of plasma cells. Identification of T-cells at present is usually accomplished by the sheep cell rosette method, and that of B-cells by immunofluorescent techniques that demon-strate immunoglobulin production in cell cytoplasm. In general, most work to date indicates that multiple myeloma and the majority of cases of chronic lymphocytic leukemia and lymphocytic lymphomas (especially the well-differentiated variety) are of B-cell origin. (A few cases of chronic lympho-cytic leukemia have been T-cell.) Childhood acute lymphoblastic leuke-mia is most frequently "null" (neither B- nor T-cell markers); one smaller subgroup is reported to possess T-cell markers. This T-cell subgroup of childhood acute lymphoblastic leukemia has many clinical features in common with a cytologically similar subgroup of the malignant lymphomas (so-called lymphoblastic lymphoma, or Sternberg's sarcoma). These fea-tures include a mediastinal mass, onset in later childhood or adolescence, predominance in males and poor prognosis. Other T-cell malignancies in-clude the so-called cutaneous lymphomas, mycosis fungoides and Sézary syndrome.

BURKITT'S LYMPHOMA. — Burkitt's lymphoma is a variant of malignant lymphoma originally reported in African children. It is now known to occur in children elsewhere in the world. About 30% have involvement of the jaw, a site which is rarely affected by other lymphomas. A tumor is fre-quently located in the abdomen; single peripheral lymph node groups are involved in about 30% of patients; widespread peripheral lymphadenop-athy is rare. Histologically, the cells are rather uniform, may be lympho-blastic or histiocytic in appearance and characteristically include scattered single cells exhibiting phagocytosis ("starry sky appearance"). Occasional patients in the United States have developed acute lymphoblastic leuke-mia. In addition, several of the U.S. patients have been young adults.

HODGKIN'S DISEASE. — Hodgkin's disease is usually considered a sub-group of the malignant lymphomas. The basic neoplastic cell is the malig-nant reticulum cell. Some of these malignant reticulum cells take on a bi-nucleated or multinucleated form with distinctive large nucleoli and are called Reed-Sternberg cells. These are the diagnostic cells of Hodgkin's disease.

Other types of cells may accompany the Reed-Sternberg cells. There-fore, Hodgkin's disease is usually subdivided according to the cell types present (Fig 6–2). Besides Reed-Sternberg cells (R-S cells), there may be

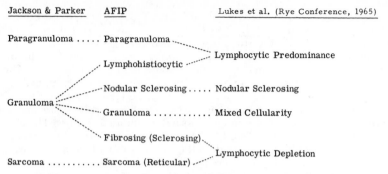

Fig 6–2.—Various histologic classifications of Hodgkin's disease.

various combinations of lymphocytes, histiocytes, eosinophils, neutrophils and reticulum cells. The main histologic forms of Hodgkin's disease are the following (using a classification developed at the Armed Forces Institute of Pathology [AFIP]):

1. Paragranuloma: Lymphocytes only (plus R-S cells).
2. Lymphohistiocytic: Lymphocytes and histiocytes (plus R-S cells).
3. Granuloma: At least 3 different cell types (plus R-S cells).
4. Nodular sclerosis: A peculiar variation of granuloma that occurs predominantly in the mediastinum and cervical lymph nodes, characterized by a nodular pattern, the nodules separated by bands of fibrous tissue.
5. Sclerosing: Rare—granuloma that is mostly replaced by spontaneous fibrosis.
6. Sarcoma: Predominantly malignant reticulum cells (including R-S cells).

The most widely accepted pathologic classification today is the one developed by Lukes and his colleagues at the Rye Conference in 1965 (see Fig 6–2). This combines certain histologic tissue patterns with similar prognosis, resulting in four groups instead of six.

Prognosis

Prognosis is relatively good for (uncured) lymphocytic predominance (9–15 years average survival). Lymphocytic depletion behaves like histiocytic lymphoma or acute leukemia, with average survival 1 year or less. Mixed cellularity has an intermediate prognosis (average 2–4 years). The nodular sclerosing category as a group falls between lymphocytic predominance and mixed cellularity, with much individual variation; a considerable number approach lymphocytic predominance survival figures. Life expectancy in Hodgkin's disease has proved quite variable, even without treatment, and some patients live for many additional years with the lymphocytic predominance, nodular sclerosing and even the mixed cellularity forms. Also of great importance, especially for therapy, is the degree of spread when the patient is first seen (Table 6–2). Localized Hodgkin's disease has some possibility of cure by adequate radiotherapy. Naturally, there is considerable correlation between the tissue histologic patterns and the clinical stage (degree of localization) of disease when first seen.

TABLE 6-2.–CLINICAL STAGING
OF THE MALIGNANT LYMPHOMAS*

Stage I	Localized in 1 group of lymph nodes
IE	Localized involvement (1 area) of 1 extralymphatic organ or site
Stage II	Localized in 2 separate groups of lymph nodes on the same side of the diaphragm
IIE	Localized in 1 group of lymph nodes plus localized involvement of 1 extralymphatic organ or site (including spleen) on the same side of the diaphragm
Stage III	Involving components of the lymphoid system (including spleen) on both sides of the diaphragm
IIIE	Involving components of the lymphoid system on both sides of the diaphragm plus localized involvement of 1 extralymphatic organ or site
Stage IV	Diffuse or disseminated involvement of 1 or more extralymphatic organs or sites with or without lymph node involvement.

In Hodgkin's disease, patients are additionally subclassified as A or B, according to whether systemic symptoms are absent (A) or present (B).

*Ann Arbor revision of Peter's classification.

Clinical Findings and Diagnosis

The diagnosis of malignant lymphoma is made by tissue biopsy, usually of lymph nodes. As a rule, the peripheral blood and bone marrow are not involved early in the disease. Later in the disease the bone marrow may become infiltrated. In some cases of lymphocytic lymphoma the lymphoma cells appear in the peripheral blood, with or without bone marrow invasion. Since lymphocytic leukemia may in the later stages involve and replace lymph nodes, there occasionally may be a problem in differentiation between lymphocytic leukemia and lymphocytic lymphoma. However, since the two are equivalent, the differentiation in such cases simply rests on the peripheral blood and bone marrow findings at the time of first diagnosis. If the marrow is diffusely involved, the disease is considered leukemia; if not involved or only focally involved, lymphoma. Histiocytic lymphoma may occasionally disseminate malignant cells into the peripheral blood; this is rare in Hodgkin's disease.

Clinically, malignant lymphoma is more common in males. The peak incidence for Hodgkin's disease is age 20–40 and for other malignant lymphomas, age 40–60. Lymph node enlargement is found in the great majority of cases but may not become manifest until later. Fever is present at some time in at least half the patients. Staging laparotomy has shown that splenic Hodgkin's disease occurs in 35–40% of cases; if this occurs, para-aortic nodes are usually involved. Liver metastasis is found in about 5–10% of cases; if so, the spleen is always invaded. In non-Hodgkin's lymphoma, laparotomy discloses splenic involvement in about 30–40% and hepatic tumor in about 10–20% of cases, with rather wide variation according to histologic classification. Splenomegaly is not reliable as a criterion for presence of splenic tumor. Bone marrow metastasis is present at the time of diagnosis in 10–60% of cases of non-Hodgkin's lymphoma and

5–30% of cases of Hodgkin's disease. Lymphocytic lymphoma has a greater tendency to reach bone marrow, liver or spleen than histiocytic lymphoma has; the nodular form is more likely to metastasize to these organs than the diffuse type. In both Hodgkin's and non-Hodgkin's lymphoma needle biopsy demonstrates bone marrow involvement more frequently than do clot sections or smears. A second biopsy increases yield by 10–20%. Anemia is found in 33–50% and is most common in Hodgkin's disease and least common in histiocytic lymphoma. Occasionally, this anemia becomes overtly hemolytic. The platelet count is usually normal unless the bone marrow is extensively infiltrated. The WBC count is usually normal in malignant lymphoma until late in the disease; in Hodgkin's disease, it is more often mildly increased, but may be normal or decreased. WBC differential counts are usually normal in malignant lymphoma unless malignant cells disseminate into the peripheral blood or, more commonly, if some other condition is superimposed, such as infection. In Hodgkin's disease, eosinophilia may occur; in late stages, leukopenia and lymphopenia may be present.

Several diseases may enter into the differential diagnosis of malignant lymphoma. Tuberculosis, sarcoidosis and infectious mononucleosis all have fever, lymphadenopathy and, frequently, splenomegaly. The atypical lymphocytes of infectious mononucleosis (p. 183) may simulate lymphocytic lymphoma cells, since both are abnormal lymphocytic forms. Usually lymphoma cells in the peripheral blood are either more immature or more distorted than the average infectious mononucleosis (virocyte) cell. Nevertheless, since infectious mononucleosis patients are usually younger persons, the finding of lymphadenopathy and a peripheral blood picture similar to infectious mononucleosis in a patient over age 40 would suggest lymphosarcoma (if some other viral illness is not present). This suspicion would be intensified if results of the Paul-Bunnell (heterophil) test (p. 184) were less than 1:28, or were 1:28–1:112 with a normal differential absorption pattern (two different determinations normal; done 2 weeks apart, to detect any rising titer). Occasionally, the rheumatoid-collagen disease group may cause a clinical picture that might suggest either an occult malignant lymphoma or its early stages. Dilantin, smallpox vaccination and certain skin diseases may produce a lymphadenopathy, which creates difficulty for both the clinician and the pathologist. Malignant lymphoma often enters into the differential diagnosis of splenomegaly, especially if no other disease is found to account for the splenomegaly.

As mentioned before, diagnosis of the malignant lymphomas is obtained by tissue biopsy. This usually means lymph node biopsy. The particular node selected is important. The inguinal nodes should be avoided, if possible, because they often contain changes due to chronic inflammation that tend to obscure the tissue pattern of a lymphoma. If several nodes are enlarged, the largest one should be selected; when it is excised, the entire node should be taken out intact. This helps to preserve the architectural pattern and allows better evaluation of possible invasion outside the node capsule, one of the histologic criteria for malignancy.

REFERENCES

Berard, C. W., and Dorfman, R. F.: Histopathology of malignant lymphomas, Clin. Haematol. 3:39, 1974.

Bloomfield, C. D.: Recognizing and evaluating non-Hodgkin's lymphomas, Geriatrics 30:56, 1975.

Brunning, R. D.: Bone marrow and peripheral blood involvement in non-Hodgkin's lymphomas, Geriatrics 30:146, 1975.

Burgert, E. O.: Nonlymphocytic leukemia in childhood, Mayo Clin. Proc. 48:255, 1973.

Byrne, G. E., and Rappaport, H.: Malignant histiocytosis, Gann Monograph on Cancer Research 15:145, 1973.

Cline, M. J., and Golde, D. W.: A review and reevaluation of the histiocytic disorders, Am. J. Med. 55:49, 1973.

Desser, R. K., et al.: Staging of Hodgkin's disease and lymphoma: diagnostic procedures including staging laparotomy and splenectomy, Med. Clin. North Am. 57: 479, 1973.

Dorfman, R. F.: Diagnosis of Burkitt's tumor in the United States, Cancer 21:563, 1968.

Dorfman, R. F., and Warnke, R.: Lymphadenopathy simulating the malignant lymphomas, Hum. Pathol. 5:519, 1974.

Ellis, J. T., et al.: The bone marrow in polycythemia vera, Semin. Hematol. 12:433, 1975.

Ellman, L.: Bone marrow biopsy in the evaluation of lymphoma, carcinoma, and granulomatous disorders, Am. J. Med. 60:1, 1976.

Gilbert, H. S.: Definition, clinical features and diagnosis of polycythemia vera, Clin. Haematol. 4:263, 1975.

Gilbert, H. S., and Dameshek, W.: The Myeloproliferative Disorders, in Dowling, H. F. (ed.): *Disease-a-Month* (Chicago: Year Book Medical Publishers, Inc., Oct. 1970).

Herbert, V.: Diagnostic and prognostic values of measurement of serum vitamin B_{12} binding proteins, Blood 32:305, 1968.

Hollander, P., and Mauer, A. M.: Myeloid leukemoid reactions in children, Am. J. Dis. Child. 105:568, 1963.

Jones, S. E.: Clinical features and course of the non-Hodgkin's lymphomas, Clin. Haematol. 3:131, 1974.

Jones, S. E., et al.: Immunologic aspects of the hematologic neoplasms, Postgrad. Med. 54:209, 1973.

Kahn, L. B., et al.: Primary gastrointestinal lymphoma: a clinicopathologic study of fifty-seven cases, Am. J. Dig. Dis. 17:219, 1972.

Kaplan, H. S., and Rosenberg, S. A.: Cure of Hodgkin's disease and other malignant lymphomas, Postgrad Med. 43:146, 1968.

Kaplan, H. S., and Rosenberg, S. A.: Hodgkin's disease: current recommendations for management, CA 25:306, 1975.

Kaplow, L. S.: Leukocyte alkaline phosphatase in disease, CRC Crit. Rev. Clin. Lab. Sci. 2:243, 1971.

Kyle, R. A., and Pease, G. L.: Basophilic leukemia, Arch. Intern. Med. 118:205, 1966.

Linman, J. W., and Saarni, M. I.: The preleukemic syndrome, Semin. Hematol. 11: 93, 1974.

Lipton, A., and Lee, B.: Prognosis of stage I lymphosarcoma and reticulum cell sarcoma, N. Engl. J. Med. 284:230, 1971.

Lutzner, M., et al.: Cutaneous T-cell lymphomas: the Sézary syndrome, mycosis fungoides, and related disorders, Ann. Intern. Med. 83:534, 1975.

Miescher, P. A., and Farquet, J. J.: Chronic myelomonocytic leukemia in adults, Semin. Hematol. 11:129, 1974.

Moran, E. M., and Ultmann, J. E.: Clinical features and course of Hodgkin's disease, Clin. Haematol. 3:91, 1974.

Morris, M. W., and Davey, F. R.: Immunologic and cytochemical properties of histiocytic and mixed histiocytic-lymphocytic lymphomas, Am. J. Clin. Pathol. 63: 403, 1975.

Nathwani, B. N., et al.: Malignant lymphoma, lymphoblastic, Cancer 38:964, 1976.

Neiman, R. S., et al.: Lymphocyte-depletion Hodgkin's disease: A clinicopathologic entity, N. Engl. J. Med. 288:751, 1973.

Pierre, R. V.: Preleukemic states, Semin. Hematol. 11:73, 1974.

Piessens, W. F., et al.: Lymphocyte surface immunoglobulins: distribution and frequency in lymphoproliferative diseases, N. Engl. J. Med. 288:176, 1973.

Prosnitz, L. R., et al.: Role of laparotomy and splenectomy in the management of Hodgkin's disease, Cancer 29:44, 1972.

Rivers, S. L., et al.: Acute leukemia in the adult male, Cancer 16:249, 1963.

Rosenthal, D. S., and Maloney, W. C.: Myeloid metaplasia: A study of 98 cases, Postgrad. Med. 45:136, 1969.

Saarni, M. I., and Linman, J. W.: Myelomonocytic leukemia: Disorderly proliferation of all marrow cells, Cancer 27:1221, 1971.

Schwartz, D. L., et al.: Lymphosarcoma cell leukemia, Am. J. Med. 38:788, 1965.

Seshadri, R. S., et al.: Leukemic reticuloendotheliosis: a failure of monocyte production, N. Engl. J. Med. 295:181, 1976.

Shaw, M., and Ishmael, D. R.: Acute lymphocytic leukemia with atypical cytochemical features, Am. J. Clin. Pathol. 63:415, 1975.

Staging in Hodgkin's Disease (Symposium), Cancer Res. 31:1707, 1971.

Takacsi-Nagi, L., and Graf, F.: Definition, clinical features and diagnosis of myelofibrosis, Clin. Haematol. 4:291, 1975.

Trujillo, J. M., et al.: General implications of chromosomal alterations in human leukemia, Hum. Pathol. 5:675, 1974.

Ultmann, J. E., and Stein, R. S.: Non-Hodgkin's lymphoma: an approach to staging and therapy, CA 25:320, 1975.

Weick, J. K., et al.: Leukoerythroblastosis: diagnostic and prognostic significance, Mayo Clin. Proc. 49:110, 1974.

Wood, N. L., and Coltman, C. A., Jr.: Localized primary extranodal Hodgkin's disease, Ann. Intern. Med. 78:113, 1973.

7 / Blood Coagulation

NORMALLY, blood remains fluid within a closed vascular system. Abnormalities of blood coagulation take two main forms – failure to clot normally (and thus to prevent abnormal degrees of leakage from the vascular system) and failure to prevent excessive clotting (and thus maintain the patency of the blood vessels). Most emphasis in clinical medicine has been on diagnosis and treatment of coagulation deficiency. To understand the various laboratory tests designed to pinpoint defects in the coagulation mechanism, it is necessary to outline the most currently accepted theory of blood coagulation (Fig 7 – 1).

BLOOD COAGULATION THEORY

The theory states that circulating blood contains two inactive proteins – prothrombin and fibrinogen. When blood comes in contact with an area of damaged blood vessel endothelium, platelets are stimulated to release a coagulation-initiating substance. In conjunction with certain factors present in normal blood (thromboplastin-generating factors), a substance called thromboplastin is formed. With the cooperation of ionized calcium, this thromboplastin catalyzes the conversion of prothrombin to thrombin. The conversion of prothrombin to thrombin is greatly speeded up by certain accelerator factors present in normal blood. Thrombin is a powerful enzyme that acts on the soluble monomer protein fibrinogen and causes it to polymerize to the insoluble product fibrin. Fibrin forms the structural framework of a blood clot. This series of reactions will be discussed in more detail, followed by consideration of laboratory tests that reflect abnormality in the various reactions. Note that many authors use only three stages in their coagulation schemes, combining stage I and II into stage I.

Stage I – The Initiator Reaction
Abnormality in this stage of coagulation concerns defects in platelets, either in number or in functional ability. Also included for purposes of discussion are intrinsic abnormalities of the capillary wall leading to abnormal permeability, either congenital or acquired. (Although this is not strictly a part of the blood coagulation sequence itself, it is inseparable from it clinically.)

Stage II – Thromboplastin Generation
The various blood factors involved will be listed and briefly discussed. The biochemistry of most is obscure, and most have not been isolated in

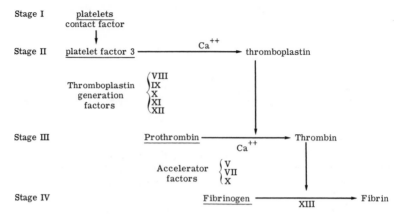

Fig 7–1. — Blood coagulation pathway.

even a relatively pure form. Knowledge of these factors derives mainly from study of persons who lack one or more of them. They are designated by roman numerals, but other names have been applied to them in the past and are still frequently used.

Factor VIII (Antihemophilic Globulin or AHG). — Deficiency of this factor causes classic hemophilia. It is inherited as a sex-linked recessive gene, so that females with the gene are usually carriers (heterozygous, xX), and males with the gene have clinical disease (xY, the hemophilic x gene not being suppressed by a normal X gene, as it would be in a female carrier). However, sporadic cases do occur without known inheritance. Hemophilia can exist in a severe (classic) form or in a mild clinical form, depending on the amount of factor VIII (AHG) the patient has. Classic (severe) hemophiliacs show 1–10% of normal factor VIII levels on assay; mild hemophiliacs have 10–35% of normal. Carrier females sometimes fall into the mild group, although usually they are completely asymptomatic.

The major clinical symptom is excessive bleeding. This classically occurs from what would be considered minor trauma or injury (sometimes almost not noticeable) in normal persons. In classic hemophilia, bleeding into joints is a characteristic finding. In mild hemophilia, there may be only an equivocal history of excessive bleeding or no history at all before severe trauma or surgery brings the condition to light. Of course, both classic and mild hemophiliacs vary somewhat in symptoms, depending on the amount of AHG they have.

Factor VIII is an unstable substance. Once blood is withdrawn from the body, there begins a slow decay of factor VIII activity, which reaches the 50% level in about 1 week. Fresh blood, fresh frozen plasma, factor VIII concentrate or cryoprecipitate are the current therapeutic sources of factor VIII. Serum does not contain factor VIII.

Factor IX (Plasma Thromboplastin Component or PTC). — Deficiency of this factor creates a condition similar to hemophilia, which has been called

Christmas disease (named after the first patient studied in detail). Clinical manifestations may show a severe or mild form, just as in hemophilia. However, although hemorrhage into joints may occur in severe cases, it is not nearly as frequent as in severe hemophilia.

Factor IX.—Found in both plasma and serum and stable in either.

Factor X (Stuart Factor).—This is the only factor that is equally important in both thromboplastin generation (stage II) and thrombin generation (stage III). Deficiency is rare and results in a disease similar to hemophilia but somewhat milder, inherited as an incompletely dominant trait. The factor is stable and is present in both serum and plasma.

Factor XI (Plasma Thromboplastin Antecedent or PTA).—Deficiency of factor XI is a mild disease. There is usually no history of excessive bleeding, which occurs only after major trauma or during surgery. It occurs in both males and females. The factor is stable and is present in plasma and in serum.

Factor XII (Hageman Factor).—This is an unusual substance whose importance derives from its role as a surface contact activator. Deficiency of factor XII markedly prolongs test-tube blood clotting time, especially in glass containers. Since most laboratory tests in hemorrhagic disease are carried out in glass test tubes, a defect in factor XII mimics the effect of the real hemorrhagic stage II factor deficiencies. Factor XII deficiency is detected only on routine laboratory screening tests, since no clinical manifestations are ever produced.

Fletcher Factor.—This substance apparently affects Hageman factor (factor XII), either by assisting in its complete activation or in its function (Fig 7–2). There is also a link to the kallikrein system, but this has not been completely worked out. Deficiency reported to date has been very rare.

Stage III—Thrombinogenesis
This involves conversion of prothrombin to thrombin in the presence of ionized calcium, aided by the accelerator factors.

Prothrombin.—This substance is synthesized by the liver. Vitamin K is necessary for its synthesis, although vitamin K is apparently not an actual precursor substance. Vitamin K is a fat-soluble vitamin manufactured by small intestinal bacteria from food precursors, which is itself present in an adequate diet and can be absorbed directly. A deficiency of vitamin K may thus result from malabsorption of fat (such as with lack of bile salts in obstructive jaundice, or the primary malabsorption of sprue—see Chapter 19) or from failure of the bacteria to synthesize this substance (due to prolonged oral antibiotic therapy). It usually takes more than 3 weeks before the body vitamin K stores are exhausted and the deficiency of available vitamin K becomes manifest. Dietary lack may be important but ordinarily does not cause a severe enough deficiency to give clinical abnormality unless other factors (such as the anticoagulant vitamin K inhibitors) are present. However, breast milk and certain infant milk formulas are relatively low in vitamin K and predispose to clinical deficiency.

Assuming normal supplies of available vitamin K, the other main limiting factor in prothrombin formation is the ability of the liver to synthesize it. In severe liver disease (most often far-advanced cirrhosis), enough parenchyma is destroyed to decrease prothrombin formation in a measurable way, eventually leading to a clinical coagulation defect. Whereas a deficiency of available vitamin K responds promptly to administration of parenteral vitamin K, hypoprothrombinemia due to liver parenchymal disease responds little, if at all, to parenteral vitamin K therapy.

Vitamin K is also necessary for synthesis of factors VII, IX, and X. The greatest effect seems to be on prothrombin and factor VII.

Factor VII (Stable Factor).—As just mentioned, vitamin K is necessary in some way for synthesis, which takes place in the liver. Factor VII is affected even more than prothrombin by lack of vitamin K and by severe parenchymal liver disease. Factor VII is present in serum or plasma, and is stable.

Factor V (Labile Factor).—This substance is apparently also synthesized by the liver, although direct proof is lacking. It is often decreased in severe parenchymal liver disease, although to a somewhat lesser degree than prothrombin and factor VII. Factor V is found only in plasma and disappears in a few days from stored blood in the blood bank.

Calcium.—Ionized calcium is essential for blood coagulation, mainly in stages II and III. Most laboratory anticoagulants, such as oxalate, citrate, and EDTA, take advantage of this by their calcium-binding action. It is very rare to have an ionized (serum) calcium level decreased enough to interfere with clotting; hypocalcemic tetany and death would probably occur first. Massive transfusion of citrated blood rarely makes this "citrate intoxication" a possibility; when bleeding difficulties are encountered in this situation, it is more likely due to the low platelets or low factor VIII and V levels of bank blood (pp. 75 and 100).

Stage IV—Fibrin Formation

This reaction features the conversion of fibrinogen to fibrin, catalyzed by previously formed thrombin. Besides catalyzing the reaction, some of the thrombin is apparently absorbed onto the clot as it forms, so that eventually not enough thrombin is left to carry the reaction further. This provides a limiting mechanism to the coagulation process.

Factor XIII.—Known as fibrin-stabilizing factor. Subclinical deficiency occurs in a variety of conditions, such as severe liver damage; clinically evident defects are rare, and the few cases reported are mostly in newborns. The results of all the usual coagulation tests are normal.

Fibrinogen.—This protein is synthesized in the liver, as so many other coagulation substances are. Apparently the production mechanism is very efficient, because hypofibrinogenemia due to liver disease is extremely uncommon. In some patients with cirrhosis there is a mild degree of fibrinolytic activity, usually not enough to be evident clinically, due to circulating fibrinolysins. Low plasma fibrinogen levels most often result from disseminated intravascular coagulation. A thromboplastin tissue substance is liberated into the bloodstream and causes fibrin deposition (clots) in small blood vessels, thus depleting the plasma of the precursor substance fibrinogen ("defibrination syndrome"). Hypofibrinogenemia may also be due to circulating fibrinolysins—enzymes which destroy fibrinogen. This most often occurs in disseminated prostate carcinoma, although other carcinomas have also been associated. Fibrinolysins have been occasionally reported after extensive surgery, most often pulmonary operations. Fibrinolysin may in rare cases accompany a wide variety of diseases, and rarely appears without any apparent cause.

Disseminated intravascular coagulation (DIC) is a much more frequent cause for hypofibrinogenemia than primary fibrinolysis is. Originally considered an obstetrical disease associated with premature separation of the placenta, DIC is now being attributed to a growing list of etiologies, among which are septicemia, surgery complicated by postoperative shock, severe burns or trauma, extensive cancer and newborn respiratory distress syndrome; and it is occasionally seen in many other conditions. Shock is the best common denominator but is not always present, nor has it been definitely proved to be either a cause or an effect. A wide range of laboratory tests have been advocated for diagnosis of DIC, many of which are being discarded as newer tests are announced or older ones reevaluated. At present, hypofibrinogenemia and thrombocytopenia are the two best-established lab findings. Cases have been reported in which either fibrinogen or platelet levels are normal. Other useful laboratory procedures are the protamine sulfate and the split-products test (p. 70).

Some persons with *dysproteinemia,* either multiple myeloma or one of the macroglobulinemias, have interference with conversion of fibrinogen to fibrin despite normal fibrinogen levels. This is manifest by poor clot stability and failure of clot retraction, and may cause a hemorrhagic tendency or purpura.

INHIBITOR SYSTEMS

Having discussed the blood coagulation substances and the blood factors involved in their activation, we should give some attention to inhibitors of various essential substances in this system. These inhibitors retard coagulation, and thus are considered anticoagulants.

DICUMAROL AND THE WARFARIN DRUGS.—These inhibit the utilization of vitamin K by the liver and therefore decrease prothrombin synthesis (as well as the other vitamin K-dependent factors). Dicumarol affects mainly stage III in the coagulation scheme. The most frequent clinical sign of warfarin (Coumadin) toxicity is hematuria.

HEPARIN.—Heparin acts primarily as antithrombin, but it also acts against some of the thromboplastin generation factors and has some effect on all stages of coagulation, with the exception of factor XII. Protamine and polybrene are specific neutralizing agents for heparin. Platelets contain a heparin-neutralizing factor (platelet factor 4). The liver affects heparin degradation and the kidney affects excretion. Severe thrombocytopenia or liver disease may increase sensitivity to heparin, while severe renal disease may delay heparin excretion.

SEVERE LIVER DISEASE. — This was discussed earlier. The main effect is on stage III of coagulation.

THE PLASMIN SYSTEM. — This is an intrinsic blood fibrinolytic system. Plasmin is a fibrinolytic enzyme that exists in blood as the inactive precursor plasminogen. A trigger mechanism is needed to set off the reaction. This may be accomplished by certain enzymes, such as streptokinase, or by other means, at present poorly understood. Note that the mechanism involved is very similar to that of coagulation stage IV, except that the activator is streptokinase (or other enzymes) instead of thrombin, and the reaction catalyzed is plasminogen to plasmin instead of fibrinogen to fibrin. There also are inhibitors of the plasmin system, just as antithrombins may inhibit stage IV coagulation development. In the plasmin system, the most effective inhibitor available is a compound called epsilon-aminocaproic acid (EACA), which provides effective therapy for many cases of circulating fibrinolytic anticoagulants. However, note that EACA would not affect a hypofibrinogenemia due to disseminated intravascular fibrin coagulation (most commonly seen in obstetrics, as mentioned earlier), where the plasmin mechanism is not involved.

MEDICATION. — Various drugs may affect coagulation. Aspirin and certain others have direct effect on clotting. Aspirin inhibits platelet adhesion and thus may potentiate a tendency to hemorrhage when a patient is receiving anticoagulant therapy. Other medications may have indirect effects by enhancing or inhibiting anticoagulants (p. 472).

TESTS IN HEMORRHAGIC DISORDERS

HISTORY. — History of easy bleeding or easy bruising should lead to further investigation.

PLATELET COUNT. — Platelet disorders will be discussed later. Using the direct count (normal values 150,000 – 300,000), a platelet count below 100,000/cu mm indicates moderate thrombocytopenia; under 50,000/cu mm means severe thrombocytopenia. Platelet number can be estimated with a reasonable degree of reliability from a well-made peripheral blood smear.

CLOT RETRACTION. — Platelets have a major role in clot retraction. The clot shrinks and pushes out serum, which was trapped within as the blood clotted. The shrunken clot is much firmer than it was originally. Normally, clot retraction begins at about 1 hour and is complete by 24 hours. With thrombocytopenia, there is deficient clot retraction.

TOURNIQUET TEST. — This demonstrates capillary fragility, due either to intrinsic defect in capillary walls (vascular purpura) or to some types of thrombocytopenia. The tourniquet test is usually positive with idiopathic thrombocytopenic purpura (ITP) and immunologic or drug-induced thrombocytopenia. It gives variable, more often negative, results with thrombocytopenia from other causes. It is usually negative in stages II, III and IV defects, but occasionally may be positive.

BLEEDING TIME. — The routine bleeding and clotting times used for pre-surgery screening tests have been shown to be highly inefficient and inaccurate. When a bleeding time is indicated, the Ivy technique is standard; many authorities now use the template (Mielke, et al.) modification of the Ivy method. The template procedure, however, utilizes a 9-mm-long (1-mm-deep) incision, which may leave a scar. The bleeding time is most helpful as an indication of platelet abnormality, whether in number or function, and provides some indication of the potential clinical severity of the function abnormality. The bleeding time may be abnormal in a variable number of patients with capillary fragility problems. In stage II defects, it is variable, often normal in mild cases. In stages III and IV defects, it is more often normal, but may be positive if the defect is severe.

PROTHROMBIN TIME (PT). — A "complete" tissue thromboplastin (which contains a platelet substitute) plus calcium is added to the patient's plasma. Formation of a fibrin clot is the end point. The PT mainly indicates defects in stage III (prothrombin and factors V, VII and X). If defects in stage IV are severe, they also will produce abnormal PT test results since the test depends on an intact stage IV to generate the clot end point. However, the fibrinogen level usually must be under 100 mg/100 ml (normal 200–400 mg/100 ml) before hypofibrinogenemia affects the PT. Stages I and II defects do not influence the PT, because a complete thromboplastin reagent is provided.

Because the "classic" coagulation theory postulated conversion of prothrombin to thrombin as the major reaction in stage III, prothrombin is commonly considered the principal agent measured by the PT. Actually, the test is more sensitive to factor VII than to prothrombin. Clinically, this makes little difference since both factor VII and prothrombin are altered by the same two major conditions affecting stage III, liver parenchymal disease and vitamin K disorders (particularly Coumadin anticoagulation).

The PT is also affected by heparin, although the degree of response is variable. To obtain a valid PT, it is necessary to wait until heparin effect has disappeared (6 hours after subcutaneous injection).

ACTIVATED PARTIAL THROMBOPLASTIN TIME (APTT). — An "incomplete" thromboplastin reagent plus calcium is added to the patient's plasma as was done for the PT. This incomplete (partial) thromboplastin (PTT) is essentially only a platelet substitute, with all the other thromboplastin factors lacking. The PTT is very sensitive to defects in stage II. It may also show abnormal results in stages III and IV defects, but only if the defects are severe. (Stages III and IV may influence the test because the test depends on fibrin clot formation as the end point.) The reason that the PTT is not as sensitive to stage III defects as the PT is that the extrinsic thromboplastin used in the PT is more powerful than the intrinsic thromboplastin generated in the PTT, thus enabling the PT to demonstrate relatively smaller defects in the substrate prothrombin or the accelerator factors. Stage I abnormalities do not influence the PTT. Also, deficiency of factor VII does not influence the PTT, for unknown reasons.

The original PTT was useful in detecting coagulation abnormalities, but was relatively insensitive to effects of heparin. Adding certain "activators" (usually chemicals or particulate matter, such as kaolin) to the PTT reagent was found to activate factor XII (contact factor) swiftly and uniformly and thus eliminate another variable in the clotting process. In addition, the activated PTT (APTT) was found to be sensitive to heparin.

Advantages of the APTT are adequate reproducibility (less than 10% variation), speed (reaction time in the neighborhood of 30–50 seconds), ease of performance and suitability for automation. Disadvantages are that blood levels of heparin that are very much above anticoagulant range cause the APTT to become nonlinear, excessively prolonged and unreliable; and the APTT is not affected by platelets, whereas platelets do influence heparin activity in vivo. In addition, the APTT is affected by Coumadin. When the PT is in Coumadin therapeutic range, the APTT is also prolonged and may even be above the APTT therapeutic range for heparin. Various techniques and equipment are used for the APTT readout (clot detection); the different machines as well as different companies' reagents may produce results which deviate significantly on the same specimen. This may cause problems in comparing values from different laboratories.

PROTHROMBIN CONSUMPTION TEST (PCT).—This is also called the serum prothrombin time or the two-stage prothrombin time. The patient's blood is drawn and allowed to clot. A standard PT is then run on the serum left after the clot. Al(OH)$_3$ absorbed normal plasma without prothrombin is added to provide an end point. If prothrombin was utilized normally when the patient's blood clotted, only a very small amount of prothrombin will remain in the serum unused, and the serum PT will be considerably prolonged. However, if a defect is present in either stage I or stage II, the utilization of prothrombin will be decreased, and a greater amount will be left in the serum, thus shortening the serum PT. The platelet defect in stage I may be either defect in platelet quantity or a normal quantity but defective function (thrombasthenia). The PCT is thus very sensitive to stage I and stage II defects, but is not influenced by stage III and stage IV defects (unless there is a circulating anticoagulant).

VENOUS CLOTTING TIME (VCT).—The Lee-White method is preferred. Technique is extremely important. When the usual three test tubes are used, tube #3 is filled first, since the last blood to enter the syringe is probably least contaminated with tissue juice. With glass syringes, start the test timing as soon as blood enters the syringe. With plastic syringes, one can wait until blood enters tube #3 (the first tube filled) to start the test timing, because clotting time in plastic is prolonged. The tubes should be incubated at 37° C. The VCT is affected mainly by defects in stages II and IV. It is not sensitive to defects in stage I and is relatively insensitive to defects in stage III, where extremely severe deficiency is required to show significant VCT abnormality. In stages II and IV, the test is only moderately sensitive, requiring considerable quantitative deficiency to cause abnormal test results. The VCT is reasonably sensitive to heparin effect, and was the original test used to monitor heparin therapy.

Disadvantages of the VCT are relative lack of reproducibility (more than 15% variation in most laboratories when the test is repeated on the same patient); necessity for 37° C incubation and careful technique (hardly ever observed by the average technologist); relatively long reaction time (5–15 minutes), the fact that each test must be done separately at each patient's bedside; and the fact that platelets do not affect the test. The VCT is being replaced in most laboratories by the APTT or some other method that is more reproducible and more easily controlled.

It might be useful to compare the results of the laboratory tests just discussed in the various stages of blood coagulation:

	STAGE I	STAGE II	STAGE III	STAGE IV
PT	no	no	VS	ins.
PTT	no	VS	ins.	ins.
PCT	VS	VS	no°	no°
VCT	no	mod. S	ins.	mod. S

°Unless circulating anticoagulants are present
VS = very sensitive; ins. = insensitive; mod. S = moderately sensitive

In hemophilia (factor VIII defect), the various tests have approximately the following sensitivity:

VCT—normal until AHG values are less than 2% of normal.
PCT—normal until AHG values are less than 10% of normal.
PTT—normal until AHG values are less than 30–35% of normal.

Note that normal persons may show 60–100% of "normal" levels on factor VIII assay.

THROMBOPLASTIN GENERATION TIME (TGT).—This is the basic reference test for pinpointing defects in stage II, and can be used to assay the degree of defect. This procedure tests the ability of the patient to generate thromboplastin (stage II). If the patient's platelets are used in the TGT instead of a platelet substitute, a sensitive assay system for stage I is added, which reflects deficiency either in number or in function of the platelets. The TGT is quite complicated and time consuming, demanding an expert technician and strict attention to a considerable number of technical details to provide reliable results. Therefore, only a relatively few research centers do this procedure. The TGT is extremely sensitive to stage II defects, detecting abnormality of AHG when less than 30% of normal levels is present. As mentioned, the TGT can also pinpoint what the stage II defect is. Stages III and IV defects can be detected, but are more easily picked up by other tests.

PLASMA FIBRINOGEN.—A fibrin clot is precipitated from plasma, either by adding thrombin or calcium. The fibrin clot is then quantitated chemically by one of several indirect methods. Mild cases of circulating fibrinolysins have normal plasma fibrinogen. However, if the fibrinolysin is potent, fibrinogen may be inactivated as well, so that a fibrin clot cannot be produced by ordinary methods, and plasma fibrinogen will appear falsely low or absent. True low plasma fibrinogen levels may be due to primary fibrinolysins or to the disseminated intravascular coagulation (DIC) syndrome (p. 65). DIC is by far the more common. A thromboplastin tissue substance or equivalent in action is liberated in the bloodstream and causes fibrin deposition (clots) in small blood vessels.

CLOT LYSIS TEST.—This is a simple yet fairly sensitive and reliable test for circulating fibrinolysins. Normally, a blood clot retracts and forms a solid, firm, hard mass. Circulating fibrinolysin in sufficient quantity attacks and dissolves the clot. This is different from the clot retraction defect of thrombocytopenia, where the clot forms and simply does not retract well, but does not dissolve. In mild cases of circulating fibrinolysins, the patient's own blood will clot, followed by clot lysis. However, if the fibrinolysin is potent, fibrinogen may be inactivated and the blood will not clot. In these cases, plasma fibrinogen level determinations will show a falsely low level, as noted above. The clot lysis test should then be done by adding the patient's plasma to a fresh blood clot from a normal person. The euglobulin lysis test, a variation of the clot lysis procedure, is considered more sensitive and accurate. However, it is not as widely available.

PROTAMINE SULFATE TEST. — Normally, thrombin catalyzes conversion of fibrinogen to fibrin monomers; fibrin monomers then polymerize with the assistance of factor XIII. Polymerized (clotted) fibrin is the scaffolding on which a blood clot forms. Fibrinolysins may attack either fibrinogen or fibrin, splitting off fragments ("split products"), which, in turn, are broken into smaller pieces. These split products may form a complex with fibrin monomers and prevent polymerization. Protamine sulfate in low concentration is thought to release fibrin monomers from the split-product complex and allow the monomers to polymerize. The test is positive in conditions producing secondary fibrinolysin and is negative with primary fibrinolysin. Primary fibrinolysin will not induce a protamine sulfate reaction because the end point of this test depends on the presence of fibrin monomers produced by action of thrombin. Primary fibrinolysin is not ordinarily associated with activation of the thrombin clotting mechanism.

Since DIC is the major condition associated with substantial production of secondary fibrinolysin, recent studies endorse protamine sulfate as a good screening test for DIC. Negative results would be strong evidence against DIC. Various modifications of the protamine sulfate method are being introduced. These vary in sensitivity, so that it is difficult to compare results in diseases other than DIC. Any condition leading to intravascular clotting may conceivably produce secondary fibrinolysin; these conditions include pulmonary embolization, venous thrombosis, infarcts and postoperative complications. Occasional positive results have been reported without good explanation.

SPLIT-PRODUCTS TESTS. — When fibrinogen is attacked by plasmin, a large fragment called X is broken off. In turn, X is split into a larger fragment Y and a smaller fragment D. Fragment Y is further broken down into another fragment D and the smallest fragment of all, called E. Therefore, intermediate products are fragments X and Y, and final products are 2 fragment Ds and 1 fragment E. The split products retain some antigenic determinants of the parent fibrinogen molecule. Antibody to certain of these fragments can be produced and, as part of an immunologic test, can detect and quantitate these fragments. Since the antibodies will react with fibrinogen, fibrinogen must be removed prior to the test, usually by clotting the blood. The earliest test of this kind in general use was the "Fi test," a slide latex agglutination procedure detecting mainly intermediate fragments X and Y, which was shown to be insufficiently sensitive. Another test, the tanned red cell hemagglutination-inhibition test (TRCHII), detected fragments X, Y and D and was sensitive enough but too complicated for most laboratories. A newer 2-minute latex agglutination slide procedure ("Thrombo-Wellcotest") has immunologic reactivity against fragments D and E and seems to have adequate sensitivity and reliability.

Most conditions that induce clotting and, therefore, an abnormal protamine sulfate test (described previously) will also result in abnormal immunologic split product tests. The Thrombo-Wellcotest seems to be replacing protamine sulfate in many laboratories.

Classic laboratory findings in DIC include hypofibrinogenemia (leading to abnormal PTT and PT) and thrombocytopenia. In mild cases these tests may be within normal limits. The protamine sulfate and split-products tests are positive, apparently even in some of the milder cases. The clot lysis test is most often negative. It is not necessary to perform both the protamine sulfate and the split-products test; both give the same information.

WORKUP FOR HEMORRHAGIC PROBLEMS

A basic workup for suspected or actual hemorrhagic problems begins with a good history. Laboratory tests include a bleeding time and a tourniquet test (to rule out capillary fragility), a platelet count (to rule out thrombocytopenia), a PT (to rule out stage III defects), and an APTT (to rule out stage II defects). For example, a normal PT with an abnormal APTT means a stage II defect only; the opposite results would point toward a pure stage III defect, while finding both tests abnormal would suggest factor X or a stage IV problem (although marked defects in prothrombin or factor V can begin to affect the APTT). Stage IV defects may then be investigated with a plasma fibrinogen level and a split-products test; if necessary, a clot lysis test may be done. In this manner, one can narrow down the problem to a manageable size. Once the problem area is isolated, the exact defect can be pinpointed using specialized procedures, such as the TGT (or PCT if the TGT is not available), details of which are listed in standard textbooks on the subject. Also, diseases present or drugs known to cause difficulty in a certain coagulation area certainly call for the selected tests referable to that problem.

If facilities for specialized coagulation tests are not available, a coagulation defect can be further isolated by means of certain simple correction experiments. Normal serum contains factors VII, IX, X, XI and XII. Therefore, one can mix an equal quantity of the patient's fresh oxalated plasma with normal serum. If the mixture of patient's plasma and normal serum corrects the coagulation defect, the defect must be due to one of the factors supplied by the normal serum. Similar procedures can be used to further isolate the individual defect, and actually are carried out as part of the TGT; however, they should be left to persons experienced in their performance and interpretation.

Anticoagulation by warfarin-type drugs is best monitored by the PT. Therapeutic range varies with each manufacturer's thromboplastin (p. 477); the most commonly desired effect is a reduction to a level of 10–20% of those clotting factors affected by Coumadin. A recent report indicates that the commonly accepted therapeutic range of 2.0–2.5 times control cannot be blindly imposed on all thromboplastins because of variability in composition and thereby in effect on clotting factors. Results in terms of seconds compared to control is preferred to percentage of normal, because percentage must be based on dilution curves, which frequently are inaccurate.

Anticoagulation by heparin is monitored by the APTT (or by one of the other procedures listed beginning on page 440). The therapeutic range is 1½ to 2½ times upper normal limits. Heparin is usually administered either by continuous intravenous infusion or by intermittent injection. With constant IV infusion, heparin anticoagulant response is theoretically uniform, and the APTT may be performed at any time. When intermittent injection is used, peak heparin response is obtained ½ to 1 hour after intravenous injection or at 3 to 4 hours after subcutaneous injection. In the average person, using a single small or moderate-sized heparin dose, anticoagulant effect decreases below the threshold of measurement by 3–4 hours after IV injection and 6 hours after subcutaneous injection. Most feel that the optimum time to monitor therapy is 1 hour before the next dose. At this time the APTT should be at least 1½ times upper normal limit. There is controversy as to whether the peak of the response should also be measured. If "low-dose" therapy is used, many clinicians do not monitor blood levels at all.

Certain technical problems affect interpretation of PT and APTT results. The labile factors are preserved better in citrate than in oxalate anticoagulant. Once exposed to air, citrated plasma is stable for only 3 hours at room temperature and 6 hours in the refrigerator at 4° C. If collected in a vacuum tube and if the top has not been opened, the plasma is stable for a longer time. Excess anticoagulant relative to amount of plasma may affect results. Insufficient blood drawn in the tube means that less plasma is available for

Fig 7–2. — Blood coagulation pathway.

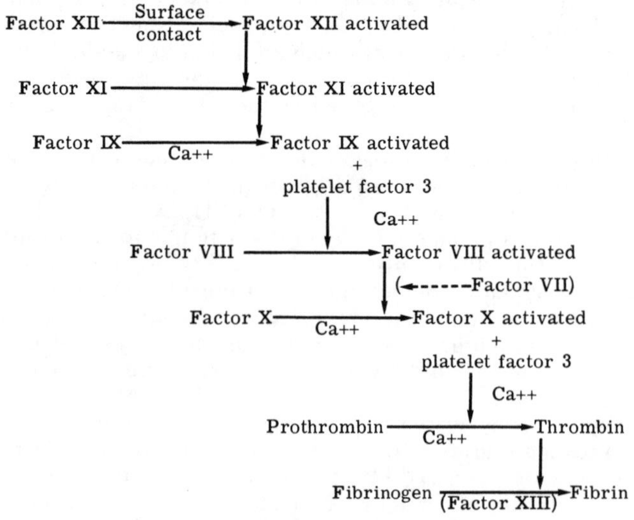

the amount of anticoagulant present, and the test results may be falsely prolonged. The same thing may occur in blood that has a high hematocrit, since in that case the excess RBC are replacing some of the plasma. One of the most frequent difficulties arises from attempts to keep intravenous lines open by heparin flushes. Usually this is not known to the phlebotomist.

Although the coagulation theory outlined in Figure 7–1 is probably the best sequence to explain coagulation test actions, it very likely is not the actual manner in which blood clots. A current and widely accepted theory is presented in Figure 7–2.

VASCULAR DEFECTS

A frequent nonhereditary type of vascular fragility problem is called "senile purpura." Localized purpuric lesions or small bruises develop on the extremities in older people. The only laboratory abnormality is a positive tourniquet test in some of the cases. A somewhat similar clinical condition is the easy bruising found in many younger adult persons, especially women. All results of standard laboratory tests are usually normal, except for an occasionally positive tourniquet test. Some of these persons have abnormal platelet function tests; in the majority, however, the reason for abnormality is not known.

It should be mentioned that continued or intermittent bleeding from a small localized area is most often due to physical agents (such as repeated trauma) or to a local condition (such as scar tissue) that prevents normal small vessel retraction and subsequent closure by thrombosis.

Allergic (anaphylactoid) purpura is characterized by small blotchy hemorrhages over the extremities and bilateral ankle swelling. The cause is allergy, but it may also appear in association with glomerulonephritis. Henoch's purpura is a subdivision of this condition, in which the bleeding is mainly in the GI tract. Schönlein's purpura features the skin manifestations without GI involvement. The tourniquet test is usually positive. Platelet counts and results of other laboratory tests are normal.

Occasional cases of purpura, most commonly on the extremities, have been reported in association with hyperglobulinemia. This may be idiopathic, secondary to various diseases (such as cirrhosis or granulomatous infection) that produce considerably elevated gamma globulin levels, or secondary to one of the "monoclonal gammopathies." (These globulins are not macroglobulins, however.) It may or may not be accompanied by cryoglobulinemia. "Purpura hyperglobulinemia" is one name given to this condition, which is not a frequent etiology for purpura. The tourniquet test is sometimes positive; most other coagulation defect tests are normal.

Finally, there is a group that simulates capillary fragility defects, but which is primarily embolic. However, some element of increased capillary fragility is often present. These diseases include subacute bacterial endocarditis, fat emboli and some cases of septicemia (although other cases of septicemia also have thrombocytopenia). The tourniquet test is often positive, and the bleeding time is variable. Other coagulation defect tests are normal (except as mentioned).

PLATELET DEFECTS

Platelet-associated abnormality is most commonly produced by decreased number (thrombocytopenia) or defective function (thrombocytopathia). A bleeding tendency may also appear when greatly increased platelet numbers are found (thrombocythemia) such as occasionally is seen in chronic myelocytic leukemia or polycythemia vera. Clinically, purpura is the hallmark of platelet abnormality. Most other types of coagulation disorders do not cause purpura.

Thrombocytopenia

Decrease in number is the most common platelet abnormality. In general, such conditions may be classified according to etiology:

1. Acquired immunologic thrombocytopenia;
2. Idiopathic thrombocytopenic purpura;
3. Hypersplenism;
4. Bone marrow hypoplasia;
5. Toxic or other causes.

ACQUIRED IMMUNOLOGIC THROMBOCYTOPENIA. — This syndrome occurs due to idiosyncratic hypersensitivity to certain drugs. This may develop either during initial, continued or intermittent use of the drug; once commencing, platelet depression occurs swiftly. The bone marrow shows most often normal or increased megakaryocytes, which often display degenerative changes. The most frequently associated drugs are quinidine, quinine and various sulfonamide derivatives, but other drugs have been incriminated in rare instances. Of course, even with the relatively frequent offenders, this effect is very uncommon. Platelet antibodies have been demonstrated in many cases.

IDIOPATHIC THROMBOCYTOPENIC PURPURA (ITP). — This syndrome may exist in either an acute or a chronic form. The acute form is usually seen in children, has a sudden onset, lasts a few days to a few weeks, and does not recur. The majority of cases follow infection, most often viral, but some do not have a known precipitating cause. The chronic form is more common in adults; onset, however, is not frequent after age 40. There are usually remissions and exacerbations over variable periods of time. No precipitating disease or drug is usually found. Platelet antibodies have been demonstrated in 80–90% of patients with chronic ITP. Some of these patients eventually are found to have systemic lupus erythematosus or other diseases.

Clinically, there is purpura or other hemorrhagic manifestations. The spleen is usually not palpable, and an enlarged spleen is evidence against the diagnosis of ITP. Bone marrow aspiration shows a normal or increased number of megakaryocytes, although not always.

HYPERSPLENISM. — This entity was discussed in Chapter 4 (see p. 136). The syndrome may be primary or secondary; if secondary, it is most commonly due to portal hypertension. There may be any combination of anemia, leukopenia or thrombocytopenia, but isolated thrombocytopenia is a fairly frequent manifestation. The spleen is usually palpable, but not always. Bone marrow megakaryocytes are normal or increased. The thrombocytopenia seen in lupus erythematosus is usually associated with anti-platelet antibodies, but there may be an element of splenic involvement, even though the spleen is often not palpable.

BONE MARROW HYPOPLASIA. — This condition and its various etiologies were discussed in Chapter 3 (see p. 16). This group forms a large and important segment of the thrombocytopenias and is the reason why bone marrow examination is nearly always indicated in a patient with thrombocytopenia.

Thrombocytopenia is a very frequent feature of acute leukemia and monocytic leukemia. This is true even when the peripheral blood WBC pattern is aleukemic. It may also occur in the terminal stages of chronic leukemia.

Aplastic anemia and extensive replacement of bone marrow by tumor often includes thrombocytopenia as an accompanying finding.

TOXIC OR OTHER CAUSES. — A miscellaneous group is left, which includes several unrelated disorders:

Neonatal Thrombocytopenia. — This may be due to ITP or idiosyncratic platelet antibodies in the mother, may follow virus infection in utero or may be idiopathic. Hemorrhagic manifestations are usually not severe, and the symptoms subside spontaneously.

Thrombotic Thrombocytopenic Purpura (Moschcowitz's Disease). — A very uncommon disorder most frequent in young adults, although it may occur at any age. There is a characteristic triad of severe hemolytic anemia, thrombocytopenia and multiple shifting neurologic symptoms. The WBC count is usually increased, although it may be normal. Fibrin and platelet thrombi occur in capillaries and small arterioles, giving rise to the symptoms. Diagnosis is through biopsy, usually of the kidney, although other tissues (even bone marrow sections) have been used.

Megaloblastic Anemia. — In untreated, well-established cases, occasionally even when clinically mild, thrombocytopenia occurs as a frequent manifestation of the B_{12} and folic acid deficiency anemias. In chronic iron deficiency anemia, platelets are normal and may at times actually be somewhat increased.

Infections. — Transient thrombocytopenia may be an uncommon manifestation of a wide variety of severe infections or septicemia. It occasionally follows various viral infections.

Massive Transfusions with Stored Bank Blood. — If given during a short period, thrombocytopenia may develop, due to the low functional platelet content of stored bank blood. This may or may not be accompanied by a bleeding tendency. However, deficiency of factors V and VIII (the unstable clotting factors) may contribute to any bleeding problem from this source. It takes at least 5 units of blood, and usually more than 10, given within 1–2 days' time. Transfusions may produce thrombocytopenia even when only 1 unit is given. Platelets have surface antigens of several types, including the HL-A system. Platelet antigens resemble univalent red cell antigens in that antibodies against these antigens do not occur normally.

Transfusion of whole blood, packed cells or nonmatched platelets may induce antiplatelet antibody formation; the more units given, the greater chance to develop these antibodies.

Platelet Function Defects

When one speaks of platelet function, what is usually meant is their role in blood coagulation. To carry out this role, platelets go through a series of changes, partially morphologic and partially biochemical. Abnormality may develop at various stages in this process, and so-called platelet function tests have been devised 'to detect abnormality in certain of these stages. These are special procedures not available in most laboratories, and include techniques designed to evaluate platelet factor release (PF-3 or serotonin), platelet aggregation (ADP, thrombin, collagen, epinephrine) and platelet adhesion (glass bead retention). These tests are mainly useful to categorize platelet action abnormality rather than to predict the likelihood of bleeding. The bleeding time is probably the best procedure to evaluate degree of clinical abnormality.

Defective platelet action with normal platelet count is uncommon, the most famous of this group being Glanzmann's disease (hereditary thrombasthenia). Platelets in Glanzmann's disease have abnormal aggregation and glass bead retention. The clot retraction test is abnormal, whereas it is normal in other thrombopathic (platelet function abnormality) disorders. Tourniquet test results are variable.

Defective platelet function has been observed in some patients with uremia or with chronic liver disease, even without the thrombocytopenia that occasionally may develop. Giant platelets may be found in certain conditions, especially in myeloid metaplasia (less often in chronic myelocytic leukemia), but this does not seem to produce a clinical bleeding tendency.

Certain drugs may interfere with platelet function. Aspirin affects platelet factor release and also platelet aggregation. Other drugs may interfere with one or more platelet function stages.

Von Willebrand's disease combines platelet abnormalities with other defects to produce a hemorrhagic disorder, sometimes quite severe. This disorder has also been called "pseudohemophilia." Although there is considerable argument as to just what this disease should include, it is generally restricted to a congenital (hereditary) disorder. These patients have an abnormal bleeding time (and, in many cases, a positive tourniquet test) with decreased platelet adhesiveness (decreased retention in a glass bead column). In addition, many display decreased platelet ability to agglutinate in vitro with the antibiotic ristocetin. Factor VIII levels are decreased in many patients (the number and degree being disputed by different investigators).

Purpura

The etiologic diagnosis of purpura should begin with a platelet count and a complete blood count (CBC), with special emphasis on the peripheral blood smear. Investigation of thrombocytopenia should include a platelet count and a bone marrow examination utilizing preferably both a clot section and a smear technique. The clot section affords a better estimate of cellularity. The smear allows better study of morphology. This is true for megakaryocytes as well as for other types of cells. Investigation of purpura without thrombocytopenia should include bleeding time (for overall platelet function) and tourniquet tests (attempting to demonstrate abnormal capillary fragility). If necessary, platelet function tests may be done. If platelet function tests are not available, a PCT or possibly a TGT (using the patient's platelets in the TGT), may assist in diagnosis of a platelet action defect. These tests are not indicated in already known thrombocytopenia, because their results would not add any useful information. The other tests for hemorrhagic disease must previously rule out abnormality in other areas. Occasional cases of nonthrombocytopenic purpura are caused by abnormal serum proteins, which may be demonstrated by serum protein electrophoresis (then confirmed by other tests, described in Chapter 21).

Usually a bleeding tendency does not develop in thrombocytopenia until the platelet count is less than 100,000/cu mm (direct method), and most often does not occur until the platelet count is below 50,000/cu mm. The 50,000 value is usually considered the critical level. However, some patients do not bleed even with platelet counts near zero, while occasionally there may be trouble with patients with counts above 50,000. Most likely there is some element of capillary fragility involved, but the actual reason is not known at this time.

BLEEDING PROBLEMS IN SURGERY

Bleeding constitutes a major concern to surgeons; problems may arise during operation or postoperatively, and bleeding may be concealed or grossly obvious. The major causes are:

1. Physical defect in hemostasis – improper vessel ligation, overlooking a small transected vessel, or other failure to achieve adequate hemostasis.

2. Unrecognized preoperative bleeding problem – one of the coagulation defects present that was not recognized prior to surgery. This may be congenital (such as the hemophilias), secondary to a disease that the patient has (such as cirrhosis) or due to drug therapy (such as anticoagulant therapy).

3. Transfusion reactions or complications from massive transfusion.

4. Unexplained bleeding difficulty.

Unusual bleeding has some correlation to the type (magnitude) of the operative procedure, the length of the operation and the particular disease involved. The more that any of these parameters is increased, the more likely that excessive bleeding may occur. In most cases, the defect can be traced by means of laboratory tests; or, retrospectively, by reestablishing physical hemostasis. However, with category number 4 (unexplained etiology), even after thorough investigation, some patients still show no real explanation. Nevertheless, this fact cannot be used as an excuse for inadequate workup, because proper therapy depends on finding the etiology. This is why some knowledge of blood coagulation mechanisms is necessary.

REFERENCES

Antithrombin (editorial), Lancet 1:1333, 1976.
Alami, S. Y., et al.: Fibrin stabilizing factor (factor XIII), Am. J. Med. 44:1, 1968.

Bachman, F.: Paradoxes of disseminated intravascular coagulation, Hosp. Practice 6:113, 1971.

Bachman, F., and Pichairut, O.: Surgical bleeding, Med. Clin. North Am. 56:207, 1972.

Bell, W. R.: Thrombocytopenia occurring during heparin therapy, N. Engl. J. Med. 295:276, 1976.

Borden, C. W.: The current status of therapy with anticoagulants, Med. Clin. North Am. 56:235, 1972.

Bowie, E. J., et al.: The spectrum of Von Willebrand's disease revisited, Mayo Clin. Proc. 51:35, 1976.

Bowie, E. J. W., and Owen, C. A.: Von Willebrand's disease, Med. Clin. North Am. 56:275, 1972.

Call, F. L., II, et al.: Fibrin-fibrinogen degradation products in cardiovascular surgery, Arch. Surg. 107:834, 1973.

Coleman, R. W., et al.: Statistical comparison of the automated activated partial thromboplastin time and the clotting time in the regulation of heparin therapy, Am. J. Clin. Pathol. 53:904, 1970.

Currimbhoy, Z., et al.: Fletcher factor deficiency and myocardial infarction, Am. J. Clin. Pathol. 65:970, 1976.

Davey, F. R.: Laboratory approach to platelet disorders, Postgrad. Med. 54:109, 1973.

Deykin, D.: Emerging concepts of platelet function. N. Engl. J. Med. 290:144, 1974.

Diamond, L. K., and Porter, F. S.: Inadequacies of routine bleeding and clotting times, N. Engl. J. Med. 259:1025, 1958.

Fung, C. H. K., and Woodson, B.: Laboratory suggestion: interpretation of the plasma protamine sulfate paracoagulation test, Am. J. Clin. Pathol. 65:698, 1976.

Gynn, T. N., et al: Drug-induced thrombocytopenia, Med. Clin. North Am. 56:65, 1972.

Hemofil and Other Factor VIII Concentrates, Med. Lett. Drugs Ther. 11:96 (Nov. 14), 1969.

Hussain, S.: Disorders of hemostasis and thromboses in the aged, Med. Clin. North Am. 60:1273, 1976.

Karpatkin, M.: Diagnosis and management of disseminated intravascular coagulation, Pediatr. Clin. North Am. 18:23, 1971.

Karpatkin, S.: Autoimmune thrombocytopenic purpura, Am. J. Med. Sci. 261:127, 1971.

Kazmier, F. J.: Current practice with vitamin K antagonist therapy, Mayo Clin. Proc. 49:918, 1974.

Kidder, W. R., et al.: The plasma protamine paracoagulation test: clinical and laboratory evaluation, Am. J. Clin. Pathol. 58:675, 1972.

Koepke, J. A., et al: Pre-instrumental variables in coagulation testing, Am. J. Clin. Pathol. 64:591, 1975.

Lackner, H., and Karpatkin, S.: On the "easy bruising" syndrome with normal platelet count, Ann. Intern. Med. 83:190, 1975.

Leslie, J., and Ingram, G. I. C.: The diagnosis of long-standing bleeding disorders, Semin. in Hematol. 8:140, 1971.

Losowsky, M. S., et al.: Coagulation abnormalities in liver disease, Postgrad. Med. 53:147, 1973.

Marder, V. J., et al.: Detection of serum fibrinogen and fibrin degradation products: comparison of six techniques using purified products and application in clinical studies, Am. J. Med. 51:71, 1971.

Miale, J. B., and Kent, J. W.: Standardization of the therapeutic range for oral anticoagulants based on standard reference plasmas, Am. J. Clin. Pathol. 57:80, 1972.

Morse, E. E.: Effects of drugs on platelet function, Ann. Clin. Lab. Sci. 7:68, 1977.

Poller, L., et al.: Measuring partial thromboplastin time: an international collaborative study, Lancet 2:842, 1976.

Post, R. M., and Desforges, J. F.: Thrombocytopenia and alcoholism, Ann. Intern. Med. 68:1230, 1968.

Prentice, C. R. M., and Ratnoff, O. D.: Genetic disorders of blood coagulation, Semin. Hematol. 4:93, 1967.

Quick, A. J.: Trait vs. disease (aspirin tolerance), J.A.M.A. 233:1260, 1975.

Quick, A. J.: The tourniquet test as a diagnostic aid for the study of telangiectasia, Am. J. Clin. Pathol. 65:199, 1976.

Rapaport, S. I.: Blood coagulation: biochemical, physiological and clinical considerations, Clin. Obstet. Gynecol. 11:207, 1968.

Ratnoff, O. D.: The interrelationship of clotting and immunologic mechanisms, Hosp. Practice 6:119, 1971.

Rosenberg, R. D.: Actions and interactions of antithrombin and heparin, N. Engl. J. Med. 292:146, 1975.

Rossi, E. C. (ed.): Symposium on hemorrhagic disorders, Med. Clin. North Am. 56:3, 1972.

Rozengvaig, S., et al.: Benign purpura hyperglobulinemia, A.M.A. Arch. Intern. Med. 99:913, 1957.

Schloesser, L. L., et al: Thrombocytosis in iron-deficiency anemia, J. Lab. Clin. Med. 66:107, 1965.

Smith, R. T., and Ts'ao, C-H: Fibrin degradation products in the postoperative period, Am. J. Clin. Pathol. 60:644, 1973.

Soloway, H. B.: Drug-induced bleeding, Am. J. Clin. Pathol. 61:622, 1974.

Soong, B. C. F., et al.: Coagulation disorders in cancer. III. Fibrinolysis and inhibitors, Cancer 25:867, 1970.

Sussman, L. N.: The clotting time: An enigma, Am. J. Clin. Pathol. 60:651, 1973.

Udall, J. A.: Human sources and absorption of vitamin K in relation to anticoagulation stability, J.A.M.A. 194:127, 1965.

Umlas, J.: In vivo platelet function following cardiopulmonary bypass, Transfusion 15:596, 1975.

Weintraub, R. M., et al.: Rapid diagnosis of drug-induced thrombocytopenic purpura, J.A.M.A. 180:130, 1962

Wilson, J. E., III, and Thornton, R. D.: Comparison of a direct latex-agglutination technique with the tanned red cell hemagglutination inhibition immunoassay (TRCHII) for semiquantitation of fibrinogen/fibrin degradation products, Am. J. Clin. Pathol. 65:528, 1976.

Yip, M. L. B., et al.: Nonspecificity of the protamine test for disseminated intravascular coagulation, Am. J. Clin. Pathol. 57:487, 1972.

Yoshikawa, T., et al.: Infection and disseminated intravascular coagulation, Medicine 50:237, 1971.

Ziegler, F. D., and Kelly, J. H.: The critical evaluation of thromboplastin, Ann. Clin. Lab. Sci. 2:16, 1972.

8 / Immunohematology: Antibodies and Antibody Tests

BEFORE DISCUSSING THIS SUBJECT, it is useful to give some definitions:

Antigen: Any substance that causes formation of antibodies to it. The most common antigens are protein, but certain carbohydrate polysaccharides may act in a similar manner. Lipid may be combined with either. Each antigen has a certain chemical configuration that gives it antibody-provoking ability. This specific chemical group may become detached from its carrier molecule and temporarily lose antigenic power; it is then called a hapten. Attachment of a hapten to another suitable molecule leads to restoration of antigenic properties.

Antibody: Serum proteins produced by the reticuloendothelial system in response to antigenic stimulation. Antibodies are globulins—most often gamma globulins. They may be specific, combining only with specific antigen molecules, or nonspecific, combining with a variety of antigens. Presumably, nonspecific antibodies attack a variety of molecules because similar hapten groups may be present even though the carrier molecule is different (so-called cross reactivity).

Agglutinogen: Antigen on the surface of a red blood cell.

Agglutinin: Antibody that attacks RBC antigens and manifests this activity by clumping the RBC.

Hemolysin: Same as an agglutinin, except that lysis of affected erythrocytes takes place.

Isoantibodies: Antibodies produced to antigens coming from outside the body; in other words, to "foreign" antigens. These antibodies do not cause disease unless red cells containing these antigens are subsequently added or exposed to these antibodies.

Autoantibodies: Antibodies produced by the body against one or more of its own tissues. These antibodies are associated with autoimmune disease and may cause clinical difficulty.

There are several types of antibodies, depending on their occurrence and laboratory characteristics:

Natural antibody: These appear without any apparent antigenic stimulus.

Immune antibody: These appear following introduction of antigen due to disease, transfusion or other mechanisms.

Complete (bivalent) antibody: These usually will directly agglutinate appropriate RBC. In vitro tests for these antibodies tend to demonstrate

80

better reaction in saline medium at room temperature (20° C) or lower. They often require complement.

Incomplete (univalent) antibody: These usually cannot directly agglutinate appropriate RBC but only coat their surface. In vitro tests for these antibodies tend to show better reaction at higher temperatures, such as 37° C, and in high-protein medium.

Warm antibody: Reacts best in vitro at 37° C.

Cold antibody: Reacts best at 4 – 10° C.

THE COOMBS TEST

There are two methods of detecting and characterizing these antibodies; these are the Coombs test and a group of procedures that demonstrate the action of the antibody under controlled conditions, so as to exhibit some of its properties.

To prepare reagents for the Coombs test, human globulin, either gamma, nongamma or mixed, is injected into rabbits. The rabbit produces antibodies to the injected human globulin. Rabbit serum containing these antihuman globulin antibodies is known as Coombs' serum. Since antibody is globulin, usually gamma globulin, the addition of Coombs' serum (antihuman globulin rabbit antibodies) to any solution containing human antibodies will result in the combination of the Coombs rabbit antibody with human antibody. Incidentally, this can be seen visually if the Coombs rabbit antibody has been tagged with a fluorescent dye.

The Coombs test may be carried out in either direct or indirect form. The *direct Coombs test* consists in adding Coombs' serum to a preparation of RBC that is coated with antibody. The Coombs reagent will attack this antibody coating the surface of the RBC and will cause the RBC to agglutinate to one another. This is a one-stage procedure. The direct Coombs test demonstrates that in vivo coating of RBC by incomplete antibody has occurred, but does not identify the antibody responsible. The direct Coombs test may be done by either a test-tube or a slide method.

The *indirect Coombs test* is a two-stage procedure. The first stage takes place in vitro and may be done in either of two ways:

1. RBC of known antigenic makeup are exposed to serum containing unknown antibodies. If the antibody combines with the RBC, as detected by the second stage, this proves that circulating antibody to one or more antigens on the RBC is present. Since the RBC antigens are known, this may help to more specifically identify that antibody.

2. Serum containing known specific antibody is exposed to RBC of unknown antigenic makeup. If the antibody combines with the RBC, as detected by the second stage, this identifies the antigen on the RBC.

The second stage consists in adding Coombs' serum to the RBC after the red cells have been washed to remove nonspecific unattached antibody or proteins. If specific antibody has coated the RBC, the Coombs serum will attack this antibody and cause the cells to agglutinate. The second stage is thus essentially a direct Coombs test done on the products of the first stage.

Therefore, the indirect Coombs test can be used either to detect free antibody in a patient's serum or to identify certain red cell antigens, depending on how the test is done.

The main indications for the direct Coombs test include the following (most of which will be discussed later in detail):

1. For the diagnosis of hemolytic disease of the newborn.

2. For diagnosis of hemolytic anemia in adults. These include many of the acquired autoimmune hemolytic anemias of both idiopathic and secondary varieties. The direct Coombs test at normal temperatures is usually negative with cold agglutinins.

3. For investigation of hemolytic transfusion reactions.

In these clinical situations the indirect test should not be done if the direct test is negative, since in these situations one is interested only in those antibodies which are affecting red cells (and thus precipitating clinical disease).

The main indications for the indirect Coombs test are:

1. Detection of certain weak antigens in RBC, such as D^u or certain red cell antigens whose antibodies are of the incomplete type, such as Duffy or Kidd (see Chapter 9).

2. Detection of incomplete antibodies in serum, usually for purposes of titration.

3. Demonstration of cold agglutinin autoantibodies.

Therefore, it should be noted that the indirect Coombs test is almost never needed routinely. In most situations, such as cold agglutinins or antibody identification, simply ordering a test for these substances will automatically cause an indirect Coombs test to be done. The indirect Coombs test should be thought of as a laboratory technique rather than as an actual laboratory test.

False positives and false negatives may occur with either of the Coombs tests due to poor technique, contamination or faulty commercial Coombs' serum. The test must be done on clotted blood or serum, since laboratory anticoagulants may interfere. A false positive direct Coombs test result may be given by increased peripheral blood reticulocytes using the test-tube method, although the slide technique will remain negative. Therefore, one should know which method the laboratory uses for the direct Coombs test. False positive direct Coombs tests are also reported after methyldopa and cephalosporin therapy and after cardiac operations.

Autoantibodies present an interesting problem, both in their clinical manifestations and in the difficulty of laboratory detection and identification (p. 34). They may be either warm or cold type, complete or incomplete.

Warm autoantibodies react at body temperature and are most often of the incomplete type. They may be idiopathic or secondary to certain diseases (causing so-called symptomatic hemolytic anemia). The main disease categories responsible are leukemias and lymphomas, particularly chronic lymphocytic leukemia and Hodgkin's disease; collagen diseases, especially disseminated lupus; and uncommonly a variety of other diseases, including cirrhosis, carcinomas and ovarian dermoids. The direct Coombs test is usually, but not always, positive, both in the secondary and the "idiopathic acquired" hemolytic anemias. If the Coombs test is negative, it becomes very difficult and often impossible to demonstrate that warm autoantibodies are present.

Cold autoantibodies react at 4–20° C and are found so frequently in normal persons that titers up to 1:64 are considered normal. They are hemagglutinating and are believed due to infection by organisms having antigenic groups similar to some of those on RBC. These antibodies mostly behave as bivalent types and require complement for reaction. In normally low titer they need icebox temperatures to attack RBC. In response to a considerable number of diseases these cold agglutinins are found in high titer, sometimes very high, and may then attack RBC in temperatures approaching body levels, causing hemolytic anemia. High-titered cold agglutinins may be found in nonbacterial infections, especially mycoplasma pneumonia (primary atypical pneumonia), influenza and infectious mononucleosis; in collagen diseases, including rheumatoid arthritis; in malignant lymphomas; and occasionally in cirrhosis. Fortunately, even in high titer there usually is no trouble, and generally only very high titers are associated with in vivo erythrocyte agglutination or hemolytic anemia. This is not always true, however. The direct Coombs test is usually negative. When cold agglutinin studies are ordered, an indirect Coombs test is generally done, with the first stage being incubation of RBC and the patient's serum at 4–10° C.

REFERENCES

American Association of Blood Banks: Seminar on problems encountered on pretransfusion tests, 1972.

Chaplin, H., Jr.: Antiglobulin (Coombs) testing (1966): How much ignorance is bliss, Transfusion 6:64, 1966.

Dacie, J. V.: *The Haemolytic Anemias, Congenital and Acquired* (2d ed.; New York: Grune & Stratton, Inc., 1960–1963).

Fayen, A. W., and Miale, J. B.: False positive antiglobulin tests in reticulocytosis, Am. J. Clin. Pathol. 39:645, 1963.

Gralnick, H. R., et al.: Drug-related positive direct Coombs test (abstr.), Am. J. Clin. Pathol. 49:241, 1968.

Griffitts, J. J., et al.: The influence of albumin in the antiglobulin crossmatch, Transfusion 4:461, 1964.

Hyland Reference Manual of Immunohematology (2d ed.; Los Angeles: Hyland Laboratories, 1964).

Kabat, E. A.: *Blood Group Substances: Their Chemistry and Immunochemistry* (New York: Academic Press, Inc., 1965).

Lau, P., et al.: Positive direct antiglobulin reaction in a patient population, Am. J. Clin. Pathol. 65:368, 1976.

Mollison, P. L.: *Blood Transfusion in Clinical Medicine* (5th ed.; Philadelphia: J. B. Lippincott Company, 1972).

Samter, M. (ed.): *Immunological Disease* (2d ed.; Boston: Little, Brown & Company, 1976).

Stratton, F.: Complement in immunohematology, Transfusion 5:211, 1965.

9 / Blood Groups and Isoimmunization

ABO BLOOD GROUP SYSTEM

THE ABO BLOOD GROUP SYSTEM is a classic example of agglutinogens and their corresponding isoantibodies. There are three of these antigens — A, B and O — whose genes are placed in one locus on each of two paired chromosomes. These genes are alleles, meaning that they are interchangeable at their chromosome location. Therefore, each of the paired chromosomes carries any one of the three antigen genes. This makes four major phenotype groups possible — A, B, AB and O — since A and B are dominant over O. A and B are strong antigens, whereas O is so weak an antigen that for practical purposes it is considered nonantigenic. Furthermore, it is a rule that when either A or B is present on an individual's RBC, the corresponding isoantibodies anti-A or anti-B will be absent from his serum; conversely, if he lacks either A or B, his serum will contain the isoantibody to the missing isoantigen. Therefore, a person who is AA or AO will have anti-B in his serum; a person who is OO will have both anti-A and anti-B, and so on. Why the body is stimulated to produce antibodies to the missing AB antigens is not definitely understood, but apparently antigens similar to ABO substances exist elsewhere in nature and somehow cause a natural type of sensitization.

Anti-A and anti-B are bivalent antibodies that react in saline at room temperature. Ordinarily, little difficulty is encountered in ABO typing. There is, however, one potentially serious situation that arises from the fact that subgroups of agglutinogen A exist. These are called A_1, A_2 and A_3. The most common and strongest of these is A_1. A_2 is troublesome because sometimes it is so weak that some commercial anti-A serums fail to pick it up. This may cause A_2B to be falsely typed as B or A_2O to be falsely typed as O. Fortunately, this situation is not frequent with present-day potent typing serums. Group A subgroups weaker than A_2 exist, but are rare. They are easily missed even with potent anti-A typing serums. The main importance of the A_2 subgroup is that these persons sometimes have antibodies to A_1 (the most common subgroup of A).

RH BLOOD GROUP SYSTEM

The next major blood group is the Rh system. There is considerable controversy over nomenclature of the genetic apparatus involved between

84

SIMPLIFIED REPRESENTATION OF WIENER AND FISHER-RACE THEORIES
(schematic)

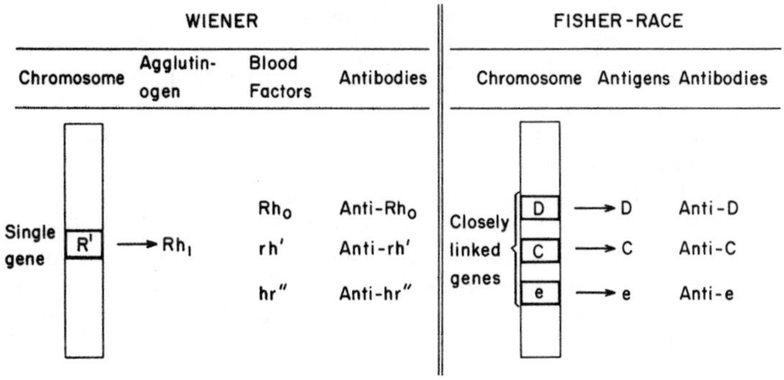

WIENER					FISHER-RACE		
Chromosome	Agglutinogen	Blood Factors	Antibodies		Chromosome	Antigens	Antibodies

Single gene R^1 → Rh_1

	Blood Factors	Antibodies
	Rh_0	Anti-Rh_0
	rh′	Anti-rh′
	hr″	Anti-hr″

Closely linked genes

	→	Antigens	Antibodies
D	→	D	Anti-D
C	→	C	Anti-C
e	→	e	Anti-e

COMPARISON OF THE WIENER MULTIPLE ALLELE THEORY
AND THE FISHER-RACE LINKED GENE THEORY

	WIENER			FISHER-RACE	
Gene	Corresponding agglutinogen	Blood factors		Genes	Corresponding antigens
r	rh	hr′ and hr″		cde	c,d,e
r'	rh′	rh′ and hr″		Cde	C,d,e
r''	rh″	rh″ and hr′		cdE	c,d,E
r^y	rh_y	rh′ and rh″		CdE	C,d,E
R^0	Rh_0	Rh_0, hr′ and hr″		cDe	c,D,e
R^1	Rh_1	Rh_0, rh′ and hr″		CDe	C,D,e
R^2	Rh_2	Rh_0, rh″ and hr′		cDE	c,D,E
R^z	Rh_z	Rh_0, rh′ and rh″		CDE	C,D,E

Fig 9–1.—Comparison of the Fisher-Race and Wiener nomenclatures. (From *Hyland Reference Manual of Immunohematology* [2d ed.; Los Angeles: Hyland Division of Travenol Laboratories, Inc., 1964], pp. 38–39.)

advocates of the English Fisher-Race CDE-cde nomenclature and the American Wiener's Rh-Hr labeling (Fig 9–1).

According to Wiener, the Rh group is determined by single genes, each chromosome of a pair containing one of these genes. In most situations, each gene would be expected to determine one antigen, to which there may develop one specific antibody. In Wiener's Rh system theory, each gene does indeed control one antigen. However, each of these antigens (agglutinogens) gives rise to several different blood factors, and it is antibodies to these factors that are the serologic components of the Rh system. There are eight of these agglutinogens, and each is associated with certain specific blood factors. In most situations, specific antibodies are produced when a person is stimulated by a specific antigen that he lacks. In the Rh system, most people respond in the usual manner to stimulation by specific Rh-system agglutinogens by producing certain specific blood factors. In a few persons, a blood factor different from the expected ones may be produced, along with some or all of the expected blood factor antibodies to one of the specific agglutinogens. Since this rare factor is inherited as one of a specific group of factors dependent on a specific agglutinogen, new antibodies can be added to Wiener's Rh system and assigned to one of the agglutinins by statistical computation of inheritance patterns.

According to the Fisher-Race theory, there are supposed to be three sets of two allelic genes, Cc, Dd and Ee; one gene from each of the three pairs is linked together in one single locus on each of two paired chromosomes. Therefore, the result is CDE, each letter of which can be either big or little, on each of the two chromosomes.

Therefore, in the Fisher-Race system a single gene controls one single antigen, which controls one single antibody. Moreover, this means that three genes would be present on each chromosome of a chromosome pair, and that the three-gene group is inherited as a unit. New antibodies are assumed to be due to mutation or defective separation of the genes (that make up the gene group) during meiosis ("crossover" rearrangement).

At present, the majority of experts believe that Wiener's theory fits the actual situation better than the Fisher-Race theory. The main drawback to the Wiener theory is its cumbersome terminology. Actually, in the great majority of situations, the much simpler Fisher-Race terminology works very adequately, because the antibodies that it names by its special letters are the same as the basic blood factors of Wiener's system. It is only when the unusual or rare situations develop that the Wiener system becomes indispensable. In other words, the Fisher-Race terminology has persisted because, for most practical work, one can use this terminology even though its underlying theory of gene inheritance is ignored. In the literature one often finds both the Fisher-Race and the Wiener nomenclatures, one of them being given in parentheses.

Of the Rh antigens, D (Rh$_o$) is by far the most antigenic, and when it is present on at least one chromosome the patient types as Rh positive. Only 20% of the population lacks D (Rh$_o$) completely and is considered Rh negative. Of the other antigens, c (hr') is the next strongest, although much less important than D.

Rh antigens lack corresponding naturally occurring antibodies in the serum. Therefore, when antibodies appear, they are of immune type, and are the result of sensitization by having received Rh antigen stimulation from the red cells of another person. This may occur by transfusion or in pregnancy. It is now well documented that red cells from the fetus escape the placenta into the blood stream of the mother. In this way the mother can develop Rh antibodies against the Rh antigen of the fetus. One exception to this occurs when the mother's serum contains antibodies against the ABO group of the fetus; for example, if the mother were group O and the fetus group B. In these cases the fetal RBC are apparently destroyed in the maternal circulation before Rh sensitization can proceed to a significant extent, although this does not always happen. The syndrome of Rh-induced erythroblastosis will be discussed later. Rh incompatibility was a major cause of blood transfusion reactions, although these reactions occur much less often than ABO transfusion reactions. Rh antibody transfusion reactions may occur by transfusion of donor blood containing Rh antibodies or by previous sensitization of a recipient, who now will have the antibodies in his own serum.

Rh antigen may be typed using commercial antiserum. Preliminary screening is only for antigen D, which establishes a person as Rh positive or negative. If a person is Rh negative, further studies with antiserum to other components of the Rh group may be done, depending on the situation and the individual blood bank. In particular, there is a weak subgroup of D (Rh$_0$) called D^u (Rh$_0$ variant) which is analogous to the weak A$_2$ subgroup of A in the ABO system. D^u blood often fails to give a positive reaction with some commercial Rh anti-D typing serums, and thus may falsely type as Rh negative. Therefore, many large blood banks screen Rh negative red cells for D^u as well as for c (hr') and E (rh''), the most antigenic of the minor Rh antigens.

Rh antibodies are usually univalent and react best in vitro at 37° C in high-protein medium. Large blood banks screen donor serum for these antibodies using a variety of techniques. When Rh antibodies attack RBC in vivo, whether in transfusion or in hemolytic disease of the newborn, they coat the surface of the red cells in the usual manner of univalent antibodies and are then positive with the direct Coombs test (until the affected RBC are destroyed).

OTHER ANTIGENIC SYSTEMS

Besides the ABO and the Rh systems there are a considerable number of other unrelated antigenic systems that have some importance, either from medicolegal parenthood studies or from sensitization leading to transfusion reactions or hemolytic disease of the newborn. The most important of these systems is Kell (K), a well-recognized blood bank problem. The Kell antibodies are similar in characteristics and behavior to the Rh system D (Rh$_0$) antibody. Fortunately, only about 10% of whites and 2% of blacks have the Kell antigen and are thus Kell-positive, so that opportunities for sensitization of a Kell-negative person are not great. Kell antibody is univalent and acts best in vitro using high-protein media at 37° C, just as Rh does. If reactions due to Kell antibodies occur, the direct Coombs test is positive (until the affected RBC are destroyed). A similar situation exists for the rare Duffy (Fy) and Kidd (jK) systems. There are other systems that resemble ABO in their antibody characteristics, and these include the MN, P, Lewis (Le) and Lutheran (Lu) systems. They are primarily bivalent antibodies, and react best in vitro with saline media at room temperature or below. They are rare causes for transfusion reactions, and even when difficulties arise they are clinically milder than the univalent antibody systems. They may, however, be dangerous, and cannot be ignored.

CROSSMATCHING

Even if major blood group typing has been done, transfusion reactions may occur due to antibodies other than ABO or Rh$_0$ (D). To prevent this, the concept of a crossmatch has evolved. There are two basic procedures: the major crossmatch, involving the serum of the recipient and the cells of the donor, and the minor crossmatch, involving the cells of the recipient and the serum of the donor. Some blood banks replace the minor crossmatch with antibody screening procedures, using the donor's serum and a panel of different RBC containing various blood group antigens. Theoretically, even if the serum of the donor contains antibodies to one or more of the red cell antigens of the recipient, the relatively large blood volume of the recipient should dilute the relatively small volume of the donor serum to a point at which it is harmless. This is the rationale for using O negative blood (the so-called universal donor) in emergencies without crossmatch. Even so, there is risk involved, since the recipient may possess antibody to some other blood group antigen of the donor (such as anti-Rh or anti-Kell). A crossmatch would pick this up. Moreover, the anti-A or anti-B in group O blood may be in high titer, and transfusion reactions may occur when these bloods are used in recipients who are of other ABO groups. Many blood banks maintain a certain amount of low-titer O negative blood for use in emergencies. Titers over 1:50 are considered too high for this purpose. In addition, A and B group specific substance (Witebsky substance) may be added to the donor blood to partially neutralize anti-A and anti-B. These substances are A and B antigen manufactured from animal sources and, being foreign antigens, may possibly sensitize the patient.

Therefore, the purpose of crossmatch compatibility tests is to detect antibodies of either person. It incidentally serves as a check on ABO typing, since antibodies to the ABO system occur naturally. The procedure will not detect errors in Rh typing if no Rh antibodies are present in donor or recipient. Since Rh antibodies do not occur naturally, either donor or recipient would have to be previously sensitized before Rh or similar antibodies would appear. Without antibodies present the crossmatch does not demonstrate antigens, and thus will not prevent immunization (sensitization) of the recipient by Rh or similar groups. This can be done only by proper typing of the donor and recipient cells beforehand.

The crossmatch is usually carried out in several steps using several techniques so as to pick up groups of antibodies that have different temperature and reaction media requirements. Occasionally the laboratory is asked to do an "emergency crossmatch." There is no such thing. Certain procedures may be eliminated to gain speed, but this correspondingly increases the risk of missing those antigens that they are designed to detect. It must be realized that emergency crossmatch blood has not been properly screened.

A word must also be said regarding a few patients whose blood presents unexplained difficulty in crossmatching. The laboratory should be allowed to solve the problem and possibly to obtain aid from a reference laboratory. During this time 5% serum albumin or saline may temporarily assist the patient. In the absence of complete crossmatching blood is given as a calculated risk.

If blood is needed for emergency transfusion without crossmatch, a frequent decision is to use group O Rh negative blood. A better method would be to use blood of the same ABO and Rh type as the patient's. ABO and Rh typing can be done within five minutes using anticoagulated specimens of the patient's blood. This would avoid interpretation problems produced by putting group O cells into a group A or B patient and subsequently attempting crossmatches for more blood.

When repeated transfusions are needed, a new specimen should be drawn from the patient (recipient) for crossmatching purposes if blood had last been given more than 24 hours previously. Some patients demonstrate marked anamnestic responses to red cell antigens that they lack, and may produce clinically significant quantities of antibody in a few hours. This antibody would not be present in the original specimen from the patient.

In summary, red cell typing is designed to show what antigens are on the RBC, and thus what blood group red cells can be given to a recipient either without being destroyed by antibodies the recipient is known to possess or without danger of sensitizing the recipient by introducing antigens that he might lack and thus against which he might produce antibodies. The cross-match procedure (comprising major and minor techniques) is designed to demonstrate unexpected antibodies in the serum (of donor or recipient) that may destroy RBC otherwise considered compatible as a result of RBC blood group typing.

WHITE BLOOD CELL ANTIGENS

The red cell ABO surface antigens are found in most tissues (except those of the central nervous system). Some of the other RBC antigens, such as the P system, may occur in some locations outside red cells. White blood cells also possess a complex antigen group that is found in other tissues; more specifically, in nucleated cells. This is called the human leukocyte-A (HL-A) system. HL-A is found in one site (locus) on chromosome number 6. Each locus is composed of four subloci. Each of the four subloci contains one gene. Each sublocus (gene) has multiple alleles (i.e., a pool of several genes), any one of which can be selected as the single gene for a sublocus. The four subloci are currently designated A, B, C and D. The two major subloci are A and B, also called segregant series A (formerly known as the first series, or LA) and B (formerly the second series, or FOUR). There are over 15 alleles in both the A and the B segregant series. The four subloci that form one locus are all inherited as a group (linked), in a manner analogous to the Fisher-Race theory of Rh inheritance. Again analogous to Rh, some HL-A gene combinations are found much more frequently than others.

The HL-A system has been closely identified with tissue transplant compatibility, to such a degree that some refer to HL-A as histocompatibility leukocyte-A. It has been shown that HL-A antigens introduced into a recipient by skin grafting stimulate production of antibodies against the HL-A antigens that the recipient lacks; also, that prior sensitization by donor leukocytes produces accelerated graft rejection. In kidney transplants from members of the same family, transplant survival was found to correlate with closeness of HL-A matching between donor and recipient. On the other hand, there is evidence that HL-A is not the only factor involved, since cadaver transplants frequently do not behave in the manner predicted by closeness of HL-A typing.

Besides their association with immunologic body defenses, certain HL-A antigens have been found to occur with increased frequency in various diseases. The B-27 (formerly W-27) antigen is associated with so-called rheumatoid arthritis (RA) variants (p. 261). In ankylosing spondylitis, Reiter's syndrome and *Yersinia enterocolitica* arthritis, HL-A B-27 occurs in

70-90% (literature range 30-95%) of cases, depending on the investigator. In juvenile rheumatoid, psoriatic and enteropathic (ulcerative colitis and Crohn's disease) arthritis, incidence of HL-A B-27 depends on the presence of spondylitis or sacroiliitis. In all "RA variant" patients, those with spondylitis or sacroiliitis have B-27 in more than 50% of cases (some report as high as 70-95%); without clinical disease in these locations, B-27 is found in less than 25%. Increased frequency of B-27 was also reported in close relatives of patients with ankylosing spondylitis.

Increased incidence of certain other HL-A antigens have been reported in celiac disease (HLA-8), chronic active hepatitis, and multiple sclerosis (as well as in various other diseases), but with lesser degrees of correlation than in the RA variants. The significance of this is still uncertain, and verification is needed in some instances.

REFERENCES

Bach, F. H., and Van Rood, J. J.: The major histocompatibility complex: Genetics and biology, N. Engl. J. Med. 295:806, 872, 927, 1976.

Dugan, C. C.: A new look at gene determinants and their controls, J. Fla. Med. Assoc. 63:29, 1976.

Dykes, D. D., and Polesky, H. F.: The usefulness of serum protein and erythrocyte enzyme polymorphisms in paternity testing, Am. J. Clin. Pathol. 65:982, 1976.

Gray, R. G., and Gottlieb, N. L.: The HL-A B27 histocompatibility antigen in rheumatoid arthritis variants, J. Fla. Med. Assoc. 63:339, 1976.

Greenwalt, T. J., and Steane, E. A.: The problem of red cell polyagglutinability, Postgrad. Med. 52:170, 1972.

Griffitts, J. J., and Schmidt, P.: Effectiveness of techniques in demonstrating the isohemagglutinins, Transfusion 2:385, 1962.

Grove-Rasmussen, M.: Routine compatibility testing, Transfusion 4:200, 1964.

Grove-Rasmussen, M.: Selection of "safe" group O blood, Transfusion 6:331, 1966.

Hyland Reference Manual of Immunohematology (2d ed.; Los Angeles: Hyland Laboratories, 1964).

Jennings, E. R., and Hindmarsh, C.: The significance of the minor crossmatch, Am. J. Clin. Pathol. 30:302, 1958.

Lalezari, P.: HL-A—transplantation antigens or genetic markers? Am. J. Med. Sci. 264:55, 1972.

Lockshin, M. D., et al.: Ankylosing spondylitis and HL-A: A genetic disease plus? Am. J. Med. 58:695, 1975.

Mannick, J. A.: Clinical kidney transplantation: areas of current interest, Postgrad. Med. 54:171, 1973.

Mollison, P. L.: *Blood Transfusion in Clinical Medicine* (5th ed.; Philadelphia: J. B. Lippincott Company, 1972).

Race, R. R., and Sanger, R.: *Blood Groups in Man* (6th ed.; Philadelphia: F. A. Davis Co., 1975).

Simmons, A., et al.: Effect of varying the crossmatch procedure upon detection of anti-D and anti-Kell, Am. J. Med. Technol. 37:83, 1971.

Stern, K.: Unusual blood types as a cause of disease, Med. Clin. North Am. 46:277, 1962.

Wiener, A. S., and Wexler, I. B.: *Heredity of the Blood Groups* (New York: Grune & Stratton, Inc., 1958).

Woodrow, J. C.: Histocompatibility antigens and rheumatic diseases, Semin. Arthritis Rheum. 6:257, 1976.

10 / Immunohematologic Reactions

TRANSFUSION REACTIONS occur in a certain percentage of blood transfusions. The three main types are: hemolytic, febrile and allergic.

HEMOLYTIC REACTIONS

Hemolytic reactions may be caused by either complete or incomplete antibodies. In those resulting from *complete* antibodies, such as occur in the ABO system, there is usually intravascular hemolysis. The amount of hemolysis depends on several factors, such as quantity of incompatible blood, antibody titer and the nature of the antibody involved. However, there is an element of individual susceptibility, for some patients die from less than 100 ml of incompatible blood, whereas others survive after several times this amount. The direct Coombs test is often positive, but this depends on whether all the RBC attacked by the complete antibody have been lysed, whether more antibody is produced and to some extent on how soon the test is obtained. If the sample is drawn more than 1 hour after the ABO transfusion reaction is completed, the chance of a positive direct Coombs test begins to become less and less. Also, a "broad-spectrum" Coombs reagent is needed; most laboratories now use this type routinely. Free hemoglobin is released into the plasma (thence into urine via the kidney), and indirect bilirubin then rises also. In reactions caused by *incomplete*-type antibodies, such as the Rh system, there is sequestration of antibody-coated cells in organs such as the spleen, with subsequent breakdown by the reticuloendothelial system. Thus, RBC breakdown is extravascular; in small degrees of reaction, plasma free hemoglobin may not rise, although indirect bilirubin eventually will. In more extensive reactions, plasma hemoglobin is often elevated, although sometimes delayed in onset. The direct Coombs test should be positive in reactions due to incomplete antibodies (unless all affected RBC have been destroyed).

Hemolytic reaction is usually caused by incompatible blood, although occasionally it may be due to partial hemolysis of the red cells before transfusion. The great majority of cases result from human error, usually mislabeled crossmatch specimens or administration to the wrong patient. Symptoms include chills, fever and pain in the low back or legs. Jaundice may appear later. Severe reactions lead to shock. Renal shutdown is common, due either to shock or to precipitation of free hemoglobin in the renal tubules. Therefore, oliguria and often hemoglobinuria develop, manifested by red urine or nearly black coffee-ground acid hematin urine color.

Tests for Hemolytic Transfusion Reaction

These tests include plasma hemoglobin ("free hemoglobin") and serum haptoglobin both immediately and at 6 hours, and serum indirect bilirubin at 6 and 12 hours. The urine should be examined for hemoglobin, hemoglobin casts, red cells and proteinuria. A direct Coombs test and crossmatch recheck studies should be performed as soon as possible. A culture should be done from the remaining blood in the donor bag. The best immediate test for plasma hemoglobin is simple visual inspection of plasma. Most complete-antibody transfusion reactions produce enough hemolysis to be grossly visible. (Artifact hemolysis from improperly drawn specimens must be ruled out.) If chemical tests are to be done, plasma hemoglobin is preferred to serum hemoglobin because less artifact hemolysis takes place before the specimen reaches the laboratory. Although hemolytic reactions due to incomplete antibodies, such as Rh, have clinical symptoms similar to those of ABO, direct signs of hemolysis (such as free plasma hemoglobin) are more variable or may be delayed for a few hours, although they become abnormal if the reaction is severe. Another drawback in the interpretation of plasma hemoglobin values is the effect of the transfusion itself. The older erythrocytes stored in bank blood die during storage, adding free hemoglobin to the plasma. Therefore, although normal values are usually stated in the range of 1–5 mg/100 ml, values between 5 and 50 mg/100 ml are equivocal if stored blood is given. Hemolysis is barely visible when plasma hemoglobin reaches the 25–50 mg/100 ml range. Frozen blood has a greater content of free hemoglobin than stored whole blood or packed cells, and may reach 300 mg/100 ml.

Hemoglobin passes the glomerular filter into the urine when plasma hemoglobin is more than 125 mg/100 ml. Therefore, since hemolysis should already be visible, the major need for urine examination is to verify that intravascular hemolysis occurred rather than artifact hemolysis from venipuncture or faulty specimen processing. Conversely, unless elevated plasma free hemoglobin is present, urine hemoglobin may represent lysed RBC of hematuria unrelated to a hemolytic reaction. However, if sufficient time passes, the serum may be cleared of free hemoglobin while hemoglobin casts are still present in urine. Hemosiderin may be deposited in renal tubule cells and continue to appear in the urine for several days.

Serum haptoglobin (pp. 23, 241) is an alpha$_2$ globulin that binds free hemoglobin. Two types of measurements are available; haptoglobin binding capacity and total haptoglobin. Binding capacity can be measured by electrophoresis or chemical methods. Total haptoglobin is usually estimated by immunologic (antibody) techniques; a 2-minute slide test is now commercially available. Haptoglobin binding capacity shows almost immediate decrease when sufficient quantity of free hemoglobin is liberated and remains low for 2–4 days. Stored bank blood, fortunately, does not contain enough free hemoglobin to produce significant changes in haptoglobin binding capacity. Total haptoglobin level decreases more slowly than binding capacity after onset of a hemolytic reaction and might not reach lowest value until 6–8 hours later. Haptoglobin assay is much less helpful when frozen red cells are being transfused, due to normally increased free hemoglobin in most frozen red cell preparations. Bilirubin determinations are not needed if haptoglobin assay is done the same day.

A pretransfusion blood specimen, if available, should be included to provide a baseline when performing the various tests for hemolysis.

Transfusion should be stopped at the first sign of possible reaction and complete studies done to recheck compatibility of the donor and recipient blood. If these are still satisfactory, and if the direct Coombs test and the studies for intravascular hemolysis are negative, a different unit can be started on the assumption that the symptoms were pyrogenic rather than hemolytic. Naturally, whatever unused blood remains in the donor bottle, the donor bottle pilot tube, and a new specimen drawn from the patient must all be sent to the blood bank for the recheck studies. Especially dangerous situations exist in transfusion during surgery, where anesthesia may mask the early signs and symptoms of a reaction. Development during surgery of a marked bleeding tendency at the operative site is an important danger signal. A transfusion reaction requires immediate mannitol therapy to protect the kidneys.

FEBRILE REACTIONS

LEUKOAGGLUTININS.— Probably the most common variety of transfusion reaction is that due to white blood cell incompatibility, produced by antibodies against leukocytes (leukoagglutinins). Before leukoagglutinins were recognized, these episodes were included with the pyrogenic reaction category. Symptoms include fever, chills, myalgia and nonproductive cough. In a small minority of cases, a syndrome is produced that includes these symptoms plus dyspnea and tachycardia; the chest x-ray has a characteristic pattern described as numerous hilar and lower lobe nodular infiltrates without cardiac enlargement or pulmonary vessel congestion. Symptoms abate in 24 – 48 hours but the x-ray abnormalities may persist for several days. Some patients have eosinophilia, but others do not. The syndrome has been called "noncardiac pulmonary edema," a somewhat unfortunate term since pulmonary edema is not present, although many clinical findings simulate this condition. Most cases of this syndrome follow transfusion of whole blood.

Most patients acquire leukoagglutinins from previous transfusion or from fetal antigen sensitization in pregnancy. The more transfusions, the more likelihood of sensitization.

Reactions due to leukoagglutinins are usually not life-threatening, but are unpleasant to the patient, physician and laboratory. Since clinical symptoms are similar to those of a hemolytic reaction, each febrile reaction must be investigated to rule out red cell incompatibility, even if the patient is known to have leukoagglutinins. Leukoagglutinin reactions may be reduced or eliminated by the use of leukocyte-poor packed cells, washed cells or frozen red cells (Chapter 11). There are specialized tests available to demonstrate leukoagglutinin activity, but most laboratories are not equipped to perform them. The diagnosis, therefore, is usually a presumptive one based on history and ruling out hemolytic reaction.

IGA ANTIGEN REACTIONS. — IgA is the principal immunoglobulin in such human secretions as saliva, bile and gastric juice. "Class-specific" anti-IgA occurs in patients who lack IgA; these persons may be clinically normal or have such disorders as malabsorption syndrome, autoimmune diseases or recurrent sinus or pulmonary infection. "Limited specificity" anti-IgA occurs in persons who have normal IgA levels but who become sensitized from exposure to human plasma proteins from blood transfusion or pregnancy. Anti-IgA antibodies produce reaction only in transfusions that include human plasma proteins. Symptoms consist of tachycardia, flush, headache, chest pain, dyspnea and fever. Severe episodes may include hypotension. Again, these are nonspecific symptoms that could be produced by leukoagglutinins or hemolytic reactions. Tests to prove IgA incompatibility are available only in a few medical centers; therefore, the diagnosis is rarely made. Reactions of this type can be avoided by eliminating plasma proteins through the use of washed cells or frozen cells.

PYROGENIC REACTIONS. — These result from contamination by bacteria, dirt or foreign proteins. One frequently quoted study estimates that nearly 2% of donor blood units have some degree of bacterial contamination, regardless of amount of care taken when the blood is drawn. Symptoms begin during or shortly after transfusion, and consist of chills and fever. The more severe cases often have abdominal cramps, nausea and diarrhea. Very heavy bacterial contamination may lead to shock. Therefore, in a patient with transfusion-associated reaction that includes hypotension, a gram-stained smear should be made from blood remaining in the donor bag without waiting for culture results.

ALLERGIC REACTIONS. — Allergic types of reaction are presumably due to substances in the donor blood to which the recipient is allergic. Symptoms are localized or generalized hives, although occasionally severe asthma or even laryngeal edema may occur. There is usually excellent response to antihistamines or epinephrine.

PLATELET REACTIONS

Blood platelets contain at least three antigen systems capable of producing a transfusion reaction. The first is the ABO (ABH) system also found on RBC; for that reason the American Association of Blood Banks recommends that single donor platelet units be typed for the ABO group before being transfused. Platelets do not contain the Rh antigen; however, since platelet units may be contaminated by red cells, it is safer to type for D (Rh_o) antigen in addition to ABO typing. The majority of investigators believe that ABO-Rh typing is useful only to avoid possible sensitization of the recipient and that recipient anti-A or anti-B antibody will not destroy ABO-incompatible platelets. There are specific platelet antigens (Pl group, also called Zw^a, and several others) that are high incidence and thus rarely cause difficulty. Finally, there is the histocompatibility leukocyte antigen (HL-A) group (p. 89). This tissue compatibility system has been incriminated when patients become refractory to repeated platelet transfusions (i.e., fail to raise the platelet count) and may develop a febrile reaction. Persons who are HL-A compatible (usually siblings) as a rule are able to donate satisfactorily. The HL-A antigens are also present on white blood cells. Finally, other types of antiplatelet antibodies may appear, such as those of chronic idiopathic thrombocytopenia (p. 74). In this situation, transfused platelets are quickly destroyed, making the transfusion of little value unless the patient is actively bleeding.

HEMOLYTIC DISEASE OF THE NEWBORN

The other major area where blood banks meet blood group hemolytic problems is that of hemolytic disease of the newborn. This may be due to ABO, Rh or (rarely) minor group incompatibility between fetal and maternal red cells. Basically, the situation results from fetal cell antigens that the maternal red cells lack. These fetal RBC antigens provoke maternal antibody formation when fetal red cells are introduced into the maternal circulation after escaping from the placenta. The maternal antibodies eventually cross the placenta to the fetal circulation and attack the fetal red cells.

Hemolytic disease of the newborn due to Rh incompatibility varies in severity from subclinical status through mild jaundice with anemia to the dangerous and often fatal condition of erythroblastosis fetalis. The main clinical findings are anemia and rapidly developing jaundice. Reticulocytosis over 6% accompanies the anemia, and the jaundice is mainly due to unconjugated (indirect) bilirubin released from the reticuloendothelial sequestration and destruction of RBC. The direct Coombs test is positive. In severe cases there are usually many nucleated RBC in the peripheral blood. Jaundice is not present at birth but develops several hours later or even after 24 hours in mild cases. Diseases that cause jaundice in the newborn, often accompanied by anemia and sometimes a few peripheral blood nucleated RBC, include septicemia, cytomegalic inclusion disease, toxoplasmosis and syphilis. Physiologic jaundice of the newborn is a frequent benign condition that may be confused with hemolytic disease or vice versa. There is, however, no significant anemia. A normal newborn has an (average) hemoglobin value of 18 gm/100 ml, and less than 15 gm/100 ml indicates anemia.

Fifty per cent or more of hemolytic disease is due to ABO incompatibility between mother and fetus. Anti-A and anti-B production begins between 3 and 6 months of age. From birth until this time, ABO antibodies in the infant's serum come from the mother. If the infant's ABO isoagglutinogens are compatible with the ABO group of the mother, everything is fine. If, however, the mother possesses antibodies to the A or B red cell antigens of the fetus, hemolytic disease of the newborn may result, just as if the newborn had received a transfusion of serum with antibodies against his red cells. This being the case, it is surprising to find that although 20–25% of all pregnancies display maternal-fetal ABO incompatibility, the great majority of these infants seem perfectly healthy. Only a small minority develop various degrees of hemolytic disease. This may be due to the fact that ABO hemolytic disease as a group is usually milder than its counterpart caused by Rh incompatibility, which was discussed earlier. In fact, many infants with ABO disease may have degrees of hemolysis too small to be detected clinically and may be apparently well. The incidence of clinically evident disease is about the same as that of Rh, although, as just said, even severe cases are relatively milder than the comparable Rh cases. Some infants, however, will die or suffer cerebral damage if treatment is not given. Therefore, the diagnosis of ABO disease and its differential diagnosis from the other causes of jaundice and anemia in the newborn are of great practical importance.

There are two types of ABO antibodies—the naturally occurring complete saline-reacting type discussed earlier, and an immune univalent (incomplete) type produced in some unknown way to fetal A or B antigen stimulation. Most cases of clinical ABO disease have a group O mother and a group A or B infant. The immune anti-A or anti-B antibody, if produced by the mother, may cause ABO disease, because it can pass the placenta. Maternal titers of 1:32 or more are considered dangerous. The saline antibodies do not cross the placenta and are not significant in hemolytic disease of the newborn.

The direct Coombs test done on the infant with ABO hemolytic disease is sometimes but not often positive. Spherocytes are often present. Good evidence for ABO disease is detection of immune anti-A or anti-B in the cord blood of a newborn whose RBC belong to the same blood group as the antibody. Detection of these antibodies only in the serum of the mother does not conclusively prove ABO disease in the newborn.

Hemolytic disease caused by Rh sensitization occurs usually in a mother who is Rh negative with a fetus who is Rh positive. The direct Coombs test on the cord or infant blood is usually positive and should be done in all cases of possible hemolytic disease of the newborn, because incomplete antibodies occasionally may coat the surface of the fetal RBC to such an extent as to interfere with proper Rh typing. Maternal serum contains immune antibodies to the Rh factor, whose titer usually rises if serial studies are done during pregnancy. The first child is usually not affected, but the mother becomes sensitized during that pregnancy. Subsequent pregnancies may show fetal hemolytic disease, although not always. For the sake of prognosis in future pregnancies, the husband should get a complete Rh typing to see if he is homozygous or heterozygous for the Rh factor involved.

Infants with hemolytic disease of the newborn can usually be saved by exchange transfusion. The indications for this procedure are:

1. Infant serum indirect bilirubin above 20 mg/100 ml or premature infant 15 mg/100 ml.

2. Cord blood indirect bilirubin over 4 mg/100 ml.

3. Hemoglobin less than 13 gm/100 ml.

4. Maternal Rh antibody titer of 1:64 or greater, although this is not an absolute indication if the bilirubin does not rise very high.

Routine prenatal tests should include ABO and Rh typing of the mother. If the mother is Rh negative, the father should be Rh typed also. If an Rh incompatibility exists, follow-up should include maternal Rh antibody titration at 3 months and 6 months, then bimonthly to detect any rising titer.

Serum bilirubin levels are considered the main parameter of severity in hemolytic disease of the newborn. Recently, amniocentesis has been advocated as a means of estimating fetal risk while still in utero. A long needle is introduced into the amniotic fluid cavity of the fetus by means of a suprapubic puncture approach in the mother. The amniotic fluid is subjected to spectrophotometric estimation of bilirubin pigments. Markedly increased bilirubin pigment strongly indicates significant degrees of hemolytic disease in the fetus. If necessary, delivery can then be induced prematurely once the 32d week of gestation has arrived. Before this, or in utero with severe disease, intrauterine exchange transfusion has been attempted, using a transabdominal approach. The indications for amniocentesis are development of significant titer of Rh antibody in the mother or a history of previous erythroblastosis. Significant maternal antibody Rh titers do not always mean serious fetal Rh disease, but absence of significant titer nearly always indicates a benign prognosis. Also, if initial amniocentesis at 32 weeks does not suggest an immediately dangerous situation, even though mild or moderate abnormalities are present, a fetus can be allowed to mature as long as possible (being monitored by repeated studies) to avoid the danger of premature birth.

Studies have now proved that a great majority of mothers with potential or actual Rh incompatibility problems can be protected against sensitization by the fetus. A "vaccine" composed of gamma globulin with a high titer of anti-Rh antibody (anti-D or Rh_o) is given to the mother during the 1–3 days following delivery of the first child with red cell Rh antigen incompatibility to the mother. This exogenous antibody seems to suppress maternal endogenous antibody production in many cases. Subsequent pregnancy in these cases would not provoke anamnestic antibody response.

REFERENCES

Alter, A. A., et al.: Direct antiglobulin test in ABO hemolytic disease of the newborn, Obstet. Gynecol. 33:846, 1969.

Andrews, A. T., et al.: Transfusion reaction with pulmonary infiltration associated with HL-A—specific leukocyte antibodies; Am. J. Clin. Pathol. 66:483, 1976.

Baker, R. J., et al.: Diagnosis and treatment of immediate transfusion reaction, Surg., Gynecol. Obstet. 130:665, 1970.

Bohnen, R. F., et al.: The direct Coombs test: Its clinical significance, Ann. Intern. Med. 68:19, 1968.

Bowman, J. M.: Hemolytic disease of the newborn, Obstet. Gynecol. 40:217, 1966.

Chan, A. C., et al.: ABO hemolytic disease, J. Pediatr. 61:405, 1962.

Cushman, P., and Maniatas, A.: Direct antiglobulin tests in narcotic addicted patients, Transfusion 15:107, 1975.

Fink, D. J., et al.: Serum haptoglobin. A valuable diagnostic aid in suspected hemolytic transfusion reactions, J.A.M.A. 199:615, 1967.

Fraser, I. D., and Tovey, G. H.: Observations on Rh isoimmunization: past, present, and future. Clin. Haematol. 5:149, 1976.

Freda, V. J., et al.: Current concepts. Prevention of Rh hemolytic disease—ten years' clinical experience with Rh immune globulin, N. Engl. J. Med. 292:1014, 1975.

Jandl, J. H., and Tomlinson, A. S.: The destruction of red cells by antibodies in man. II. Pyrogenic, leukocytic, and dermal responses to immune hemolysis, Medicine 43:207, 1964.

Javid, J.: Human serum haptoglobins—A brief review, Semin. Hematol. 4:35, 1967.

Jennings, E. R.: Recent Advances in Diagnosis, Treatment, and Prevention of Hemolytic Disease of the Newborn, in Stefanini, M. (ed.): *Advances in Clinical Pathology* (New York: Grune & Stratton, Inc., 1966), vol. 1, p. 458.

Kahan, B. D.: Single donor, HL-A matched platelet transfusions for thrombocytopenic patients undergoing surgery, Surgery 77:241, 1975.

Mollison, P. L.: *Blood Transfusion in Clinical Medicine* (5th ed.; Philadelphia: J. B. Lippincott Company, 1972).

Moncrieff, R. E., et al.: Delayed hemolytic transfusion reaction with four antibodies undetected by pretransfusion tests, Am. J. Clin. Pathol. 64:251, 1975.

Odell, G. B., et al.: Exchange transfusion, Pediatr. Clin. North Am. 9:605, 1962.

Pineda, A. A., et al.: Transfusion reactions associated with anti-IgA antibodies: report of four cases and review of the literature, Transfusion 15:10, 1975.

Polesky, H. F., et al.: Positive antiglobulin tests in cardiac surgery patients, Transfusion 9:43, 1969.

Transfusion Reaction Workshop, American Association of Blood Banks, 1973.

Ward, H. W.: Pulmonary infiltrates associated with leukoagglutinin transfusion reactions, Ann. Intern. Med. 73:689, 1970.

11 / Blood Transfusions

BLOOD TRANSFUSIONS may consist of whole blood or various blood fractions.

WHOLE BLOOD

Whole blood is collected in a citrate anticoagulant with either ACD or CPD formulations. Acceptable storage life in ACD is 21 days and in CPD, 28 days, both maintained at 4° C; at the end of this time there is approximately 70% red cell viability. There are certain problems involving stored bank blood. After approximately 2 weeks' storage, some of the RBC lose vitality and become spherocytes. Since spherocytosis is a feature of certain isoimmune and autoimmune hemolytic anemias, transfusion of such blood prior to diagnostic investigation may cause confusion. Potassium concentration slowly rises during storage as it escapes from devitalized RBC. After 15 days' storage, plasma levels reach approximately 25 mEq/L, roughly 5–6 times normal (1 unit of whole blood equals about 500 ml; normal blood volume is equivalent to roughly 8–10 whole blood units; normal plasma volume is about 3 L; and 3 units of whole blood together equal about 1 L of plasma). Although the hyperkalemia of stored blood seems to have little effect on most persons, even when many units are transfused, it may be undesirable if the patient already has elevated serum potassium, as seen in uremia or acute renal shutdown. Ammonium levels of stored blood also increase, and may reach values of 10–15 times normal. Large volumes of such blood may be dangerous in severe liver disease. The citrate anticoagulant may cause difficulty with really massive transfusions. Its calcium-binding actions may lead to hypocalcemia if substituted for a large portion of the blood volume. This is the so-called citrate intoxication and fortunately is rare. In addition, citrate in large quantities does have a depressant effect on the myocardium. Platelets disintegrate rapidly on storage and are physiologically useless after 1–2 days. Bank blood, therefore, essentially has no functioning platelets, even though the platelet count may be normal. This may produce difficulty in massive transfusions using stored bank blood, although there is usually no problem when administration takes place over longer periods of time.

Massive blood transfusion is defined by the American Association of Blood Banks (AABB) as replacement of the patient's blood volume (equivalent to 8–10 units of whole blood) in 12 hours. Such volumes present special difficulties of various types, depending on the substances being transfused and the rate of administration. Potassium and ammonium have been mentioned; they usually do not cause problems in massive transfusion except for uremic patients (potassium) and patients with severe liver disease(ammonium). After total blood volume replacement, the platelet count may reach 50,000/cu mm or less, and not all of these are functional. In addition, the labile coagulation factors V and VIII are depleted. Some advocate 1 unit of fresh blood (or fresh frozen plasma) for every 10 units of bank blood.

Citrate anticoagulant may cause difficulty when large volumes of blood are given in very short periods of time. Citrate has calcium-binding activity that may lead to hypocalcemia and also has a potential depressant effect on the myocardium. Fortunately, most patients are able to tolerate a large amount of citrate if liver function is adequate. One investigator states that the average person could receive 1 unit of blood every 5 minutes without requiring calcium supplements. Others have used 10 ml of a 10% calcium gluconate solution for every 2 units of citrated blood if more than 2 units are given in less than 20 minutes. Another recommendation is 1 ampule (1 gm) of calcium gluconate for every 3–5 units of citrated blood. Calcium chloride has 4 times as much calcium as calcium gluconate, so that dosage using calcium chloride must be reduced proportionately. Large amounts of rapidly administered cold blood increases the possibility of ventricular fibrillation. Ordinarily blood can be allowed to warm in room air; if this is not possible, one can use a water bucket (30° C) for unopened blood containers or special warming devices (37° C) through which the blood passes via tubing while being administered. Transfusion of blood at ordinary speed does not require warming.

Under usual circumstances, AABB recommends that 1 unit of whole blood or packed cells be administered in 1½–2 hours. The infusion rate should be slower during the first 15 minutes (100 ml/hour), during which time the patient is observed for signs and symptoms of transfusion reaction. One unit of whole blood or packed cells raises hemoglobin approximately 1 gm and HCT approximately 3 percentage units. (Various factors could modify these average values.) Red blood cells will hemolyze when directly mixed with 5% dextrose in either water or 0.25% saline or with Ringer's solution.

Stored blood may carry the organisms of hepatitis, syphilis, and malaria. The spirochete of syphilis will die in 4–5 days under usual storage conditions, but the others survive.

Whole blood is used for restoration of blood volume due to acute simultaneous loss of both plasma and red blood cells. This is most frequently seen in acute hemorrhage, both external and internal. Stored blood is adequate for this in most cases.

Fresh whole blood is used within 2 days and preferably 1 day after collection. Platelets are still viable, and certain other substances, such as factor VIII (antihemophilic globulin) and factor V, are still at least partially active. The other disadvantages of prolonged storage are absent. Obviously, donor and administrative problems greatly limit use and availability of fresh blood.

Since the use of blood transfusion has increased dramatically over the years, maintenance of adequate donor sources has been a constant problem. In Russia, cadaver blood has apparently been utilized. If collected less than 6 hours post mortem, it does not differ significantly from stored (bank) blood, except that anticoagulation is not required. A few experimental studies have been done in the United States, with favorable results.

Autotransfusion avoids all problems of reaction and is useful in those whose religious beliefs preclude receiving blood from others. Depending on the circumstances, 1 or more units may be withdrawn at appropriate intervals before elective surgery and either preserved as whole blood or as frozen RBC.

PACKED RED CELLS

Packed red cells consist of bank blood with about three fourths of the plasma taken out. Packed cells help avoid the problem of overloading the patient's blood volume and throwing him into pulmonary edema. This is especially useful in anemias due to destruction or poor production of red cells, when the plasma volume does not need replacement. In fact, when anemia is due to pure red cell deficiency, plasma volume becomes greater than usual, because extracellular fluid tends to replace the missing RBC volume to maintain total blood volume. Packed cells are sometimes used when the donor red cells type satisfactorily but antibodies are present in donor plasma. Packed cell administration also helps diminish some of the other problems of stored blood, such as elevated plasma potassium or ammonium. Packed RBC retain about 20–25% of the plasma and most of the WBC and platelets.

Leukocyte-Poor Packed Cells

Techniques are available to remove 80–90% of the WBC, depending on the method used. The RBC have normal preservation, but nearly 20% of them are lost in processing. This type of preparation is indicated when a patient has reactions due to leukoagglutinins (p. 93).

Washed Red Cells

Washed RBC are packed cells that have received 1 or more washes with saline. This removes about 85% of the WBC and most of the platelets and plasma proteins. About 20% of the RBC are lost. After washing, the RBC must be administered within 24 hours. Indications for washed cells are relatively few; removal of donor antibody in IgA immune problems, paroxysmal nocturnal hemoglobinuria, and possibly in certain instances when extraordinary precautions are necessary to avoid hepatitis and when frozen red cells are not available.

Frozen Red Cells

Fresh citrate-anticoagulated red cells may have their storage life greatly prolonged by freezing. Glycerol is added to packed red cells to protect them during freezing; this substance prevents intracellular fluid from becoming ice. The blood is slowly frozen, and is maintained at below-zero temperatures until ready for use. Thereafter it must be thawed, after which the glycerol is removed (to avoid osmotic hemolysis), and the cells are resuspended in saline. This technique will maintain packed red cells for up to 5 years. Advantages to the blood bank include the ability to maintain a much greater inventory of rare blood types without fear of outdating and better control over temporary fluctuations in donor supply or recipient demand. Advantages to the patient include approximately 95% elimination of leukocytes, platelets and plasma proteins, thus removing sources of immunization and febrile reactions; removal of most potassium, ammonium, and citrate, three substances that might be undesirable in large quantities; and possibly the elimination or marked reduction of hepatitis contamination. Disadvantages include greater cost; significant time lost in thawing and preparing the RBC (1 hour or more), together with equipment limitation on the number of units that can be prepared simultaneously, which might cause difficulty in emergencies; the fact that once thawed, the cells must be used within 24 hours (by current AABB rules; some data suggest this could be extended); and the presence of variable amounts of free hemoglobin, which might be present in sufficient quantity to be troublesome if tests are needed for possible hemolytic transfusion reaction.

Frozen red cells are becoming more widely used as larger blood banks acquire the necessary equipment. Besides use for persons with rare blood types, current use tends to favor those circumstances with greater risk of hepatitis or immunohematologic sensitization. These include repeated transfusions or exposure to blood, as is frequently necessary in leukemia, chronic hemolytic anemias, bone marrow suppression, patients undergoing renal dialysis, elective multiple unit transfusion (such as cardiac surgery), and patients with leukoagglutinins.

PLATELETS

Platelet transfusions are most commonly used when bleeding or high risk of bleeding occurs and the patient is severely thrombocytopenic (less than 50,000 platelets/cu mm). Repeated transfusion carries the risk of inducing antiplatelet antibody formation (p. 94). In serious acute bleeding episodes there is clear indication for transfusion. When the patient has thrombocytopenia but has very minor bleeding or is not bleeding, the question of prophylactic platelet transfusion may arise. The decision is usually based on degree of risk and the type of disorder being treated. According to some authorities, high-risk patients are those with platelet counts less than 10,000/cu mm; moderate risk (transfusion only if clinically indicated), those with counts of 10,000 – 30,000/cu mm; and low risk, those over 30,000/cu mm. In patients with chronic bone marrow depression, an additional factor is the probability of developing antiplatelet antibodies that would interfere with therapy if actual bleeding developed later. In idiopathic thrombocytopenic purpura (ITP) antiplatelet antibodies that destroy donor platelets are already present, so that transfusion is useless unless the patient is actively bleeding. In drug-induced thrombocytopenia, transfusion is useless if the drug is still being given; after discontinuing the medication, transfusion can be helpful since a normal platelet count will usually return in about 1 week and transfused platelets survive about 1 week.

GRANULOCYTES

White blood cell transfusions have been used in a few centers for treatment of infection not responding to antibiotics in patients with severe leukopenia due to acute leukemia or to bone marrow depression. Clinical improvement has been reported in some of these patients, but not all. Most blood banks do not have the equipment to offer granulocyte transfusion as a routine procedure.

PLASMA

Plasma itself may be either stored or fresh frozen. Stored plasma, until recently, was the treatment of choice for blood volume depletion in burns and proved very useful as an initial temporary measure in hemorrhagic shock while whole blood was being typed and crossmatched. It was also useful in some cases of shock not due to hemorrhage. Stored plasma may be either from single donors, in which case it must be crossmatched prior to transfusion, or more commonly from a pool of many donors. Pooled plasma dilutes any dangerous antibodies present in any one of the component plasma units, so that pooled plasma may be given without crossmatch. For many years it was thought that hepatitis virus in plasma would be inactivated after storage for 6 months at room temperature. For this reason, pooled stored plasma was widely used. In 1968 a study reported a 10% incidence of subclinical hepatitis even after prescribed lengths of storage. The National Research Council Committee on plasma and plasma substitutes now recommends that 5% albumin solution be used instead of plasma whenever possible. Purified plasma protein fraction is also available and considered satisfactory.

Fresh frozen plasma used to be the treatment of choice in factor VIII deficiency (hemophilia). Since large volumes were often required, methods were devised to concentrate factor VIII. Concentrated factor VIII solutions and cryoprecipitate are both available commercially and have mostly superseded the use of fresh frozen plasma in hemophilia. All of these products, unfortunately, may transmit hepatitis.

FIBRINOGEN

Fibrinogen is a blood fraction that is essential for clotting. It is decreased in 2 ways, both relatively uncommon: (1) by intravascular deposition of fibrin in the form of small clots (disseminated intravascular coagulation, DIC) and (2) by inactivation in the presence of primary fibrinolysin. Most commonly, DIC is seen in the obstetric condition of premature placental separation (abruptio placentae) and in medical or surgical conditions associated with shock. Primary fibrinolysins are rare; they occasionally are seen with widespread cancer, especially from the prostate. The most useful diagnostic procedures are the plasma fibrinogen level and serum "split products." These conditions and laboratory tests are discussed more extensively in Chapter 7. Fibrinogen solutions are associated with an even greater risk of hepatitis than plasma.

BLOOD VOLUME MEASUREMENT

The most frequent indication for transfusion therapy is to replace depleted blood volume. This most commonly arises in association with surgery or from nonsurgical blood loss, acute or chronic. Immediately after an acute bleeding episode, the hemoglobin and HCT are unchanged (because whole blood has been lost), even though total blood volume may be greatly reduced, even to the point of circulatory collapse (shock). With the passage of time, extracellular fluid begins to diffuse into the vascular system to partially restore total blood volume. Since the HCT is simply the percentage of red cells compared to total blood volume (total blood volume being the red cell mass plus the plasma volume), this dilution of the blood by extracellular fluid means that the HCT begins eventually to decrease, even while total blood volume is being increased (by extracellular fluid increasing plasma volume). Hemodilution (and thus the HCT drop) may be hastened if the patient has been receiving intravenous fluids. Serial HCT determinations (once every 2–4 hours) may thus be used as a rough indication of blood volume changes. It usually takes at least 2 hours after an acute bleeding episode for a significant drop in HCT to be demonstrated. Sometimes it takes longer—even as long as 6–12 hours. The larger the extracellular blood loss, the sooner a significant HCT change (over 2%) is likely to appear.

Previous dehydration and/or low plasma protein level will tend to delay a hematocrit drop. Besides the uncertainty of time lag, other conditions may affect the hematocrit and thus influence its interpretation as a parameter of blood volume. Anemias due to red cell hemolysis or blood factor deficiencies such as iron may decrease red cell mass without decreasing plasma or total blood volume. Similarly, plasma volume may be altered in many situations involving fluid and electrolyte imbalance without changing the red cell mass. Obviously, a need exists for more accurate methods in measuring blood volume.

The first widely used direct blood volume measurement technique was Evans blue dye (T-1824). After intravenous injection of the dye, the amount of dilution produced by the patient's plasma was measured, and from this the plasma volume was calculated. At present, radioisotopes are the procedure of choice. These methods also are based on the dilution principle. Chromium-51 can be used to tag RBC; a measured amount of the tagged red cells is then injected into the patient. After equilibration for 15 minutes, a blood sample is obtained and radioactivity is measured. Since the tagged RBC have mixed with the patient's RBC, comparison of the radioactivity in the patient's RBC with the original isotope specimen that was injected gives the amount that the original isotope specimen has been diluted by the patient's red cells; thus the patient's total RBC mass (RBC volume) may be calculated. Knowing the RBC mass, plasma volume and total blood volume may be obtained using the HCT value of the patient's blood. Another widely used method is that using serum albumin labeled with radioactive iodine (RISA). This substance circulates in the plasma along with the other plasma proteins. Again, a measured amount is injected, a blood sample is withdrawn after a short period of equilibration and the dilution of the original injected specimen is determined by counting the radioactivity of the patient's plasma. Plasma volume is given by RISA; red cell volume must be calculated using the patient's HCT. There is no doubt that isotope techniques are much more accurate than the HCT for estimating blood volume. Nevertheless, there are certain limitations to isotope techniques in general and specific limitations to both ^{51}Cr and RISA. The main drawback of blood volume techniques is the lack of precise normal values. Attempts have been made to establish normal values for males and females in terms of height, weight or surface area, or from lean body mass. Unfortunately, when one tries to apply one of these formulas to an individual patient, there is never any guarantee that the patient fits whatever category of normal persons that the formula was calculated from. The only way to be sure is to have a blood volume measurement from a time when the patient was healthy, or prior to the bleeding episode. Unfortunately, this information is usually not available. Another drawback is the fact that any dilution method will not detect bleeding that is going on during the test itself. This is true because whole blood lost during the test contains the isotope in the same proportion as the blood remaining in the vascular system (a diminished isotope dose in a diminished blood volume) contrasted to the situation which would prevail if bleeding were not going on, when the entire isotope dose would remain in a diminished blood volume. Fortunately, such active bleeding would have to be severe for test results to be materially affected. Another problem is dependence on HCT when results from RISA are used to calculate RBC mass or data from ^{51}Cr are used to obtain plasma volume. It is well established that HCT from different body areas or different size vessels can vary considerably—and disease may accentuate this variation. The venous HCT may therefore not be representative of the average vascular HCT.

All authorities in the field agree that blood volume determination combining independent measurement of RBC mass by ^{51}Cr and plasma volume by RISA is more accurate than the use of either isotope alone. Nevertheless, because both isotopes must be counted separately with special equipment, most laboratories use only a single isotope technique. Most authorities concede that ^{51}Cr has a slightly better overall accuracy than RISA, although some dispute this strongly. However, most ^{51}Cr techniques call for an extra venipuncture to obtain RBC from the patient for tagging, plus an extra 30-minute wait for the actual tagging of the cells. In addition, tagged RBC (and their radioactivity) remain in the circulation during the life span of the cells. The main advantages of RISA are the need for one less venipuncture than ^{51}Cr, and the fact that RISA procedures can be done in less than half the time of ^{51}Cr. The expected error with RISA blood volume reaches 300 ml in some studies, although the majority of determinations come much closer to double isotope results. In patients with markedly increased vascular permeability significant quantities of RISA may be lost from blood vessels during the test, and thus lead to even greater errors. Severe edema is an example of such a situation. Nevertheless, even under adverse conditions RISA (and ^{51}Cr) represent a decided advance over use of HCT for estimating blood volume.

Central venous pressure (CVP) is frequently used as an estimate of blood volume status. However, CVP is affected by cardiac function and by vascular resistance as well as by blood volume. Circumstances in which CVP does not accurately reflect the relationship between blood quantity and vascular capacity include pulmonary hypertension (emphysema, embolization, mitral stenosis), left ventricular failure and technical artifacts due to defects in catheter placement and maintenance.

REFERENCES

Ahn, Y. S., and Harrington, W. J.: Platelet Transfusions in Clinical Medicine, in Stollerman, G. H. (ed.): *Advances in Internal Medicine* (Chicago: Year Book Medical Publishers, Inc., 1975), vol. 20, p. 379.

Bailey, D. N., and Bove, J. R.: Chemical and hematological changes in stored CPD blood, Transfusion 15:244, 1975.

Bick, R. L., et al.: Disseminated intravascular coagulation and blood component therapy, Transfusion 16:361, 1976.

Boyan, C. P.: Cold or warmed blood for massive transfusions, Ann. Surg. 160:282, 1964.

Collins, J. A.: Massive blood transfusion, Clin. Haematol. 5:201, 1976.

Connell, R. S., and Swank, R. L.: Pulmonary microembolism after blood transfusions, Ann. Surg. 177:40, 1973.

Cove, H., et al.: Autologous blood transfusion in coronary artery bypass surgery, Transfusion 16:245, 1976.

Gump, F. E.: Physiological measurements and their interpretation, Med. Clin. North Am. 55:1141, 1971.

Hoak, J. C., and Koepke, J. A.: Platelet transfusions, Clin. Haematol. 5:69, 1976.

Ingram, G. I. C.: The bleeding complications of blood transfusion, Transfusion 5:1, 1965.

Jacobs, R. G., et al.: Serial microhematocrit determinations in evaluating blood replacement, Anesthesiology 22:342, 1961.

Lowenthal, R. M., et al.: Granulocyte transfusions in treatment of infections in patients with acute leukemia and aplastic anaemia, Lancet 1:353, 1975.

McCullough, J.: Blood component therapy, Geriatrics 29:85, 1974.

Merritt, J. A.: Complications related to blood replacement, Am. J. Surg. 116:333, 1968.

Mollison, P. L.: *Blood Transfusion in Clinical Medicine* (5th ed.; Philadelphia: F. A. Davis Co., 1972).

Moore, C. J., et al.: Present status of cadaver blood as transfusion medium, Arch. Surg. 85:364, 1962.

Morse, E. E.: Platelet transfusions, Lab. Med. 1:37, 1970.

Pepper, D. S.: Frozen red cells, Clin. Haematol. 5:53, 1976.

Rizza, C. R.: Coagulation factor therapy, Clin. Haematol. 5:113, 1976.

Robertson, H. D., and Polk, H. C.: Blood transfusions in elective operations: Comparisons of whole blood versus packed red cells, Ann. Surg. 181:778, 1975.

Ryden, S. E., and Oberman, H. A.: Compatibility of common intravenous solutions with CPD blood, Transfusion 15:250, 1975.

Symposium on Blood Volume, Am. Surg. 30:347, 1964.

Umlas, J., and Sakhuja, R.: The effect on blood coagulation of the exclusive use of transfusions of frozen red cells during and after cardiopulmonary bypass, J. Thorac. Cardiovasc. Surg. 70:519, 1975.

Wright, R. R., et al.: Blood volume, Semin. Nucl. Med. 5:63, 1975.

Zucker, M. B.: Unexplained bleeding in operations for neoplasias, Ann. NY Acad. Sci. 115:225, 1964.

12 / Urinalysis and Renal Disease

URINALYSIS

URINALYSIS is an indispensable part of clinical pathology. It may reveal pathology anywhere in the urinary tract. Also, it may afford a semiquantitative estimate of renal function and furnish clues to the etiology of dysfunction. Finally, systemic diseases may be revealed by quantitative or qualitative alterations of urine constituents or by the presence of abnormal substances, quite apart from their direct effects on the kidneys. Contrariwise, urinary tract disease may produce striking systemic symptoms.

The standard urinalysis includes appearance of the specimen, pH, specific gravity, protein semiquantitation, presence or absence of glucose and ketones, and microscopic examination of the centrifuged urinary sediment.

Appearance
The appearance of the specimen is usually reported only if abnormal.

Red color:	Blood; porphyria; occasionally urates, phenophthalein or Dorbane (laxative use)
Brown color:	Blood (acid hematin); alkaptonuria (urine turns brownish on standing); melanin (may be brown and turn black on standing)
Dark orange:	Bile, pyridium (a urinary tract disinfectant)

pH
A determination of pH is of little importance in the usual case. Normal urine is usually acid; it may be alkaline in alkalosis or in those rare instances when the acidifying mechanism of the kidney fails (renal acidosis syndrome) or is poisoned (carbonic anhydrase inhibitors). Proteus infections characteristically alkalinize. Finally, urine standing at room temperature will slowly become alkaline due to bacterial growth.

Specific Gravity
Specific gravity will be considered also under renal function. It is important for several reasons: (1) It is one parameter of renal tubular function. (2) Inability to concentrate may accompany certain diseases with otherwise relatively normal tubular function, such as diabetes insipidus or occasionally in severe hyperthyroidism and sickle cell anemia. (3) It affects other urine tests: a concentrated specimen may give higher results (for protein, etc.) than a dilute specimen, since the amount excreted per 24 hours is usually quantitatively the same in both cases; that is, the same amount of substance tested in a small quantity of fluid (high specific gravity) may

107

appear more than if present in a larger dilute urine volume (low specific gravity).

Protein

In health the glomerular membrane prevents most of the relatively large protein molecules of the blood from escaping into the urine. A small amount does get through, of which a small fraction is reabsorbed by the tubules, and the remainder (up to 0.1 gm/24 hours) is excreted. These amounts are normally not detected by routine clinical methods. One of the first responses of the kidney to a great variety of clinical situations is an alteration in glomerular filtrate. To a lesser extent, mere increase in glomerular filtration rate may increase normal protein excretion. Since albumin has a relatively small molecular size, it tends to become the dominant constituent in proteinuria, but rarely so complete as to justify the term "albuminuria" in a pure sense. Depending on the clinical situation, the constituents of "proteinuria" may or may not approach the constituents of plasma. Besides excess of normal plasma proteins, at times abnormal proteins may appear in the urine, notably Bence Jones (up to 50% of multiple myeloma patients).

To interpret proteinuria, one needs to know not only the major conditions responsible, but also the reason for production of excess urine protein. A system such as the following one is very helpful in this respect; proteinuria is classified according to the relationship of its etiology to the kidney and also to the mechanism involved.

A. Functional: not associated with easily demonstrable systemic or renal damage
   1. Severe muscular exertion
   2. Pregnancy (p. 125)
   3. Orthostatic proteinuria (This term designates slight to mild proteinuria associated only with the upright position; the exact etiology is poorly understood, with usual explanations tending to revolve around local factors causing renal passive congestion when in the upright position. It is easily diagnosed by comparing a specimen of early morning urine, produced entirely while asleep, with one taken late in the day. This is probably the most common cause of "functional" proteinuria.)
B. Organic: associated with demonstrable systemic disease or renal pathology
   1. Prerenal proteinuria: not due to primary renal disease
      a) Fever, or a variety of toxic conditions (This is the most common etiology for "organic" proteinuria and is quite frequent.)
      b) Venous congestion (This is most often produced by chronic passive congestion due to heart failure; also, occasionally, by intraabdominal compression of the renal veins.)
      c) Relative anoxia (Such situations may be produced by severe dehydration, shock, severe acidosis, acute cardiac decompensation or severe anemias—all leading to a decrease in renal blood flow or possibly hypoxic renal changes. Very severe hypoxia, especially if acute, may lead to renal tubular necrosis.)

    d) Hypertension (moderate or severe chronic hypertension, malignant hypertension or eclampsia)

    e) Myxedema

    f) Bence Jones protein of multiple myeloma

2. Renal proteinuria: primarily kidney disease

    a) Glomerulonephritis

    b) Nephrotic syndrome, primary or secondary

    c) Destructive parenchymal lesions (tumor, infection, infarct)

    d) Poisoning with certain nephrotoxic drugs or chemicals

3. Postrenal proteinuria: protein added to the urine at some point farther down the urinary tract from the renal parenchyma

    a) Infection of the renal pelvis or ureter

    b) Cystitis

    c) Urethritis or prostatitis

    d) Contamination with vaginal secretions

Postrenal proteinuria is usually relatively small. Thus, by testing the supernate of a centrifuged specimen for protein, it can tentatively be assumed that pus mainly originated in the lower urinary tract, if pyuria occurs in the absence of proteinuria.

There are several clinically acceptable methods for semiquantitative protein testing. Those most used are heat with acetic acid, sulfosalicylic acid (3, 10 or 20%) and Robert's reagent. Sulfosalicylic acid is slightly more sensitive than the heat and acetic acid method. Sulfosalicylic acid false positive reactions may occur, notably with tolbutamide (Orinase), urates, hemoglobin (RBC or hemolysis), massive penicillin dose, dextran, occasionally salicylates and various radiopaque x-ray substances. Bence Jones protein is also positive. Results are expressed as 1+ to 4+; this correlates very roughly to the amount of protein present (Table 12–1).

The Kingsbury-Clark procedure is a quantitative sulfosalicylic acid method using a series of permanent standards, each representing a different but measured amount of protein. After adding sulfosalicylic acid to the unknown specimen, a precipitate is formed that is compared with the standards and reported as the amount in the particular standard that it matches. Besides these traditional methods, there are two newer tests that are widely used. One is a tablet procedure (Albutest) and the other is a paper dipstick (Albustix). The sulfosalicylic acid method is sensitive to as little as 10 mg/100 ml protein. Albutest and Albustix are not reliable for

TABLE 12–1.—RELATIONSHIP OF QUALITATIVE AND
QUANTITATIVE URINE PROTEIN RESULTS

QUALITATIVE	PROTEIN	ROUGH QUANTITATIVE CORRELATION, GM/L
Light cloud	Trace	0.1–0.5
Medium cloud	1+	0.5–1.0
Heavy cloud	2+	3.0
Light coagulum	3+	5.0
Heavy coagulum	4+	10.0 (or more)

less than 25–30 mg/100 ml. Both will react with hemoglobin, but will not give the other false positives occasionally found with sulfosalicylic acid that were listed earlier. Behavior with Bence Jones is erratic; many cases are positive, but some unaccountably give negative test results. Urine with very alkaline pH may give false positives with the dipstick but not the tablet test. In addition, the readings are often difficult to quantitate, especially with the dipstick, and vary widely when the amount of protein is large.

Because individuals often vary in their interpretations, it is sometimes useful to determine 24-hour urine protein excretion. It should also be noted that degree of concentration may influence results on random urine specimens; a 24-hour specimen may also be affected, but to a lesser extent.

In summary, not all proteinuria is pathologic (p. 108); even if so, it may be transient; often the kidney is also indirectly involved; individual interpretations of turbidity tests may vary widely; and occasionally protein may be added to the urine beyond the kidney.

Glucose

The most common and important glucosuria occurs in diabetes mellitus. A normal renal threshold is usually about 180 mg/100 ml blood glucose level; beyond that, enough glucose is filtered to exceed the usual tubular transfer maximum for glucose reabsorption, and the surplus remains in the urine. However, individuals vary in their tubular transfer reabsorptive capacities; if this happens to be low, that individual may spill sugar at lower blood levels than the average person ("renal" glucosuria). Certain uncommon conditions may elevate blood sugar levels in nondiabetic persons. A partial list of the more important conditions associated with glucosuria includes the following (discussed more fully in Chapter 27):

Glucosuria without hyperglycemia
1. Renal glucosuria
2. Glucosuria of pregnancy (lactosuria may occur as well as glucosuria)
3. Certain inborn errors of metabolism (Fanconi syndrome)
4. After certain nephrotoxic chemicals (carbon monoxide, lead, mercuric chloride)

Glucosuria with hyperglycemia
1. Diabetes mellitus
2. Alimentary glucosuria (Hyperglycemia is very transient.)
3. Increased intracranial pressure (tumors, intracerebral hemorrhage, skull fracture)
4. Certain endocrine diseases or hormone-producing tumors (Cushing's disease, pheochromocytoma)
5. Hyperthyroidism (Graves' disease), occasionally
6. Occasionally, transiently, after myocardial infarction
7. After certain types of anesthesia, such as ether
8. Emotional (infrequent)

The most commonly used tests are Benedict's method and Clinitest, which depend on copper sulfate reduction of potentially reducing substances and, therefore, are not specific for glucose or even sugar; and glucose oxidase enzyme papers (Clinistix and Tes-Tape), which are specific for glucose. In several reported comparisons of these tests, Tes-Tape proved most sensitive but also gave occasional false positives. Clinistix gave few false positives, but also gave equivocal results or missed a few positive results that Tes-Tape picked up. The copper reduction tests included about 10% positive results from reducing substances other than glucose. Clinitest is a copper reduction tablet test that seemed to have median sensitivity, whereas Benedict's, which is a standard type of chemical procedure, was least sensitive, missing 10–15% positive by glucose oxidase, but with very few false positives apart from other reducing substances. Some feel that Benedict's is equally sensitive; the difficulty seems to lie in different criteria for what constitutes a trace reaction as opposed to a negative reaction. Benedict's method, the traditional reference procedure of the past, is time-consuming and is not commonly used today, since the tablet and dipstick tests are much faster and easier.

Although specific and relatively sensitive, the enzyme papers are not infallible. False positive results have been reported due to hydrogen peroxide and to hypochlorites (found in certain cleaning compounds). These substances give negative copper reduction test results. False negative results using Clinistix (but not Tes-Tape) have been reported from homogentisic acid (alkaptonuria), L-dopa, and large doses of aspirin. Also, the enzyme papers may unaccountably miss an occasional positive result that is picked up by copper reduction techniques.

Reducing sugar (copper reduction) false positives include sugars besides glucose (galactose, lactose) and homogentisic acid (alkaptonuria). Other potentially troublesome substances are para-aminosalicylic acid (PAS), methyldopa (Aldomet), heavy salicylate therapy (salicyluric acid excreted), heavy concentrations of urates, high doses of streptomycin or cephalothin (Keflin) and occasionally of penicillin or of Terramycin. An important technical consideration is to keep Clinitest tablets (and the enzyme papers) free from moisture before use.

The original methodology for Clinitest used 5 drops of urine. When urine contains large amounts of sugar, the color change typical of a high concentration may be unstable and quickly change to another color, which could be misinterpreted as an endpoint produced by smaller amounts of sugar ("pass-through" phenomenon). Many laboratories now use a 2-drop specimen, which avoids the "pass-through" effect. However, the color changes that represent different concentrations of reducing substances are not the same with 5 drops as with 2 drops. Knowledge of the method used in essential for correct interpretation by the patient or the physician.

Microscopic Examination of Sediment

Microscopic examination is routinely done on centrifuged urine sediment. There is no widely accepted standardized procedure for this, and the varying degrees of sediment concentration that result make difficult any strict interpretation of quantitative reports. It is fairly safe to say, however, that normally so few cellular elements are excreted that results of examinations fall within normal clinical values no matter how much the specimen is centrifuged. Normal range means fewer than 1 red blood cell (RBC) or 5 white blood cells (WBC) per high-power field and only an occasional cast.

The main pathologic elements of urinary sediment include RBC, WBC, casts and other less important findings, such as yeast, crystals or epithelial cells.

RBC. — Gross urinary bleeding is usually associated with stones, tumors, tuberculosis and acute glomerulonephritis, although these may (less often) present only as microscopic hematuria. There are conditions that usually give significant microscopic hematuria but occasionally approach gross bleeding. Some of the more important include: bleeding and clotting disorders (such as purpura or anticoagulants); blood dyscrasias (including sickle cell anemia or leukemia); renal infarction; malignant hypertension; subacute bacterial endocarditis (SBE); collagen diseases (especially lupus and periarteritis nodosa); Weil's disease; and various bladder, urethral and prostatic conditions, including necrotizing cystitis and acute prostatitis. Red cell casts are the only means of localizing the source of bleeding to the kidney. In the female, vaginal blood or leukocytes may contaminate ordinary voided specimens; finding significant numbers of squamous epithelial cells in the urinary sediment suggests such contamination. Yeast may simulate RBC (discussed later).

WBC. — These may be from any point in the urinary tract. Hematogenous spread of infection to the kidney usually first localizes in the renal cortex. Isolated cortical lesions may be relatively silent. Retrograde invasion from the bladder tends to involve calyces and medulla initially. Urinary tract obstruction is often a factor in retrograde pyelonephritis. Generally speaking, pyuria of renal origin is usually accompanied by significant proteinuria. That originating from the lower urinary tract may have proteinuria, but it tends to be relatively slight.

Urinary tract infections tend to be accompanied by bacteriuria. Tuberculosis of the kidney, besides producing hematuria, is said characteristically to have pyuria without bacteriuria. Naturally, ordinary urine cultures would be negative in tuberculosis. White cell casts are definite evidence localizing WBC to renal origin (discussed later); WBC in clumps are strongly suggestive, but are not conclusive.

CASTS. — Casts are protein conglomerations outlining the shape of the renal tubules in which they were formed. Factors involved in cast formation include:

1. pH: Protein casts tend to dissolve in alkaline medium.
2. Concentration: Casts tend to dissolve in considerably dilute medium. Concentration also has a considerable role in formation of casts; it favors precipitation out of protein.
3. Proteinuria: Protein is necessary for cast formation, and significant cylindruria (cast excretion) is most often accompanied by proteinuria. Proteinuria may be of varied etiology (p. 108). The postrenal type is added beyond the kidneys and obviously cannot be involved in cast formation.
4. Stasis: Stasis is usually secondary to intratubular obstruction and thus allows time for protein precipitation within tubules.

Mechanisms of cast formation are better understood if one considers the normal physiology of urine formation. The substance filtered at the glomerulus is essentially an ultrafiltrate of plasma. In the proximal tubules, up to 85% of filtered sodium and chloride is reabsorbed, with water passively accompanying these ions. In the thick ascending loop of Henle, sodium is actively reabsorbed; however, since the membrane here is impermeable to

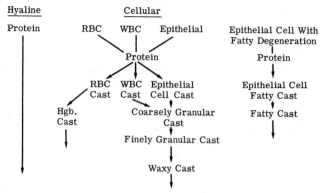

Fig 12–1. – Formation of casts.

water, an excess of water (free water) remains. As water passes along the distal tubules, some may be reabsorbed with sodium ions; and in the collecting tubules, up to 5% of the glomerular filtration rate is osmotically reabsorbed due to the relatively high osmolarity of the renal interstitial cells. Water reabsorption in distal and collecting tubules is under the control of antidiuretic hormone (ADH). At this point, the urine reaches its maximum concentration and proceeds to the bladder relatively unchanged. Thus, cast formation takes place ordinarily in the distal and collecting tubules, where acidification takes place and concentration reaches its height.

There are two main types of casts – cellular and hyaline – depending on their main constituents.

Cellular Casts. – Either RBC, WBC, desquamated renal epithelial cells or any combination of these may conglomerate together in a protein matrix. The cast is basically cellular in content (Fig 12–1).

As the cellular cast moves slowly down the nephron, the cells begin to disintegrate. Eventually, all that is left of the cells are relatively large fragments, chunks or granules. This has now become a *coarsely granular cast.* The cast is now composed entirely of large irregular or coarse solid granules.

If disintegration is allowed to continue, the coarse granules break down to small granules, and a relatively homogeneous *finely granular cast* is formed.

The end stage of this process is the production of a homogeneous refractile material still in the shape of the tubule, known as *waxy cast.* Now the cast is translucent, without granules and reflects light, giving a somewhat shiny, semisolid appearance. What stage of cast finally reaches the bladder depends on how long the cast takes to traverse the nephron and thus how long it remains in the kidney, where the forces of disintegration may work. A waxy cast is thus indicative of fairly severe localized stasis in the renal tubules.

Hyaline Casts. – Hyaline casts are composed almost exclusively of protein alone. They pass almost unchanged down the urinary tract. They are dull, nearly transparent material and reflect light poorly in contrast to waxy casts; thus, hyaline casts are often hard to see, and the microscope condenser usually has to be turned down to give better contrast.

Sometimes cellular elements may be trapped within hyaline casts; if hyaline material still predominates, the result is considered a hyaline cast with cellular inclusions. Degenerative changes can take place just as with regular cellular casts, with the production of *hyaline coarsely granular* and *hyaline finely granular casts*.

Fatty Casts. — These are a special type of cellular cast. In certain types of renal tubular damage fatty degeneration of the tubular epithelial cells takes place. These cells desquamate and are incorporated into casts. The epithelial cells contain fatty droplets; as the cells themselves degenerate, the fatty droplets remain and even may coalesce somewhat. The end result is a cast composed mainly of fatty droplets and protein. Sometimes either renal epithelial cells with fatty degeneration or the remnants thereof containing fat droplets are found in the urine floating free and are called *oval fat bodies*.

When present in significant number, this kind of picture is seen mainly in diseases that produce the nephrotic syndrome, such as primary lipoid nephrosis or secondary to Kimmelstiel-Wilson syndrome, lupus, amyloid, subacute glomerulonephritis, the nephrotic stage of chronic glomerulonephritis, certain tubule poisons, such as mercury, and rare hypersensitivity reactions to such things as insect bites. Oval fat bodies have essentially the same significance as fatty casts. Fat droplets have a "Maltese cross" appearance in polarized light but are identifiable without this.

Broad Casts. — In cases where severe stasis takes place, irrespective of the type of cast involved, cast formation may take place in the larger collecting tubules, where large ducts drain several smaller collecting tubules. If this occurs, a *broad cast* is formed, several times wider than ordinary sized casts. This is always indicative of severe localized renal stasis, and is most often found when the kidney is bordering on renal shutdown. These broad casts may be of any cast type, and due to their peculiar mode of formation are sometimes spoken of as "renal failure casts." This is not entirely accurate, for the kidney may often recover from that particular episode.

Hemoglobin Casts. — These are derived from RBC casts that degenerate into granular (rarely even waxy) material but still have the peculiar orange-red color of hemoglobin. Not all casts derived from RBC retain this color. Strongly acid urine changes the characteristic color of hemoglobin to the nonspecific gray-brown color of acid hematin. Also, one must differentiate the brown or yellow-brown coloring derived from bile or other urine pigments from the typical color of hemoglobin.

The significance of casts in the urine is a difficult question. Fatty casts and RBC and WBC casts are always significant. In all honesty, the only general statement one can make about ordinary hyaline or granular casts is that their appearance in significant numbers has some correlation with the factors involved in cast formation — proteinuria, concentration and stasis. Of these, the most general correlation is with stasis, although one cannot tell whether this is generalized or merely localized. It is common for showers of casts to clear dramatically once the underlying cause of their formation is corrected. On the other hand, significant numbers of casts that persist for some time despite therapeutic efforts may suggest serious intrarenal derangement. In this respect, granular casts in the late stages of their development will be seen. Generally speaking, hyaline casts alone are of little practical importance and are usually only an acute, mild and temporary phenomenon. Thus, to have any meaning, appearance of casts must be correlated with other findings and with the clinical situation. A few hyaline or granular casts in themselves have no importance.

CRYSTALS.—These are often overemphasized in importance. They may, however, be a clue to calculus formation and certain metabolic diseases. Crystals tend to be pH-dependent:

Acid urine: uric acid, cystine, calcium oxalate.

Alkaline urine: phosphates, as triple phosphate (magnesium ammonium phosphate), which comprises many staghorn calculi. *Note:* Alkaline urine is most often produced by *(Proteus)* infection.

Amorphous crystalline sediment: If pH is acid, urates; if alkaline, phosphates. Rarely one might find sulfa crystals in acid urine, since sulfadiazine is still sometimes used. Most sulfas resemble needle-like crystals in bunches, but this appearance can be mimicked by certain nonpathologic crystals.

MISCELLANEOUS.—*Trichomonas* is fairly common; often associated with slight proteinuria, WBC and epithelial cell sediment. Diagnosis is by motility (and thus, a fresh specimen is essential); when nonmotile, it resembles a large WBC or small tubular epithelial cell. Trichomonas is found occasionally in the male. Spermatozoa may appear in the urine of males and, occasionally, in that of females.

Yeasts are important; the usual type is Candida (Monilia). Yeast cells are often misdiagnosed as RBC. Differential points are budding (not always noticed without careful search); ovoid shape (not always pronounced); an appearance slightly more opaque and homogeneous than RBC; insolubility in both acid and alkali. If the cells are numerous and still in doubt, a chemical test for blood is recommended.

Note: The most common mistake in microscopic examination is failure to mix the specimen sufficiently before putting it into the centrifuge tube. This is most important.

Other Examinations

BILE (DIRECT-ACTING BILIRUBIN).—Bile typically appears in urine secondary to hepatic obstruction, either extrahepatic (common duct obstruction) or intrahepatic (obstruction phase of hepatitis). Typically, in infectious hepatitis bile appears in urine a few days before the icteric stage, clearing swiftly once this begins.

In pulmonary infarction, there often occurs some elevation in serum (indirect-acting) bilirubin but not in the urine.

Tests for bile include Fouchet's reagent or Ictotest. The simple foam test (yellow foam after shaking) may be all that is necessary (false positive: pyridium). The commercial tablet test, Ictotest, is fairly sensitive, detecting as little as 0.1 mg/100 ml. It also is reasonably specific.

UROBILINOGEN. — This substance appears classically as a secondary product from intravascular RBC breakdown (hemolytic processes). It may also be present in hepatitis, presumably due to inability of damaged hepatic parenchyma to handle normal amounts of urobilinogen produced by the intestine.

Tests for urobilinogen include an Ehrlich's reagent semiquantitative method, or a 24-hour quantitative determination.

For routine specimens, it is of the greatest importance that the test be done within one-half hour after voiding. Urobilinogen rapidly oxidizes in air to nondetectable urobilin, and, without special preservatives, will decrease significantly after about one-half hour. It is probably this unrecognized fact that accounts for the test's poor reputation. If the procedure cannot be done relatively soon after voiding, it is probably better to get a 24-hour specimen with preservatives.

ACETONE AND DIACETIC ACID (ALSO CALLED KETONE BODIES). — These are classic findings of diabetic acidosis. However, acetonuria may also be found in starvation, many normal pregnancies and especially in severe dehydration from many causes (vomiting, diarrhea, severe infections). In children, ketone bodies are prone to appear on what, by adult standards, would be very slight provocation. A weakly positive test for acetone is usually of little significance.

In fatty acid metabolism, acetyl-CoA formed from fat breakdown may, under appropriate conditions, condense to form acetoacetic (diacetic) acid and thence convert to acetone.

There are some reports that acetone formation from diacetic acid does not take place as much as is generally thought, and that even in only moderate degrees of ketonuria, the amount of diacetic acid in the urine is several times that of acetone. This evidence supports the fact that, clinically, there is little need to distinguish between acetone and diacetic acid. Both have essentially the same significance. Most tests for acetone employ a nitroprusside reagent, and since nitroprusside will detect both, there seems no real reason to test for diacetic separately. Among widely used tests, Acetest tablets will detect concentrations of 5 mg/100 ml of diacetic acid as well as react with acetone, and can be used with either urine, serum or plasma. There is a new dipstick-type method called Ketostix, which is specific for diacetic acid, and detects 10 mg/100 ml. This method is incorporated into certain multiple-test dipsticks from the same manufacturer. These give false positive results with L-dopa. For the reasons just mentioned, the Acetest tablet is preferable.

Finally, it must be emphasized that diabetes is practically the only disease in which ketonuria has real diagnostic importance. Slight to moderate degrees of ketonuria are fairly common in other conditions, as mentioned earlier, but are only incidental. In diabetes the presence of large amounts of ketones is one of the major indications of diabetic acidosis or impending acidosis. In real diabetic acidosis the serum or plasma acetone test will always be positive. (However, cases of hyperosmolar or lactic acidosis coma rarely occur.) In fact, the amount of ketones present, estimated by testing dilutions of plasma, is a good indication of the severity of acidosis and the amount of insulin needed. In the urine of diabetic acidosis, nitroprusside tests usually will be strongly positive. In most cases, there will be glucosuria as well as strong ketonuria. The only major exception is the presence of renal insufficiency with oliguria, due to severe renal disease, shock or exceptionally severe acidosis with secondary renal shutdown. The BUN is frequently elevated in diabetic acidosis; even so, there usually will be strong ketonuria. If there is any question, a plasma or serum acetone test should be done.

In summary, the urine ketone level in diabetic acidosis usually is very strongly positive and the plasma acetone is positive. However, if *symptoms* of diabetic acidosis are present, lack of strongly positive urine ketones does not rule out the diagnosis, since a few patients with renal shutdown may be unable to filter the elevated blood ketones through the kidney.

CALCIUM. — Urine is tested for calcium with Sulkowitch reagent; it is a semiquantitative method reported 0 – 4+ (normal being 1+) or as negative, moderately positive and strongly positive. (For interpretation, see p. 377.) Excessively concentrated or diluted urine may produce unreliable results, just as it will for protein.

PORPHOBILINOGEN. — Porphobilinogen is diagnostic of acute porphyria (p. 235) (episodes of abdominal crampy pain with vomiting and leukocytosis, etc.). Porphobilinogen is colorless and is easily identified by rapid screening tests, such as the Watson-Schwartz procedure.

URINARY COPROPORPHYRINS. — These substances show increased urinary excretion in lead poisoning (p. 431), providing a relatively simple means to help detect this condition. Type III is the coproporphyrin involved. (Actually it is not specific for lead poisoning alone.)

PHENYLPYRUVIC ACID. — Phenylpyruvic acid is excreted in phenylketonuria (p. 413). A ferric chloride test is the classic means of detection. There is a dipstick ("Phenistix") method for the diagnosis of phenylketonuria, which depends on the reaction between ferric ions and phenylpyruvic acid, much like the classic ferric chloride test. It is more sensitive than ferric chloride, detecting as little as 8 mg/100 ml or trace amounts of phenylpyruvic acid in urine. False positives occur if large amounts of ketone bodies are present. Reactions will take place with salicylates, PAS and phenothiazine metabolites, but the color is said to be different from that given by phenylpyruvic acid.

BLOOD. — Three simple procedures are on the market for detecting hemoglobin in urine. Occultest is an orthotolidine tablet test for which sensitivity has been adjusted to approximately 1:100,000 (about that of the old benzidine method). This is reported to detect less than 5 RBC/HPF. Hematest is another tablet test with the same basic reagents but adjusted to approximately 1:20,000 sensitivity — slightly more than the guaiac method. Experimentally, this will not reliably detect less than 200 RBC/HPF, unless some of the cells have hemolyzed. It is much more sensitive to free hemoglobin, where it can detect amounts produced by hemolysis of only 25 – 30 RBC/HPF. It has been used for feces as well as urine, although at this sensitivity there are appreciable false positives. Hemastix is a dipstick method that is otherwise identical to Hematest. The usefulness of these tests lies in their ability to detect hemoglobin even after some or all of the RBC have disintegrated and are no longer visible microscopically. Red cell lysis is particularly likely to occur in dilute urine. However, these tests cannot be used as a substitute for microscopic examination.

Points to remember when interpreting results of a urinalysis:

1. Laboratory reports usually err in omission, rather than commission (except occasionally in RBC vs. yeast). If technicians cannot identify something, they usually will not mention it at all.

2. Certain diagnostic findings, such as RBC casts, may not appear in every high-power (or even every low-power) field. If one finds hematuria, one should look for them, and, similarly, for WBC casts and other such structures in the appropriate sediment settings.

3. If laboratory personnel know what you are after, they usually will give more than a routine glance. Otherwise, the pressure of routine work may result in examination that is not sufficient to detect important abnormalities.

4. In many laboratories, reports will include only items specifically requested, even when other abnormalities are grossly visible (such as bile).

5. One fact that should be stressed when using commercial tests of any type is to *follow all the directions exactly.* Many dipstick methods require a certain length of time in contact with the specimen; when this is true, a quick dip-and-read technique may lead to false results. The time interval of reading may be crucial in tablet tests or other procedures.

THE KIDNEY IN DISEASE

Primary glomerular renal disease for a long time was subdivided into glomerulonephritis (acute, subacute, chronic) and the nephrotic syndrome, based on clinical and light microscope findings. With the advent of renal biopsy, electron microscopy and immunoglobulin fluorescent staining of tissue sections, the clinical categories are being reclassified on the basis of ultrastructure and immunologic characteristics. Some of the immunohistopathologic subdivisions have different prognoses (and, in some cases, different responses to certain therapeutic agents) and, therefore, could logically be regarded as separate entities. Nevertheless, I have chosen to describe laboratory findings in terms of the original clinical syndromes, since this is the way most clinicians will encounter primary renal disease. A morphologic classification is included on page 480.

Glomerulonephritis

ACUTE GLOMERULONEPHRITIS (AGN). – In the classic form, this disease corresponds to a subcategory of proliferative glomerulonephritis that is considered a hypersensitivity reaction, usually associated with concurrent or recent infection. The most common organism incriminated is the beta hemolytic Lancefield group A streptococcus. Only a relatively small number of specific group A strains are known to cause AGN, in contrast to the large number that may initiate acute rheumatic fever.

Clinically, onset of the disease is usually manifested by hematuria. The urine may be red or may be "coffee-ground" color (due to breakdown of hemoglobin to brown acid hematin). In mild cases, gross hematuria may be less evident, or hematuria may be microscopic only. Varying degrees of peripheral edema, especially of the upper eyelids, are often present. Varying degrees of hypertension are frequent initially.

Laboratory features are a usually elevated erythrocyte sedimentation rate and frequently a mild-to-moderate normocytic-normochromic (or slightly hypochromic) anemia. There is mild to moderate proteinuria (0.5–3.0 gm/24 hours). The urinary sediment contains varying degrees of hematuria, often with WBC also present. Red cell casts are characteristic and are the most diagnostic laboratory finding. They may be present only intermittently, sometimes may be few in number, and may be degenerated enough to make recognition difficult. Although RBC casts are not specific for AGN, the number of diseases consistently associated with RBC casts are relatively few. They include AGN, subacute and occasionally chronic glomerulonephritis, subacute bacterial endocarditis, some of the collagen diseases (especially lupus) and hemoglobinuric acute tubular necrosis.

Prolonged azotemia is not common in poststreptococcal AGN (5–10% of cases), despite hypertension, although as many as 50% have some BUN elevation initially. Renal function tests are said to be essentially normal in nearly 50% of patients; the rest have varying degrees of impairment for varying time intervals, and a small percentage show renal insufficiency with uremia. Urine-concentrating ability is generally maintained for the first few days; in some, it may then be impaired for considerable time intervals. Function tests in general tend to reflect (although not exclusively) the primarily glomerular lesion found in AGN, manifested on light microscopy by increased glomerular cellularity, swelling and proliferation of capillary endothelial cells and on electron microscopy by subepithelial "humps." In addition to urinalysis, the antistreptolysin-O (ASL or ASO) titer may be helpful, since a significant titer (over 200 Todd units) means recent or relatively recent group A streptococcal infection. However, since up to 20% of AGN patients have normal range ASO titers, a negative ASO titer does not rule out the diagnosis nor does a "positive" titer guarantee that the condition is indeed AGN. Measurement of other streptococcal enzyme antibodies, such as anti-NADase, in addition to ASO will improve sensitivity of the test. Several commercial kits now have combined reagents active against several of the antistreptococcal antibodies. The third component (C3) of serum complement is nearly always depressed in streptococcal AGN and returns to normal in 6–8 weeks. Consistently normal early C3 levels are evidence against streptococcal etiology; and failure to return to normal in 8 weeks also suggests a different etiology.

It is interesting that AGN is a relatively benign disease in childhood; the mortality is only about 1%, and fewer than that seem to have permanent damage. In adults, the incidence of the disease is much less, and 25–50% of the patients develop chronic renal disease.

RAPIDLY PROGRESSIVE GLOMERULONEPHRITIS.—This may follow the acute stage but much more commonly appears without any previous clinical or serologic evidence of AGN. It is more common in older children and adults. The original term "subacute" was misleading; it referred to the duration of the clinical course, longer than that of the average AGN patient but much shorter than chronic glomerulonephritis. Histologically, the glomeruli show marked epithelial cell proliferation with resultant filling in of the space between Bowman's capsule and the glomerular tuft (epithelial crescent). The urine sediment includes many casts of hyaline and epithelial series; RBC, and often WBC, are present in varying numbers, often with a few RBC casts. There is moderately severe to marked proteinuria, and both the degree of proteinuria and the urinary sediment may sometimes be indistinguishable from the nephrotic syndrome, even with fatty casts present. Clinically, rapidly progressive glomerulonephritis behaves as a more severe form of acute glomerulonephritis and generally leads to death in weeks or months. It is not the same process as the nephrotic episodes that may form part of chronic glomerulonephritis. In addition to urinary findings, anemia is usually present. Renal function tests demonstrate both glomerular and tubule destruction, although clinically there is usually little additional information gained by extensive renal function studies. Serum complement C3 is temporarily depressed in those cases of poststreptococcal origin, but otherwise is usually normal.

CHRONIC GLOMERULONEPHRITIS. — This infrequently is preceded by AGN, but usually has no antecedent clinical illness or etiology. It most often runs a slowly progressive or intermittent course over several or many years. During the latent phases there may be very few urinary abnormalities, but RBC are generally present in varying small numbers in the sediment. There is almost always proteinuria, generally of mild degree, and rather infrequent casts of the epithelial series. Progression is documented by slowly decreasing ability to concentrate the urine, followed by deterioration in clearance or PSP tests. Intercurrent streptococcal upper respiratory infection or other infections may occasionally set off an acute exacerbation. There may be one or more episodes of the nephrotic syndrome, usually without much, if any, hematuria. The terminal or azotemic stage produces the clinical and laboratory picture of renal failure. Finely granular and waxy casts predominate, and broad casts are often present. There is moderate proteinuria.

Nephrotic Syndrome

The criteria for diagnosis of the nephrotic syndrome include high proteinuria (over 3.5 gm/24 hours), edema, hypercholesterolemia and hypoalbuminemia. However, one or occasionally even more of these criteria may be absent. The level of proteinuria is said to be the most consistent criterion. In addition, patients with the nephrotic syndrome often have a characteristic serum protein electrophoretic pattern, consisting of greatly decreased albumin and considerably increased $alpha_2$ globulin. However, in some cases, the pattern may not be marked enough to be characteristic. The nephrotic syndrome is one of a relatively few diseases in which the serum cholesterol may add a substantial contribution toward establishing the diagnosis, especially in borderline cases.

The nephrotic syndrome has nothing to do with hemoglobinuric nephrosis (so-called lower nephron nephrosis), despite the unfortunate similarity in names. Hemoglobinuric nephrosis is a distinct clinical entity seen in some cases of acute renal shutdown, most commonly due to marked intravascular hemolysis. The term "nephrotic syndrome" as it is currently used is actually a misnomer, and dates from the time when proteinuria was thought primarily to be due to a disorder of renal tubules. The word nephrosis was then used to characterize such a situation. It is now recognized that various glomerular lesions form the actual basis for proteinuria in the nephrotic syndrome, either of the primary or the secondary type. The nephrotic syndrome as a term is also confusing because it may be of two clinical types.

PRIMARY (OR "LIPOID") NEPHROSIS. — This is the idiopathic form, usually found in childhood. The etiology of primary (idiopathic or "lipoid") nephrosis is still not definitely settled. Renal biopsy has shown various glomerular abnormalities, classified most easily into basement membrane and focal sclerosis varieties. In most children the basement membrane changes may be so slight (null lesion) as to be certified only by electron microscopy (manifested by fusion of the footplates of epithelial cells applied to the basement membrane). The null lesion is associated with excellent response to steroids, a great tendency to relapse and eventual relatively good prognosis. Focal sclerosis most often is steroid-resistant and has a poor prognosis.

In lipoid nephrosis, the urine contains mostly protein; the sediment may display relatively small numbers of fatty and granular casts, and there may be small numbers of RBC. Greater hematuria or cylindruria suggests greater severity, but not necessarily a worse prognosis. Renal function tests are normal in most; the remainder have various degrees of impairment.

NEPHROTIC SYNDROME. — Although lipoid nephrosis may be found in adults, nephrotic syndrome is more common and may be either idiopathic or secondary to a variety of diseases. The most common idiopathic lesions include a diffuse light microscope "wire loop" basement membrane thickening, which has been termed "membranous glomerulonephritis," and a type that has been called "membranoproliferative." Prognosis in these is worse than in childhood lipoid nephrosis.

The most common etiologies of secondary nephrotic syndrome are chronic glomerulonephritis, Kimmelstiel-Wilson syndrome, lupus, amyloid and renal vein thrombosis. In the urine, fat is the most characteristic element, appearing in oval fat bodies and fatty casts. Also present are variable numbers of epithelial and hyaline series casts. Urine RBC are variable — usually only few, but sometimes many. Significant hematuria suggests lupus; the presence of diabetes and hypertension, Kimmelstiel-Wilson syndrome; a history of previous proteinuria or hematuria, chronic glomerulonephritis; and the presence of chronic long-standing infection, amyloid. About 50% of cases are associated with chronic glomerulonephritis. Renal function tests in lupus, Kimmelstiel-Wilson and amyloid generally show diffuse renal damage. The same is true for chronic glomerulonephritis in the later stages; however, if the nephrotic syndrome occurs relatively early in the course of this disease, changes may be minimal, reflected only in impaired concentrating ability. Histologically, renal glomeruli in the nephrotic syndrome exhibit lesions that vary according to the particular disease responsible.

Membranoproliferative glomerulonephritis occurs in older children and teenagers, and displays some features of AGN as well as nephrotic syndrome. Hematuria and complement C3 decrease occur, but C3 decrease usually is prolonged beyond 8 weeks (60% or more cases). However, C3 levels may fluctuate during the course of the disease.

Malignant Hypertension (Accelerated Arteriolar Nephrosclerosis)

This disease is most common in middle age, the great majority of patients being between ages 30 and 60. There is a tendency toward males, and an increased incidence in blacks. The majority of patients have a history of preceding mild or "benign" hypertension, most often for 2–6 years, although the disease can begin abruptly. The syndrome may also be secondary to severe chronic renal disease of several varieties. Clinical features are markedly elevated systolic and diastolic blood pressure levels, the presence of papilledema, and evidence of renal damage. Laboratory tests show anemia to be present in most cases, even in relatively early stages. Urinalysis in the early stages shows most often a moderate proteinuria and hematuria, usually without RBC casts. It thus may mimic to some extent the sediment of acute glomerulonephritis. Later, the sediment may show more evidence of tubular damage. There usually develops a moderate-to-high proteinuria (which uncommonly may reach 5–10 gm/24 hours) accompanied by considerable microscopic hematuria and often many casts, including all those of the hyaline and epithelial series—even fatty casts occasionally. In the terminal stages, late granular or waxy casts and broad renal failure casts predominate. The disease produces rapid deterioration of renal function tests; most cases terminate in azotemia. Nocturia and polyuria are common due to the progressive renal damage. If congestive heart failure is superimposed, there may be decreased urine volume plus loss of ability to concentrate urine.

Pyelonephritis

Acute pyelonephritis often elicits a characteristic syndrome (spiking high fever, costovertebral angle tenderness, dysuria, back pain, etc.). Proteinuria is mild, rarely exceeding 2 gm/24 hours. Pyuria (and often bacteriuria) develops. Presence of WBC casts is diagnostic, although they may have to be carefully searched for or may be absent. Urine culture may establish the diagnosis of urinary tract infection but cannot localize the area involved. Hematogenous spread of infection to the kidney tends to localize in the renal cortex and may give fewer initial urinary findings; retrograde ascending infection from the lower urinary tract reaches renal medulla areas first and shows early pyuria.

In chronic low-grade pyelonephritis, the urine may not be grossly pyuric, and sediment may be scanty. In some cases, even random urine culture may be negative. Very frequently, however, there is a significant increase in pus cells; they often, but not invariably, occur in clumps when the process is more severe. Casts other than the WBC type are usually few or absent in pyelonephritis until the late or terminal stages, and WBC casts themselves may be absent.

A urine culture should be obtained in all cases of suspected urinary tract infection, to isolate the organism responsible and determine antibiotic sensitivity.

Tuberculosis is a special type of renal infection. It involves the kidney in possibly 25% of patients with chronic or severe pulmonary tuberculosis, although the incidence of clinical disease is much less. Hematuria is frequent; it may be gross or only microscopic. Pyuria is also common. Characteristically, pyuria should be present without demonstrable bacteriuria (of ordinary bacterial varieties), but this is not reliable due to a considerable frequency of superinfection by ordinary bacteria in genitourinary tuberculosis. Dysuria is also present in many patients. If hematuria (with or without pyuria) is found in a patient with tuberculosis, genitourinary tract tuberculosis should be suspected. Urine cultures are said to be positive in about 7% of cases with significant pulmonary tuberculosis. At least three specimens, one each day for 3 days, should be secured, each one collected in a sterile container. A fresh early morning specimen has been recommended rather than 24-hour collections. If suspicion of renal tuberculosis is strong, an IVP should be done in order to assess the extent of involvement.

Renal papillary necrosis should be mentioned here as a possible complication of acute pyelonephritis, particularly in diabetics.

Renal Papillary Necrosis (Necrotizing Papillitis)

As the name suggests, this condition results from necrosis of a focal area in one or more renal pyramids. Papillary necrosis is most frequently associated with infection, but may occur without known cause. It is much more frequent in diabetics. A small minority of cases are associated with sickle-cell hemoglobin diseases or phenacetin toxicity. The disease usually is of an acute nature, although some patients may have relatively minor symptoms or symptoms overshadowed by other complications or disease. The patients are usually severely ill and manifest pyuria, hematuria and azotemia, especially when renal papillary necrosis is associated with infection. A drip-infusion intravenous pyelogram is the diagnostic test of choice. Naturally, urine culture should be done.

Renal Embolism and Thrombosis

Renal artery occlusion or embolism most often affects the smaller renal arteries or the arterioles. Such involvement produces renal infarction in that vessel's distribution; usually manifested by hematuria and proteinuria. Casts of the epithelial series may also appear.

Acute Tubular Necrosis (Lower Nephron Nephrosis)

This syndrome may result from acute or sudden renal failure from any cause, most often secondary to hypotension, although marked intravascular hemolysis from blood transfusion reactions is probably the most famous etiology. It begins with a period of oliguria or near anuria, and manifests subsequent diuresis if recovery ensues. Urinalysis demonstrates considerable proteinuria with desquamated epithelial cells and epithelial and hyaline casts. There are usually some RBC (occasionally many), and often large numbers of broad and waxy casts (indicative of severe urinary stasis in the renal parenchyma). Hemoglobin casts are usually present in those cases due to intravascular hemolysis. Specific gravity is characteristically fixed at 1.010 after the first hours, and the BUN begins rising shortly after onset. In those cases not due to intravascular hemolysis, the pathogenesis is that of generalized tubular necrosis, most often anoxic.

Congenital Renal Disease

POLYCYSTIC KIDNEY.—There are two clinical forms, one fatal in early infancy and the other (adult type) usually asymptomatic until the third or fourth decade. The urinary sediment is highly variable; microscopic intermittent hematuria is common, and gross hematuria may occasionally take place. Cysts may become infected and produce symptoms of pyelonephritis. In general, the rate of proteinuria is minimal or mild, but may occasionally be higher. Symptoms may be those of hypertension (50–60% cases) or renal failure. If the condition does progress to renal failure, the urinary sediment is nonspecific, reflecting only the presence of end-stage kidneys of any etiology. Diagnosis may be suggested by family history and the presence of bilaterally palpable abdominal masses and confirmed by radiologic procedures, such as the IVP.

RENAL DEVELOPMENTAL ANOMALIES.—This category includes horseshoe kidney, solitary cysts, reduplication of a ureter, renal ptosis, etc. There may be no urinary findings or, sometimes, a slight proteinuria. In children, urinary tract anomalies are a relatively frequent predisposing cause for repeated urinary tract infection. Recurrent urinary tract infection, especially in children, should always be investigated for the possibility of either urinary tract obstruction or anomalies. Diagnosis is by IVP.

Renal Neoplasia

The most common sign of carcinoma anywhere in the urinary tract is hematuria. A neoplasm should be suspected if this finding is not explained by other conditions known to frequently produce hematuria. Even if such diseases are present, this would not rule out genitourinary carcinoma. The workup of a patient with hematuria is discussed elsewhere (p. 135). The detection of renal cell carcinoma is included in Chapter 32.

Lupus Erythematosus or Periarteritis Nodosa

About two thirds of lupus patients show renal involvement. Generally, there is microscopic hematuria; otherwise, there may be a varying picture. In the classic case of lupus (much less often in periarteritis), one finds a "telescoped sediment," containing the characteristic sediment elements of all three stages of glomerulonephritis (acute, subacute, chronic—manifested by fatty, late granular and RBC casts). Usually, hematuria is predominant, especially in polyarteritis. In lupus RBC casts are more commonly found. Up to one third of lupus patients develop the nephrotic syndrome. Complement C3 levels are frequently decreased in active lupus nephritis.

Embolic Glomerulonephritis

Scattered small focal areas of necrosis are present in glomerular capillaries, most often due to subacute bacterial endocarditis. There is some uncertainty whether the lesions are embolic, infectious or allergic in origin. Since the glomerular lesions are sharply focal, there usually is not much pyuria. Hematuria usually is present and may be pronounced. If localized tubular stasis occurs in addition, *RBC casts* may appear with resultant simulation of latent or acute glomerulonephritis. The rate of proteinuria often remains relatively small, frequently not over 1 gm/24 hours.

Diabetes

The kidney may be affected by several unrelated disorders, including (1) a high incidence of pyelonephritis; sometimes renal papillary necrosis. (2) A high incidence of arteriosclerosis with hypertension. (3) Kimmelstiel-Wilson syndrome (intercapillary glomerulosclerosis). Urinary findings may produce the nephrotic syndrome in late stages of this syndrome. Otherwise, only varying degrees of proteinuria are manifest, perhaps with a few granular casts.

Pregnancy

Several abnormal urinary findings are associated with pregnancy.

"BENIGN" PROTEINURIA. — Proteinuria may appear in up to 30% of otherwise normal pregnancies during the time of labor. Of these, only about 3% are reported to surpass 100 mg/100 ml. It is unclear whether proteinuria must be considered pathologic if it occurs in uncomplicated pregnancy before labor. Some authorities believe that proteinuria is not found in normal pregnancy; others report an incidence of up to 20%, which is ascribed to abdominal venous compression.

ECLAMPSIA. — This condition, also known as toxemia of pregnancy, denotes a syndrome of severe edema, proteinuria, hypertension and convulsions associated with pregnancy. This syndrome without convulsions is called preeclampsia. In most cases, onset occurs either in the last trimester or during labor, although uncommonly the toxemic syndrome may develop after delivery. The etiology is unknown, despite the fact that delivery usually terminates the signs and symptoms. Pronounced proteinuria is the rule; the most severe cases may have oval fat bodies and fatty casts. Other laboratory abnormalities include principally an elevated serum uric acid in 60–70% of cases and a metabolic acidosis. The BUN is usually normal. Diagnosis at present depends more on the physical examination, including ophthalmoscopic observation of spasm in the retinal arteries and blood pressure changes, than on the laboratory (except for proteinuria). Gradual onset of eclampsia may be confusing, since some degree of edema is common in pregnancy, and proteinuria (although only slight or mild) may appear during labor.

GLUCOSURIA. — Glucosuria is found in 5–35% of pregnancies, mainly in the last trimester. Occasional reports state an even higher frequency. It is not completely clear whether this is due to increased glucose filtration resulting from increased glomerular filtration rate, decreased renal tubular transport maximum (reabsorptive) capacity for glucose, a combination of the two or some other factor. As noted elsewhere, lactosuria may also occur in the last trimester and may be mistaken for glucosuria when using copper sulfate reducing tests for urine sugar.

RENAL FUNCTION TESTS. — Glomerular filtration rate is increased during pregnancy. Because of this, BUN is apparently somewhat decreased and clearance tests somewhat increased. Concentration tests may be falsely decreased because of edema fluid excretion that takes place during sleep. Since ureteral dilatation usually occurs in the last trimester, PSP excretion may be falsely decreased because of stasis in the dilated upper urinary tract.

INFECTION.—Bacteriuria has been reported in 4–7% of pregnant patients, whereas the incidence in nonpregnant healthy women is approximately 0.5%. It is believed that untreated bacteriuria strongly predisposes to postpartum pyelonephritis.

URINALYSIS IN MISCELLANEOUS DISEASES

FEVER.—This is the most common cause of proteinuria (up to 75% of febrile patients). If severe, it may be associated with an increase in hyaline casts (etiology unknown; possibly dehydration?).

CYSTITIS-URETHRITIS.—These are lower urinary tract infections, often hard to differentiate from renal infection. Clumping of WBC is suggestive of pyelonephritis, but not absolutely specific, as WBC casts are. Necrotizing cystitis may cause hematuria. The two-glass urine test helps to differentiate urethritis from cystitis. After cleansing the genitalia, the patient voids about 10–20 ml into container #1 and the remainder into container #2. Significant increase in container #1 cell count suggests urethral origin.

GENITOURINARY TRACT OBSTRUCTION.—Neuromuscular disorders of the bladder, congenital urethral strictures and valves, intrinsic or extrinsic ureteral mechanical compressions and intraluminal calculi produce no specific urinary changes but predispose to stasis and infection. Obstruction (whether partial or complete) is a frequent etiology for recurrent GU infections.

AMYLOIDOSIS.—Renal involvement usually leads to proteinuria. In a minority of cases, when the process severely affects the kidney, there may be high proteinuria and sediment typical of the nephrotic syndrome. The urinary sediment, however, is not specific, and RBC casts are not present. Renal amyloidosis is usually associated with chronic diseases, such as long-standing osteomyelitis or infection, or multiple sclerosis.

URINARY CALCULI.—These often cause hematuria of some type and may be associated with excess excretion of calcium, uric acid, cystine, phosphates or urates in the urine even when calculi are not clinically evident. Frequent complications are infection or obstruction, and infection may occur even in the absence of definite obstruction. Ureteral stone passage gives hematuria, often gross. An IVP is the best means of diagnosis; some types of calculi are radiopaque, and others may be localized by finding a site of ureteral obstruction.

SICKLE-CELL ANEMIA.—Kidney lesions may result from intracapillary RBC plugs, leading to congestion, small thromboses and infarctions. Also, at times of hematologic crises, hematuria is frequent. Hematuria may be present even without crises in sickle-cell disease or sickle-cell variants. Sickle-cell patients may lose urine-concentrating ability for unknown reasons—this happens even with sickle-cell variants, but is less common.

CHRONIC PASSIVE CONGESTION (CPC).—A result of cardiac failure or inferior vena caval obstruction. It produces mild diffuse tubular atrophy and hyperemia, leads to proteinuria (usually mild to moderate) and hyaline casts, and sometimes also elicits epithelial casts and a few RBC. Occasionally, but not commonly, severe CPC may simulate the nephrotic syndrome to some extent, including desquamated epithelial cells containing fat plus many casts of epithelial series. In CPC of strictly cardiac origin without significant previous renal damage, there is decreased urine volume but usually retained urine-concentrating ability. No anemia is present unless due to some other systemic etiology.

BENIGN ARTERIOSCLEROSIS.—This involves the renal parenchyma secondarily to decreased blood supply. In the majority of cases in the earlier stages, there are few urinary findings, if any; later, there is often mild proteinuria (0.1–0.5 gm/24 hours) and a variable urine sediment, such as a few hyaline casts, epithelial cells, and perhaps occasional RBC. If the condition eventually progresses to renal failure, there will be significant proteinuria and renal failure sediment with impaired renal function tests.

WEIL'S DISEASE.—A classic combination of hepatitis and hematuria. Characteristically, there are also high fever and severe muscle aching, and there may be associated symptoms of meningitis.

INFECTIOUS MONONUCLEOSIS.—Renal imvolvement with hematuria occurs in 5–6% of cases.

PURPURA AND HEMORRHAGIC DISEASES.—These diseases should be recognized as a cause of hematuria, either by itself or in association with glomerular lesions. The Henoch-Schönlein syndrome (anaphylactoid purpura) is a rare condition that often is concurrent with hematuria and nephritis.

HYPERSENSITIVITIES.—These may lead to proteinuria (usually slight) with hematuria and perhaps a moderate increase in casts. Kidney involvement may occur due to mercurials, sulfas, etc.

FAT EMBOLISM.—Most commonly, fat embolism occurs after trauma, especially fractures. Cerebral or respiratory symptoms develop the second or third day after injury, usually associated with a significant drop in hemoglobin values. Fat in the urine is found in 50% or more of patients and is a very valuable diagnostic test (p. 232). Unfortunately, an order for a test of fat in the urine will usually produce microscopic examination of the sediment. Whereas this is correct procedure for nephrotic syndrome, where fat is located in renal epithelial cells and casts, this is worthless for fat embolism diagnosis, where free fat is the item to be located. Since free fat tends to float, a simple procedure is to fill an Ehrlenmeyer (thin-neck) flask with urine up into the thin neck, agitate gently to allow fat to reach the surface, skim the surface with a bacteriologic loop, place the loop contents on a slide and then stain with a fat stain such as Sudan IV.

HEMOCHROMATOSIS.—This condition presents hepatomegaly, gray skin pigmentation and proteinuria in a diabetic patient. Proteinuria may exceed 1 gm/24 hours, but sediment may be scanty and fat is absent. In severe cases yellow-brown coarse granules of hemosiderin are seen in cells, in casts and lying free. Prussian blue (iron) stains in this material are positive. Distal convoluted tubules are the areas primarily involved. Since hemo-chromatosis does not invariably involve the kidney until late, a negative urine does not rule out the diagnosis. False positives (other types of urinary siderosis) may occur in pernicious anemia, hemolytic jaundice and in patients who have received many transfusions.

THYROID DYSFUNCTION. — *Myxedema.* — Proteinuria is said to occur without other renal disease; its incidence is uncertain, especially since some reports state that proteinuria is actually not common, and usually persists after treatment.

Hyperthyroid. — The kidney may lose its concentrating ability so that specific gravity may remain low even in dehydration; this is reversible with treatment and return to euthyroid. Glucosuria occurs in occasional patients.

REFERENCES

Adams, E. C., et al.: Hemolysis in hematuria, J. Urol. 88:427, 1962.

Berman, L. B., and Schreiner, G. E.: Clinical and histologic spectrum of the nephrotic syndrome, Am. J. Med. 24:249, 1958.

Beskow, A.: A survey of tuberculosis of the kidney in relation to tuberculosis in general, Acta Tuberc. Scand., Suppl. 31, 1952.

Brough, A. J., and Zuelzer, W. W.: Renal vascular disease, Pediatr. Clin. North Am. 11:533, 1964.

Dornfeld, L., and Narins, R. G.: Pre- and postoperative renal failure, Urol. Clin. North Am. 3:363, 1976.

Gifford, H., and Bergerman, J.: Falsely negative enzyme paper tests for urinary glucose, J.A.M.A. 178:423, 1961.

Hayslett, J. P., et al.: Glomerulopathy, in Stollerman, G. H. (ed.): *Advances in Internal Medicine* (Chicago: Year Book Medical Publishers, Inc., 1975), vol. 20, p. 215.

Kimmelstiel, P., et al.: Chronic pyelonephritis, Am. J. Med. 30:589, 1961.

Kincaid-Smith, P., et al. (eds.): *Glomerulonephritis: Morphology, Natural History and Treatment* (New York: Wiley-Interscience, 1973), vol. 1.

Lee, C. T., Jr.: Renal disease in diabetes mellitus, Med. Clin. North Am. 47:1069, 1963.

Letteri, J. M.: The urinary sediment in renal disease, Med. Clin. North Am. 47:887, 1963.

Levitt, J. I.: The prognostic significance of proteinuria in young college students, Ann. Intern. Med. 66:685, 1967.

Lewy, P. R.: How to determine the specific nephritis when the child's kidneys may be at stake, Mod. Med. 42:26, 1974.

Lippman, R. W.: *Urine and the Urinary Sediment* (2d ed.; Springfield, IL: Charles C Thomas, Publisher, 1957).

Maxon, W. T.: Benign proteinuria of childhood and adolescence: A survey, Clin. Pediatr. 2:662, 1963.

McDonald, B. M., and McEnery, P. T.: Glomerulonephritis in children, Pediatr. Clin. North Am. 23:691, 1976.

Mostofi, F. K., et al.: Lesions in kidneys removed for unilateral hematuria in sickle cell disease, Arch. Pathol. 63:336, 1957.

O'Sullivan, J. B., et al.: Comparative value of tests for urinary glucose, Diabetes 11:53, 1962.

Pollak, V. E., and Kark, R. M.: The toxemias of pregnancy and the renal lesion of pre-eclampsia, Am. J. Med. 30:181, 1961.

Pollak, V. E., et al.: Renal vein thrombosis, Postgrad. Med. 40:282, 1966.

Rance, C. P., et al.: Management of the nephritic syndrome in children, Pediatr. Clin. North Am. 23:735, 1976.

Reikers, H., and Miale, J. B.: Ketonuria: An evaluation of tests and some clinical implications, Am. J. Clin. Path. 30:530, 1958.

Reynolds, T. B., and Edmondson, H. A.: Chronic renal disease and heavy use of analgesics, J.A.M.A. 184:435, 1963.

Salomon, M. I., et al.: Renal lesions in hepatic disease, Arch. Intern. Med. 115:704, 1965.

Strauss, M. B., and Welt, L. G., (eds.): *Diseases of the Kidney* (Boston: Little, Brown & Company, 1963).

Velosa, J. A., et al.: Focal sclerosing glomerulopathy: A clinicopathologic study, Mayo Clin. Proc. 50:121, 1975.

West, C. D.: Serum complement and chronic glomerulonephritis, Hosp. Practice 5: 75, 1970.

Wilson, R. M., et al.: Lupus nephritis, Arch. Intern. Med. 111:429, 1963.

13 / Renal Function Tests

THE MEASUREMENT OF RENAL FUNCTION is fully as evasive as that of hepatic function. In both the kidney and the liver, a multiplicity of enzyme and transport systems coexist—some related, others both spatially and physiologically quite separate. Processes going on in one section of the nephron may or may not directly affect those in other segments. Like the liver, the kidney has not one but a great many "functions" that may or may not be affected in a given pathologic process. By measuring the capacity to perform these individual functions, one hopes to extrapolate anatomical and physiologic information. Unfortunately, the tests available to the clinical laboratory are few and gross compared to the delicate network of systems at work. It is often difficult to isolate individual functions without complicated research setups, and even more so to differentiate between localized and generalized damage, between temporary and permanent malfunction, and between primary and secondary derangements. One can measure only what passes into and out of the kidney. What goes on inside is all-important, but must be speculated on by indirect means. One can accurately interpret renal function tests only by keeping these facts in mind, by learning the physiologic basis for each test and by careful correlation with other clinical and laboratory data.

Proteinuria almost invariably accompanies serious renal damage. Its severity does not necessarily correlate with the amount of damaged renal parenchyma or the status of any one renal function or group of systems. Its presence and degree may, in association with other findings, aid in the diagnosis of certain syndromes or disease entities whose renal pathologic findings are known. Its presence may be secondary to benign or even extrarenal etiologies.

Renal function tests fall into three general categories: (1) tests predominantly of glomerular function; (2) tests reflecting severe glomerular or tubular damage or both, and (3) tests of predominantly tubular function.

TESTS PREDOMINANTLY OF GLOMERULAR FUNCTION (CLEARANCE TESTS)

Clearance is a theoretical concept defined as that volume of plasma from which a measured amount of substance could be completely eliminated (cleared) into the urine per unit time. This depends on the plasma concentration and excretory rate, which, in turn, involve the glomerular filtration rate (GFR) and renal plasma flow (RPF). Clearance tests in general are the best available for estimating mild-to-moderate diffuse glomerular damage (e.g., acute glomerulonephritis). Serum levels of urea or creatinine reveal only extensive renal disease. Note, however, that many "extrarenal" conditions (shock, hyponatremia, etc.) cause vasoconstriction and will reduce RPF, and thus possibly reduce clearance values.

UREA CLEARANCE. — Urea is filtered at the glomerulus, and approximately 40% is reabsorbed in the tubules by passive back-diffusion. Thus, under usual conditions, urea clearance values parallel the true GFR at about 60% of it. However, several factors may adversely influence this situation. (1) The test is dependent on rate of urine flow. At low levels (less than 2 ml/minute), the values are very inaccurate, even with certain "correction" formulas. (2) Levels of blood urea vary considerably during the day and according to diet and other conditions.

CREATININE CLEARANCE. — Creatinine is a metabolic product of creatine-phosphate dephosphorylation in muscle. It has a relatively constant hourly and daily production, and fairly stable blood levels. Excretion is by a combination of glomerular filtration (70–80%) and tubular secretion. It usually parallels true GFR by ± 10%. However, at low filtration rates (less than 30% of normal), creatinine rates become increasingly inaccurate due to the relatively higher proportion of the secreted fraction. Advantages are constancy of production, allowing larger time interval collections — also freedom from dependence on urine flow. The main disadvantage is the moderate technical difficulty of laboratory analysis, which may magnify small errors when dealing with the small amounts of substance usually present. In general, creatinine clearance is definitely a better test than urea clearance and, for clinical purposes, affords adequate estimation of GFR.

A major drawback is that normal values (90 – 120 ml/minute) were established for young adults. The GFR has been shown to decrease with age; one report states 4 ml/minute decrease for each decade after age 20. Several studies found creatinine clearances as low as 50 ml/minute in the elderly, and one study found values between 40% and 70% of normal. Creatinine excretion also diminishes, although serum creatinine remains within established normal range. Whether age-related normal values should be applied depends on whether these changes are regarded as physiologic (because they occur frequently in the population) or pathologic (because they are most likely due to arteriolar nephrosclerosis).

TESTS REFLECTING SEVERE GLOMERULAR OR TUBULAR DAMAGE OR BOTH (BUN, NPN, SERUM CREATININE)

In azotemia BUN and NPN are equally satisfactory in most cases. BUN is easier to perform technically. In chronic diffuse types of renal disease, significant azotemia usually heralds the end-stage kidney. In other renal diseases, azotemia may be only transient or permanently reversible. It may occur in many conditions:

Prerenal azotemia
1. Traumatic shock (head injuries; postsurgical hypotension)
2. Hemorrhagic shock (varices, ulcer, postpartum hemorrhage, etc.)
3. Severe dehydration or electrolyte loss (severe vomiting, diarrhea, diabetic acidosis, Addison's disease)

4. Acute cardiac decompensation (especially after extensive infarction)
5. Overwhelming infections or toxemia
6. Excess intake of proteins or extensive protein breakdown. (Usually other factors are also involved, such as the normally subclinical slight functional loss from aging.)

Renal

1. Chronic diffuse bilateral kidney disease or bilateral severe kidney damage (e.g., chronic glomerulonephritis or bilateral chronic pyelonephritis)
2. Acute tubular necrosis (lower nephron nephrosis: glomerular or tubular injury; due to shock with renal shutdown, crush injuries, transfusion or allergic reactions, certain poisons and precipitation of uric acid or sulfa crystals in renal tubules)
3. Severe acute glomerular damage (e.g., acute glomerulonephritis)

Postrenal (obstruction)

1. Ureteral or urethral obstruction by strictures, stones, external compression (pelvic tumors, etc.)
2. Obstructing tumors of bladder; congenital defects in bladder or urethra
3. Prostatic obstruction (tumor or benign hypertrophy; a very common cause in elderly males)

In azotemia due to excess protein, some of the more common clinical situations are high protein tube-feedings or gastrointestinal tract hemorrhage (where protein is absorbed from the GI tract); a low-calorie diet (as in patients on intravenous fluids, leading to endogenous protein catabolism); and adrenocortical steroid therapy (since these substances have a catabolic action).

Thus, in general, prerenal azotemia etiologies can be divided into two main categories: (1) decreased blood volume or renal circulation, and (2) increased protein intake or endogenous protein catabolism.

In primary renal disease, azotemia may be due to either primarily glomerular or tubular destructive conditions or to diffuse parenchymal destruction. It must be remembered that rarely would one get glomerular damage to the point of severe azotemia (5–10% of AGN cases) without some effect on the tubules, and vice versa. Therefore, BUN must be correlated with other clinical observations before its significance can be estimated. There is nothing etiologically distinctive about the terminal manifestations of chronic kidney disease, and it is most important to rule out treatable diseases that may simulate the uremic laboratory or clinical picture. Anuria (less than 100 ml/24 hours) *always* suggests urinary obstruction.

Terminal azotemia, sometimes to uremic levels, occurs in the last hours or days of a significant number of seriously ill patients with a variety of diseases, including cancer. Often no clinical or pathologic cause is found, even microscopically. Urine specific gravity may be relatively good.

Two screening methods for BUN, called Urograph and Azostix, are commercially available. Evaluations to date indicate that both of these methods are useful as emergency or office screening procedures to separate normal persons (BUN less than 20 mg/100 ml) from those with mild azotemia (20–50 mg/100 ml) and those with considerable BUN elevation (over 50 mg/100 ml). If accurate quantitation is desired, one of the standard quantitative BUN procedures should be done.

Serum creatinine determination has much the same significance as BUN but tends to rise later. Significant creatinine elevations thus suggest chronicity without being diagnostic of it. It has been reported that ketone bodies and cephalosporin antibiotics may give false elevation of creatinine in serum or urine.

The question sometimes is raised as to the degree of BUN increase that is possible in short periods of time. In one study daily increase after onset of acute renal failure ranged from 10–50 mg/100 ml during the first week, with the average daily increase being 25 mg/100 ml. After the first week, the amount of increase tended to be less.

TESTS OF PREDOMINANTLY TUBULAR FUNCTION (PSP, CONCENTRATION AND DILUTION)

Phenolsulfonphthalein (PSP) is excreted mainly by the renal tubules (p. 442). In general, results give about the same clinical information as creatinine clearance since glomerular and tubular dysfunction usually occur together in acute and chronic kidney damage. Creatinine clearance seems to be increasingly replacing PSP in the relatively few situations in which this type of information is needed.

Specific gravity is important in the evaluation of chronic diffuse parenchymal disease (chronic glomerulonephritis, chronic pyelonephritis, etc.). As such conditions progress, tubular ability to concentrate urine is often affected relatively early and slowly decreases until the urine has the same specific gravity as the plasma ultrafiltrate—1.010. This usually, but not always, occurs in advance of final renal decompensation. Concentration tests, to be accurate, must deprive the patient of water over a long period to exclude influence from previous ingestion. The usual test should run 16–17 hours; after previous forced fluids, a longer time may be necessary. This may be impossible in patients with cardiac disease, those with renal failure, aged persons, or those with electrolyte problems. Under these test conditions, the average person should concentrate up to 1.025; at least to 1.020. Concentration tests are also impaired in diabetes insipidus, the diuretic phase of acute tubular necrosis; and occasionally in hyperthyroidism, severe salt-restricted diets and sickle cell anemia. These diseases may result in failure to concentrate without the presence of irreversible renal tubular damage. Abnormal urinary substances may raise specific gravity to a small extent; for 10 gm protein/L subtract .003; for 1% glucose, subtract .004. In addition, the radiopaque contrast media used for intravenous pyelograms (IVP) considerably increase urine specific gravity; this effect may persist for 1–2 days. Ability to concentrate urine does not rule out many types of active kidney disease, nor does absence of ability to concentrate necessarily mean closely approaching renal failure. Adequate ability to concentrate is, however, decidedly against the diagnosis of chronic severe diffuse renal disease. A relatively early manifestation of chronic diffuse bilateral renal disease is often impairment of concentrating ability (on a concentration test), which becomes manifest before changes in other function tests appear. (This refers to beginning impairment, not to fixation of specific gravity.)

Clinically, fixation of specific gravity is usually manifested by nocturia and a diminution of the day-night ratio (normally 3 or 4:1) approaching 1:1. Other causes must be considered: diabetes mellitus and insipidus, hyperparathyroidism, renal acidosis syndrome, beginning of congestive heart failure and occasionally hyperthyroidism. True nocturia or polyuria must be distinguished from urgency, incontinence or enuresis.

One improvement on the standard concentration procedure is to substitute for water deprivation a single injection of Pitressin tannate in oil. Five units of this long-acting preparation are given intramuscularly in the late afternoon, and urine collections for specific gravity are made in the early morning and 2 times thereafter at 3-hour intervals. One danger of this procedure is the possibility in certain patients, such as infants on liquid diet, of water intoxication.

A relatively recent innovation is to measure the *urine osmolality* (sometimes incorrectly called osmolarity) instead of conventional specific gravity. Osmolality is a measure of the osmotic strength or number of osmotically active ions or particles present per unit of solution. Specific gravity is defined as the weight or density per unit volume of solution compared to water. Since the number of molecules present in a solution is a major determinant of its weight, it is obvious that there is a relationship between osmolality and specific gravity; since the degree of ionic dissociation is very important in osmolality but not in specific gravity, values of the two for the same solution may not always correspond closely. The rationale for using this concept is that specific gravity is a rather empirical observation and does not measure the actual ability of the kidney to concentrate electrolytes or other molecules relative to the plasma concentration; also, certain substances are of relatively large molecular weight and tend to disproportionately affect specific gravity. The quantity of water present may vary, even in concentration tests, and influence results.

Osmolality is defined in terms of milliosmoles (mOsm) per kilogram of solution and can be easily and accurately measured by determining the freezing point depression of a sample in a specially designed machine (in biologic fluids, such as serum or urine, water makes up nearly all of the specimen weight; since water weighs 1 gm/ml, osmolality may be approximated clinically by values reported in terms of milliosmoles per liter rather than per kilogram). Normal values for urine osmolality after 14-hour test dehydration are 800–1300 mOsm/L. Most osmometers are accurate to less than 5 mOsm, so the answer thus has an aura of scientific exactness that is lacking in the relatively crude specific gravity method. Unfortunately, having a rather precise number and being able to use it clinically are often two different things. Without reference to the clinical situation, osmolality has as little meaning as specific gravity. In most situations, they have approximately the same significance. Both vary and depend on the amount of water excreted with the urinary solids. In some cases, however, such as when the specific gravity is fixed at 1.010, osmolality after dehydration may still be greater than that of the serum, suggesting that it is a more sensitive measurement. Also, osmolality does not need correction for glucosuria, proteinuria, or urine temperature.

Intravenous pyelogram (IVP), a radiologic technique, uses iodinated contrast media, most of which are tubular-secreted. To appear radiographically, once secreted they must also be concentrated. Thus, incidental to delineating calyceal and urinary tract outlines and revealing postrenal obstruction, IVP also affords some information as to kidney concentrating ability or ability to excrete the dye — two tubular "functions." These are not sufficient for visualization with BUN over 50 mg/100 ml using ordinary (standard) IVP technique. New methods (drip-infusion IVP) can be used with higher BUN levels, but these are not routine and usually must be specifically requested. Radioisotope techniques using the scintillation camera are frequently able to demonstrate the kidneys when IVP fails.

Another renal tubule activity is the handling of electrolytes, such as sodium (p. 285). This may be of clinical value in certain situations (pp. 141, 444) and can be estimated by measurement of the urine levels of these electrolytes. A variety of research techniques not generally available can measure one or another of the many kidney "functions," such as tubular secretion of various substances, glomerular filtration of nonreabsorbed materials (such as inulin), and renal blood flow by clearance of substances (such as PAH) that are both filtered and secreted.

SELECTION AND INTERPRETATION OF TESTS

Next we shall discuss the interpretation of certain tests and also some suggestions on how to select them. Most of the time only a few tests are needed to get all the useful information available.

One question that continually arises is the significance of small degrees of proteinuria. Textbook normal values are usually stated as 10 mg/100 ml (0.1 gm/L). Generally speaking, values of up to 30 mg/100 ml are within normal range; 30–40 mg/100 ml may or may not be significantly abnormal. It should be noted that normal values in terms of total urinary protein output per 24 hours may be up to 100 mg (0.1 gm) per 24 hours. Values stated in terms of mg/24 hours may not coincide with values expressed in terms of mg/100 ml, due to varying quantities of diluent water. It must be stressed that duration of proteinuria is even more important than quantity, especially at low values. As an example, 60 mg/100 ml or even more may have minor or little importance on an admission urine if this subsequently clears up, whereas 40 mg/100 ml may possibly be significant if this level persists. This becomes clear by examining the list of possible causes of proteinuria. Intrinsic renal disease usually has proteinuria which persists, whereas many of the extrarenal types will quickly disappear if the primary disease is successfully treated. However, this does not always hold true, and one must remember that a single disease may cause permanent damage to more than one organ. In arteriosclerosis or hypertension, for example, functioning kidney tissue may be reduced or destroyed to varying degrees by arteriolar nephrosclerosis, although cardiac symptoms due to heart damage may overshadow the clinical picture.

The problem of hematuria is somewhat different from that of proteinuria. One must always remember that hematuria is the most frequent symptom of urinary tract cancer — often the only one. If no disease is present to account for the hematuria, which can be either gross or microscopic, the patient should get an IVP. If this is negative, and if the hematuria persists or there is some other reason to suspect a neoplasm, the IVP should be followed by cystoscopy to detect bladder carcinoma. It must also not be forgotten that the patient may have hematuria due to carcinoma of kidney or bladder and at the same time have other diseases, such as hypertension, which themselves are known causes of hematuria. Generally speaking, however, the diseases that cause significant hematuria are in a minority and can usually be diagnosed and evaluated without too much difficulty. Hypertension most often is at least moderately severe for really significant hematuria (e.g., over 5 RBC/high-power field) to be present. Finding RBC casts means that the hematuria is from the kidney and that the problem is a medical disease rather than a surgical one or cancer. Also, the age of the patient is important; in a child, a neoplasm of the urinary tract would be very unlikely. In adults, most bladder and renal carcinomas develop in patients over age 40. (Many other diseases do likewise, unfortunately.)

Clearance tests may be needed occasionally, and this usually happens in three situations; (1) in acute glomerulonephritis (AGN), to follow the clinical course and as a parameter of therapeutic response; (2) to demonstrate the presence of acute, strictly glomerular disease in contrast to more diffuse chronic structural damage, and (3) as a measurement of overall renal functional impairment. In AGN, there is frequently, but not always, a decrease in glomerular filtration due to primary glomerular involvement. When this is true, the clearance tests have been used to evaluate the length of time that bed rest and other therapy are necessary. However, the erythrocyte sedimentation rate gives the same information in a manner that is cheaper, simpler and probably more sensitive. Therefore, the ESR seems preferable in most cases. Concerning the second category, it is not so easy to demonstrate strictly glomerular disease because many diseases will reduce renal blood flow and thus glomerular filtration rate. Also, some patients with AGN may have some degree of tubular damage. One situation in which clearance tests may be used to diagnostic advantage is the rare case of a young person with sudden gross hematuria but without convincing clinical or laboratory evidence of AGN. Since in a young person one would expect normal clearance values, finding reduced creatinine clearance would be in favor of nephritis.

Clearance as a measurement of overall renal function impairment demonstrates roughly the same information as is obtained from the PSP and has mostly replaced it in practice. Clearance tests are reliable in detecting mild-to-moderate diffuse renal disease, but they depend on completely collected specimens and accurate recording of the time the specimens were collected and presuppose adequate renal blood flow. If a patient is incontinent of urine, one must use either a short period of collection or a catheter, or else use some other test. Of course, if a Foley catheter is already in place, there is no problem. The clearance range of 60–80% of normal is usually taken to represent mild diffuse renal function impairment. Values between 40% and 60% of normal are considered moderate decrease, and between 20% and 40% of normal are considered severe, since about half the patients in this group have elevated BUN. As long as the BUN is elevated, clearance tests are usually not helpful.

In the classic case of chronic diffuse bilateral renal disease, the first demonstrable test abnormality is a decrease in urine-concentrating ability shown by the concentration test. As the disease progresses, the creatinine clearance becomes reduced. Then the specific gravity becomes fixed and the creatinine clearance demonstrates considerable decrease. Finally, clearance becomes markedly decreased and the BUN starts to rise, followed shortly by the serum creatinine.

Renal function tests may be useful in the evaluation of hypertension. There are many causes of hypertension and the kidneys are involved in several (discussed further in Chapter 29). The kidney is damaged secondarily by essential hypertension. The kidney may itself be the primary source, since a small but significant number of hypertension cases are due to unilateral renal disease, most commonly renal artery stenosis, and these can often be cured by removal of the ischemic kidney or surgical repair of the stenotic renal artery. One method of diagnosis is an IVP, but the standard IVP is not very satisfactory for this purpose, and a special modification called the "minute-sequence" IVP should be ordered. Films are made every minute for 5 minutes after injection of the contrast medium, whereas the standard IVP has films at only 5, 10 and 15 minutes after injection. Unilateral lack of dye concentration or a small kidney on one side only is strongly suspicious. The minute-sequence IVP is reported to pick up 70–90% of cases. However, a positive minute-sequence IVP means only that the patient has unilateral renal disease, and does not tell the etiology or whether any hypertension is actually due to the renal disease. For example, it cannot differentiate unilateral renal disease due to renal artery stenosis from unilateral renal disease due to chronic pyelonephritis; and if the patient has hypertension, it cannot show whether the hypertension is due to the renal lesion or to some other cause. Therefore, the minute-sequence IVP is classed as a screening test.

Radioisotope techniques provide another good screening test for unilateral renal disease. The earliest versions were the so-called radiorenogram (isotope-labeled Hippuran) and the chlormerodrin uptake (labeled mercury chlormerodrin), in which two radiation detector probes were placed over the kidney areas and a curve obtained from serial radiation counts. Although a considerable number of investigators obtained 80–90% sensitivity, enough false positive (5–10%) and negative (10–30%) results occurred to throw the technique into disrepute. Current nuclear medicine techniques that use a scintillation camera are much more informative. Serial 1- or 2-minute photographs of the kidneys are obtained after injection of an isotope-labeled substance, such as Hippuran or DTPA, that is excreted by the kidney. The difference between the old and the new renograms is that in the new, one can actually see what is happening in each kidney rather than blindly relying on changes in count rate. There is enough difference between the two techniques to cast doubt on the current validity of statistics based on the old radiorenograms. Information about cortex function can be obtained, as well as comparison of the two kidneys. In addition, renal blood flow can be estimated (flow study) by injecting various radioisotopes and obtaining serial 1-2 second photographs. This gives additional information about function and also helps confirm differences between the kidneys. Finally, a renal scan can be done, which may demonstrate size differences and also focal lesions. The flow study may be able to predict degree of vascularity of focal lesions if the lesion is of sufficient size.

Unfortunately, radioisotope studies cannot prove whether any hypertension present is due to the renal disease or to some other cause, or if the hypertension is potentially curable. Therefore, just as with the minute-sequence IVP, there will be some "positive" results in patients with renal disease but with hypertension from some other etiology.

A third procedure useful to demonstrate unilateral renal disease is the Howard test. The Howard test (or one of its modifications, such as the Stamey test) is based on the fact that renal water and electrolyte excretion may be utilized to diagnose and pinpoint the affected kidney in hypertension due to unilateral renal disease. Bilateral ureteral catheters are placed, and the urine from each kidney is analyzed separately for electrolyte content and volume. In the Howard test, unilateral reduction in volume during the test period over 50%, and/or reduction of sodium content over 15%, is considered strong evidence of unilateral renal disease. Again, this does not exactly pinpoint the type of lesion present, although this pattern is more common with renal artery stenosis. Some believe that this pattern can be used to predict whether nephrectomy will benefit the patient with hypertension. The main drawback with the test is technical difficulty. Bilateral ureteral catheterization is not a simple procedure, and proper wedging of the catheters so that no urine escapes is somewhat difficult. For screening purposes, the Howard test has been largely replaced by the radioisotope techniques, which by comparison are relatively simple to perform.

None of the previously mentioned tests, with the possible exception of the Howard test, can predict whether surgery will cure the hypertension. Some medical centers catheterize both renal veins and take blood samples for renin assay (p. 362). A ratio greater than 2.0 is reported to have 90–95% chance of cure by surgical treatment of the diseased kidney. However, almost 50% of those whose ratio did not predict cure were nevertheless improved by surgery.

The other useful technique in hypertension due to unilateral renal disease is renal angiography. This is a diagnostic test for renal artery stenosis since, when technically well done, it will not only demonstrate the lesion but will localize it anatomically. This technique involves direct injection of radiopaque dye into the abdominal aorta or renal arteries and then photographing its passage through the renal arteries with x-ray techniques. Again, this is not a simple procedure and carries with it some risk, although not great. Also, some people with renal artery stenosis do not have hypertension, so that demonstration of a lesion does not in itself prove that the lesion is affecting the kidney. Because of this, most use the renal arteriogram as a confirmatory test for proving renal artery stenosis after screening tests have demonstrated renal abnormality.

Hypertension due to unilateral renal disease is often curable, and it should be ruled out as a cause of hypertension when the patient is relatively young or the hypertension is of recent onset. A suggested sequence of action is to obtain a minute-sequence IVP and, if available, a radioisotope procedure, such as the renogram. If the results of both are negative, chances that the patient has unilateral renal disease are slight. If either result is positive, a renal arteriogram should be obtained to demonstrate renal artery lesions.

A suggested sequence for proper workup of patients with actual or suspected renal problems of a medical type follows. One of the most common situations is the patient who has asymptomatic proteinuria, or exhibits it in association with a disease in which it is not expected. The first step is to repeat the test after a couple of days or when the presenting disease is under control, using an early morning specimen to avoid orthostatic proteinuria. If proteinuria persists, the microscopic report should be analyzed for any diagnostic hints. The presence and degree of hematuria suggests a certain number of diseases, and pyuria does likewise; if either is present, there should be a careful search for RBC or WBC casts. A careful history may elicit information of previous proteinuria or hematuria, suggesting chronic glomerulonephritis or previous kidney infection or calculi, which would be in favor of chronic pyelonephritis. Uremia due to chronic bilateral renal disease often has an associated hypertension. (Of course, hypertension may itself be the primary disease and cause extensive secondary renal damage.) In addition, a low-grade or moderate anemia, either normochromic or slightly hypochromic and without evidence of reticulocytosis or blood loss, is often found with severe chronic diffuse renal disease. The next step is to note the random specific gravities taken. If one is normal (i.e., over 1.020), renal function is probably adequate. If all are lower, one can proceed to a concentration or creatinine clearance test, since low random specific gravities may simply mean high water excretion rather than lack of urine-concentrating ability. If the creatinine clearance is mildly or moderately reduced, the patient most likely has only mild or possibly moderate functional loss. If the creatinine clearance is markedly abnormal and the BUN is normal with no hypertension or anemia present, this is most likely severe diffuse bilateral renal disease, but not a completely end-stage situation. When the BUN is elevated with these other signs present, the prognosis is generally very bad, although some patients with definite uremia may live for years with proper therapy. There will be exceptions to the situations just outlined, but not too many.

Two other procedures have been advocated for use in renal diagnosis: the Addis count and renal biopsy.

The Addis count is used in suspected subclinical cases of chronic glomerulonephritis to demonstrate 12-hour abnormally increased rates of RBC and cast excretion too small to exceed the normal range in ordinary random specimen microscopies. If the random urine specimen already shows hematuria or pyuria, and if contamination can be ruled out by catheter or clean catch collection technique, then the Addis count cannot do anything more than show the same abnormality. Addis counts should very rarely be necessary with a good history and adequate workup.

Renal biopsy is now widely used. It may be the only way to find which disease is present, but it should be reserved for patients whose treatment depends on exact diagnosis. Most renal disease entities could be inferred by routine methods. Biopsies, because of their random sample nature, more often than not show only nonspecific changes reflecting the result rather than the etiology of the disease process, and frequently are requested only for academic rather than practical diagnostic or therapeutic reasons. In children, electron microscopy and immunofluorescent techniques are more useful than light microscopy.

The patient with an already elevated BUN often presents a diagnostic problem. In general, if the BUN is elevated but the serum creatinine is normal, this suggests a prerenal etiology for azotemia (or, alternatively, acute onset of renal failure). The same is true, to a lesser extent, if the BUN is disproportionately elevated (higher than 10:1 ratio) in relationship to serum creatinine.

Many use the term "uremia" as a synonym for azotemia, although uremia is a syndrome and should be defined in clinical terms. A BUN of approximately 100 mg/100 ml is usually considered to separate the general category of acute reversible prerenal azotemias from the more prolonged acute episodes and chronic uremias. In general, this holds true, but there is a small but important minority of cases that do not follow this rule. Thus, some uremics seem to stabilize at a lower BUN level until their terminal episode, while a few persons with acute transient azotemia may show a BUN close to 100 mg/100 ml and rarely over 125 mg/100 ml, which rapidly falls to normal levels after treatment of the primary systemic condition responsible. It must be admitted that easily correctable prerenal azotemia with appreciable BUN level is almost always superimposed on kidneys that have previous subclinical damage or function loss. While not severe enough to cause symptoms, the functional reserve of these kidneys has been eliminated by aging changes, pyelonephritis, or similar conditions. The same is usually true for azotemia of mild levels (30–50 mg/100 ml) occurring with dehydration, high protein intake, cardiac failure, and other important but not life-threatening situations. After the BUN has returned to normal levels, a creatinine clearance will allow adequate evaluation of the patient's renal status.

Normal adult urine volume is 500–1600 ml/24 hours (upper limit depends on fluid intake); less than 400 ml/24 hours is considered oliguria, if all urine produced has actually been collected. Incomplete collection or leakage around a catheter may give a false impression of oliguria. Occasionally, a patient develops oliguria and progressive azotemia, and it becomes necessary to differentiate between prerenal azotemia (which is correctable by improving that patient's circulation) and acute renal tubular necrosis (which must be promptly treated by mannitol diuresis to preserve tubular function). This problem most frequently occurs after a hypotensive episode or after surgery. If the patient's renal function is known to be adequate, then, in the presence of oliguria, if the urine osmolality (p. 134) is less then 400 mOsm/L, acute tubular necrosis is a good possibility. However, in elderly persons or others who may have significantly decreased renal function, a low osmolality is not helpful, since it may simply reflect the patient's poor concentrating ability, which he had before the episode of oliguria. If the urine osmolality is over 500 mOsm/L, this demonstrates a significant ability to concentrate and would be evidence against acute tubular necrosis. (A specific gravity over 1.015 would have the same significance, but is affected by other variables, such as proteinuria.) Urine sodium less than 20 mEq/L or over 100 mEq/L is strong evidence against acute tubular necrosis.

If the urine contained many RBC, and especially if hemoglobin or RBC casts were present, this would suggest hemoglobinuric nephrosis. If the serum creatinine is normal or only slightly elevated, this suggests relatively acute onset of the BUN elevation. The finding of many broad and waxy casts tends to suggest severe prolonged renal damage.

Urine excretion of electrolytes may be utilized as a renal function test. Normally, the kidney is very efficient in reabsorbing urinary sodium, which is filtered at the glomerulus. In acute tubular necrosis, renal ability to reabsorb sodium is impaired. Therefore, in severe diffuse bilateral renal damage (acute or chronic), renal excretion of sodium is fixed between 30–90 mEq/L and chloride between 30–100 mEq/L. Finding urine sodium or chloride concentration more than 10 mEq/L above or below these limits would be evidence against acute tubular necrosis or renal failure. Evaluation is assisted when serum electrolytes are abnormal. Hyponatremia, for example, normally would force the kidney to reabsorb more sodium ions, dropping the urine sodium to very low values, usually well below the 20 mEq/L level. Therefore, urine sodium of 30–90 mEq/L in the presence of hyponatremia would suggest severe renal damage.

Measurement of urinary urea nitrogen may be helpful. In severe diffuse bilateral renal damage (acute or chronic), urine urea nitrogen tends to be fixed at 300–500 mg/100 ml or 3–10 gm/24 hours. If the kidneys are able to produce urine concentrations significantly above these values in the presence of elevated serum BUN, this would suggest that prerenal causes (pp. 131–132) may be the etiology rather than primary renal failure. A 24-hour collection is more helpful than a random specimen, since a random specimen is affected more by the amount of water output.

Radioisotope studies with a scintillation camera may sometimes be helpful. Bilateral poor uptake, poor cortex-pelvis transit, and decreased blood flow suggest chronic diffuse renal disease. Good cortex uptake, poor cortex-pelvis transit, and good blood flow are more indicative of acute tubular necrosis or prerenal azotemia. Isotope techniques can demonstrate postrenal obstruction and frequently can visualize the kidneys when the IVP fails.

In a patient with uremia (chronic azotemia), there is no good way to determine prognosis by laboratory tests. The degree of azotemia does not correlate well with the clinical course in uremia except in a very general way.

REFERENCES

Blahd, W. H. (ed.): *Nuclear Medicine* (2d ed.; New York: McGraw-Hill Book Company, 1971).

Dean, R. H., et al.: Split renal function studies and renal vein renin assays: Comparative analysis, Surg. Forum 25:257, 1974.

Dornfeld, L., and Narins, R. G.: Pre- and postoperative renal failure, Urol. Clin. North Am. 3:363, 1976.

Dosseter, J. B.: Creatinemia versus uremia, Ann. Intern. Med. 65:1287, 1966.

Drayer, J. I., et al.: The reliability of the measurement of plasma renin activity by radioimmuno assay, Clin. Chim. Acta 61(3):309, 1975.

Friedman, S. A., et al.: Functional defects in the aging kidney, Ann. Intern. Med. 76:41, 1972.

Galambos, J. T., et al.: Specific-gravity determination: Fact or fancy? N. Engl. J. Med. 270:506, 1964.

Greenhill, A., and Gruskin, A. B.: Laboratory evaluation of renal function, Pediatr. Clin. North Am. 23:661, 1976.

Jacobson, M. H., et al.: Urine osmolality, Arch. Intern. Med. 110:121, 1962.

Jamison, R. L.: The urinary concentrating mechanism, N. Engl. J. Med. 295:1168, 1232, 1976.

Kirkendal, W. M., et al.: Renal hypertension – Diagnosis and treatment, N. Engl. J. Med. 276:479, 1967.

Lyon, R. P.: The measurement of urine chloride as a test of renal function, J. Urol. 85:884, 1961.

Marks, L. S., and Maxwell, M. H.: Renal vein renin: Value and limitation in the prediction of operative results, Urol. Clin. North Am. 2:311, 1975.

Marks, L. S., et al.: Renovascular hypertension: Does the renal vein renin ratio predict operative results? J. Urol. 115:365, 1976.

Maxwell, M. H., and Lupu, A. N.: Excretory urogram in renal arterial hypertension, J. Urol. 100:395, 1968.

Paster, S. B., et al.: Errors in renal vein renin collections, Am. J. Roentgenol. Radium Ther. Nucl. Med. 122(4):804, 1974.

Phillips, E. J., et al.: Renal vein renin and renovascular hypertension, J. Urol. 112:417, 1974.

Rosenthal, L.: Radiotechnetium renography and serial radiohippurate imaging for screening renovascular hypertension, Semin. Nucl. Med. 4:97, 1974.

Rowe, J. W., et al.: Age-adjusted standards for creatinine clearance, Ann. Intern. Med. 84:567, 1976.

Sargent, F., II, and Johnson, R. E.: The effects of diet on renal function in healthy men, Am. J. Clin. Nutr. 4:466, 1956.

Schaeffer, A. J., et al.: Comparison of split function ratios with renal vein renin ratios in patients with curable hypertension caused by unilateral renal artery stenosis, J. Urol. 112:697, 1974.

Schwartz, W. B., et al.: Intravenous urography in the patient with renal insufficiency, N. Engl. J. Med. 269:277, 1963.

Siemsen, A. W.: The differential diagnosis of azotemia in the surgical patient, Surg. Clin. North Am. 50:457, 1970.

Sigler, M. H.: Oliguric renal failure and acute tubular necrosis, Med. Clin. North Am. 47:1023, 1963.

Slotkin, E. A., and Madsen, P. O.: Complications of renal biopsy: Incidence in 5000 reported cases, J. Urol. 87:13, 1962.

Stamey, T. A.: Unilateral renal disease causing hypertension, J.A.M.A. 235:2340, 1976.

Strauss, M. B., and Welt, L. G. (eds.): *Diseases of the Kidney* (Boston: Little, Brown & Company, 1963).

Tobias, G. J., et al.: Endogenous creatinine clearance, N. Engl. J. Med. 266:317, 1962.

Viamonte, M., Jr., et al.: Renal angiography, South. Med. J. 56:1335, 1963.

Wesson, L. G., Jr.: Clinical evaluation of renal function, Med. Clin. North Am. 47:861, 1963.

Wolf, A. V.: Urinary concentrative properties, Am. J. Med. 32:329, 1962.

14 / Bacterial Infectious Diseases

PROPER THERAPY for infectious disease depends on knowledge of the etiologic agent. This is accomplished in two ways: directly, by isolation and identification by culture, or indirectly, by serologic tests that demonstrate antibodies in the patient's blood against an organism. Certain problems arise when interpreting culture or serologic test results. If a culture is positive, one must determine whether the organism reported has actual clinical significance. It may be a fortuitous "contaminant," an ordinarily nonpathogenic species that has become infectious under the prevailing circumstances, or a recognized pathogen that is a normal inhabitant of the area and whose presence may be entirely harmless. If a culture is negative, one must weigh the chances of having missed a diagnosis because the laboratory was not given a proper specimen, the specimen was obtained at an unfavorable moment during the disease or special culture techniques or media were needed.

Therefore, to evaluate laboratory data, the clinical situation has at least as much importance as considerations of laboratory methodology. It seems desirable to provide a brief survey of the major infectious agents, the diseases and circumstances in which they are most often found and the conditions under which the appearance of these organisms may be confusing. There is an element of classification because of the way laboratory reports are usually worded. Techniques of diagnosis in the area of infectious disease are discussed here, in relation to specific organisms, specific clinical situations or general laboratory methods.

LABORATORY CLASSIFICATION OF BACTERIA

The most useful laboratory classification of bacteria involves a threefold distinction: the Gram stain characteristics (gram positive or negative), morphology (coccus or bacillus) and growth oxygen requirements (aerobic or anaerobic). Species exist which are morphologic exceptions, such as spirochetes; others are intermediate in oxygen requirements; still others are identified by other techniques, such as the acid-fast stain. Reaction to Gram's stain has long been correlated with bacterial sensitivity to certain classes of antibiotics. A classic example is the susceptibility of most gram-positive organisms to penicillin. Morphology, when added to this primary reaction, greatly simplifies identification of large bacterial groups, and oxygen growth requirements narrow the possibilities still further. The interrelationship of these characteristics also helps to control laboratory error. For example, if cocci were seen to be gram negative instead of gram positive, it would call for a laboratory recheck of the decolorization step in the Gram procedure; if the staining technique were verified, the possibility of a small bacillus (coccobacillus) or a diplococcus would have to be considered.

Gram-Positive Cocci

STREPTOCOCCI. — These are gram-positive cocci which are classified in several ways. The three most useful depend on bacterial oxygen requirements, on colony appearance on blood agar and on specific carbohydrate within the organism. Depending on oxygen requirements, streptococci are aerobic, microaerophilic, or anaerobic. Most streptococci are aerobic. The microaerophilic organisms sometimes cause a chronic resistant type of skin ulcer, and occasionally are isolated in deep wound infections. The anaerobic streptococci are discussed on page 152.

According to usual colony appearance on sheep blood agar (p. 445), streptococci are divided into three types — alpha, beta, and gamma. Alpha streptococci have an incomplete type of hemolysis surrounding the colony. This incomplete hemolysis usually has a green appearance, and streptococci producing green hemolysis are often called viridans. The beta type has complete clear hemolysis. Gamma streptococci do not produce hemolysis on blood agar. These groupings have clinical value. Alpha streptococci of the viridans subgroup are one of the most frequent causes of subacute bacterial endocarditis. Beta streptococci produce several different types of infection and syndromes, as will be discussed later, and account for the great majority of disease associated with streptococci. Gamma streptococci are of lesser importance, but some of the so-called enterococci belong to this category. The enterococci have several unusual features that set them apart from other streptococci, such as resistance to heating and growth in certain media such as bile-esculin. Enterococci may produce either alpha or beta hemolysis or be gamma nonhemolytic. Their main importance is the fact that they are resistant to penicillin and sulfa.

The third classification is that of Lancefield, who discovered antibodies produced to a somatic carbohydrate of hemolytic streptococcal organisms. Hemolytic streptococci can be divided into groups depending on the particular carbohydrate they possess. These groups are given a capital letter name. Lancefield group A organisms are beta hemolytic, and the particular strains of organisms that cause acute rheumatic fever and acute glomerulonephritis are all in this group. Enterococci that are hemolytic are all in Lancefield group D, which not only demonstrates their common properties but also emphasizes that Lancefield grouping does not depend on type of hemolysis, since the enterococci in group D can be either alpha or beta hemolytic. It is an accident that Lancefield group A is all beta hemolytic. This accident is useful clinically, since by identifying an unknown streptococcus as group A, one can know it belongs to a potentially dangerous group known to cause certain important diseases. Lancefield grouping is done with appropriate group-specific antiserum. Clinically, since group A organisms seem to have an unusually marked susceptibility to the antibiotic bacitracin, presumptive identification of group A is accomplished by demonstrating inhibition of growth around a disk impregnated with a standardized concentration of bacitracin. Group A organisms may be further separated into subgroups (strains) by use of special antiserum against surface antigens (M antigens). Strain typing is mostly useful in epidemiologic work, especially in acute glomerulonephritis, and is not helpful in most clinical situations.

Certain strains of beta streptococci are associated with specific diseases, covered in more detail elsewhere, such as acute glomerulonephritis and acute rheumatic fever. Beta streptococci also produce various infections without any strain specificity. The most common is acute tonsillitis (pharyngitis). Wound infections and localized skin cellulitis are relatively frequent. Other diseases that are much less common, although famous historically, include scarlet fever, erysipelas (vesicular cellulitis) and puerperal fever.

STAPHYLOCOCCI. — These are gram-positive cocci which typically occur in clusters. They originally were divided into three groups, depending on colony characteristics on blood agar. These were *Staphylococcus albus (S. epidermidis)*, with white colonies; *S. aureus*, with yellow; and *S. citreus*, with pale green. In that classification, *S. aureus* was by far the most important; they were generally hemolytic, and the pathogenic species were coagulase positive. The newer classification recognizes the fact that coagulase activity (the ability to coagulate plasma) is a better indication of pathogenicity than colony color, since a few coagulase-positive organisms are not yellow on blood agar. Therefore, all coagulase-positive staphylococci are now called *Staphylococcus aureus;* all coagulase-negative ones are called *Staphylococcus epidermidis.* Many forms of *S. aureus* are resistant to antibiotics that normally are effective against gram-positive cocci.

Staphylococci, as well as the enteric gram-negative rod organisms and some of the clostridia gram-positive anaerobes (to be discussed later), are normal inhabitants of certain body areas. In the case of staphylococci, their habitat is the skin. Therefore, a diagnosis of staphylococcic infection should not be made solely on the basis of *S. aureus* isolation from an external wound; there should be evidence that *S. aureus* is actually causing clinical disease. Besides the skin, about half of all adults outside the hospital carry staphylococcus in the nasopharynx; this reportedly increases to 70–80% if these persons have cultures performed repeatedly over a long period. More than 50% of hospitalized persons have positive nasopharyngeal cultures. Exactly what factors induce these commensal organisms to cause clinical disease is not completely understood. Staphylococci are typically associated with purulent inflammation, and characteristically are abscess-formers. The most common site of infection is the skin, most frequently confined to minor lesions, such as pustules or possibly small carbuncles, but occasionally producing widespread impetigo in children and infants. The most frequent type of serious staphylococcic disease (other than childhood impetigo) is wound infection or infection associated with hospital diagnostic or therapeutic procedures.

In a small but important number of cases, staphylococci produce certain specific infections. Staphylococcic pneumonia may occur, especially in debilitated persons or following a viral pneumonia. Meningitis and septicemia are also occasionally found; again, more commonly in debilitated persons or those with decreased resistance — often without any apparent portal of entry. Staphylococci are the most common cause of acute (rather than subacute) bacterial endocarditis. They are the most common (but not the only) etiology for a serious gastrointestinal infection called pseudo-membranous enterocolitis, caused by suppression of normal bacterial flora by oral broad-spectrum antibiotics, with resultant overgrowth of pathogens. Finally, staphylococci may cause a type of food poisoning that is different from the infectious variety; symptoms result from ingestion of bacterial toxins rather than from actual enteric infection by living organisms.

PNEUMOCOCCI. — *Streptococcus pneumoniae* (pneumococci) are gram-positive diplococci, which are still the most common cause of bacterial pneumonia in adults. They also produce many pediatric cases of middle ear infection and are an important etiology of meningitis, most commonly in debilitated persons. All strains are very sensitive to penicillin. Pneumococci usually produce alpha (green) incomplete hemolysis on blood agar and thus mimic viridans streptococci. Morphologic differentiation from streptococci may be difficult, especially in cultures, since streptococci may appear singly or in pairs (instead of chains), and pneumococci often do not have the typical "lancet" shape or diplococcic pattern. In the laboratory, differentiation is readily made because of the special sensitivity of pneumococci to a compound known as optochin. A disk impregnated with optochin is placed on the culture plate; inhibition of an alpha-hemolytic coccus denotes pneumococci.

Gram-Negative Cocci

Gram-negative diplococci include *Neisseria* organisms, such as the meningococcic and gonococcic families. Meningitis due to meningococci is still the most common type, although the incidence varies with age group (p. 201). Incidentally, nonpathogenic *Neisseria* organisms are common normal inhabitants of the nasopharynx, and it takes special subculturing to differentiate these from the meningococcic variety which are not normally present.

GONOCOCCI. — Gonococci are the cause of gonorrheal urethritis and the majority of cases of acute salpingitis, so-called pelvic inflammatory disease (PID). Chronic salpingitis (chronic PID) may occur either as residual effects of one or more episodes of acute gonorrheal salpingitis or from tubal infection by other organisms (mainly streptococcus or *E. coli*) after the original gonorrheal infection has disappeared. A presumptive diagnosis of gonorrhea can often be made from a cervical smear or male urethral discharge smear prepared by Gram stain. The organisms appear as gram-negative intracellular diplococci, located within the cytoplasm of polymorphonuclear neutrophils. Extracellular organisms are not considered reliable for diagnosis. Certain other organisms (Mima species) may have a similar morphologic appearance to the gonococcus; the Mima bacteria are usually extracellular, but can be intracellular. Nevertheless, the consensus seems to be that diagnosis of gonorrhea can be made from a urethral smear with reasonable confidence if there are definite organisms having characteristic morphology within neutrophils. In males if a urethral exudate is present, a smear is usually all that is required. The patient can wait while the smear is processed; and if the smear is negative or equivocal, a culture can be obtained. In females, although a gram-stained smear can be prepared from the endocervix, the number of positive diagnoses from such a smear are much less frequent. Cultures should therefore be taken, both to supplement the smear as a screening technique and to provide a definitive diagnosis. A study from the U.S. Communicable Disease Center indicates that in females the endocervical canal (after removal of mucus) is the single best site for culture; about 82% of cases will be detected. Surprisingly, in that study about 50% of patients had positive rectal cultures (swab culture using an anoscope, taking care to avoid fecal contamination). The combination of endocervical and rectal culture raised the percent detected to 92–94%. Culture of other sites did not increase the yield. The remaining 6–8% of cases were discovered on repeat culture 1 week later.

Although it is well known that gonorrhea in females is often not clinically evident, several studies have demonstrated positive urethral cultures in a small but significant percentage of asymptomatic males.

All the *Neisseria* have to be cultured on special media, such as Thayer-Martin (which is replacing the less selective chocolate agar), and usually grow best in high carbon dioxide atmospheres. A modification of the Thayer-Martin medium, called Transgrow, is being used for immediate specimen inoculation to keep organisms alive while transporting the culture to a laboratory.

CHLAMYDIA.—Nongonococcal urethritis is being reported frequently, and some believe that it is more frequent than gonorrhea, especially in males. *Chlamydia trachomatis* (p. 187) is the most commonly reported organism. T mycoplasmas are frequently cultured, but their relationship to disease is not yet proved. Reiter's syndrome might also be mentioned. Other diseases include lymphogranuloma venereum (p. 188, caused by another *Chlamydia* organism closely related to *C. trachomatis*), syphilis, granuloma inguinale (p. 150), trichomonas (p. 195), chancroid, herpesvirus type 2, molluscum contagiosum and condylomata acuminata. In females, infection of the vaginal region by *Candida* organisms and by *Corynebacterium* organisms (*Hemophilus vaginalis*) are fairly common, but venereal transmission is disputed.

Enteric Bacilli (Enterobacteriaceae)

These organisms form a large family of gram-negative rods. As their name implies, the majority of these bacteria are found primarily in the intestinal tract. These include salmonellae, shigellae, *E. coli*, *Enterobacter*, *Klebsiella* organisms, *Proteus* organisms and the paracolons. Many are normal inhabitants and cause disease only if they escape to other locations or if certain pathogenic types overgrow; others are introduced from contaminated food or water. Salmonellae and shigellae are not normal gastrointestinal inhabitants and always mean a source of infection from the environment.

SALMONELLA.—These organisms cause several clinical syndromes. Typhoid fever is produced by *S. typhosa* (*S. typhi*). The classic symptoms are a rising fever during the first week, a plateau at 103–104°F for the second week, then a slow fall during the third week, plus gastrointestinal symptoms and splenomegaly. There is a mild leukopenia with a lymphocytosis and monocytosis. Despite fever, the pulse rate tends to be slow (bradycardia). This picture is often not present in its entirety. During the first and second weeks of illness, blood cultures are the best means of diagnosis; thereafter, the incidence of positive specimens very rapidly declines. During the latter part of the second week to the early part of the fourth week, stool cultures are the most valuable source of diagnosis. However, stools may occasionally be positive in the first week; in carriers, positive stool cultures may persist for long periods. (About 3–5% of typhoid patients become carriers—persons with chronic subclinical infection.) Urine cultures may be done during the third and fourth weeks, but are not very effective. At best, blood cultures will miss at least 20% of cases, stool cultures at least 25% and urine cultures at least 75%. Repeated cultures increase the chance of diagnosis. Besides cultures, serologic tests may be performed. There are three major antigens in the *Salmonella typhosa*—the H (flagellar), O (somatic), and Vi (capsule or envelope). Antibody titers against these antigens constitute the Widal test. Most authorities agree that of the three antibodies, only that against the O antigen is meaningful for diagnosis. Vaccination causes a marked increase in the anti-H antibodies; the anti-O antibodies rise to a lesser degree and return much more quickly to normal. The Widal test (anti-O) antibodies begin to appear about 7–10 days after onset of illness. The highest percentage of positive tests is reported to be in the third and fourth weeks. As in any serologic test, a rising titer is more significant than a single determination. There has been considerable controversy over the usefulness of the Widal test in diagnosis of *Salmonella* infections. It seems to have definite, but limited, usefulness. Drawbacks of the Widal test include the following: (1) antibodies do not develop early in the illness, and may be suppressed by antibiotic therapy; (2) antibody behavior is often variable and often does not correlate with the severity of the clinical picture; (3) an appreciable number of cases (15% or more) do not have a significantly elevated anti-O titer, especially if only one determination is done. To summarize: in typhoid fever, blood cultures during the first and second weeks and stool cultures during the second, third, and fourth weeks are the diagnostic tests of choice. The Widal test may also be helpful.

Paratyphoid fever (enteric fever) is produced by salmonellae other than *S. typhosa;* the clinical picture is similar to typhoid fever, but milder. *Salmonella schottmülleri* and *S. paratyphi* are the most common causes in the United States. Diagnosis is similar to that of typhoid fever.

In the United States, salmonella gastroenteritis is probably next in frequency after typhoid or enteric fever. The gastroenteritis syndrome has a short incubation, features abdominal pain, nausea and diarrhea, and is most commonly produced by *S. typhimurium.* There is usually a leukocytosis with a minimal increase in neutrophils, in contrast to the usual finding in typhoid fever. Blood cultures are said to be negative; stool cultures are usually positive.

In addition to these syndromes, salmonellae may cause other types of disease. Septicemia may occasionally be found, and salmonellae may rarely cause focal infection in various organs, resulting in pneumonia, meningitis and endocarditis. Salmonella osteomyelitis has been associated with sickle cell anemia, for unknown reasons.

SHIGELLA.—The shigellae are the next most important sources of intestinal infection after the salmonellae. *Shigella* organisms cause so-called bacillary dysentery. Shigellae usually remain localized to the colon and do not enter the peripheral blood; blood cultures are therefore negative, in contrast to early *Salmonella* infection. Stool culture is the main diagnostic test. Besides salmonellae and shigellae, certain other bacteria (such as staphylococci and certain strains of *E. coli*) may cause gastrointestinal infection; these will be covered elsewhere.

ENTEROBACTER AND KLEBSIELLA.—These organisms are normal gastrointestinal inhabitants. Nomenclature has been particularly confusing in relation to these organisms. *Enterobacter* was formerly called *Aerobacter*. *Enterobacter (Aerobacter)* and *Klebsiella* have differences in reaction to certain test media, but are similar enough that previous classification included both in the same group. According to previous custom, if infection by these organisms was in the lungs it was called *Klebsiella* (Friedländer's pneumonia); if it was in the urinary tract, it was called *Aerobacter*. *Klebsiella* produces a resistant necrotizing pneumonia, which often cavitates and which is characteristically found in alcoholics and debilitated patients. *Enterobacter* causes one of the more frequent urinary tract infections, which is often resistant to therapy and occasionally produces septicemia.

Present classification differentiates *Enterobacter* from *Klebsiella*. Sources of confusion include the family name Enterobacteriaceae, which is similar to the name of one component genus. Enterobacteriaceae is a group of several tribes, each of which contains a genus or genera. One tribe, Klebsiellae, has a similar name to one of its three component genera, Klebsiella, and also includes the genus Enterobacter. A further source of difficulty is that the predominant species of Klebsiella is *K. pneumoniae*—which, in spite of the name, is found more frequently in the urinary tract than the lungs.

ESCHERICHIA COLI.—This organism is the most common cause of urinary tract infection. As with any urinary tract pathogen, this organism may occasionally reach the bloodstream and cause septicemia. This is more frequent with urinary tract obstruction. *Escherichia coli* is one of the most common etiologies for severe infections, especially meningitis, in the newborn. In addition, certain strains of *E. coli* have caused epidemic diarrhea in infants. However, since *E. coli* is a normal intestinal organism, a stool culture growing *E. coli* is of uncertain significance unless one of these special subtypes is present.

PROTEUS.—This is a gram-negative rod probably second to *E. coli* for frequency in urinary tract infection.

THE PARACOLONS.—The paracolons comprise a sort of dumping ground for gram-negative rods that have certain laboratory characteristics similar to *E. coli* although cultural behavior in other respects resembles that of other enteric bacteria groups. There are four main subgroups of paracolons; *Bethesda (Citrobacter)*, *Providencia*, *Arizona*, and *Serratia*. Originally, it was thought that members of the paracolon group were nonpathogenic and that their importance was only in the necessity for differentiation from more pathogenic enteric organisms such as *Salmonella*. Now, however, it is recognized that these organisms produce disease, especially urinary tract infections, septicemia and pulmonary infections, so that the organisms have been reclassified according to predominant culture characteristics. *Serratia* is usually considered the most dangerous of these organisms.

Other Gram-Negative Organisms

PSEUDOMONAS. — This gram-negative rod is not classified with the Enterobacteriaceae, although it may be found normally in the gastrointestinal tract. Infection is less common than with any of the Enterobacteriaceae, but becomes more frequent in certain special situations. In human disease, *Pseudomonas* has many aspects similar to "opportunistic fungi," in that infection is most often superimposed on serious underlying diseases, such as leukemia. *Pseudomonas* is relatively resistant to many of the standard antibiotics, such as penicillin, sulfa and tetracycline, and thus assumes importance as a secondary invader after antibiotic therapy of the original infection. This is most frequent in urinary tract infections. *Pseudomonas* may be found normally on the skin (as well as in the gastrointestinal tract), and thus is a very important and frequent problem in severe burns. *Pseudomonas septicemia* is not common, but is increasing as a complication or a terminal event in the conditions just mentioned.

CALYMMATOBACTERIUM GRANULOMATIS (DONOVANIA GRANULOMATIS). Granuloma inguinale is a venereal disease caused by a gram-negative rod bacterium that has some antigenic similarity to the *Klebsiella* group. Infection is transmitted by sexual contact. After incubation, an elevated irregular flattened granulomatous lesion develops, usually in or around the medial aspect of the inguinal area or on the labia. The organism is difficult to culture and requires special media, so that culture is not usually done. Diagnosis is accomplished by demonstration of the organisms in the form of characteristic "Donovan bodies," found in the cytoplasm of histiocytes. The best technique is to take a punch biopsy of the lesion, crush the fresh tissue between two glass slides, and make several smears with the crushed tissue. These smears are air-dried and stained with Wright's stain. (It is possible to process a biopsy in the routine manner and do special stains on tissue histologic sections, but this is not nearly as effective.) Granuloma inguinale is sometimes confused with lymphogranuloma venereum, a totally different disease, because of the similarity in names and the fact that both are venereal diseases.

HEMOPHILUS GROUP. — These are small gram-negative bacilli, of which the most important are *Hemophilus influenzae* and *Bordetella pertussis*. *Hemophilus influenzae* infection is not very frequent, but is an important cause of meningitis between the ages of 2 months and 2 years. Occasionally, *H. influenzae* may produce a serious type of laryngitis (croup) known as acute epiglottitis. These organisms require substances called X and V factor. Therefore, *Hemophilus* culture plates contain blood agar (supplying X factor) within which is a small area previously inoculated with *S. aureus* ("staph streak"), which supplies V factor. *Bordatella pertussis* is the etiologic agent of whooping cough. This is best isolated from nasopharyngeal cultures, preferably on the special Bordet-Gengou medium (cough plate).

Anaerobic Bacteria

CLOSTRIDIA. — These gram-positive anaerobic rods include several important organisms. *Clostridium perfringens (C. welchii)* is the usual cause of gas gangrene. It is a normal inhabitant of the gastrointestinal tract, and reportedly can be isolated from the skin in about 20% of patients and from the vagina and female genitalia in about 5%. Therefore, just as with *S. aureus,* culture reports of *C. welchii* from an external wound do not necessarily mean that the organism is producing clinical infection. *Clostridium tetani* is the etiology of tetanus. This organism is only rarely found in the human gastrointestinal tract. Clinical disease is produced by release of bacterial exotoxin after local infection in a manner analogous to diphtheria. The third important clostridia organism is *C. botulinum.* Botulism, a severe food poisoning, is precipitated by ingestion of bacterial endotoxin already formed in contaminated food, rather than from actual infection of the patient by the bacterium. Clostridial infection, with the exception of *C. tetani* and *botulinum,* is associated with certain clinical situations. Wound infection is the most frequent, although in the majority of cases the clostridia coexist with other organisms and do not produce gangrene. The other major area of concern is septic (criminal) abortion.

Botulism is frequently confused with other types of "food poisoning." *Clostridium botulinum* produces a powerful neurotoxin and is usually associated with canned food, especially home-canned. Vegetables are the most frequently involved home-canned food, but any variety of canned food may become contaminated. Fortunately, the disease is not common. Although the endotoxin is preformed, symptoms most often appear 12–36 hours after ingestion and commonly include nausea, vomiting, vision difficulties and cranial nerve signs, such as dysarthria and dysphagia, usually without fever or vomiting. Diarrhea is either absent or a very minor component. *Staphylococcus aureus* may grow in certain foods (typically custards, creams, potato salad and ham, usually when allowed to remain warm), and produce a preformed exotoxin. Symptoms usually occur less than 7 hours after ingestion of the food (average 3 hours), and consist of nausea, vomiting, abdominal cramps and diarrhea. *Clostridium perfringens* occasionally may contaminate food, typically meat or gravy, that has been cooked and then allowed to cool slowly. Symptoms are due to exotoxin formed within the intestine, occur about 12 hours after eating, and consist of simultaneous abdominal cramps and diarrhea without fever or vomiting. *Vibrio parahaemolyticus* is ingested with raw or poorly cooked fish or shellfish. The organism may invade tissue or may produce an exotoxin. Average onset of symptoms is 12–24 hours after ingestion; symptoms of vomiting, nausea, cramps, diarrhea, chills and fever. *Escherichia coli* may be transmitted via contaminated food or water but also by personal contact. The organism may invade tissue or may produce an exotoxin. Symptoms occur 10–12 hours after contact, and consist of vomiting, nausea, cramps, diarrhea, chills and fever. *Salmonella* or *Shigella* gastroenteritis is due to tissue infection by the organisms, although *Shigella* is capable of toxin production. *Shigella* dysentery symptoms ordinarily occur 36–48 hours after infection, but the time is variable. *Salmonella* gastroenteritis (due to species other than *S. typhosa*) is most frequently associated with poultry, eggs and egg products, powdered milk and fresh pork. Symptoms most often become manifest in 8–48 hours, with an average onset time of 24 hours. Symptoms of both *Shigella* and *Salmonella* gastroenteritis are similar to those of *E. coli*. *Salmonella* dysentery should be differentiated from typhoid and paratyphoid fever, which have considerably longer incubations and different emphases in symptoms.

Some differential points include the incubation period; less than 7 hours suggests *S. aureus*, and about 12 hours, *C. perfringens*. Blood, mucus or segmented neutrophils in the stool are not found with *C. perfringens* and *V. parahaemolyticus*. Pus in the stool suggests *Shigella*, although this may also occur with *E. coli* and *Salmonella*. *Clostridium perfringens* usually does not induce vomiting; *C. botulinum* illness frequently does not include significant diarrhea but does have neurologic abnormalities.

Laboratory diagnosis usually involves stool culture and culture of the contaminated food. *Clostridium botulinum* can be confirmed by special tests for botulinus toxin on serum (preferably before treatment), although gastric contents and feces can also be used. The specimens or potential specimens should be kept in the refrigerator, since the toxin is heat labile. The mouse-toxin neutralization test is the standard procedure used. State Public Health laboratories or the Communicable Disease Center, Atlanta, Georgia, should be contacted for details.

BACTEROIDES. — Anaerobic infections usually center on three groups of organisms — clostridia, bacteroides, and the anaerobic streptococci. The clostridia are discussed above. Bacteroides species are anaerobic gram-negative rods normally found in the mouth, the intestine and the female genital tract. Isolation of these organisms often raises the question of their significance or pathogenicity. It seems well established that bacteroides occasionally cause serious infection, which frequently results in abscess or gangrene. The most commonly associated clinical situations include septic abortion, aspiration pneumonia, and focal lesions of the gastrointestinal tract (such as carcinoma or appendicitis).

ANAEROBIC STREPTOCOCCI. — These are frequently associated with *Bacteroides* infection but may themselves produce disease. They are normally present in the mouth and gastrointestinal tract. Septic abortion and superinfection of lesions in the perirectal area seem to be the most commonly associated factors. Anaerobic streptococci are also part of the fusiform bacteria-spirochetal synergistic disease known as Vincent's angina.

LISTERIA MONOCYTOGENES. — This is a gram-positive rod like the clostridia, but an aerobic (rather than anaerobic) organism that sometimes causes stillbirths, as well as septicemia or meningitis in newborns, especially in premature infants. Culture of the mother's lochia has been suggested as an aid in diagnosis, as well as blood cultures from the infant.

Uncommon Bacterial Diseases

DIPHTHERIA. — This disease is now uncommon, but cases appear from time to time, some of them fatal. Contrary to usual belief, the laboratory cannot make the diagnosis from gram-stained smears. Heat-fixed smears stained with methylene blue are better, but, although helpful in demonstrating organisms resembling diphtheria, they still are not considered reliable enough for definite morphologic diagnosis. Nonpathogenic diphtheroids are normal nasopharyngeal inhabitants and may resemble *Corynebacterium diphtheriae* closely. To be certain, one must culture the organisms on special media and do virulence (toxin production) studies. Direct gram-stained and methylene blue smears are of value, since other causes of pharyngeal inflammation and pseudomembrane formation, such as fungus and Vincent's angina, can be demonstrated. Therefore, two or three pharyngeal swabs should be obtained, if possible, to provide smears *and* cultures.

BRUCELLOSIS.—An uncommon disease, brucellosis sometimes must be considered in the differential diagnosis of fever of unknown origin. The brucella organism is a gram-negative coccobacillus with three main subgroups: one that infects cattle, one, goats; and one, swine. Classical brucellosis was most often transmitted to man via infected milk or milk products. However, workers in the meat-processing industry, especially those working with swine, are currently the main sufferers from brucellosis in the United States. Blood culture is the best means of isolation, but a special culture medium is required. A serologic slide agglutination test is the most frequent method of diagnosis (p. 161).

TULAREMIA.—Although uncommon, tularemia occasionally should be considered in fever of unknown origin. The organism is a small gram-negative coccobacillus. Small wild animals, such as the rabbit, constitute the main reservoir of infection, and most people who acquire tularemia are persons who handle raw game. Culture from lymph nodes or local lesions on special media is the best means of isolation but is not ordinarily done because of an unusually high rate of laboratory worker infection. A serologic slide agglutination test is the standard method for diagnosis (p. 161).

Spirochetal Diseases

Only three members of this large group of diseases will be mentioned. Vincent's angina is an infection of the mouth caused by an interesting synergistic group of organisms, including anaerobic streptococci, a fusiform gram-negative bacillus, and a spirochete. Gram-stained smears demonstrating all three organisms are usually sufficient for diagnosis. Syphilis is a very important disease and is discussed separately in Chapter 31. Weil's disease is caused by a spirochete of the *Leptospira* genus. Transmission is usually through accidental contamination by infected rat urine. The most striking findings are a combination of hepatitis and glomerulonephritis, clinically manifested by jaundice with hematuria. Therefore, the disease is sometimes considered in the differential diagnosis of jaundice of unknown etiology. In classic cases after an incubation period there is abrupt onset of high fever, severe malaise, conjunctivitis, headache and muscle ache. Chills may be present. Toward the end of the first week the fever starts to subside and a new set of symptoms begins to develop, including hepatitis and nephritis. This stage lasts about a week and is followed by improvement or death. Milder cases may lack one or many of these signs and symptoms. Symptoms of meningitis may occasionally predominate. Laboratory findings include a leukocytosis with a shift to the left. A mild normocytic-normochromic anemia usually develops by the second week. Platelet counts are normal. After jaundice develops, liver function test results are similar to those in viral hepatitis. After onset of kidney involvement, the BUN is often elevated, and hematuria is present with proteinuria. Cerebrospinal fluid examination shows normal sugar but increased cell count, which varies according to the severity of the case; initially, these are mainly neutrophils, but later on the lymphocytes predominate. Cultures on ordinary bacterial media are negative.

Diagnosis often depends on isolating the organisms, or demonstrating specific antibodies in the serum. During the first week (days 1–8), spirochetes may be found in the blood by darkfield in about 8% of the cases and can be cultured from the blood in many more. Instead of ordinary blood cultures, 1–3 drops of blood are inoculated into a special culture medium (Fletcher's), since larger quantities of blood inhibit the growth of leptospires. The cerebrospinal fluid may be cultured toward the end of the first week. During the second week the blood quickly becomes negative. During the third week (days 14–21) the spirochetes may often be recovered from the urine of those patients with nephritis. Animal inoculation is the most successful method. Antibodies start to appear at about the seventh day and are present in the majority of cases by the twelfth day. Antibodies persist for months and years after cure. A titer of 1:300 is considered diagnostic, although, without a rising titer, past infection could not be ruled out completely. If a significant titer has not developed by the twenty-first day, it would be very rare for it to do so later. In summary, blood cultures during the first week and serologic tests during the second and third weeks are the diagnostic methods of choice.

Tuberculosis

Tuberculosis is still very important and common despite advances in drug therapy. The disease usually begins in the chest; in this location the most important symptoms are cough, fever and hemoptysis. (The most important diseases to rule out are lung carcinoma and bronchiectasis.) The kidney is involved in a significant percentage of advanced cases, with the main symtom being hematuria (p. 122). The laboratory findings in tuberculosis depend to some extent on the stage and severity of the disease.

Chest x-rays.—These are often the first evidence to suggest tuberculosis, and provide a valuable parameter of severity, activity and response to therapy. Depending on the situation, there are a variety of possible roentgen findings. These may include one or more of the following:

1. Enlargement of hilar lymph nodes.
2. Localized pulmonary infiltrates. These occur characteristically in upper lobe apical location or, less commonly, the superior segment of the lower lobes. Cavitation of lesions may occur.
3. Miliary spread (small punctate lesions widely distributed). This pattern is not common, and occasionally may be missed on routine chest films.
4. Unilateral pleural effusion. The most common causes are tuberculosis, carcinoma, and congestive heart failure. Tuberculosis causes 60–80% of so-called idiopathic pleural effusions.

Sputum smear.—These provide a rapid presumptive diagnosis. They are stained by one of the acid-fast (AFB) procedures (usually Ziehl-Neelsen's method). Fluorescent staining methods are also available, and many feel they are more sensitive. The more advanced the infection, the more likely it is to yield a positive smear. Therefore, the rate of positive findings is low in early, minimal or healing tuberculosis. A substantial minority of advanced cases may also be negative. Culture is more reliable for detection of tuberculosis, and also is necessary for confirmation of the diagnosis, for differentiation of *Mycobacterium tuberculosis* from the "atypical" mycobacteria and for sensitivity studies of chemotherapeutic agents. Sputum specimens should be collected (for culture and smear of the concentrated specimen) once a day for at least 3 days. If the smear is definitely positive, it will not be necessary to have more smears done. Also, this means a probable positive culture on the specimens already collected, and it would not be necessary to collect more than 3 specimens or to proceed to more complicated diagnostic procedures. If smears are negative, then one has to consider the possibility that the culture may also be negative, and cultures take from 3 to 8 weeks to demonstrate growth. Therefore, other procedures may be considered for diagnosis so as not to lose so much time.

Culture.—Sputum is preferred for pulmonary tuberculosis (gastric aspiration if sputum is not satisfactory); urine for renal involvement; bone marrow in miliary tuberculosis. Reports indicate that an early morning specimen produces as many positive results as a 24-hour specimen, either of sputum or urine, and has much less contamination. Special culture media are needed. The necessity for adequate sputum culture specimens, regardless of the concentrated smear findings, has already been mentioned. Several reports indicate that aerosol techniques will produce a significantly greater yield of positive culture than will ordinary sputum collection. The aerosol mixture irritates the bronchial tree and stimulates sputum production. At any rate, it is necessary to get a "deep cough" specimen; saliva will not be adequate. If sputum cultures are negative, or the patient is unable to produce adequate sputum samples, gastric aspiration may be used. Note that gastric contents are suitable for culture only; nontuberculous acid-fast organisms may be found normally and cannot be distinguished from *M. tuberculosis* on AFB smear. If renal tuberculosis is suspected, urine culture should be done (this is discussed in chapter 12). Even with urine specimens on 3 consecutive days, only about 30% of cases are positive.

Skin test (Mantoux test).—This is performed with PPD or old tuberculin (Table 14–1). A positive result is an area of induration at least 5 mm in diameter by 48 hours. A positive skin test is a manifestation of hypersensi-

TABLE 14–1.—COMPARISON OF TUBERCULOSIS SKIN TESTS°

Tuberculin units (TU)	1	10	250
Micrograms of PPD	0.02	0.2	5.0
"Strength" of PPD	1st	Intermediate	2d
OT equivalent	1:10,000	1:1,000†	1:100
Milligrams of OT	0.01	0.1	1.0

°Old tuberculin (OT) and purified protein derivative (PPD).

†Some use the equivalent of a 1:2,000 intermediate strength (5 TU or 0.1 μg of PPD).

tivity to the tubercle bacillus. This reaction usually develops about 6 weeks after infection, although it may take several months. A positive reaction means previous contact and infection with tuberculosis; the positive reaction does not itself indicate whether the disease is currently active or inactive. However, in children under 3 years of age it usually means active tuberculosis infection. Apparently, once positive, the reaction persists for many years or for life, although there is evidence that a significant number of persons revert to negative if the infection is completely cured early enough. A few apparently never develop a positive test. The Mantoux test may revert to negative or fail to become positive in the following circumstances:

1. Occasionally but not frequently in old age or cachexia.
2. High percentage of patients with miliary tuberculosis.
3. High percentage of patients with overwhelming pulmonary tuberculosis.
4. A considerable number of patients who are on steroid therapy.
5. Many persons who also have sarcoidosis or Hodgkin's disease.

The standard procedure for skin testing is to begin with an intermediate-strength PPD (or the equivalent). If the person has serious infection, it is wise to begin with a first-strength dose, to avoid necrosis at the injection site. A significant minority of patients with tuberculosis (9–17%) fail to react with intermediate strength PPD; a second-strength dose is then indicated.

Biopsy. — Miliary tuberculosis is usually widely disseminated in the body via hematogenous spread. When routine clinical and culture methods fail, biopsy of bone marrow or liver may be useful. Liver biopsy shows a fairly good positive yield, considering that a needle biopsy specimen is such a tiny random sample of a huge organ. However, it is usually difficult to demonstrate acid-fast organisms on liver biopsy, even when tubercles are found — and without organisms, the diagnosis is not absolutely certain. Bone marrow aspiration is probably the best procedure is such cases. It yields much better results for mycobacterial culture than for demonstration of tubercles. Routine marrow (Wright-stained) smears are worthless for histologic diagnosis in tuberculosis. Aspirated material may be allowed to clot in the syringe, then Formalin-fixed and sent through as a regular biopsy specimen for histologic slides. Before clotting some of the aspirate is inoculated into suitable tuberculosis culture media. It should be emphasized that bone marrow aspiration or liver biopsy is not indicated in pulmonary tuberculosis (since this disease is relatively localized), only in miliary tuberculosis.

ATYPICAL MYCOBACTERIA. — Besides *M. tuberculosis*, there are other mycobacteria which are pathogenic for man. These have been termed the "atypical" mycobacteria (sometimes also called "unclassified" mycobacteria). At present, the most useful classification is that of Runyon, which subdivides the atypical mycobacteria into 4 groups, depending on growth and colony characteristics (Table 14–2). These divisions have clinical value. Group III (Battey strains) cause the majority of significant "atypical" infections, followed by group I. These organisms produce a disease similar to pulmonary tuberculosis, although often milder or more indolent. They

TABLE 14-2.—CLASSIFICATION OF THE
ATYPICAL MYCOBACTERIA

Group I	Photochromogens	(M. Kansasii)
Group II	Scotochromogens	(M. scrofulaceum)
Group III	Nonphotochromogens	(Battey)
Group IV	Rapid growers	(M. fortuitum and others)

are much more frequent in adults. Group II organisms are more frequent in children, and clinically tend to cause cervical lymphadenopathy. Diagnosis of the "atypical" mycobacteria is essentially the same as for M. tuberculosis. Skin tests (OT or PPD) for M. tuberculosis will also cross-react with the atypical mycobacteria. In general, the atypical mycobacteria tend to give less reaction to standard tuberculin skin tests than does M. tuberculosis infection. In fact, several studies claim that the majority of positive intermediate strength tuberculin skin tests that are less than 10 mm (reaction diameter) are due to atypical mycobacterial infection rather than tuberculosis. Skin test antigens are available for each of the atypical mycobacterial groups, although some reports challenge the specificity of these preparations. The main clinical importance of these "atypical" organisms is the fact that many are resistant to one or more of the standard antituberculous chemotherapeutic agents.

OTHER BACTERIAL INFECTIONS.—Coverage of bacterial infections in this chapter has been limited to the common organisms in clinical practice and a few that enter the differential diagnosis of certain common situations, such as hepatitis or fever of unknown origin. Many others here been omitted, such as those which cause plague, cholera, relapsing fever, and chancroid. In general, most of these are diagnosed through culture of appropriate specimens, such as stool for cholera and blood culture for plague. In addition, common laboratory contaminants, such as the diphtheroids and Bacillus subtilis, have not been mentioned. The reader is referred to standard textbooks on microbiology for consideration of these organisms and for more information on those which are discussed briefly.

GENERAL ISOLATION AND IDENTIFICATION TECHNIQUES

It is useful to know certain technical information involved with isolation and identification of bacteria. These facts may be of assistance to aid communication between the physician and the microbiology laboratory, for the benefit of each. It usually takes at least 48 hours, and often longer, for definitive diagnosis, 1 day to culture the organism, 1 to isolate it and often 1 or more days extra to identify it. A technician uses knowledge of the site and source of culture material in deciding what media or techniques (such as anaerobic conditions) to use for isolation. Some organisms are normal inhabitants of certain body areas but pathogens in other areas, so that an experienced technician knows to some extent what to subculture from a mixture of organisms growing in a specific location and also what special media to use for the pathogens usual in that anatomic location. This knowledge can easily save a day's time. Information that a certain specific organism is suspected may save even more, by allowing original inoculation of the culture material onto special test media. Even if definitive isolation is not yet accomplished, the technicians can often provide useful information or even a presumptive diagnosis. For example, among the enteric gram-negative rods, *E. coli, Aerobacter,* and *Klebsiella* ferment lactose, while most of the other pathogens do not. Therefore, a lactose-fermenter cannot be *Salmonella* or *Shigella.* The *Pseudomonas* group, in addition, does not ferment glucose, while most of the other pathogens do. Some of these organisms have characteristic appearances on isolation media. Some of the gram-positive aerobic bacteria produce a fairly typical appearance on original blood agar culture plates; combining this with gram stain morphology may yield a rapid presumptive diagnosis.

Taking a Culture

When any culture is taken, three things should be done. First, the culture must be taken to the laboratory as soon as possible, since many organisms die on prolonged exposure to air or drying. This is especially true for swab preparations. Swab kits are available that contain a "carrier" medium into which the specimen is placed. This is a great help in preserving most bacteria, but the medium may not be ideal for some organisms. Second, the source of the culture should be written on the request form. Finally, if a specific organism is suspected, this information should also be written on the request, so that if special culture methods are required for that organism, the requisite techniques will be anticipated and used.

BLOOD CULTURE.—To obtain material for blood culture, not only must proper aseptic techniques be followed, but extra precautions must be taken to avoid contamination by skin bacteria. Iodine should be used, if possible, because it has the most efficient bactericidal effect of the common solutions available. However, since iodine is irritating to the skin, it must be removed shortly after application with less-powerful antiseptics, such as alcohol or benzalkonium chloride.

URINE CULTURE.—For urine cultures, contamination with vaginal or labial bacteria is a serious problem. Catheterization is one way to solve this, but approximately 2% of patients develop urinary tract infection following a single catheterization. Therefore, a "midstream" voided specimen is the next best procedure. The urinary opening is cleansed. The labia are held apart in the female and the foreskin pulled back in the male. The first portion of urine is allowed to pass uncollected; then the sterile container is quickly introduced into the urine stream to catch the specimen. Quantitative urine cultures have now replaced simple cultures, since it has been shown that a titer of 100,000 or more organisms per ml has excellent correlation to clinical infection, whereas less than 10,000 organisms per ml very rarely proves significant. However, in some cases of pyelonephritis, cultures may be positive at some times but not at others, depending on the fluctuations of the disease and its anatomic location. A culture containing fewer than 10,000 organisms per ml is considered negative, but it may have to be repeated if clinically indicated. On the other hand, although this dilution procedure is supposed to compensate for small degrees of unavoidable contamination, contamination can easily be severe enough to give a positive result. Therefore, good technique in collecting the specimen is essential. Also essential is getting the specimen to the laboratory as soon as possible after collection. Urine is an excellent culture medium, and specimens which stand for more than 1 hour allow bacterial incubation and proliferation to the point at which quantitative counts are not reliable. If delivery to the laboratory must be delayed, the specimen should be refrigerated. The specimen can be preserved up to 12 hours in a refrigerator (4°C).

Kits with agar-coated slides are now available that not only yield quantitative urine culture results but also act as a culture medium for the organisms. These are reported to have 90–98% accuracy in various university hospital laboratories compared to standard quantitative culture methods. The average is about 95% reliability. There is a question whether office laboratories can approach this figure, and what provision would be made to identify the organisms.

Quantitative urine culture has two other drawbacks. Culture involves trained technical personnel and relatively expensive media, thus curtailing use for mass screening to detect urinary tract infection. Culture takes 24 hours to determine bacterial quantity and another 24–48 hours to identify the organism, thus delaying treatment in suspected infection. Therefore, several screening tests have been introduced for rapid detection of significant degrees of bacteriuria. Gram stain of uncentrifuged urine roughly indicates a good probability of a positive quantitative culture, if organisms are seen; the same is said to be true of direct examination of unstained centrifuged urine sediment. Gram-stained centrifuged sediment apparently gives too many false positives. Gram-stained uncentrifuged urine and unstained urine sediment examination are said to give relatively few false positives. Several chemical methods have been advocated; the most successful include the triphenyl tetrazolium chloride (TTC) test, the Greiss nitrate test and the catalase test. Best results have been reported with the TTC. Nevertheless, reports vary as to its accuracy, with a range of 70–90% correlation with quantitative culture, including both false positive and false negative results. The Greiss technique gives similar results, although slightly less good. The catalase test is considerably less reliable. Positive tests by any of these methods must be confirmed with quantitative culture; negative tests do not completely rule out urinary tract infection.

Although quantitative culture is widely considered the most reliable index of urinary tract infection, there are at least five major limitations.

1. A positive culture has reduced, but has not entirely eliminated, the possibility of contamination (as noted earlier).

2. A positive culture does not localize the actual area involved.

3. Bacteremia from many causes, even if transient, is filtered by the kidney and may give a temporarily positive quantitative culture.

4. Tuberculosis of the urinary tract will give a negative result on ordinary culture media.

5. Some cases of urinary tract infection may give negative cultures at various periods. In several studies, a sizable minority of patients required repeated cultures before 1 became positive. This may be due to the location of the infection in the kidney and to its degree of activity.

In summary, two cautions are required when a quantitative urine culture report is received. If the report is positive, the physician must be sure the specimen was properly collected, especially in the female; if the report is negative, this does not rule out chronic pyelonephritis. The problem of pyelonephritis and bacteriuria was discussed in Chapter 12.

SPUTUM CULTURE. — The usefulness of sputum culture has been questioned. This method of diagnosis has evoked the same spectrum of emotions and suffers from most of the same potential drawbacks as Gram's stain of sputum. Various studies have demonstrated that either sputum or bronchoscopic specimens are frequently contaminated by upper respiratory tract bacteria. Some of the contaminants, such as *S. aureus, Diplococcus pneumoniae, H. influenzae* and *Candida* organisms, are potential lower respiratory tract pathogens. In addition, bronchoscopy may introduce local anesthetic into the specimen. Transtracheal aspiration (insertion of a needle into the trachea) or direct needle aspiration of the lung have been shown to produce relatively uncontaminated specimens. However, these techniques have potential complications. While there is general agreement on contamination, there is difference of opinion in the literature about the possibility that sputum culture may sometimes fail to detect the bacteria responsible for pneumonia. The importance of a specimen from the lower respiratory tract rather than the mouth or nasopharynx must be reemphasized, especially in seriously ill, uncooperative or mentally clouded patients. As mentioned previously, a "pure culture" or marked predominance of one organism enhances suspicion of pathogenicity.

Gram's Stain

Hopefully, this method provides a presumptive diagnosis and some indication of the organism involved without waiting for culture results. On occasion, Gram's stain may reveal organisms that (for technical reasons) do not grow when cultured. Best information is obtained from normally sterile specimens. The Gram method of staining is considered a routine procedure for cerebrospinal fluid in possible meningitis, for urethral smears in possible venereal disease and for material from abscesses or effusions. (This is especially true when anaerobes may be present. These may fail to grow since "anaerobic" culture is often suboptimal, but the organisms might be seen on a Gram stain). In certain other types of specimens, such as urine or stool, a Gram stain need not be done routinely, but should be performed in special circumstances, such as on stool specimens when pseudomembranous enterocolitis is suspected or on urine specimens if quantitative culture is not available.

In several other areas use of a Gram stain is controversial. The most important example is sputum. One can find opinions in the literature on usefulness of a sputum Gram stain ranging from "essential" to "worthless and misleading." One major problem is contamination by normal organisms from the mouth and nasopharynx. Certain pathogens, such as pneumococci or *S. aureus* may be located in the upper respiratory tract of many clinically normal persons, and these may gain entry into the sputum. Another difficulty is occasional discovery of opportunists in the lower respiratory tract, organisms not normally present but not apparently causing disease. Another problem is the morphologic similarity frequently displayed by pneumococci and streptococci, among others. Finally, and most important, so-called sputum may, in reality, be only saliva.

There are certain maneuvers which may help to circumvent some of these drawbacks. The number of organisms may provide a clue to their significance. Marked predominance or heavy growth of one organism suggests true abnormality. Many polymorphonuclear leukocytes would be in favor of acute infection. Significant quantities of squamous epithelial cells (more than 10 per low power field) usually means oral contamination. The patient should be instructed how to produce a "deep cough" and, if possible, should be observed while this is done. In some cases aerosol therapy may be helpful.

Febrile Agglutinins

Febrile agglutinins are serologic tests for a group of unrelated infectious diseases that are sometimes responsible for so-called fever of unknown origin (FUO). They include typhoid and enteric *(Salmonella)* fever, certain rickettsial diseases, brucellosis and tularemia. Since these organisms are the ones most frequently considered in FUO situations, and since relatively simple slide agglutination serologic techniques are available for each, most laboratories automatically include the same selection of tests when "febrile agglutinins" are ordered. Typhoid or enteric ("paratyphoid") fever may be caused by several organisms of the *Salmonella* gram-negative rod family (p. 147). The more common salmonellae are separated into groups on the basis of antigens prepared from these organisms; these antigens are used to detect antibodies in the patient's serum (Widal test). The groups are given a letter designation; for example, S. *typhosa (S. typhi)* is included in *Salmonella* D (p. 482). The Widal agglutination test involves antibodies produced to the somatic (O) and flagellar (H) antigens of *Salmonella* organisms. These antibodies appear approximately 7–10 days after onset of illness. In nonvaccinated individuals or most of those vaccinated over 1 year previously, a titer of 1:40 for the H antigen and 1:80 for the O antigen are suspicious; 1:80 for the H antigen and 1:160 for the O antigen are definitely significant. However, recent (less than 1 year) vaccination may cause greatly increased titer of either or both the O and the H antigen. The O antigen is more significant for diagnosis than the H antigen.

Antibody-antigen agglutination tests for brucellosis and tularemia are also included. Again, titers of 1:80 are suspicious and 1:160 are definitely indicative. Antibodies appear 2–3 weeks after onset of the illness. Similar slide agglutination tests for rickettsia (Weil-Felix reaction) complete the febrile agglutinin battery. Interpretation of Weil-Felix results is given on page 186.

GENERAL CONCEPTS IN BACTERIAL INFECTION

The main systemic signs and symptoms of severe bacterial infection in general are fever and weakness; the most characteristic laboratory finding is a leukocytosis with an increase in number and immaturity of the neutrophils. However, in overwhelming infection, sometimes leukocytosis may be minimal or even absent; occasionally fever may be minimal or may not be present. This is not frequent, but happens more often in infants and the elderly. It is also more frequent in debilitated persons, especially those with other severe diseases that may impair the ability of the body to respond normally to infection. Overwhelming infection may be focal, such as massive pneumonia, or generalized, such as septicemia.

Septicemia and Bacteremia

The concept of *septicemia* should probably be separated from that of *bacteremia*. In many focal infections, a few bacteria escape from time to time into the peripheral blood. However, the main focus remains localized, and symptoms are primarily those that are secondary to the particular organ or tissues involved. In septicemia there is widespread and relatively continuous peripheral blood involvement; characteristically, the symptoms are systemic, such as marked weakness, shock or near shock. This is usually accompanied by high fever and leukocytosis, although, as mentioned earlier, sometimes leukocytosis may be absent and occasionally even fever may be slight. Any bacteria may cause septicemia. The most common types are gram-negative rod organisms, with *S. aureus* probably next most frequent. Of the gram negatives, *E. coli* and *Aerobacter* are the most numerous. The portal of entry of the gram negatives is usually from previous urinary tract infection. Many cases follow surgery or instrumentation. The source of *Staphylococcus* is often very difficult to trace, even at autopsy. However, pneumonia and skin infections (sometimes very small) are the most frequent findings. Blood cultures are the mainstay of septicemia diagnosis. They should be drawn before antibiotic therapy is begun, although they may often be positive despite antibiotics. If penicillin has previously been given, this should be noted on the request slip, so that the antipenicillin enzyme penicillinase may be added to the culture media. (There is, however, some controversy over this technique. Some authorities believe that penicillinase is of little value and might actually be a source of contamination.) Strict aseptic technique should be used in obtaining cultures, since contamination from skin bacteria may give false or confusing results. In cases of bacteremia or in septicemia with spiking types of fever, the best time to draw blood cultures is just before or at the rise in temperature. Three cultures, one drawn every 3 hours, are a reasonable compromise among the widely diverging recommendations in the literature.

Subacute Bacterial Endocarditis

This disease falls about halfway between the concepts of bacteremia and septicemia. Bacteria grow in localized areas on damaged heart valves and seed the peripheral blood; this may be infrequent, intermittent or relatively continuous, with gradations between the two extremes. Classic signs and symptoms include fever, heart murmurs, petechial hemorrhages in the conjunctivas, small "splinter hemorrhages" in the fingernail beds and splenomegaly. Hematuria is very frequent, and red cell casts are a common and very suggestive finding. There often, but not always, is a normocytic and normochromic anemia. Leukocytosis is often present, but it too may be absent. Signs and symptoms are fairly variable in many individual patients, and the diagnostic problem is often that of a fever of unknown origin. The most frequent organisms responsible are alpha streptococci *(S. viridans)* and enterococci ("heat-resistant" streptococci). Some areas report that staphylococci are almost as common. However, almost any pathogenic bacteria may be the cause, and under certain special conditions (such as severe debilitation), even some ordinarily nonpathogenic organisms. For specific diagnosis, blood cultures must be obtained; the methods used are the same as those described under septicemia. Repeated cultures are much more necessary, because of the often intermittent nature of the blood involvement, and avoidance of culture contamination becomes even more important. About 15% of patients (literature range 2.5–31%) do not provide any positive blood cultures. Uremia is especially apt to be associated with negative cultures.

In some patients with subacute bacterial endocarditis (SBE) whose symptoms persist despite treatment, it is important to know whether antibiotic therapy really is effective in vivo. Also, some antibiotics, such as gentamycin, have a therapeutic range close to the toxic range. Blood levels of some antibiotics can be measured by radioimmunoassay. For estimate of in vivo effectiveness, a Schlichter test may be performed. A patient blood specimen is obtained just before the next antibiotic dose is to be given. A standard suspension of the organisms previously cultured from the patient is placed in serial dilutions of patient serum and incubated overnight. If the lowest serum dilutions do not inhibit growth of the organism, therapy is probably not effective. (There is some dispute on exact dilution level; Schlichter accepted 1:2, but others require 1:8.)

Pneumonia

Among other bacterial syndromes, gastrointestinal infection has been covered earlier, and meningitis is discussed in Chapter 18. Pneumonia, however, has not been examined as a separate entity. Although the term "pneumonia" denotes only inflammation of the lung, which could result from noninfectious sources, such as a chemical inflammation secondary to aspiration, the great majority of cases are due to bacterial or nonbacterial infectious agents. Except for the newborn, in the early pediatric age group viruses are the most common etiology, followed by *Staphylococcus* infections. In older children and young adults, viruses still markedly predominate, but pneumococci become more prevalent. In middle-aged and older adults, pneumococci assume considerable importance, although viruses still are more frequent numerically. In debilitated persons, alcoholics, those persons with depressed immunologic defenses and the elderly, pneumococci are still very important, but other bacteria become much more common, especially *Staphylococcus* and *Klebsiella*. Staphylococcic pneumonia is particularly likely to occur following a viral pneumonia, such as influenza. The most important nonbacterial agents are respiratory syncytial virus, influenza virus and *Mycoplasma pneumoniae* (Eaton agent). Diseases caused by viruses and mycoplasma are discussed in Chapter 16.

Intra-abdominal Abscess

Intra-abdominal abscess is a recurrent problem that deserves attention. Most use the term "subphrenic" synonymously with "intra-abdominal," although some use the term "subphrenic" to refer only to abscess just below the diaphragm. The most common etiologies are postoperative complications of biliary tract or peptic ulcer surgery, penetrating abdominal trauma and perforated appendix. From 80 to 90% occur intraperitoneally. The spaces above and below the liver are the most common locations. About 25% are located on the left side. The percentage of multiple abscesses ranges from 5–40%. *Bacteroides*, *E. coli*, *S. aureus* and streptococci are the most frequent organisms.

X-ray shows pleural effusion in about 60–80% (range 43–89%), elevated diaphragm in about 70% (range 34–82%) and gas in the abscess in about 25–50% (range 9–61%). Atelectasis and pneumonia are frequent in the closest lung base.

B-mode ultrasound, gallium scanning, and lung-liver junction scanning (for suprahepatic abscess) may assist in diagnosis and localization of focal intra-abdominal infection. Computerized axial tomography may also help in some cases. Of these, gallium probably furnishes the most information. Gallium-67 has over 90% accuracy for locating abscesses and has the additional advantage of detecting osteomyelitis or localized inflammation within organs or elsewhere in the body, such as pyelonephritis, acute arthritis, acute cholecystitis, or dental infection. Disadvantages are excretion in fecal material beginning about 12 hours after injection, so that bowel cleansing may be a problem when infection occurs in areas near the colon. Pneumonia and SBE sometimes are detected, but not consistently. Intrahepatic abscess may be missed if normal liver uptake is too intense or if the focus is too small. Lung-liver junction scanning involves injection of two radionuclides, one of which localizes in the liver and the other in the lungs. The lung and liver images are obtained without moving the patient, and the normal lung-liver overlap is inspected to find a separation due to abscess between the two organs. Right pleural effusion or ascites may interfere with interpretation. B-mode ultrasound (especially with gray scale) is excellent for detection of abscess. Disadvantage is mainly the possibility of interference by air within the intestines.

Iatrogenic Infection

Intravenous catheters or fluid therapy may produce infection, either from contamination by skin bacteria, by introduction of organisms via material delivered to the intravenous lines, or by attracting organisms from bacteremia originating elsewhere. Aseptic technique in catheter introduction, proper catheter placement, adequate inspection and care of the insertion site, and extra care in maintaining sterility when fluid or other materials are added to the system are the major steps to prevent catheter-related infection. Current recommendations are (1) relocate intravenous lines to another site every 48 hours, if possible (central venous pressure catheters or patients with very poor veins are obvious exceptions); (2) avoid irrigating or manipulating occluded or infiltrating catheters; (3) use scalp vein needles instead of plastic catheters, when possible; (4) inspect dressings covering the catheter site at least once daily and change if wet; (5) change bottles and intravenous administration sets at least every 24 hours. Recommended preparation of the intended site of skin puncture includes adequate scrubbing of the skin, followed by 1% iodine solution allowed to dry 30–60 seconds, followed by 70% alcohol. (If iodophor antiseptic is used instead of iodine solution, the iodophor should not be washed off.) Puncture and catheter insertion should be done with sterile technique, when possible.

Some of the data supporting these recommendations include several reports indicating 3–18% bacterial contamination in IV fluid lines after injection of medications or additives. In addition, one study found 3% contamination in IV sets in use less than 48 hours and 15% in those used longer than 48 hours, that some organisms can proliferate to pathogenic levels in several types of IV solutions by 24 hours, and that plastic catheters were associated with septicemia in 2–5% of cases after 48 hours.

ANTIBIOTIC SENSITIVITY PROCEDURES

Finally, a word should be said about antibiotic sensitivity procedures. Two techniques are employed; tube-dilution and agar diffusion. Of these, agar diffusion is by far the more common, and the Kirby-Bauer modification of this technique is becoming standard. Kirby-Bauer involves (1) isolating a bacterial colony from original growth media, (2) allowing the bacteria to grow in broth medium to a certain predetermined visual density, (3) covering the entirety of a Mueller-Hinton agar plate with the bacterial isolate, (4) placing antibiotic sensitivity disks at intervals on the surface, (5) incubating 18–20 hours, (6) examining for clear areas around individual disks representing bacterial growth inhibition by the antibiotic-impregnated disk and (7) measuring the diameter of these inhibition zones. Results are reported as resistant, sensitive, or intermediate, depending on previously established values for zone size based on tube-dilution studies most often furnished by the disk manufacturer. Consistent results will depend on strict adherence to good technique at each step, as well as the quality of the antibiotic disks and agar used. Variation in potency of antibiotic disks from different shipments and disk or agar deterioration during storage necessitate a good quality control program. The Kirby-Bauer technique has limitations. To be accurate, it can only be used when the bacterium to be tested is aerobic and grows rapidly (produces colonies within 24 hours) on the agar growth medium (this includes Enterobacteriaciae, *Pseudomonas* organisms, staphylococci, and streptococci).

Most organisms, fortunately, may be classified as sensitive or resistant. Intermediate sensitivity is a controversial area. In general, many feel that "intermediate" zones should be considered resistant, although certain organisms, such as enterococci, may be exceptions. The test should be repeated to rule out technical variation or error. Interpretation may be influenced by location of the infection source, if the antibiotic in question can reach this area readily. Antibiotic treatment dose may occasionally be increased, especially in subacute bacterial endocarditis. Another subject of dispute is the need for sensitivity testing in those bacteria which almost always are sensitive to certain antibiotics. These organisms include Group A aerobic streptococci, pneumococci, *Neisseria* organisms and *C. diphtheriae*.

An occasional laboratory problem is requests by physicians to include additional sensitivity disks in sensitivity panels. Laboratories frequently include only one representative of an antibiotic family in sensitivity test panels because sensitivity differences between antibiotic family members (e.g., the various tetracycline derivatives) are usually very minor.

REFERENCES

Barnett, R. N., et al.: Conference on the medical usefulness of microbiology, Am. J. Clin. Pathol. 54:521, 1970.
Bartlett, J. G., et al.: Should fiberoptic bronchoscopy aspirates be cultured? Am. Rev. Resp. Dis. 114:73, 1976.

Cammerer, R. C., et al.: Clinical spectrum of pseudomembranous colitis, J.A.M.A. 235:2502, 1976.

Cannady, P. B., and Sanford, J. P.: Negative blood cultures in infective endocarditis: A review, South. Med. J. 69:1420, 1976.

Caplan, E. S., and Kluge, R. M.: Gas gangrene: Review of 34 cases, Arch. Intern. Med. 136:788, 1976.

Chow, A. W.: Genital infection with type 2 herpes simplex virus: A common venereal disease, Postgrad. Med. 58:66, 1975.

Davidson, M., et al.: Bacterologic diagnosis of acute pneumonia: Comparison of sputum, transtracheal aspirates and lung aspirates, J.A.M.A. 235:158, 1976.

Drachman, R. H.: Acute infectious gastroenteritis, Pediatr. Clin. North Am. 21:711, 1974.

Eschenbach, D. A.: Acute pelvic inflammatory disease: Etiology, risk factors, and pathogenesis, Clin. Obstet. Gynecol. 19:147, 1976.

Everett, E. D., and Hirschmann, J. V.: Transient bacteremia and endocarditis prophylaxis: A review, Medicine 56:61, 1977.

Fields, B. N., et al.: The so-called paracolon bacteria—a bacteriologic and clinical reappraisal, Am. J. Med. 42:89, 1967.

Findlay, C. W.: Sepsis in the surgical intensive care unit, Med. Clin. North Am. 55: 1331, 1971.

Finegold, S. M.: Intestinal bacteria—the role they play in normal physiology, pathologic physiology, and infections, Calif. Med. 110:455, 1969.

Finegold, S. M., and Rosenblatt, J. E.: Practical aspects of anaerobic sepsis, Medicine 52:318, 1973.

Flick, M. R., and Cuff, L. E.: Pseudomonas bacteremia: Review of 108 cases, Am. J. Med. 60:501, 1976.

Galton, M. M.: Methods in the laboratory diagnosis of leptospirosis, Ann. N.Y. Acad. Sci. 98:675, 1962.

Gangarosa, E. J., and Barker, W. H.: Cholera: Implications for the United States, J.A.M.A. 227:170, 1974.

Gardner, P., et al.: Nonfermentative gram-negative bacilli of nosocomial interest, Am. J. Med. 48:735, 1970.

Garvey, G. J., and Neu, H. C.: Infective endocarditis, Postgrad. Med. 58:107, 1975.

Goodman, J. S.: Bacteroides sepsis: Diagnosis and therapy, Hosp. Practice 6:121, 1971.

Gray, M. L.: Listeria monocytogenes and listeric infection in the diagnostic laboratory, Ann. NY Acad. Sci. 98:686, 1962.

Guckian, J. C., et al.: *Arizona* infection of man, Arch. Intern. Med. 119:170, 1967.

Habiban, M. R., et al.: Gallium citrate Ga 67 scans in febrile patients, J.A.M.A. 233: 1073, 1975.

Hable, K. A., et al.: Bacterial and viral throat flora, Clin. Pediatr. 10:199, 1971.

Huckstep, R. L.: *Typhoid Fever and Other Salmonella Infections* (Edinburgh: E. & S. Livingstone, Ltd., 1962).

Hughes, W. T.: Infectious disease in children with cancer, Pediatr. Clin. North Am. 21:583, 1974.

Kalis, P., et al.: Listeriosis, Am. J. Med. Sci. 271:159, 1976.

Konvolinka, C. W., and Olearczyk, A.: Subphrenic Abscess, in Ravitch, M. M. (ed.): *Current Problems in Surgery* (Chicago: Year Book Medical Publishers, Inc., Jan. 1972).

Kumar, B., et al.: Gallium citrate Ga 67 imaging in patients with suspected inflammatory processes, Arch. Surg. 110:1237, 1975.

Jones, F. L., Jr.: The relative efficacy of spontaneous sputa, aerosol-induced sputa, and gastric aspirates in the bacteriologic diagnosis of pulmonary tuberculosis, Dis. Chest 50:403, 1966.

Jones, R. C.: Tetanus and gas gangrene: Present attitudes, Postgrad. Med. 41:641, 1967.

Kazal, H. L.: Laboratory diagnosis of foodborne diseases, Ann. Clin. Lab. Sci. 6:381, 1976.

Kent, D. C., and Schwartz, R.: Active pulmonary tuberculosis with negative tuberculin skin reactions, Am. Rev. Respir. Dis. 95:411, 1967.

Kestle, D. G., and Kubica, G. P.: Sputum collection for cultivation of mycobacteria. An early morning specimen or the 24-to-72 hour pool? Am. J. Clin. Pathol. 48:347, 1967.

Koenig, M. G.: Diagnosis of bacterial endocarditis, Hosp. Med. 5:80, 1969.

Lang, G. R., and Levin, S.: Diagnosis and treatment of urinary tract infections, Med. Clin. North Am. 55:1439, 1971.

Lerner, P.: Infective endocarditis: A review of selected topics, Med. Clin. North Am. 58:605, 1974.

Lester, W.: Unclassified Mycobacterial Diseases, in DeGraff, A. C., and Creger, W. P. (eds.): Annual Review of Medicine (Palo Alto, CA: Annual Reviews, Inc., 1966), vol. 17, p. 351.

Maki, D. G., et al.: Infection control in intravenous therapy, Ann. Intern. Med. 79: 867, 1973.

Martin, W. J., et al.: Epidemiologic significance of Klebsiella pneumoniae, Mayo Clin. Proc. 46:785, 1971.

McCormack, W. M.: Sexually transmissible diseases, Postgrad. Med. 58:179, 1975.

McCracken, G. H., Jr.: Neonatal septicemia and meningitis, Hosp. Practice 11:89, 1976.

McHenry, M. C., et al.: Hospital-acquired pneumonia, Med. Clin. North Am. 58:565, 1974.

McHenry, M. C., et al.: Bacteremia caused by gram-negative bacilli. Med. Clin. North Am. 58:623, 1974.

Mostow, S. R.: Pneumonias acquired outside the hospital: recognition and treatment, Med. Clin. North Am. 58:555, 1974.

Nolan, C. M., and Beaty, H. N.: Staphylococcus aureus bacteremia: current clinical patterns, Am. J. Med. 60:495, 1976.

O'Neil, F. S.: Salmonellosis: Review of 124 cases, Postgrad. Med. 38:269, 1965.

Pryles, C. V., and Lustik, B.: Laboratory diagnosis of urinary tract infection, Pediatr. Clin. North Am. 18:233, 1971.

Rein, M. F., and Chapel, T. A.: Trichomonas, candidiasis, and the minor venereal diseases, Clin. Obstet. Gynecol. 18:73, 1975.

Ryan, J. A., Jr., et al.: Catheter complications in total parenteral nutrition, N. Engl. J. Med. 290:757, 1974.

Schmale, J. D., et al.: Observations on the culture diagnosis of gonorrhea in women, J.A.M.A. 210:312, 1969.

Schroeter, A. L., and Lucas, J. B.: Gonorrhea: Diagnosis and treatment, Obstet. Gynecol. 39:274, 1972.

Segura, J. W., et al.: Anaerobic bacteria in the urinary tract, Mayo Clin. Proc. 47:30, 1972.

Taylor, A., et al.: Outbreaks of waterborne diseases in the United States 1961–1970, J. Infect. Dis. 125:329, 1972.

Thorsteinsson, S. B., et al.: The diagnostic value of sputum culture in acute pneumonia, J.A.M.A. 233:894, 1975.

Tillotson, J. R., and Lerner, A. M.: Pneumonias caused by gram-negative bacilli, Medicine 45:65, 1966.

Tilton, R. C., et al.: The bacteriologic examination of sputum, Ann. Clin. Lab. Sci. 4: 60, 1974.

Vaisrub, S.: The nondiscriminant gonococcus, J.A.M.A. 228:875, 1974.

Wallace, C. K.: Enteric infections, Hosp. Med. 6:72, 1970.

White, A., and Crowder, J. G.: Pseudomonas Diseases, in Stollerman, G. H. (ed.): *Advances in Internal Medicine,* Vol. 20 (Chicago: Year Book Medical Publishers, Inc., 1975).

Young, E. J.: Human brucellosis, Clin. Med. 83(5):9, 1976.

15 / Mycotic Infections

"Systemic" Fungi

CERTAIN FUNGI, known as the "deep" or "systemic" fungi, are characterized by involvement of visceral organs or penetrating types of infection. *Actinomycosis* is caused by a gram-positive nonacid-fast anaerobic organism that often produces deep-seated abscesses. A gram-stained smear of aspirated material from the lesion will often show typical organism colonies (sometimes called "sulfur granules" from their gross appearance). Biopsy material gives similar information. Culture on special media provides definitive diagnosis. *Nocardia* organisms may produce a somewhat similar clinical picture. These fungi are also gram positive and may resemble actinomycosis in histologic appearance. *Nocardia* organisms, however, are aerobic and partially acid-fast.

Blastomycosis may primarily involve either the skin or visceral organs. Granulomatous lesions form that are somewhat similar histologically to those of tuberculosis. There are four helpful means of diagnosis: (1) a skin test, which shows infection by the organism, either past or present; (2) demonstration of typical organisms by direct wet-mount examination of material aspirated from a lesion or by histologic examination of a biopsy specimen; (3) culture of a lesion for definitive organism isolation; and (4) serologic tests (but the complement fixation procedure is relatively insensitive, detecting fewer than 50% of cases).

Coccidioidomycosis is most often contracted in the San Joaquin Valley of California, but occasionally appears elsewhere in the Southwest. It has a predilection for the lungs and hilar lymph nodes, but occasionally may become systemic to varying degrees. Clinical symptoms are most often pulmonary, manifested usually by mild or moderate respiratory symptoms and sometimes by fever of unknown origin. Rarely, overwhelming infection much like miliary tuberculosis develops. Diagnosis is made by the same combination of methods outlined under blastomycosis. Serologic tests, however, have more to offer, since the complement fixation procedure is reliable and reasonably sensitive; while a latex agglutination slide test is said to be very sensitive, although declining rapidly in positivity by 2–3 months after onset of symptoms.

Cryptococcosis (torulosis) is a fungal disease with a marked predilection for the brain. Certain birds, especially pigeons, seem to be the most frequent vectors. Persons with illnesses that induce decreased immunologic resistance (e.g., Hodgkin's disease and acute leukemia) or those undergoing therapy with steroids or immunosuppressive agents are particularly susceptible. Diagnosis can be obtained by culture, by microscopic examination of cerebrospinal fluid (CSF), using an India ink preparation (in those patients with meningitis, p. 201), and by serologic tests. Both antigen and antibody can be detected. Antibody is usually not present in CSF and is frequently absent during the acute phase of the illness. (In the very early stages, however, antibody may be present, which later disappears). In addition, some of the antibody-detection systems cross-react with histoplasmosis antibody. *Cryptococcus* antigen-detection systems do not react when the patient is infected by other fungi. The most widely used serologic test is the slide latex agglutination procedure, which detects antigen. Although latex agglutination is usually performed on serum, investigators have used the test directly on CSF and detected some cases that were missed when India ink was used. Patient serum must be heat-inactivated and tested with a control for rheumatoid factor and for nonspecific agglutinins. The latex agglutination test is said to be very sensitive. Evaluations in the literature are difficult to interpret, however, since kits by different manufacturers apparently produce different results, and some investigators used their own reagents. The variety of reagents may account for certain conflicting reports, one of which demonstrated many false positive and negative CSF results with one particular kit, while others indicated that the procedure is more reliable than classic India ink in CSF. As noted previously, the latex test may be nonreactive in the very early stage of the disease. It tends to decrease in reactivity if treatment is successful, and, in addition, may be nonreactive in low-grade chronic infections. A complement fixation test is also available. This is said to be more specific than the latex procedure, although not as sensitive.

Histoplasmosis is the most common of the systemic fungal infections. It is most often encountered in the Mississippi and Ohio Valley areas, but may appear elsewhere. Certain birds, especially chickens and starlings, are the most frequent vectors in the United States. In endemic areas, 60% or more of those infected are asymptomatic. The remainder manifest a variety of illness patterns, ranging from mild or severe acute or chronic pulmonary forms to disseminated infection. Histoplasmosis begins with a small primary focus of lung infection much like the early lesion of pulmonary tuberculosis. Thereafter, the lesion may heal or progress or reinfection may occur. Mild acute pulmonary infection with influenza-like symptoms may develop. The illness lasts only a few days, and skin tests, cultures and chest x-rays are usually negative. More severe acute pulmonary involvement produces a syndrome resembling primary atypical pneumonia. Chest x-rays may show hilar adenopathy and single or multiple pulmonary infiltrates. Histoplasmin skin tests and complement fixation or latex agglutination tests eventually convert to positive, but remain negative until after the first 2–3 weeks of illness. Sputum culture may be positive, but not often. Chronic pulmonary histoplasmosis resembles chronic pulmonary tuberculosis clinically. Cavitation sometimes develops. Skin tests and complement-fixation tests usually are positive by the time the disease is chronic. Sputum is the most accessible material for culture, although reportedly negative in 50–60% of cases. Histoplasmosis is a localized pulmonary disease in the great majority of patients, so there is usually little help from cultures obtained outside the pulmonary area. In the small group that does have disseminated histoplasmosis, either acute or chronic, there is a range of symptoms from a febrile disease with lymphadenopathy and hepato-splenomegaly to a rapidly fatal illness closely resembling miliary tuberculo-sis. Bone marrow aspiration is the diagnostic method of choice; it is useful both for cultures and for histologic diagnosis of the organisms within mac-rophages on Wright-stained smear or clot section. Occasionally lymph node biopsy may be helpful; if performed, a culture should also be taken from the node before it is placed in fixative.

Skin test and serologic test results in histoplasmosis depend on the dura-tion of illness. They may especially be negative in the acute disseminated form, just as tuberculin skin test anergy may develop in miliary tuberculo-sis. A skin test may itself convert the serologic tests from negative to posi-tive. In histoplasmosis endemic areas, many persons have positive skin or serologic tests from past infection. Therefore, a (fourfold) rising titer is much more significant than a single positive result.

Complement fixation tests are available for all of the "systemic" fungi except *Actinomyces* and *Nocardia* organisms. If no local or state health laboratory can do these tests, serum specimens may be sent to the USPHS National Communicable Disease Center, Atlanta, Georgia 30333. As was mentioned, skin tests are available. These have the same general applica-tion and limitations as the tuberculin skin test; i.e., they do not separate past or recent infection, and take several weeks after initial infection to become positive. Also, conversion of a negative to a positive reaction is highly significant. There is a good deal of cross-reaction between skin tests of these fungal diseases. The histoplasmin skin test reacts with about 30% of patients who actually have blastomycosis and about 40% of those with coccidioidomycosis. However, only about 2% of patients with histoplas-mosis give a positive coccidioidomycosis skin test; since blastomycosis infection is relatively rare, performing the different skin tests simulta-neously helps to overcome this drawback.

In serious localized infection or widespread dissemination of these fun-gi, there is often a normocytic-normochromic or slightly hypochromic anemia. The anemia is usually mild or moderate in localized infection.

"Opportunistic" Fungi

Other fungi may, under certain circumstances, produce visceral or sys-temic infection. The most common of these conditions are candidiasis, aspergillosis and mucormycosis. Persons predisposed to infection include aged persons; cachetic or debilitated patients; persons with diseases such as leukemia, which affect the body's immunologic mechanisms; and, most commonly, persons under treatment with certain drugs that impair the same immunologic mechanisms. Such drugs include many types of anti-leukemic or anticancer chemotherapeutic agents and sometimes adreno-cortical steroids if use has been heavy or prolonged. Occasionally, over-growth of *Candida* may be caused by prolonged oral antibiotic therapy that destroys normal gastrointestinal bacterial flora. *Candida fungemia* may be associated with indwelling intravenous catheters. Mucormycosis is charac-teristically but not exclusively associated with diabetics. Diagnosis in many of these patients is difficult, since the original underlying disease usually overshadows advent of the fungal infection. If the patient has a condition that predisposes to infection by fungi, culture of a fungus from an area where it is normally absent should not be disregarded as mere contamination, but should be investigated further.

Respiratory infection by *Aspergillus* organisms may appear in several forms: localized or disseminated infection (usually superimposed on iatrogenic [therapeutic] or disease-associated crippling of immunologic defense mechanisms), aspergilloma (fungus ball which may develop in lung parenchymal cystic spaces), and allergic bronchopulmonary aspergillosis. The latter condition is marked by hypersensitivity to *Aspergillus* antigen and produces symptoms of asthma with fever. In classic cases there is expectoration of golden-brown sputum plugs that contain *Aspergillus* hyphae. These patients have eosinophilia in peripheral blood and sputum, high serum IgE levels (p. 245), and positive skin and serologic tests for *Aspergillus* organisms.

Fungal Cultures

When fungal culture is indicated, the laboratory must be notified, because bacterial culture media are not generally suitable for fungi. All-purpose fungal culture media, such as Sabouraud's, under aerobic conditions, are satisfactory for most of the "systemic" fungi, except for *Actinomyces* and *Nocardia* organisms.

The *dermatophytes* include a number of fungi that attack the nails and skin. A presumptive etiologic diagnosis may be made by examining scrapings of the affected area microscopically in a wet mount of 10% potassium hydroxide. Definitive diagnosis is by culture, usually on all-purpose media, such as Sabouraud's. Skin, mucous membrane, or female vaginal infection by *Candida (Monilia)* is a fairly common fungus problem. This is more frequent in diabetics. Diagnosis is by essentially the same methods as those used for the dermatophytes.

REFERENCES

Buechner, H. A.: Clinical Aspects of Fungus Disease of the Lungs Including Laboratory Diagnosis and Treatment, in Banyai, A. L., and Gordon, B. L. (eds.): *Advances in Cardiopulmonary Disease* (Chicago: Year Book Medical Publishers, Inc., 1966), vol. 3, p. 123.

Butler, W. T., et al.: Diagnostic and prognostic value of clinical and laboratory findings in cryptococcal meningitis, N. Engl. J. Med. 270:60, 1964.

Conn, H. F. (ed.): Symposium on efficacy of antibiotic and antifungal agents, Med. Clin. North Am. 54:1077, 1970.

Dolan, C. T.: Specificity of the latex-cryptococcal antigen test, Am. J. Clin. Pathol. 58:358, 1972.

Furcolow, M. L.: Tests of immunity in histoplasmosis, N. Engl. J. Med. 268:357, 1963.

Goldstein, E., and Hoeprich, P. D.: Problems in the diagnosis and treatment of systemic candidiasis, J. Infect. Dis. 125:190, 1972.

Harding, S. A., et al.: Three serologic tests for candidiasis: diagnostic value on distinguishing deep or disseminated infection from superficial infection or colonization, Am. J. Clin. Pathol. 65:1001, 1976.

Hendry, W. S., and Patrick, R. L.: Observations on thirteen cases of pneumocystis carinii pneumonia, Am. J. Clin. Pathol. 38:401, 1962.

Littman, M. L., and Walter, J. E.: Cryptococcosis: Current status, Am. J. Med. 45:922, 1968.

Louria, D. B., et al.: Fungal infections in otherwise healthy patients, Patient Care 6(20):74, 1972.

Louria, D. B., et al.: Disseminated moniliasis in the adult, Medicine 41:307, 1962.

Louria, D. B., et al.: Fungemia caused by "nonpathogenic" yeasts, Arch. Int. Med. 119:247, 1967.

Murray, P. R., et al.: Should yeasts in respiratory secretions be identified? Mayo Clin. Proc. 52:42, 1977.

Negroni, P.: *Histoplasmosis* (Springfield, IL: Charles C Thomas, Publisher, 1965).

Quie, P. G., and Chilgren, R. A.: Acute disseminated and chronic mucocutaneous candidiasis, Semin. Hematol. 8:227, 1971.

Reeves, D. L., et al.: Phycomycosis (mucormycosis) of the central nervous system, J. Neurosurg. 23:82, 1965.

Slavin, Raymond G.: Immunologically mediated lung disease: extrinsic allergic alveolitis and allergic bronchopulmonary aspergillosis, Postgrad. Med. 59:137, 1976.

Utz, J. P.: Pulmonary Infection Due to Opportunistic Fungi, in Stollerman, G. H., et al. (eds.): *Advances in Internal Medicine* (Chicago: Year Book Medical Publishers, Inc., 1970), Vol. 16, p. 427.

Winslow, D. J., and Steen, F. G.: Considerations in the histologic diagnosis of mycetoma, Am. J. Clin. Pathol. 42:164, 1964.

Young, R. C., et al.: Aspergillosis – The spectrum of the disease in 98 patients, Medicine 49:147, 1970.

16 / Viral, Rickettsial and Miscellaneous Infectious Diseases

THIS CHAPTER will deal with the laboratory procedures available for diagnosis of viral and rickettsial infection, and will also include certain other organisms which are not bacterial but are not truly viral or rickettsial. In some cases the etiologic agent is unknown or in dispute.

VIRAL DISEASES

Viral diseases form a large heterogeneous group. A general classification (including only the most important viruses) is presented in Table 16–1. In general, diagnostic methods depend on the type of illness produced. In the great majority of situations, including infection by enterovirus, respiratory viruses, and arboviruses, the only available laboratory methods are culture and serologic tests. Culture techniques have made significant advances in the past few years but, unfortunately, still must be described as difficult and expensive. Culture is done in living cell preparations or in living tissues. This fact in itself rules out "mass production" testing. Partly because of this, facilities for work of this kind are limited, and are available mainly at sizable medical centers or large Public Health laboratories. Recent application of fluorescent antibody techniques may simplify some of the procedures and possibly provide rapid screening tests in some situations; at present, these techniques are not routine. In addition to culture, serologic tests are available for most viruses. There are several different techniques; although they are considerably less exacting than culture, most are still rather tedious and time-consuming, with the result that, again, these tests are not immediately available except at reference laboratories. Serologic tests have the additional disadvantage that antibodies usually take 1–2 weeks to develop after onset of illness and, unless a significantly (fourfold) rising titer is demonstrated, do not prove current activity of the viral agent in question. Nevertheless, it is considered good practice to attempt specific etiologic diagnosis of viral diseases to provide the community with information that may alert it to an epidemic, as well as to confirm the clinical impression and perhaps rule out other etiologies that would call for different therapy.

VIRAL RESPIRATORY DISEASE.—Respiratory disease may take several

174

TABLE 16-1.—CLASSIFICATION OF VIRUSES

TAXONOMIC CLASSIFICATION
RNA viruses
Arenavirus	Lassa fever; lymphocytic choriomeningitis
Coronavirus	Acute upper respiratory infections
Myxovirus	Influenza
Paramyxovirus	Canine distemper, measles (rubeola), mumps, Newcastle disease, parainfluenza, respiratory syncytial virus, rubella
Picornavirus	Enterovirus (coxsackie, ECHO [enteric cytopathic human orphan], poliomyelitis), rhinovirus
Reovirus	"Respiratory enteric orphan virus" of common cold
Rhabdovirus	Rabies
Togavirus	Arbovirus (arthropod-borne virus): Dengue, equine encephalitis, St. Louis encephalitis, yellow fever)

DNA viruses
Adenovirus	Acute upper respiratory infections
Herpesvirus	Cytomegalic inclusion virus, Epstein-Barr virus, herpes simplex, herpes zoster-varicella
Papovirus	Polyomavirus
Poxvirus	Molluscum contagiosum, vaccinia, variola

CLINICAL CLASSIFICATION (characteristic organ systems involved clinically)
Central nervous system
Arbovirus
Enterovirus
Rabies
Gastrointestinal
Enterovirus
Respiratory
Adenovirus
Myxovirus
Reovirus
Rhinovirus
Liver
Hepatitis viruses
Yellow fever
Skin
Poxvirus
Salivary glands
Cytomegalic inclusion virus
Mumps

forms, and the predominant etiologies are different in different age groups. Statistics also vary depending on the geographic area and the population selected. Of the known viruses, rhinoviruses seem to be predominantly associated with acute upper respiratory disease (including the common cold) in adults, while in children, rhinovirus, adenovirus, parainfluenza and the enteroviruses are important. Acute bronchitis in children is most often due to parainfluenza and respiratory syncytial virus. In croup, parainfluenza is said to be the most important virus. Respiratory syncytial virus is the predominating etiology of pediatric pneumonia, followed by adenovirus or parainfluenza. In adults, nonbacterial pneumonia is most often associated with *Mycoplasma pneumoniae* (Eaton agent); among viral agents known to cause pneumonia, the most common cause is probably influenza. In any study, a large minority of cases did not yield a specific etiologic agent.

VIRAL MENINGITIS. — Viruses are an important cause of meningitis, especially in children. They produce the laboratory picture of aseptic meningitis, with cerebrospinal fluid (CSF) findings of variable but often mildly increased protein, increased cell counts with mononuclears predominating and normal sugar. It should be remembered, however, that tuberculous meningitis gives similar findings, except for decreased CSF sugar, and also will show a sterile culture on ordinary bacterial culture media. Some patients with mumps meningoencephalitis may have decreased CSF glucose, in addition to CSF lymphocytosis. Enteroviruses form the largest etiologic group causing aseptic meningitis. Among the enteric viruses, poliomyelitis used to be the most common organism, but since the advent of widespread vaccination programs, echovirus and coxsackievirus have replaced polio in terms of frequency.

After the enterovirus group, mumps is most important. A small but significant number of patients with mumps develop clinical signs of meningitis, and a large number will show CSF changes without demonstrating enough clinical symptoms to warrant a diagnosis and workup for meningitis. Changes in CSF or the clinical picture of meningitis may occur in patients without parotid swelling or other evidence of mumps. Lymphocytic choriomeningitis and leptospirosis are uncommon etiologies for aseptic meningitis.

Encephalitis is a syndrome which presents CSF alterations similar to those of meningitis. The two cannot always be separated, but the main difference is clinical; encephalitis features depression of consciousness (lethargy, coma) over a prolonged period, whereas meningitis usually is a more acute episode, including fever, headaches, physical signs of central nervous system irritation and possibly convulsions. In severe bacterial infection, encephalitis may be the sequel of meningitis. Encephalitis is most frequently caused by mumps and measles. Meningitis cases of unknown etiology are the next largest group. Arbovirus is third in frequency. Sometimes encephalitis appears as a complication of vaccination.

VIRAL GASTROENTERITIS. — Viruses are likely to be blamed for diarrhea that cannot be explained otherwise. In most cases, definitive evidence is lacking because enteric virus is present in a significant number of apparently healthy children. In those studies where strong evidence of a viral etiology is presented, echovirus is by far the most frequent organism. Bacterial infection should always be carefully ruled out.

VIRAL INFECTIONS IN PREGNANCY. — By far the most dangerous viral disease during pregnancy is rubella. Statistics are variable, but they suggest about a 15–25% risk of fetal malformation when rubella infection occurs in the 1st trimester. The true incidence is not certain; estimates and studies generally fall within 10–15%, although some report as high as 80%. Besides this, 5–15% of fetuses probably die in utero. Risk in the 2d trimester is about 5%. After the 4th month of pregnancy, there is no longer any danger to the fetus. Most viral diseases other than rubella (e.g., cytomegalic inclusion virus) exert ill effects in the 3d trimester. Many viruses are thought to have potential to cause neonatal disease or malformation, but evidence is somewhat inconclusive as to exact incidence and effects. Herpes simplex and infectious hepatitis have some documentation.

Diagnosis of Viral Diseases

These are investigated by two main types of laboratory procedures – direct isolation by culture, and demonstration of antibodies in the patient's blood to specific organisms. Serologic test results without isolation of an organism by culture allow only a presumptive diagnosis, and cultural isolation of certain viruses without serologic confirmation does not absolutely prove that the virus is causing current disease, since many viruses are quite prevalent in the general population. If possible, both techniques should be done together, since they supplement each other. Since culture methods are still rather difficult and expensive, serologic tests are probably more widely used. One serum specimen is obtained as early in the disease as possible ("acute" stage), and a second sample is obtained 2–3 weeks later ("convalescent" stage). Blood should be collected in sterile tubes or vacutainer tubes and serum processed aseptically to avoid bacterial contamination. Hemolyzed serum is not acceptable; to help prevent hemolysis, serum should be separated from blood clot as soon as possible. The serum should be frozen as soon as possible after collection to minimize bacterial growth and sent still frozen (packed in dry ice) to the virus laboratory. Here a variety of serologic tests can be done to demonstrate specific antibodies to the various organisms. A fourfold rise in titer from acute to convalescent stage of the disease is considered diagnostic. If only a single specimen is taken, an elevated titer could be due to previous infection rather than currently active disease. A single negative test is likewise difficult to interpret, since the specimen might have been obtained too early, before antibody rise occurred.

In any kind of meningitis with negative spinal fluid cultures or severe respiratory infection of unknown etiology, it is a good idea to freeze a specimen of serum as early in the disease as possible. Later on, if desired, another specimen can be drawn and the two sent off for virus studies. As noted, serum specimens are generally drawn 2 weeks apart.

There is one notable exception to the rule of acute and convalescent serologic specimens. In some circumstances, it is desirable to learn whether a person has an antibody titer to a particular virus sufficient to prevent onset of the disease. This is especially true for a woman in early pregnancy who might be exposed to rubella. A significant antibody titer to rubella would suggest immunity to the virus.

When obtaining specimens for viral culture, the type of specimen depends on the type of illness. In aseptic meningitis, CSF should be obtained. In addition, stool culture for virus should be done, since enteroviruses are frequent etiologies of meningitis. In enterovirus meningitis, stool culture is 2–3 times more effective than CSF culture.

In suspected cases of (nonbacterial) encephalitis, whole blood should be collected for virus culture during the first 2 days of illness. During this short time there is a chance of demonstrating arbovirus viremia. This procedure is not useful in aseptic meningitis. Spinal fluid should also be sent for virus culture; even though the yield is relatively small in arbovirus infections, the specimen sometimes is positive, and also helps to rule out other organisms, such as enterovirus. In upper respiratory illness, throat or nasopharyngeal swabs are preferred. These should be placed in trypticase broth (a standard bacterial medium). Swabs without some type of media such as trypticase or Hank's solution are usually not satisfactory, since they dry out quickly and most viruses are killed by drying. Throat washings or gargle material can be used but are difficult to obtain properly. In viral pneumonia sputum or throat swabs are needed. If throat swabs are used they should be placed in acceptable collection solutions. Whether throat swabs or sputum, the specimen must be frozen immediately and sent to the virus laboratory packed in dry ice. In addition, a sputum specimen (or throat swab) should be obtained for mycoplasma culture (p. 187). In possible viral gastroenteritis stool culture is the logical procedure. In any situation where a stool culture for virus is needed actual stool specimens are preferred rather than rectal swabs, since there is a better chance of isolating an organism from the larger sample. The stool specimen should be frozen in the same manner as the serum samples. It is better to mail any virus specimens early in the week, so as to avoid arrival on weekends. An insulated container helps to prolong effects of the dry ice.

In any case an adequate clinical history with pertinent physical and laboratory findings should accompany any virus specimen, whether for culture or serologic studies. As a minimum, the date of clinical illness onset, collection date of each specimen and clinical diagnosis must be included. The most likely organism should be indicated. This information helps the virus laboratory in determining what initial procedures or techniques to use. For example, certain tissue culture cell types are better adapted than others for certain viruses. Considerable time and effort can be saved and a meaningful interpretation of results can be provided.

Certain specific viruses deserve individual discussion. The method of diagnosis or type of specimen required for some of these organisms is different from the usual procedure. In others it is desirable to emphasize certain aspects of the clinical illness which suggest the diagnosis.

German Measles (Rubella)

German measles (rubella) is especially important in pregnancy. The "rubella syndrome" includes one or more of the following: congenital heart disease, cataract, deafness and cerebral damage. Diagnosis is made by documenting active rubella infection in the mother during early pregnancy or by proving infection of the infant after birth. A significant (fourfold) rise in antibody titer using one of several varieties of serologic tests is the easiest way to demonstrate maternal infection. At present, the hemagglutination inhibition (HI or HAI) and complement fixation (CF) serologic tests form the backbone of diagnosis. HI antibodies appear during the first week after onset of rash; they are often detectable after only 2–3 days. Peak levels are reached during the second week. An elevated titer persists for many years or for life. Complement fixation antibodies develop in the more conventional time of 7 – 14 days after onset of rash and generally disappear in a few years. Absence of HAI antibody indicates susceptibility to rubella, since it usually persists, whereas CF antibody titer returns to normal. Presence of HI antibody means either past or recent infection. In a person who is clinically well, this means immunity to subsequent infection. In a person with suspected clinical rubella, an immediate serum specimen and a second one drawn at least 7 days later must be obtained, the standard procedure with all serologic tests. A fourfold rise in titer confirms very recent (active) infection. However, if the first serum specimen was not obtained until several days after onset of rash, the HI peak may already have been reached. In some of these cases, a significant (fourfold titer or 2-tube dilution) rise in CF antibody may be demonstrated, since these antibodies develop later than HI. If both antibodies are at peak, there is no way to distinguish recent infection from one occurring months or even years previously.

In the neonatal period congenital rubella can best be established by virus culture of nasopharyngeal swab material. Infant serum antibodies come from the mother. By 6 – 8 months, maternal antibody in the child has disappeared, so that persistence of antibody past this time indicates congenital or neonatal infection. For some reason, however, at least 20% of children with congenital rubella lose their HI titer by age 5.

The HI test at the present time takes considerable experience to produce reliable results. Therefore, since false positive results may occur, it is probably wise to obtain the CF test at the same time. If the patient is pregnant and test results may lead to some action, it may be advisable to split each sample, keeping part of each frozen, in case a recheck is desired.

Measles (Rubeola)

Measles (rubeola) is still important, even though widespread vaccination has begun. The two main complications are encephalitis and pneumonia. Encephalitis is, fortunately, rare, the incidence being 0.01 – 0.2%; due to the great frequency of the disease, however, the total number of cases is appreciable. About a third of those with encephalitis die, about a third recover completely and the remainder survive but show moderate-to-severe residua. This encephalitis is considered postinfectious, because it develops 4 – 21 days after onset of rash. Measles involves lymphoid tissue and respiratory epithelium early in the illness. Therefore, pneumonia is fairly frequent. The majority of pneumonia cases are due to superimposed bacterial infection (staphylococci, pneumococci, streptococci), but some occur from primarily viral effects. For diagnosis, culture and serologic tests are available. Culture depends on the stage of disease. For a period of 1 week ending with the first appearance of the rash, blood, nasopharyngeal swabs or urine provide adequate specimens. After appearance of the rash, urine culture is possible up to 4 days. Beyond this, culture is not useful, and serologic tests must be employed.

Mumps

Mumps is a disseminated virus infection, although the main clinical feature is salivary gland enlargement. Evidence of nonsalivary gland involvement is most commonly seen in adults. In adult males, orchitis (usually unilateral) is reported in about 20% of cases. Adult females occasionally

develop oophoritis. Any age group may be affected by meningoencephalitis, the most serious complication of mumps. This is reported in 0.5–10%
of patients. Many persons with CSF changes are asymptomatic. Females
are affected five times more frequently than males. Complications of
mumps may appear before, during or after parotitis, sometimes even
without clinical parotitis. Diagnosis is made by culture or serologic tests.
Saliva is probably best for culture; mouth swabs or CSF can be used.

Viral Hepatitis

Viral hepatitis is one of the major problems in diagnostic virology. At
least two major groups of hepatitis viruses seem evident: (1) short-incuba-
tion hepatitis (hepatitis A), with an incubation period of 2–6 weeks, and (2)
long-incubation hepatitis (hepatitis B), whose incubation period is from 6
weeks to 6 months. At one time hepatitis B was thought to be transmitted
only by blood transfusion and was called "serum hepatitis"; hepatitis A
was known as "infectious hepatitis." This concept changed when a geneti-
cist discovered an antigen in the blood of an Australian native (Australia
antigen) that was found to occur in many patients with hepatitis B but not
with hepatitis A. Studies have shown that the probable virus of hepatitis B
has a double-shell structure (Dane particle) with an inner core (HB_c) and
an outer envelope (HB_s), and that the Australia antigen corresponds to the
outer coat. To correspond to these findings, Australia antigen underwent a
name change to hepatitis associated antigen (HAA) and then to hepatitis B
surface antigen (HB_sAg). The HB_sAg is found in a significant percentage
(more than 5%) of persons with diseases other than hepatitis (hemophilia,
mongolism, Hodgkin's disease, leukemia, lepromatous leprosy, chronic
hepatitis), in hemodialysis patients, in drug addicts, in homosexuals and in
inhabitants of various South Pacific and Asian countries. Some of these instances could be due to blood or blood component transfusion, some to
close-contact transmissal, and some to intrauterine infection; many are unexplained.

In hepatitis B, HB_sAg can often be detected 4–8 weeks after exposure
(range 2–24 weeks) and 2–4 weeks before a rise in serum transaminases
(serum glutamic-oxaloacetic transaminase [SGOT] or serum glutamic-pyruvic transaminase [SGPT]. By onset of hepatitis symptoms, HB_sAg titer is
already falling; it may become nondetectable in as little as 1 or 2 days from
onset of clinical illness, but more often persists for 1–6 weeks with the
average between 2 and 3 weeks. About 10% of patients are still positive
after 6 months (and are then considered "carriers"). Various test systems
have been devised to detect HB_sAg. Sensitivity in patients with HB_sAg is
variable: immunodiffusion, about 30%; counterimmunoelectrophoresis,
about 40%; CF, 50–60%; radioimmunoassay (RIA), more than 75% (p.
483). Interpretation of HB_sAg results thus must take into account (1) the
knowledge that less than half the cases of hepatitis-virus hepatitis are due
to hepatitis B and, therefore, potentially detectable by HB_sAg; (2) the type
of test used, and (3) how early in the clinical course the specimen was obtained.

Prior to HB_sAg testing, posttransfusion hepatitis incidence is recorded as
high as 33%. Using HB_sAg donor screening by RIA and excluding high-
risk donor population groups, incidence is reported as 5% or less. How-

ever, the majority of this improvement was obtained by donor population selection, not from HBsAg testing.

After transfusion with blood found negative to HBsAg by RIA, some patients have developed hepatitis that clinically and histologically simulated hepatitis B but without evidence of hepatitis B antigen or antibody. This has been termed "hepatitis C" or "non-AB."

Antigenic subgroups of HBsAg exist; the most important to date are adw, ayw, adr and ayr, but others are being discovered. These are thought to indicate possible subgroups (strains) of hepatitis B virus.

An additional antigen system "e" has been described that is associated with hepatitis B but is serologically distinct from either surface or core antigen. Some evidence exists that patients with detectable "e" antigen are more likely to develop chronic hepatitis and that carriers with "e" antigen are more likely to prove infectious to others.

Antibody (HBsAb) to HBsAg is found in 80–90% of patients, usually first appearing 2–13 weeks after HBsAg is first detectable, roughly at a point in time when HBsAg titer has begun to decline (assuming HBsAg does not persist). The HBsAb remains detectable for a variable period of time, usually for several years, but it may decline earlier. Not all patients manifest detectable or persistent HBsAb. Presence of HBsAb has been employed for epidemiologic studies and as an indication of decreased risk for those who must be in a high-risk area. Presence of HBsAb, however, does not guarantee immunity from hepatitis, since no protection is conferred against hepatitis A or C. Antibody to the core antigen (HBcAb) appears during the peak of HBsAg titer, and persists for months or years; in general, however, it becomes nondetectable while HBsAb still remains.

Practical clinical laboratory tests for hepatitis A virus are not yet available for routine use, but a CF test and an immune adherence procedure have been developed.

Hepatitis A virus is excreted in stool and usually transmitted via fecal-oral routes (in adults, by contaminated water or food). Hepatitis B is found in blood and body secretions, such as saliva and semen, and is usually transmitted by introduction of these fluids into a patient's skin or mucous membranes through small breaks in the lining epithelium. This may occur from transfusion of blood or certain blood products; injury with contaminated needles; contaminated blood on the skin in the presence of breaks in the skin; contaminated material in the mouth where small breaks in the gums and oral membranes permit viral entry, and sexual intercourse.

In about 10% of hepatitis B patients chronic hepatitis develops. Approximately two thirds of these patients have a form termed "chronic persistent hepatitis." These persons have persistent mild elevation of enzymes sensitive to hepatocellular damage (SGOT, SGPT, p. 210) and minimal changes on liver biopsy. About one third of chronic hepatitis patients have a more severe form, termed "chronic active hepatitis," which demonstrates a spectrum of severity on liver biopsy (with corresponding abnormalities in liver function tests) and which may progress to cirrhosis. Of the patients with chronic hepatitis 20–30% remain HBsAg-positive. In all, 5–10% of hepatitis B patients become carriers; 80–85% of these have chronic hepatitis, with the rest being asymptomatic and demonstrating normal transaminases.

Nearly all hepatitis A patients recover completely within several weeks. According to current opinion, hepatitis A does not have a carrier state. In general, 4 or 5 patients with hepatitis B are nonicteric for each one who develops jaundice; nonicteric hepatitis is even more frequent in hepatitis A.

Although many use "viral hepatitis" as a synonym for infection by hepatitis viruses A and B, a wide range of viruses may infect hepatic cells with varying frequency and severity. The most common (but not the only) examples are infectious mononucleosis (Epstein-Barr virus) and the cytomegalic inclusion virus.

The antigen HB_sAg has been associated with some cases of polyarteritis nodosa, membranous or membranoproliferative glomerulonephritis and serum sickness, the latter occurring as the initial phase of hepatitis clinical illness. Some type of autoimmune mechanism is believed to be responsible.

Cytomegalic Inclusion Virus Disease

Cytomegalic inclusion virus may cause localized infection of the salivary glands without any clinical symptoms. If it becomes disseminated, a variety of manifestations may be produced, depending on the age of the patient, the presence of underlying diseases, which might alter the patient's immunologic response to the virus, or the visceral organs affected.

In the newborn the disseminated disease may appear in two forms:

1. A subacute form with predominantly cerebral symptoms, manifested by the picture of cerebral palsy or mental retardation.

2. An acute form with various combinations of hepatosplenomegaly, thrombocytopenia, hepatitis with jaundice and cerebral symptoms, such as convulsions. There usually is anemia, and there may be nucleated RBC and a shift to the left on peripheral blood smear.

In young children, the most common manifestation is probably mild fever or a febrile illness; one report indicates that hepatitis (usually mild, often nearly asymptomatic) is frequent.

In older children and adults clinical disease is very uncommon. It is most often superimposed on preexisting malignancy, such as leukemia or malignant lymphoma, and has predominantly pulmonary or hepatic involvement, which usually is overshadowed by the preexisting nonviral disease. Steroid or immunosuppressive therapy also predisposes to infection. In adults, cytomegalic inclusion virus disease may mimic infectious mononucleosis and is an important cause for postperfusion (posttransfusion) syndrome. This condition occurs after transfusion or extracorporeal circulation pump priming with whole blood, and consists of a febrile illness with liver function test abnormalities and atypical lymphocytes in the peripheral blood.

In the newborn periventricular cerebral calcification is demonstrable by x-ray in about 25%; this is highly suggestive, although the same pattern may be found in congenital toxoplasmosis. Characteristic inclusion bodies may be demonstrated within renal epithelial cells in stained smears of the urinary sediment in about 60% of cases; this may be an intermittent finding, which may require specimens on several days. A fresh specimen is preferable to a 24-hour collection, since the cells tend to disintegrate on standing. Probably the best procedure, when available, is virus culture of a urine specimen. For best results, this must reach the virus culture laboratory within 1–2 days. The specimen should not be frozen, as freezing progressively inactivates the virus; this is in contrast to most other viruses, where quick freezing is the procedure of choice for preserving specimens. The specimen should be refrigerated without actual freezing. In this way it may be preserved up to a week. It should be sent to the virus laboratory packed in ordinary ice (not dry ice); if possible, in an insulated container. Isolation of the cytomegalic virus may take several weeks.

In older children and adults the kidney is not often severely affected, so that urine specimens for cytomegalic inclusion bodies usually are not helpful. Urine, sputum or mouth swab culture for the virus is the method of choice. Fresh specimens are essential. If virus culture cannot be performed, serologic tests may be substituted. Complement fixation is the usual method available. Since antibody levels may persist for years, acute and convalescent specimens are necessary to demonstrate current infection. The method is not invariably abnormal in newborns. Immunofluorescence techniques have also been described; these have the additional advantage that infant IgM antibodies can be differentiated from maternal IgG antibodies. However, reaction to IgM globulins is not absolutely specific for cytomegalic inclusion disease.

Infectious Mononucleosis

The Epstein-Barr virus is now considered responsible for infectious mononucleosis. The same virus is also thought to be associated with a peculiar type of malignant lymphoma called Burkitt's lymphoma. Infectious mononucleosis patients are most often young adults, but a good percentage are children, and some are older adults. The most common features are fever, pharyngitis and adenopathy, with lymph node enlargement being the most frequent. It may be localized or generalized. The posterior cervical nodes are the most commonly enlarged. Soft-palate petechiae are found in 10–30% of the cases. Jaundice due to mild hepatitis is found in approximately 5% of the large patient series. Uncommon symptoms are skin rashes and supraorbital edema. The spleen is enlarged in about 40%. Laboratory data show normal hemoglobin and platelets, although rare cases of thrombocytopenia are reported. Incidentally, normal hemoglobin values help in differentiation from lymphoma and leukemia, which the clinical symptoms may resemble, as these two usually have anemia. There is a leukocytosis, usually by the second week or by the time lymphadenopathy is well established. However, during the first week there may be leukopenia. The differential white count is characteristic and includes two of the three criteria for diagnosis (serologic tests being the third). There is usually lymphocytosis with lymphocytes making up more than 50% of the total WBC; of these lymphocytes, a significant number (amounting to more than 20%) must be atypical. These so-called atypical lymphocytes are of three main types: type I has vacuolated or foamy blue cytoplasm and rounded nucleus; type II has an elongated flattened nucleus and large amounts of pale cytoplasm with sharply defined irregular borders; and type III has an immature irregular nucleus, which may have a nucleolus or show folding. All three types are larger than normal mature lymphocytes, and their nuclei are somewhat less dense. These atypical lymphocytes are not specific for infectious mononucleosis, but may be found in small-to-moderate numbers in a variety of viral diseases, including cytomegalic inclusion disease and infection by hepatitis virus. Many choose to call these cells virocytes. In addition, some of the type II variety may be created artificially by crushing and flattening normal lymphocytes near the edge of the blood smear. Infectious mononucleosis cells are sometimes confused with those of acute leukemia or lymphosarcoma, although in the majority of cases there is no problem.

The serologic test for infectious mononucleosis known as the Paul-Bunnell test is based on the discovery that the antibody produced in infectious mononucleosis will agglutinate sheep RBC. Dilutions are set up for 1:7, 1:14, 1:28, 1:64, 1:112, and so on serially, and the last tube dilution to show agglutination is reported as the titer. Normally, the titer is less than 1:112 and most often is almost or completely negative. The Paul-Bunnell test is also known as the "presumptive test," because later it was found that certain antibodies different from those of infectious mononucleosis will also attack sheep RBC. This is true of antibodies produced to the so-called Forssman antigen found naturally in man and certain other animals. Thus, if the Paul-Bunnell test is elevated, one does not know if this means infectious mononucleosis antibody or a nonspecific Forssman antibody. Fortunately, Forssman antibodies are usually not produced in high titers, so this fact may help in many cases. Eventually, the so-called differential absorption test (Davidsohn differential test) was developed.

It seems that guinea pig kidney is a good source of Forssman antigen. Therefore, if a serum containing Forssman antibody is allowed to come in contact with guinea pig kidney material, the Forssman antibody will combine with the kidney antigen and be removed from the serum when the serum is taken off. The serum will then show either a very low or a negative titer, whereas before it had been strongly positive. The infectious mononucleosis antibody will not be significantly absorbed by guinea pig kidney, but will be nearly completely absorbed by beef RBC, which do not significantly affect the Forssman antibody. The only other antigen that may be involved is that produced in serum sickness, and this will absorb both with beef RBC and guinea pig kidney. In the absorption test, there must be at least a three-tube decrease in titer to be considered significant absorption. In other words, true infectious mononucleosis antibody will not drop more than 3 tubes dilution when treated with guinea pig kidney, whereas Forssman antibody will. The height of the titer after absorption has no diagnostic value. However, the original presumptive test must have at least a 1:28 titer to allow the differential to be done at all. The Paul-Bunnell test remains elevated for several weeks or months after clinical symptoms have disappeared. The level of Paul-Bunnell titer does not correlate well with the clinical course of infectious mononucleosis. Titer is useful only in making a diagnosis, and should not be relied on to follow the clinical course of the disease or to assess results of therapy.

In suspected mononucleosis, the presumptive test should be done first; if necessary, it can be followed by a differential absorption procedure. The Paul-Bunnell and differential tests are usually positive by 3 weeks after onset of symptoms. Most cases are positive during the 2d week, although the Paul-Bunnell titer may not yet have risen to its full height. Many cases have such high presumptive titers that a differential is not necessary. Some never reach 1:112, and it is in these patients and those with only moderate titer elevation that the differential absorption is most helpful.

False positive differential results have been reported but are extremely rare. Elevated titer from infectious mononucleosis may persist for months, and it is possible that even the few reported false positive cases had subclinical mononucleosis sometime earlier. On the other hand, there are reports describing outbreaks of a disease that clinically was identical to infectious mononucleosis with typical blood changes, but with the Paul-Bunnell test negative in many or even all cases. A similar situation has been reported following blood transfusions; some of these posttransfusion patients prove to have cytomegalic inclusion virus on culture. This raises a question as to what criteria to use in differentiating infectious mononucleosis. When all three criteria are satisfied, there is no problem. When the Paul-Bunnell test and/or differential absorption are positive, most authors believe that the diagnosis can be made, although there are reports that viral infections occurring after infectious mononucleosis can cause anamnestic "false positive" heterophil reelevations. When the blood picture is characteristic both regarding number and type of lymphocytes, but the Paul-Bunnell test is negative as late as 3 weeks after onset, most believe that the diagnosis can be considered probable but not established. Parenthetically, many articles in the literature give only the results of the presumptive test; as mentioned, one can have a presumptive test within normal range (which is less than 1:112) and still have a positive differential absorption (if the titer is at least 1:28).

"Spot" tests have been devised in which the Paul-Bunnell and differential absorption tests are converted to a rapid slide procedure without titration. Citrate-preserved horse RBC are used instead of sheep RBC. The antigen-antibody reactions and absorptions are carried out visually by adding drops of reagents to areas on a slide or piece of paper, rather than by titration in test tubes. If properly done, preliminary reports indicate that the method is as sensitive and nearly as specific as the classic procedure. However, at least one report indicates that false positives may occur in malignant lymphoma when this particular technique is used.

A rapid modification of the heterophil procedure called Mono-Test uses formalin-fixed RBC without differential absorption. The Mono-Test has been reported to have almost the same specificity as the differential absorption technique. Burkitt's lymphoma may produce a false positive reaction.

In summary, the three criteria for the diagnosis of infectious mononucleosis are:

1. Lymphocytosis more than 50% of total WBC count.
2. Atypical lymphocytes more than 20% of the total lymphocytes.
3. Significantly elevated Paul-Bunnell test or differential absorption test. A positive Mono-Test or spot test, from current reports, satisfies this criterion.

Work has been done using antibodies to Epstein-Barr virus for diagnosis, but this has not proved very useful clinically.

Reye Syndrome

This is a childhood disease that usually begins a few days after onset of a viral illness, the reason for including it here. There is protracted vomiting;

then an encephalitis without focal neurologic signs accompanied by hepatitis with marked derangement of SGOT, SGPT, and lactic dehydrogenase (LDH). Although jaundice is not prominent, liver function is decreased to the extent that blood ammonia and prothrombin time are usually elevated. Creatine phosphokinase is markedly abnormal and phosphorus is decreased, indicating muscle involvement. Fatty liver is frequently found on biopsy or autopsy. Although exact etiology is not known, influenza A and B, especially B, have been associated with the majority of cases, with chickenpox next most frequent and other viruses also implicated on occasion.

RICKETTSIAL DISEASES

The rickettsiae to some extent resemble small bacteria, but are not stained with gram stain and cannot be cultured on artificial media. These organisms are spread only by insect vectors that have fed on blood from a patient with the disease—not from personal contact with a patient. Blood culture is the method of definitive identification for rickettsiae, especially in Rocky Mountain spotted fever. The blood specimen should be frozen and sent to the virus laboratory packed in dry ice. However, chick embryo or live animal inoculation must be done, since artificial culture medium is not available, and thus serologic tests by far overshadow culture as diagnostic aids. The most commonly used procedure is the Weil-Felix reaction. This test takes advantage of the fact that certain rickettsial diseases produce antibodies that also react (or cross-react) with antigen contained in certain strains of *Proteus* bacteria. These *Proteus* groups are called OX-19 and OX-K. Titers of 1:80 are suspicious, and 1:160 are definitely significant. Antibodies appear 7 – 10 days after onset of illness. Rickettsial diseases that may be diagnosed by means of the Weil-Felix reaction are the following:

DISEASE	PROTEUS STRAIN	VECTOR	ORGANISM
Epidemic typhus	OX-19	body louse	R. prowazekii
Endemic (murine) typhus	OX-19	rat flea	R. mooseri
Scrub typhus	OX-K	mite	R. tsutsugamushi
Rocky Mountain spotted fever	OX-19	tick	R. akeri

Unfortunately, there are certain limitations to the Weil-Felix test. First, there are a fairly large number of borderline false positive results as well as occasional outright false positives. Since the Weil-Felix reaction depends on *Proteus* antigen, urinary tract infection by *Proteus* should be ruled out if the Weil-Felix test is positive. Second, about two thirds of patients with Rocky Mountain spotted fever and Brill's disease (recrudescent typhus) give false negative reactions. In these two diseases, serologic CF tests are preferred to the Weil-Felix. The serum specimens should be frozen and sent to the laboratory packed in dry ice.

Rocky Mountain spotted fever occurs in spring and summer, predominantly in the eastern two thirds of the United States (the area east of the Rocky Mountains). Fever and rash are the most characteristic clinical findings, with the rash typically including the palms and soles. Since antibodies do not appear until 10 – 14 days after onset of illness, serologic tests are not useful during acute illness, the time when therapy must be instituted. The disease is transmitted through the bite of an infected tick; if the tick can be recovered intact, it is reported that examination of the tick hemolymph (p. 446) can demonstrate whether the tick actually is infected. However, the test is not widely available.

NONVIRAL, NONBACTERIAL INFECTIOUS AGENTS

Several unrelated groups of organisms will be discussed.

Mycoplasma

Primary atypical pneumonia is a name describing pulmonary infection by a variety of viruses and viruslike organisms that, nevertheless, produce a fairly characteristic syndrome. It consists of cough, fever, headache and malaise lasting about 10 days. Chest x-ray shows mottled infiltrates, which are most pronounced in the hilar areas of the lower lobes and are more often unilateral. Despite the symptoms and x-ray findings, there is characteristically very little abnormal on physical examination. The blood count is either normal or close to it. About half the cases have been found due to *Mycoplasma pneumoniae*, the so-called Eaton agent, a pleuropneumonialike organism (PPLO). The PPLO group is intermediate in size and other characteristics between viruses and bacteria. In primary atypical pneumonia due to mycoplasma, there is an abnormal CF test in 60–70% of cases and cold agglutinins are present in 50–60%.

Cold agglutinins are antibodies that are able to agglutinate type O RBC at icebox temperatures but not at room temperature. They are found in other diseases, and thus are nonspecific, but in adults with an acute respiratory syndrome, their presence in significant titer is usually associated with Eaton agent pneumonia. Cold agglutinins elevated over 1:32 are abnormal and can be found during the second week of illness, reaching a peak in the third or fourth week. A rising titer is more significant than a single determination. The PPLO can be cultured on special media, but this takes about a week. Sputum or pharyngeal swabs may be used. If preservation is necessary, specimens should be frozen and transported with dry ice.

T-strain mycoplasma have been cultured from a considerable percentage of patients with nongonococcal urethritis, but direct causation is still in doubt. *Mycoplasma hominis* has been associated with some cases of gynecologic infection.

The Chlamydiae

Chlamydiae (formerly called Bedsoniae) are tiny bacteria midway between viruses and rickettsiae in size. They cause psittacosis, lymphogranuloma venereum and trachoma. They also are probably responsible for a considerable proportion of nongonococcal urethritis. Psittacosis organisms are contracted from birds, most commonly parakeets. Two syndromes may be produced: (1) a typhoid-like picture or (2) a respiratory illness. Pulmonary involvement is more frequent, resembling a viral bronchopneumonia or influenza syndrome. White blood counts are usually normal or subnormal. Diagnosis is usually made through serologic (antibody) tests and a history of contact with birds. The antibodies of psittacosis cross-react with those of lymphogranuloma venereum.

Lymphogranuloma venereum (LGV) is transmitted by sexual contact. After an incubation period, the inguinal lymph nodes become swollen and tender in males; in females, the lymphatic drainage is usually to the intra-abdominal, perirectal and pelvic lymph nodes. In a considerable number of cases, the perirectal nodes develop abscesses and the nearby wall of the rectum is involved, eventually leading to scar tissue and constriction of the rectum. In either male or female, in the acute stage of lymphatic involvement, there may be fever, malaise and headache with sometimes joint aching – but all these may be absent. In the majority of cases the main findings are acute inguinal node enlargement in the male and chronic rectal stricture in the female. Laboratory findings in active disease include mild anemia, moderate leukocytosis and serum protein disturbances with considerable hyperglobulinemia and hypoalbuminemia.

The elevated globulin gives a high diffuse gamma elevation on serum protein electrophoresis, similar to that seen with far-advanced tuberculosis. Laboratory diagnosis includes a skin test called the Frei test, and serologic CF studies. Complement fixation is currently the test of choice since it is more sensitive than the Frei test. The CF reaction becomes positive about a month after infection and will remain elevated for years. Acute and convalescent serum should be obtained to demonstrate a rising titer. The Frei test is an intradermal skin injection of lymphogranuloma antigen giving a papule after 48 – 72 hours. This becomes positive in 2 – 3 weeks after the lymph node inflammation and remains positive for years. Either the serologic tests or the Frei test crossreact with psittacosis, although this usually is not a problem. Lymph node biopsy shows a characteristic histologic pattern which, however, is also seen with tularemia and cat-scratch fever. There is a relatively high incidence of syphilis serology biologic false positive reactions (p. 386) in LGV. This may cause confusion because, due to the venereal nature of transmission, syphilis may also be present, and early syphilis can give inguinal lymph node enlargement similar to LGV.

The Chlamydia and PPLO groups were included among the viruses for a long time. In the older literature there is frequent reference to them as "large viruses."

REFERENCES

Cesario, T. C.: Viral infections that affect the fetus, Postgrad. Med. 59:66, 1976.

Chanock, R. M., and Purcell, R. H.: Role of mycoplasmas in human respiratory disease, Med. Clin. North Am. 51:791, 1967.

Cheever, F. S.: Viral agents in gastrointestinal disease, Med. Clin. North Am. 51: 637, 1967.

Chin, T. D. Y.: Diagnosis of infectious mononucleosis, South. Med. J. 69:654, 1976.

Corey, L., et al.: Dealing with possible rabies exposure, Postgrad. Med. 59:87, 1976.

Corey, L., et al.: A nationwide outbreak of Reye's syndrome: Its epidemiologic relationship to influenza B, Am. J. Med. 61:615, 1976.

Coriell, L. L.: Clinical syndromes in children caused by respiratory infection, Med. Clin. North Am. 51:819, 1967.

Curnen, E. C.: The Coxsackie viruses, Pediatr. Clin. North Am. 7:903, 1960.

Davidsohn, I., and Lee, C. L.: The laboratory in the diagnosis of infectious mononucleosis, Med. Clin. North Am. 46:225, 1962.

DeVivo, D. C., et al.: Acute encephalopathy with fatty infiltration of the viscera, Pediatr. Clin. North Am. 23:527, 1976.

Dupont, J. R., and Earle, K. M.: Human rabies encephalitis, Neurology 15:1023, 1965.

Evans, A. S.: Clinical syndromes in adults caused by respiratory infection, Med. Clin. North Am. 51:803, 1967.

Gifford, H.: Cat scratch disease, Pediatr. Clin. North Am. 2:33, 1955.

Gitnick, G. L.: The liver and the antigens of hepatitis B, Ann. Intern. Med. 85:488, 1976.

Gocke, D. J.: Viral hepatitis, Postgrad. Med. 58:137, 1975.

Gocke, D. J.: Extrahepatic manifestations of viral hepatitis, Am. J. Med. Sci. 270:49, 1975.

Grady, G. F., et al.: Relation of e antigen to infectivity of HB$_s$Ag-positive inoculation among medical personnel, Lancet 2:492, 1976.

Gwaltney, J. M., Jr., and Jordon, W. S., Jr.: The present status of respiratory viruses, Med. Clin. North Am. 47:1155, 1963.

Holder, W. R., and Duncan, W. C.: Lymphogranuloma venereum, Clin. Obstet. Gynecol. 15:1004, 1972.

Holland, P. V., and Alter, H. J.: The clinical significance of hepatitis B virus antigens and antibodies, Med. Clin. North Am. 59:849, 1975.

Hoofnagle, J. H., et al.: Hepatitis B virus and hepatitis B surface antigen in human albumin products, Transfusion 16:141, 1976.

Kennedy, C., and Wangle, P.: Encephalitis: A variable syndrome in response to viral infection, Pediatr. Clin. North Am. 14:809, 1967.

Koretz, R. L., et al.: Post transfusion chronic liver disease, Gastroenterology 71:797, 1976.

Krugman, S.: Hepatitis: current status of etiology and prevention, Hosp. Practice 10: 39, 1975.

Krugman, S.: Varicella and herpes virus infections, Pediatr. Clin. North Am. 7:881, 1960.

Krugman, S., et al.: Viral hepatitis, type A: Identification by specific complement fixation and immune adherence tests, N. Engl. J. Med. 292:1141, 1975.

Langmuir, A.: Medical importance of measles, Am. J. Dis. Child. 103:224, 1962.

Lennette, E. H.: Rubella: technical problems in the performance of hemagglutination-inhibition (HI) tests, Calif. Med. 111:351, 1969.

Marymount, J. H., Jr., and Herrmann, K. L.: Rubella in pregnancy: Review of current problems, Postgrad. Med. 56:167, 1974.

McAllister, R. M.: ECHO virus infections, Pediatr. Clin. North Am. 7:927, 1960.

McChesney, J. A., et al.: Acute urethritis in male college students, J.A.M.A. 226:37, 1973.

Medical News: Clues tantalizing in efforts to link mycoplasmas, infertility, J.A.M.A. 226:263, 1973.

Murray, E. S.: Rocky Mountain spotted fever: A life-saving diagnostic problem. Clin. Med. 83(8):9, 1976.

Rifkind, D.: Cytomegalovirus mononucleosis, Ann. Intern. Med. 69:842, 1968.

Robinson, W. S., and Lutwick, L. I.: The virus of hepatitis, type B, N. Engl. J. Med. 295:1168, 1232, 1976.

Sadoff, L., and Goldsmith, O.: False-positive infectious mononucleosis spot test in pancreatic carcinoma, J.A.M.A. 218:1297, 1971.

Schachter, J., et al.: Are chlamydial infections the most prevalent venereal disease? J.A.M.A. 231:1252, 1975.

Scott, T. F. M.: Postinfectious and vaccinal encephalitis, Med. Clin. North Am. 51: 701, 1967.

Seitanides, B.: A comparison of the Monospot with the Paul-Bunnell test in infectious mononucleosis and other diseases, J. Clin. Pathol. 22:321, 1969.

Sever, J. L.: Viral teratogens: A status report, Hosp. Practice 5:75, 1970.

Snydman, D. R., et al.: Prevention of nosocomial viral hepatitis, type B (Hepatitis B), Ann. Intern. Med. 83:838, 1975.

Stevens, D. P., et al.: Asymptomatic cytomegalovirus infection following blood transfusion in tumor surgery, J. A.M.A. 221:1341, 1970.

Trepo, C. G., et al.: Detection of e antigen and antibody: Correlations with hepatitis B surface and hepatitis B core antigens, liver disease, and outcome in hepatitis B infections, Gastroenterology 71:804, 1976.

Weller, T. H.: The cytomegaloviruses: Ubiquitous agents with protean clinical manifestations, N. Engl. J. Med. 285:203, 267, 1971.

Ziring, P. R., et al.: The diagnosis of rubella, Pediatr. Clin. North Am. 18:87, 1971.

17 / Medical Parasitology

Toxoplasmosis

THIS DISEASE is caused by a protozoan organism, *Toxoplasma gondii*. The disease is transmitted via raw or poorly cooked meat, and possibly in some cases by oocysts in feces of infested cats. There may be a congenital form transmitted to the fetus during the early stages of pregnancy or an acquired form. The congenital form is manifested most often by chorioretinitis (usually bilateral); other frequent findings include brain damage (mental retardation, microcephalus or hydrocephalus and convulsions), and intracerebral calcifications on x-ray. Cerebrospinal fluid (CSF) is abnormal in about two thirds of patients, containing xanthochromia, mononuclear pleocytosis and elevated protein. There may also be a neonatal disseminated type whose clinical picture is similar to bacterial septicemia. The acquired form is usually seen in adults, where the most common manifestations are lymphadenopathy and low-grade fever. In addition, there is an acquired disseminated type that is associated with deficient immunologic defense mechanisms, either from immunologic suppression therapy or a disease such as leukemia. Diagnosis includes isolation of the organisms and serologic tests for antibody formation. Culture has proved to be very difficult, and most laboratories are not equipped to do this. Lymph node biopsy often shows a histologic pattern that is nonspecific but still characteristic enough to be suggestive, although not diagnostic, of the disease.

Serologic tests form the backbone of diagnosis. The Sabin-Feldman dye test was the original standard procedure. The dye test involves working with live *Toxoplasma* organisms, but is very sensitive and demonstrates specific antibody to *Toxoplasma*. Usually it begins to become positive as early as the 10th day after infection, although some cases may take considerably longer. The titer climbs rapidly and remains elevated for months, eventually falling to a stable low level of less than 1:256, which persists for years or life. To make a diagnosis of acute infestation requires a change from negative to positive, a rapid fourfold or greater rise in titer (preferably from a low level) or a very high stable titer. The dye test has the disadvantage just mentioned that antibody levels tend to persist. Therefore, it is often difficult to be certain whether an elevated titer from a single specimen represents recent or old infestation. This is made worse by the fact that exposure to *Toxoplasma organisms* is very common. Surveys have shown positive dye studies in 20–70% of the various populations studied. Also, the antibody crosses the placenta and will appear in the fetus if the mother

191

has an elevated titer either from old or recent infestation. Therefore, to make a diagnosis of congenital toxoplasmosis, it is necessary to have either very high titer in both mother and infant, or to demonstrate a rising titer in the infant from specimens taken in the 1st and 6th weeks of life. If no active organisms were present and antibody was only passively acquired from the mother, instead of rising, the titer should fall during this time. In acute acquired toxoplasmosis the diagnosis is made as described earlier. If the toxoplasmosis is chronic, titer levels may be relatively low, as mentioned previously, so clinical findings may be more important than the laboratory results.

The Sabin-Feldman dye test is being replaced by the Indirect Fluorescent Antibody (IFA) procedure, which detects the same antibody as the dye test, has the same sensitivity, rises at about the same time and remains elevated in similar fashion. False positive reactions may occur in patients who display antinuclear antibodies, such as those found in rheumatoid-collagen diseases. A complement fixation (CF) test has been described that reacts with a different but still specific antibody. This test becomes positive a few weeks after the dye or IFA tests in a dilution greater than 1:2 (some require 1:8), rapidly rises and then gradually falls to negative, usually within 2–4 years. An indirect hemagglutination test has also been used. It also becomes abnormal later than the dye or IFA tests, but persists nearly as long.

Malaria

This widespread cause of serious infection in Asia and Africa may be acquired by travelers or military personnel. Diagnostic procedures were discussed under Anemia (p. 35).

Gastrointestinal Parasites

Ascaris, hookworm, *Strongyloides,* the tapeworms and the amebas form the majority of gastrointestinal parasites that have clinical significance in the United States. Diagnosis usually depends on examination of the feces for larvae or eggs. In most situations (except for amebiasis) 3 routine stool specimens, collected 1 every other day and sent for "ova and parasites," is adequate.

ENTAMEBA HISTOLYTICA. — This etiologic agent of amebiasis is acquired by ingestion of ameba cysts from contaminated food or water. Waterborne invasion is frequently associated with a water supply in close proximity to sewer material. Clinically, there are several forms of acute amebiasis: a severe acute colitis which may resemble severe ulcerative colitis (sometimes with blood and mucus in the stool) or shigellosis; chronic diarrhea similar to milder ulcerative colitis; intermittent mild diarrhea; asymptomatic carriers; and even a group with constipation. Acutely ill patients are usually afebrile and have normal WBC and hemoglobin, although patients with severe amebic colitis or hepatic abscess frequently have low-grade fever, leukocytosis between 10,000 and 20,000/cu mm, and mild anemia. *Entameba histolytica* is more difficult to diagnose than most of the common intestinal parasites and requires special precautions. If the specimen for amebas is soft or liquid, it should be sent to the laboratory immediately, with the time of collection noted, because fresh specimens are essential to demonstrate the trophozoite stage. Well-formed stools usually contain only cysts, and may be refrigerated temporarily. For collection routine, 3 specimens, 1 specimen collected every other day, are more reliable than a single specimen. Multiple specimens collected the same day are not much better than a single specimen. If the stools on 3 alternate days are all negative, and if strong clinical suspicion is still present, a saline purge should be used. After a saline purge (such as Fleet Phosphosoda), the patient should be passing liquid stools within a few hours. Oily laxatives (such as mineral oil or magnesia) make the stools useless for examination. Enema specimens are not advisable, because they are too dilute to be of much value and, in addition, may destroy the trophozoites. Barium, if present, also makes the preparation unfit to read. If stool specimens for ameba must be sent by mail, they should be placed in a preservative (1 part specimen to 3 parts of 10% Formalin). If possible, a second portion using a special polyvinyl alcohol fixative (PVA) as a preservative (in the same proportions) should be included along with the Formalin-fixed portion of the specimens. (Formalin preserves ameba cysts, and also eggs and larvae of other parasites; PVA preserves ameba trophozoites, although ameba cysts are often distorted.)

The preceding discussion was concerned with the usual type of amebiasis — amebiasis localized to the colon. Visceral amebiasis is not common. Liver involvement with abscess formation constitutes a majority of these cases. Clinical hepatic amebiasis is always associated with chronic rather than acute ameba infestation. Only 30–50% of patients provide a history of diarrhea. Only about 25% of patients will have amebae detectable in the stool. Classic cases have hepatomegaly, right upper quadrant pain, elevation of the right hemidiaphragm, leukocytosis as high as 20,000/cu mm and fever. Alkaline phosphatase surprisingly is normal in more than half of the patients. Liver scan is often very helpful, both for detection and localization of a lesion.

Serologic tests for amebiasis are now becoming available in reference laboratories. The most important of these are CF, indirect hemagglutination (IHA), gel diffusion (GD) and slide latex agglutination (LA). Of these methods, all are positive in 80–100% of those with hepatic abscess, with IHA and LA probably more consistently abnormal. For intestinal amebiasis, IHA and LA are reported to detect 80–90% of clinically evident amebiasis patients, considerably more than the other methods. The more serious cases are more likely to be positive. Antibody development has some correlation to tissue invasion, and the majority of asymptomatic carriers are nonreactive. Antibody levels persist for some time, so that a positive test does not necessarily mean active infestation.

SCHISTOSOMA MANSONI. — *Schistosoma* is sometimes encountered in the United States because it is endemic in Puerto Rico. Routine stools for parasite ova are often not sufficient, because the adult lays its eggs in the venous system, and the ova must penetrate the intestinal mucosa in order to appear in the stool. In difficult cases, proctoscopic rectal biopsy with a fresh unstained crush preparation of the biopsy specimen has been advocated. A CF test with 90% sensitivity has been reported, but this is not widely available.

PINWORM (*Enterobius* or *Oxyuris vermicularis*). — Infestation with pin-worms is fairly common in children. The female worm lays her eggs at night around the anal region. The best diagnostic procedure, therefore, is some method to swab the anal region thoroughly with an adhesive sub-stance such as transparent celluloid tape ("Scotch tape"). The sticky sur-face with the eggs can then be directly applied to a microscope glass slide and later examined for the characteristic pinworm ova. Such slides can also be sent through the mail, if necessary. The best time for obtaining speci-mens is early in the morning, before the child gets up. Stool samples are not satisfactory for diagnosis of enterobiasis. Since the worms do not lay eggs every night, repeated specimens may be necessary.

HOOKWORM. — A problem in some areas of the southern United States, hookworm occasionally may be the etiology of an iron-deficiency anemia in children. Routine stool examinations for ova and parasites are usually ade-quate for diagnosis.

TAPEWORM. — The fish tapeworm *Diphyllobothrium latum (Dibothrio-cephalus latus)* is only rarely a problem in the United States. The organ-isms are ingested with raw pike fish from the Great Lakes area. Usually very few symptoms are produced, but occasionally the syndrome of mega-loblastic anemia may result from ingestion of dietary vitamin B_{12} by the parasite. Diagnosis consists of stool examinations for ova.

Tapeworm infestation in man ordinarily occurs when the intermediate host (animal or fish) ingests tapeworm eggs or prolarvae, the egg (or prolar-va) evolves to a larval form within the intermediate host, man eats flesh from the intermediate host that contains the larva and the larva develops into an adult worm in the lumen of the patient's intestine. If man ingests ova or prolarva rather than the larva, larva may develop within the patient's intestine, proceed through the intestinal wall, and reach the bloodstream, capable of producing abnormality in various organs or tissues.

The most publicized tapeworm larval diseases are echinococcus or hydatid cyst (*Echinococcus granulosus*, the dog tapeworm); cysticercosis (*Taenia solium*, the swine tapeworm), and sparganosis (a dog or cat tape-worm of the *Spirometra* genus related to the fish tapeworm *D. latum*). No good laboratory method is available for diagnosis of cysticercosis or sparga-nosis. The laboratory may be helpful in echinococcus (hydatid) disease, although this condition is rare in the United States. The primary host is the dog; the ova are ingested by man or sheep (or other animals), who act as intermediate hosts, from material contaminated by dog feces. Larva emerge from the ova, penetrate the intestinal wall, and travel to the liver. Cystic structures (hydatid cysts) containing brood capsules filled with sco-lices grow in the liver (75% of cases) but may appear in the lungs or other locations. Diagnostic aids include the liver scan, a skin test known as the Casoni test, a hemagglutination test, and immunoelectrophoresis (IEP). The Casoni and hemagglutination tests are said to be positive in 90% of those patients with hepatic lesions but abnormal in less than half of those with cysts elsewhere. False positive results in the Casoni test are said to occur with some frequency. The most specific technique is said to be IEP by the method of Capron.

TRICHINELLA SPIRALIS. — This organism is usually ingested with raw or insufficiently cooked pork, or insufficiently cooked meat products contaminated by infected pork. During the first week after ingestion, symptoms consist of nausea and diarrhea; this may be minimal or absent. Seven to 8 days after ingestion, there is onset of severe muscle pain, which sometimes begins in the face. Bilateral periorbital edema often develops. Eosinophilia may begin as early as 10 days after ingestion, and, with muscle pain and periorbital edema, forms a very suggestive triad. The eosinophilia reaches its peak during the 3d week. The most helpful laboratory test is a skin test; this becomes positive near the end of the 3d week after ingestion. A positive result consists of a wheal and erythema reaction within 15 minutes. A delayed reaction after 24 hours has been described, but this is apparently less specific. A negative result does not rule out the diagnosis. A positive result does not guarantee that symptoms are due to trichinosis, because a skin test remains positive for many years. Some commercial skin test antigen has been reported to be insufficiently sensitive. All antigens may cross-react with *Trichuris* organisms. Muscle biopsy is occasionally useful; it is considered best to wait until at least 3 weeks after ingestion to do this procedure, to allow the larvae time to encyst. A painful area of a skeletal muscle has been recommended as the preferred site for biopsy.

A latex agglutination slide test is now available: 20–30% of cases are positive by 7 days after onset of symptoms and 80–90% in 4–5 weeks. False positive results have been recorded in polyarteritis nodosa (also in tuberculosis, typhoid and infectious mononucleosis, but these would ordinarily not be considered in differential diagnosis).

Trichomonas Vaginalis

This protozoan parasite infests the vagina and labial area in the female and occasionally produces urethritis in the male. The diagnosis is accidentally made in many cases by a microscopic examination of a fresh urine centrifuged sediment. The living organism has a typical appearance and motility. However, on dying, the parasite assumes a round shape and resembles a large white blood cell or small epithelial cell; therefore, a fresh specimen is essential. The urine specimen must be taken without cleansing the genitalia, since the organism is actually a contaminant. A more reliable method consists of a vaginal swab, which is immediately placed into a small amount of 0.9% saline. A wet preparation is then made from this material and examined microscopically. Swabs from the ectocervix and endocervix are unreliable, although the organism may sometimes be found in a cervical PAP smear.

REFERENCES

Barrett-Connor, E.: Amebiasis, today, in the United States, Calif. Med. 114:1, 1971.
Faust, E. C., and Russell, P. F.: *Clinical Parasitology* (7th ed.; Philadelphia: Lea & Febiger, 1964).
Feldman, H. A.: Toxoplasmosis, N. Engl. J. Med. 279:1370, 1431, 1968.
Feldman, H. A.: Toxoplasma and toxoplasmosis, Hosp. Practice 4:64, 1969.
Harrison, E. G., et al.: Human and canine dirofilariasis in the United States, Mayo Clin. Proc. 40:906, 1965.
Healy, G. R.: Laboratory diagnosis of amebiasis, Bull. NY Acad. Med. 47:478, 1971.

Jacobs, L., et al.: A comparison of the toxoplasma skin tests, the Sabin-Feldman dye
    tests, and complement fixation tests in various forms of uveitis, Bull. Johns Hop-
    kins Hosp. 99:1, 1956.
Jones, T. C., et al.: Acquired toxoplasmosis, NY J. Med. 69:2237, 1969.
Kagan, I. G.: Evaluation of routine serologic testing for parasitic diseases, Am. J.
    Pub. Health 55:1820, 1965.
Kean, B. H., and Kimball, A. C.: The complement-fixation test in diagnosis of con-
    genital toxoplasmosis, Am. J. Dis. Child. 131:21, 1977.
Markell, E. K., and Voge, M.: Diagnostic Medical Parasitology (3d ed.; Philadel-
    phia: W. B. Saunders Company, 1971).
Maynard, J. E., and Kagan, I. G.: Intradermal test in the detection of trichinosis, N.
    Engl. J. Med. 270:1, 1964.
Salfelder, K., and Schwarz, J.: Pneumocystosis, Am. J. Dis. Child. 114:693, 1967.
Schantz, P. M.: Testing for hydatid disease, Lancet 2:1022, 1976.
Smith, M. H. D., and Beaver, P. C.: Visceral larva migrans due to infection with dog
    and cat ascarids, Pediatr. Clin. North Am. 2:163, 1955.
Sterman, M. M.: Amebae of man: Classification and practical laboratory diagnosis,
    Ann. NY Acad. Sci. 98:725, 1962.
Stoll, N. R.: For hookworm diagnosis, is finding an egg enough? Ann. NY Acad. Sci.
    98:712, 1962.
Taylor, R. L.: Sparganosis in the United States, Am. J. Clin. Pathol. 66:560, 1976.
Turner, J. A., et al.: Amebiasis—A symposium, Calif. Med. 114:44, 1971.

18 / Cerebrospinal Fluid Examination

Pressure

NORMAL VALUES FOR CEREBROSPINAL FLUID (CSF) are 100–200 mm of water. Elevations are due to increased intracranial pressure. The two most common causes are meningitis and subarachnoid hemorrhage. Brain tumor and brain abscess will, in most cases, cause increased intracranial pressure, but only after a varying period —days or even weeks. An increase is present in many cases of lead encephalopathy. Cerebrospinal fluid pressure varies directly with venous pressure but has no constant relationship to arterial pressure. The Queckenstedt sign makes clinical use of this information; increased venous pressure via jugular vein compression increases CSF pressure at the lumbar region, whereas a subarachnoid obstruction above the lumbar will prevent this effect.

Appearance

Normally CSF is clear. It may be pink or red with many RBC present, or white and cloudy if there are many WBC or especially high protein content. Usually there have to be more than 500 WBC/cu mm before cloudiness can begin to appear. When blood has been present in the CSF for more than 4 hours, xanthochromia (yellow color) may occur, although the RBC may eventually disappear due to lysis. Severe jaundice may give false xanthochromic appearance.

Sugar

Normal values are 50 mg/100 ml or higher (Somogyi or "true glucose" methods). Values of 40–50 mg/100 ml are equivocal, although it is rare to find values below 45 mg/100 ml. normally. The CSF level depends on the blood glucose values and is usually one half to two thirds of the blood level. The main pathologic significance of the CSF sugar level occurs when it decreases, as it does classically in bacterial and tuberculous meningitis. It is important to know, however, that when seen very early, the patient may still have normal CSF glucose level, although later it begins to decrease. Since elevated blood sugar levels may mask a decrease in CSF values, it is helpful to secure a blood glucose determination at the same time that the CSF specimen is obtained, especially if intravenous glucose therapy is being given. In addition, a low level of CSF glucose may be due to peripheral blood hypoglycemia, especially if the CSF cell count is normal. Other conditions which may cause a decrease are metastatic carcinoma of the meninges and also, sometimes, subarachnoid hemorrhage, probably due to release of glycolytic enzymes from the red cells and dying tissue. In most other central nervous system diseases, including viral meningitis, enceph-

197

alitis, brain abscess and syphilis, CSF sugar levels typically are normal when bacterial infection of the meninges is not present. However, decreased levels are sometimes found in mumps meningoencephalitis and lymphocytic choriomeningitis.

Protein

Protein concentration in CSF is normally 15–40 mg/100 ml. As a general but not invariable rule, increased protein is roughly proportional to the degree of leukocytosis in the CSF; protein concentration is also increased by the presence of blood. There are, however, certain diseases in which mild to moderate protein increase with relatively slight leukocytosis may be present; these include brain tumor, multiple sclerosis, chronic infections and similar conditions. Diabetics with peripheral neuropathy frequently have elevated CSF protein levels of unknown cause. A marked protein elevation without corresponding cell increase is known as albuminocytologic dissociation; this is found classically in the Guillain-Barré syndrome.

Protein may be measured in the laboratory quantitatively by any of several methods. A popular semiquantitative bedside method is Pandy's test, in which CSF is added to a few drops of saturated phenol agent. This agent reacts with all protein, but apparently much more with globulin. Chronic infections or similar conditions, such as (tertiary) syphilis or multiple sclerosis, tend to accentuate globulin elevation and thus may give positive Pandy test results, although the total CSF protein may not be tremendously increased. Contamination by blood will often give false positive test results.

The technical method used can influence results. The two most common methods use sulfosalicylic acid and trichloracetic acid. Sulfosalicylic acid is influenced by the ratio of albumin to globulin, whereas trichloracetic acid is not.

In some CNS diseases there is a disproportionate increase in gamma globulin compared to albumin or total protein. Several investigators have noted that increased CSF gamma globulin occurs in approximately 70–85% (literature range 50–88%) of patients with multiple sclerosis, whereas total protein is elevated only in about 25% of the patients (range 13–34%). Various other acute and chronic diseases of the brain may elevate CSF gamma globulin, and this fraction may also be affected by serum hyperglobulinemia. The latter artifact may be excluded by comparing gamma globulin quantitation in serum and CSF. Specificity of CSF gamma globulin may be improved by quantitation of the immunoglobulin components of the gamma fraction (IgG, IgA and IgM, p. 245). Multiple sclerosis is associated with isolated CSF IgG (or IgG/albumin) increase, which helps rule out certain other conditions (e.g., bacterial meningitis, which is associated with elevation of all three Ig components). Neurosyphilis, subacute sclerosing panencephalitis and postvaccinal encephalitis have an IgG pattern similar to multiple sclerosis. For screening purposes, immunoglobulin fractionation is reported to improve sensitivity of the test in multiple sclerosis and to provide greater specificity.

The colloidal gold test (p. 447) also depends on changes in CSF globulins and for some time was considered very helpful in diagnosis of multiple sclerosis. The classic pattern associated with multiple sclerosis was a "first-zone" curve; however, only about 25% of patients actually displayed a first-zone curve, while about 25% produced a second-zone pattern. Therefore, fewer than 50% showed an abnormal colloidal gold curve. The typical "multiple sclerosis pattern" was found in a distinct minority of cases, and the pattern is actually not specific, since it is also found in general paresis and occasionally in a variety of other disorders. Immunoglobulin quantitation by CSF electrophoresis or immunodiffusion is replacing the colloidal gold test.

Cell Count

As a general rule, any conditions that affect the meninges will cause CSF leukocytosis; the degree will depend on the type of irritation, its duration and its intensity. Usually, the highest WBC counts are found in severe acute infections. The classic variety is the acute bacterial infection. One important thing to keep in mind is that if the patient is seen very early, leukocytosis may be minimal or even absent, just as CSF sugar level may be normal. However, in a few hours a repeat lumbar puncture usually finds steadily increasing WBC counts. Normal initial counts are not frequent but may occur and can be very misleading. Another general rule is that in bacterial infections polymorphonuclear neutrophils usually are the predominating cell type, whereas in viral infections, chronic nervous system diseases and tertiary syphilis, lymphocytes or mononuclears ordinarily predominate. The main exception is tuberculous meningitis, which combines a bacterial with a chronic type of infection; in this case, the cells are

TABLE 18–1.—PATTERNS OF CSF ABNORMALITY: CELL TYPE
AND GLUCOSE LEVEL

Polymorphonuclear: low glucose
  Acute bacterial meningitis
Polymorphonuclear: normal glucose
  Early phase acute bacterial meningitis (some cases)
  Brain abscess
  Early phase coxsackievirus and echovirus meningitis
  Amebic meningitis
  Early phase *Leptospira* meningitis
  Acute bacterial meningitis with intravenous glucose therapy
Lymphocytic: low glucose
  Tuberculosis meningitis
  Cryptococcal (*Torula*) meningitis
  Mumps meningoencephalitis (some cases)
  Meningeal carcinomatosis (some cases)
  Meningeal sarcoidosis (some cases)
Lymphocytic: normal glucose
  Viral meningitis
  Viral encephalitis
  Postinfectious encephalitis
  Lead encephalopathy
  CNS syphilis
  Brain tumor (occasionally)
Leptospira meningitis (after the early phase)

predominantly lymphocytes (although frequently combined with some increase in neutrophils). On the other hand, coxsackievirus and echovirus infections may have a predominance of neutrophils in the early stages; in most of these patients, the CSF subsequently shifts to lymphocytosis. Uremia is said to produce a mild lymphocytosis in about 25% of patients. Partial treatment of bacterial meningitis may cause a shift in cell type toward lymphocytosis.

In cases of subarachnoid hemorrhage or traumatic spinal fluid taps, approximately 1 WBC is added for every 500 RBC, and approximately 1 mg/100 ml of protein for every 1,000 RBC. Also, the presence of blood may sometimes cause moderate meningeal irritation, with subsequent increase in polymorphonuclear leukocytes. Another exception is so-called aseptic meningeal reaction that is secondary to either a nearby infection or sometimes to acute localized brain destruction. In these cases, which actually are not too common, there may be a wide range of WBC values with neutrophils often predominating. When this occurs, however, CSF sugar level should be normal, since the meninges are not directly infected. Aseptic meningitis is not the same as aseptic meningeal reaction. Aseptic meningitis is due to direct involvement of the meninges by nonbacterial organisms. Viruses cause most cases, but organisms such as *Leptospira* sometimes do also. Bacterial CSF cultures are negative. Sugar is usually normal. Protein is usually, but not always, increased. The WBC count is elevated to varying degree; the predominant type of cell depends on the etiology.

Serology

Serology is discussed in Chapter 31. Nevertheless, some of that discussion will be repeated here for the sake of continuity. The standard serologic tests for syphilis (STS), such as the Venereal Disease Research Laboratory Test (VDRL), usually, but not always, yield positive results in the blood when results in CSF are positive. A lack of relationship is most often found in the tertiary stage, when the blood VDRL sometimes reverts to normal. Conversely, CSF tests very often yield negative results when peripheral blood STS results are positive, since central nervous system (CNS) syphilis is usually a tertiary form in which symptoms develop only after years of infection. In many cases of syphilis, the CNS is not clinically involved at all. The more specific tests, such as the treponemal immobilizing test (TPI) or fluorescent treponemal antibody-absorption test (FTA-ABS) usually yield positive results in the blood if CNS syphilis exists. Increased CSF white cell counts and protein concentrations are better guides to actual syphilitic activity than the CSF serology, and they may be present as early as the secondary stage. A positive serology alone, either in the blood or the CSF, does not indicate if the disease is currently active. Results of CSF serology are usually negative in patients with so-called biologic false positive blood reactions. The three most important forms of CNS syphilis are general paresis, tabes dorsalis, and vascular neurosyphilis. In general paresis, the STS on spinal fluid almost always yields positive results in untreated cases. In tabes, the VDRL on spinal fluid is said to yield usually positive results in early untreated cases, but negative results may appear in up to 50% of late, or so-called burnt-out, cases. In vascular neurosyphilis, there are positive results in approximately 50% of cases. The FTA-ABS is more sensitive than the VDRL, but there is no agreement on the clinical significance of a reactive FTA-ABS and nonreactive VDRL on spinal fluid.

Bacteriology

The diagnosis of acute bacterial meningitis often depends on the isolation of the organisms in the spinal fluid. In children, there is some regularity of the types of infection most commonly found. In infants under the age of 6 months, gram-negative coliform organisms are most frequent (in neonatal meningitis, group B streptococci, *S. aureus*, and *Listeria* should also be mentioned). In children from 6 months to 5 years of age, *Hemophilus influenzae* and *Meningococcus* are the two most common organisms, and *Pneumococcus* is the third. In older children and adolescents, *Meningococcus* is first and *Pneumococcus* second. In adults, *Meningococcus* and *Pneumococcus* are still dominant, but *Pneumococcus* is more prevalent in some reports. In old age, there may be practically any type of organism, including an increasing number of fungi. Also, in patients who are debilitated or have underlying serious diseases such as leukemia or carcinoma, fungi are not uncommon. In many cases, a centrifuged spinal fluid sediment can be smeared and gram stained so that the organisms can be seen easily. A (bacterial) culture should be done in all cases where bacterial meningitis is suspected or in any cases where bacterial meningitis could be even a remote possibility. Special provision should be made for spinal fluid to reach the laboratory as quickly as possible, and if any particular organism is suspected, the laboratory should be informed so that special media can be used if necessary. For example, meningococci grow best in a high CO_2 atmosphere, and *H. influenzae* should be planted on media provided with a staph. streak.

When meningitis or brain abscess due to *Cryptococcus* is suspected, an India ink spinal fluid preparation is the classic diagnostic test. *Cryptococcus* is a yeastlike (fungus) organism (also known as *Torula*) whose peculiarity is a thick gelatinous capsule. This capsule shows up well in the dark background of black India ink. Sometimes this organism is demonstrated only after repeated spinal fluid examinations and some reports indicate that as many as 50% never demonstrate *Torula*. A culture should also be done. Fungi require different culture media than bacteria, so the laboratory must be notified that fungi are suspected. Meningitis due to *Cryptococcus* produces a CSF pleocytosis consisting predominantly of mononuclears. The protein concentration is elevated; the sugar level frequently is decreased. As noted above, cultures on ordinary bacterial (or tuberculosis) culture media will be negative. Serologic tests such as the latex slide procedure (p. 170) are now available for serum and CSF and are said to be more sensitive than India ink. There is some controversy over accuracy of the latex test when performed on CSF.

CEREBROSPINAL FLUID FINDINGS IN BRAIN DISEASES

Brain Abscess

Apparently the CSF findings in brain abscess are not significantly influenced by the causative organism or the location of the lesion. The spinal fluid is most often clear, and about 70% of patients are said to have increased pressure. Protein levels are normal in nearly 25% of patients, with about 55% of the values between 45 and 100 mg/100 ml and the remaining 20% over 100 mg/100 ml. Sugar level is normal. Cell counts are variable; about 30% are between 5 and 25, about 25% between 25 and 100, and about 25% between 100 and 500/cu mm. Lymphocytes generally predominate, but a significant percentage (5–25%) of polymorphonuclear neutrophils are said to be nearly always present. In occasional cases, an abscess breaks through to the subarachnoid space and results in purulent meningitis.

Brain Tumor

In primary cortical brain tumor, the CSF usually is clear and colorless, although xanthochromia may be present. Spinal fluid pressure is elevated in 70% of patients. Seventy percent show increased protein levels, with about half of these over 100 mg/100 ml. Levels of CSF sugar are normal. The majority (70%) of brain tumor patients have normal cell counts. Of the remainder, about two thirds have counts less than 25/cu mm, mostly lymphocytes. In the few patients with high cell counts, there may be appreciable numbers of neutrophils, and the spinal fluid pattern would then resemble that of brain abscess. Other methods of diagnosis are discussed in Chapter 32. Most metastatic tumors behave like primary neoplasms. In occasional instances, metastatic carcinoma may spread widely over the meninges. In such cases, the findings are similar to those of tuberculous meningitis (high cell count, lymphocytes predominating, elevated protein, and decreased sugar). Cell blocks and cytologic smears of spinal fluid sediment are helpful for diagnosis. These would not be useful in the ordinary case of metastatic carcinoma or in primary intracranial neoplasms, where the meninges are not directly involved.

Lead Encephalopathy

Lead poisoning is discussed elsewhere (p. 430). Lead encephalopathy occurs mainly in children (adults are more likely to develop peripheral neuropathy), and it is more common in acute than in chronic poisoning. Clinical signs and symptoms include visual disturbances, delirium, convulsions, severe headaches, hypertension, and sometimes papilledema. CSF usually displays increased pressure. Cell count varies from normal to several thousand; the majority of patients have mild to moderate pleocytosis. Mononuclears usually predominate, but polymorphonuclears may occasionally be high, especially in those patients with the more elevated cell counts. Protein level may be normal or increased; sugar level is normal. These findings may indicate a variety of conditions, such as meningitis or meningoencephalitis due to virus or fungus, or early bacterial meningitis.

CSF Puncture Artifacts

One or two other subjects should be mentioned. Too often, unfortunately, during a lumbar puncture, the question is brought up whether blood has been introduced into the spinal fluid by the spinal needle, resulting in a so-called traumatic tap. There are several useful differential points. Xanthochromia, if present, suggests previous bleeding. However, a nonxanthochromic supernatant fluid does not rule out the diagnosis, since xanthochromia may be absent even when subarachnoid bleeding has occurred many hours before. A second point utilizes the fact that the standard method for collecting CSF involves catching the specimen in three consecutively numbered tubes. If blood was introduced by a traumatic tap, more blood should appear in the first tube, less in the second, and least in the third, as the bleeding decreases. Previous CSF bleeding should distribute the RBC equally throughout the spinal fluid and characteristically show approximately equal numbers of RBC in each of the three tubes. Therefore, RBC counts can, if necessary, be requested for all three tubes. However, sometimes traumatic taps, if severe, can have roughly equal numbers of RBC in each tube. As noted previously, blood in the CSF may falsely alter the various chemical tests.

SPECIAL PROCEDURES IN BRAIN DISEASES

Radioisotope Studies

Radioisotope studies include brain scan, cerebral blood flow study and isotope cisternography. Scanning the brain is similar to scanning any other organ. An appropriate compound labeled with a radioactive isotope is injected. Later, a radioactivity counting device surveys ("scans") various areas of the brain, producing an overall pattern of radioactivity in those areas. A special device translates focal variations in cerebral radioactivity into a visual picture of light and dark areas.

The brain scan has become an important screening technique in certain brain disorders. Brain scanning originated from the observation that certain radioactive isotopes seemed to localize in brain tumors. It is not certain whether this phenomenon is due to focal alterations of cerebral vascular permeability ("blood-brain barrier"), to the increased vascularity of most tumors or to both. In subsequent experience, it was shown that subdural hematomas and cerebral infarctions also displayed increased isotope pickup compared with normal brain tissue, so that brain scanning was useful for diagnosis of these conditions. Unfortunately, brain scanning cannot differentiate with certainty between tumor and cerebral infarct. Brain scanning is also helpful in diagnosis of brain abscess.

In brain tumors, best results are obtained with meningiomas and the higher-grade astrocytomas. Grade I astrocytomas, histologically very similar to normal cerebral tissue, often do not concentrate the isotopes enough to stand out from normal surrounding tissue. In addition, scanning with present equipment will miss the majority of tumors under 2 cm in size, regardless of type. Posterior fossa tumors are difficult to detect and require special techniques. Pituitary tumors frequently are not detected because of high vascularity in surrounding structures. Scanning is less useful for spinal cord tumors. Despite these limitations, brain scanning is a good screening test for either primary or metastatic brain tumors, since it can be done with negligible risk on an outpatient basis. Accuracy in diagnosis is quoted as 80–90%. Cerebral arteriography can have a similar success rate, but requires a neuroradiologist for best results and is more complicated and dangerous to perform. If both cerebral arteriography and brain scanning are to be done, the brain scan should be performed first. Angiography causes cerebral vessel dilatation, and may produce a false positive brain scan. It is necessary to wait at least 48 hours after cerebral arteriography to do a brain scan.

In cerebral infarction, fewer than half of the patients have a positive brain scan if the scan is done before the end of the second week after cerebral damage occurs. During the second to fourth week postinfarction, 75% or more of the patients have abnormal scans. After 6 weeks, the abnormal findings often disappear. The optimal time for scanning to detect cerebral infarction is during the third week after onset of symptoms. Cerebral arteriography can detect lesions soon after damage occurs, but it carries a definite risk.

A helpful alternative to angiography is available to those institutions that possess a stationary radioactive imaging device such as the Anger scintillation camera. Certain isotopes can be injected intravenously and followed through major arteries by means of rapid-sequence photography. Results do not have the same degree of detail as x-ray angiography, but complete or nearly complete large-vessel occlusion can be visualized.

Cerebral isotope angiography ("flow study") of the carotid and major cerebral vessels is frequently abnormal in the early stage of a cerebral vascular accident or subdural hematoma when brain scan is normal. Both of these lesions very often give a similar pattern; occasionally a subdural does have characteristic features. Arteriovenous malformations are frequently diagnosable.

Subdural hematoma is frequently a diagnostic problem. According to one study, 20% of patients did not have any history of head trauma and 30% had no localizing neurologic signs. Textbook CSF findings of protein increase and xanthochromia were present in only 50% of subacute and chronic cases. In subdural hematoma, cerebral isotope "dynamic flow study" is a good screening procedure, and cerebral arteriography is the procedure of choice for diagnosis during the first 2 weeks after onset. Brain scans most often do not become positive until after 2 weeks. It is thought that increased isotope pickup is not due to the hematoma itself but to the "membrane" that develops around the hematoma, consisting of highly vascular granulation tissue. Therefore, brain scanning is not very accurate for diagnosis of acute subdural hematoma but is very useful in detecting chronic subdural hematoma. The blood flow study increases accuracy in detection of the chronic form and in addition is more sensitive than the scan in acute subdural hematoma.

An abnormal scan must be interpreted with the aid of skull x-rays, since lesions of bone (such as hyperostosis and Paget's) or scalp (hematoma or laceration) may concentrate the isotope.

Intracerebral abscess can be seen on brain scans in 80–100% of cases. Although lesions may be detected soon after onset of symptoms, some feel that sensitivity of the scan is increased after an additional several days. A gallium scan (p. 164) may improve detection in early or equivocal cases.

Brain scanning can aid the diagnosis and management of hydrocephalus. A small amount of special isotope-tagged material can be injected into the lumbar spinal fluid, and sequential scans can follow the distribution of this material throughout the CSF ("cisternogram"). This is especially valuable in patients with normal-pressure hydrocephalus (Hakim's syndrome). These are predominantly older patients with progressive dementia. The classic triad includes dementia, incontinence and lower extremity weakness. When cisternography displays classic findings of lateral ventricle filling plus inability of CSF to reach the superior sagittal sinus by 48 hours, ventricular shunting frequently produces dramatic improvement.

Computerized Axial Tomography

Computerized axial tomography (CAT; p. 468) is now a very important aid in screening for abnormality in the CNS. It can visualize the ventricular system as well as detect mass lesions both within CNS tissue and outside. In addition, the nature of the lesion can frequently be deduced from density characteristics. The CAT technology has been changing rapidly, and assessment of its capabilities relates to data currently available. Detection of brain tumors is to some extent influenced by location and type of tumor as well as technical factors such as use of intravenous x-ray contrast media. Reports indicate abnormality in approximately 90–95% of patients. Statistics from CAT are not always comparable to radionuclide brain scans, since data from the scans will vary according to the number of head positions employed, the isotope preparation used, the time between administration of isotope and scanning and whether a blood flow study was included. In general, CAT is about 10–15% more sensitive than the brain scan in cerebral tumor, or about 5–10% when brain scanning is performed with optimal technique. It is somewhat more reliable than brain scanning in posterior fossa lesions. In chronic subdural hematoma, detection with CAT is about equal to that achieved when brain scanning is combined with cerebral blood flow study. In acute subdural or epidural hematoma, CAT is significantly better than radionuclide brain scanning. An important advantage over radionuclide techniques in either acute or chronic subdural hematoma is that CAT can frequently permit an exact diagnosis, whereas abnormalities found by radionuclide techniques are often not specific. In cerebral infarct, both techniques are affected by the time interval after onset. During the first week, CAT is somewhat more sensitive than scanning without blood flow study but still detects only 50–60% of infarcts. The sensitivity of both techniques increases to the 80% range by 3–4 weeks. Intracerebral hematoma is much better seen on CAT regardless of the time interval. Neither CAT nor radionuclide studies are perfect. In most of the various focal lesion categories, a certain percentage will be detected by one technique but not the other. When Hakim's syndrome is a possibility, CAT can rule out the disorder by displaying normal ventricular size. If ventricular dilatation is seen, cerebral atrophy may be inferred in some cases, but in many the differentiation between atrophy and normal pressure hydrocephalus cannot be made with adequate certainty.

Overall advantages of CAT over standard radionuclide procedures are ability to visualize the ventricular system, a relatively small but definite increase in detection rate for brain tumors, more specificity in the appearance of many lesions and better delineation of CNS anatomy. Advantages of radionuclide procedures are elimination of need for x-ray contrast media (which many CAT patients must receive), lower cost for equipment and for the patient and ability to inspect major blood vessels via blood flow studies.

REFERENCES

Ansari, K. A., et al.: Quantitative estimation of cerebrospinal fluid globulins in multiple sclerosis, Neurology 25:688, 1975.
Blahd, W. H. (ed.): *Nuclear Medicine* (2d ed.; New York: McGraw-Hill Book Co., Inc., 1971).

Bossak, H. N., et al.: A quantitative turbidimetric method for the determination of spinal fluid protein, J. Vener. Dis. Inform. 30:100, 1949.

Brain, R. W.: *Diseases of the Nervous System* (6th ed.; London: Oxford University Press, 1962).

Brown, R., et al.: Dynamic/static brain scintigraphy: An effective screening test for subdural hematoma, Radiology 117:355, 1975.

Butler, I. J., et al.: Central nervous system infections, Pediatr. Clin. North Am. 21: 649, 1974.

Butler, W. T., et al.: Diagnostic and prognostic value of clinical and laboratory findings in cryptococcal meningitis, N. Engl. J. Med. 270:59, 1964.

Christie, J. H., et al.: Computed tomography and radionuclide studies in the diagnosis of intracranial disease, Am. J. Roentgenol. Radium Ther. Nucl. Med. 127:171, 1976.

DeJesus, P. V., Jr., and Poser, C. M.: Subdural hematomas, a clinicopathologic study of 100 cases, Postgrad. Med. 44:172, 1968.

Deland, F. H.: Nuclear medicine in diseases of the central nervous system, Hosp. Practice 6:57, 1971.

Dolan, C. T.: Specificity of the latex-cryptococcal antigen test, Am. J. Clin. Pathol. 58:358, 1972.

Duncan, W. P., et al.: Fluorescent treponemal antibody-cerebrospinal fluid (FTA-CSF) test: A provisional technique, Br. J. Vener. Dis. 48:97, 1972.

Feigin, R. D., and Dodge, P. R.: Bacterial meningitis: newer concepts of pathophysiology and neurologic sequellae, Pediatr. Clin. North Am. 23:541, 1976.

Ganrot, K., and Laurell, C.-B.: Measurement of IgG and albumin content of cerebrospinal fluid, and its interpretation, Clin. Chem. 20:571, 1974.

Glasgow, J. L., et al.: Brain scans at varied intervals following cerebrovascular accidents, J. Nucl. Med. 6:902, 1965.

Gondos, B.: Cytology of cerebrospinal fluid: Technical and diagnosis considerations, Ann. Clin. Lab. Sci. 6:152, 1976.

Hooshmand, H., et al.: Neurosyphilis: A study of 241 patients, J.A.M.A. 219:726, 1972.

Hyslop, N. E., Jr., and Swartz, M. N.: Bacterial meningitis, Postgrad. Med. 58:120, 1975.

Jacobs, L., et al.: "Normal pressure" hydrocephalus: Relationship of clinical and radiological findings to improvement following shunt surgery, J.A.M.A. 235:510, 1976.

Katz, S. L., and Griffith, J. F.: Slow virus infections, Hosp. Practice 6:64, 1971.

Kieffer, S. A.: Normal pressure hydrocephalus, Geriatrics 29:77, 1974.

Madonick, M. J., and Margolis, J.: Protein content of spinal fluid in diabetes mellitus, A.M.A. Arch. Neurol. & Psychiat. 68:641, 1952.

Massanari, R. N.: Purulent meningitis in the elderly: When to suspect an unusual pathogen, Geriatrics 32(3): 55, 1977.

Merritt, H. H., and Fremont-Smith, F.: *The Cerebrospinal Fluid* (Philadelphia: W. B. Saunders Company, 1937).

Riley, H. D.: Neonatal meningitis, J. Infect. Dis. 125:429, 1972.

Rosenthal, M. S.: Viral infections of the central nervous system, Med. Clin. North Am. 58:593, 1974.

Shackelford, P. G., et al.: Countercurrent immunoelectrophoresis in the evaluation of childhood infection, J. Pediatr. 85:478, 1974.

Sodeman, T. M., and Dock, N.: Laboratory diagnosis of parasitic and fungal diseases of the central nervous system, Ann. Clin. Lab. Sci. 6:47, 1976.

Waxman, A. D., and Siemsen, J. K.: Gallium scanning in cerebral and cranial infections, Am. J. Roentgenol. Radium Ther. Nucl. Med. 127:309, 1976.

Wehrle, P. F., et al.: Seminar on infectious diseases: Infections of the central nervous system, J. Florida M. A. 57:15, 1970.

19 / Liver and Biliary Tract Tests

LIVER FUNCTION

LIVER FUNCTION TESTS form a very important segment of laboratory medicine, since both primary and secondary liver diseases are common. Since none of these tests are specific, they must be intelligently selected and interpreted to provide maximum useful information and prevent unnecessary loss of time and expense to the patient.

Serum Bilirubin

Bilirubin is formed from breakdown of hemoglobin molecules by the reticuloendothelial system. Bilirubin is carried in plasma to the liver, where it is extracted by hepatic parenchymal cells, conjugated with two glucuronide molecules to form bilirubin diglucuronide and then excreted in the bile. It has been well documented that the addition of a certain diazo compound, discovered by van den Bergh, in the presence of conjugated bilirubin results in the development of color maximal within 1 minute. If alcohol is then added, additional color development takes place for up to 30 minutes. This second component, which precipitates with alcohol, corresponds to unconjugated bilirubin. Actually it is true that color continues to develop slowly up to 15 minutes after the simple van den Bergh reaction maximal at 1 minute, and this extra fraction used to be known as the delayed or biphasic reaction. It has since been shown that a considerable proportion of the substance involved is actually unconjugated bilirubin. Since this is measured more completely in the 30-minute alcohol precipitation technique, most laboratories do not report the biphasic reaction. The 1-minute van den Bergh is also called the "direct reaction," and the conjugated bilirubin it measures is known as "direct-acting bilirubin," whereas the 30-minute alcohol measurement of unconjugated bilirubin is called the "indirect reaction" and its substrate "indirect bilirubin." Normal values for total bilirubin are less than 1.5 mg/100 ml and for 1-minute bilirubin less than 0.5 mg/100 ml.

Visible bile staining of tissue is called jaundice. Three major causes predominate — hemolysis, biliary obstruction and liver cell damage.

Hemolysis causes increased breakdown of RBC and thus increased formation of unconjugated bilirubin. If hemolysis is severe enough, more unconjugated bilirubin may be present in the plasma than the liver can handle. Therefore, the level of total bilirubin will rise, with most of the rise due to the indirect-acting fraction. The direct-acting fraction stays normal or is only slightly elevated. Certain congenital diseases of the bilirubin conjugation system show similar values without hemolysis, since ability to conjugate bilirubin is decreased. Elevated serum indirect (nonconjugated) bilirubin is a classic finding in hemolytic anemia but may occur in many other conditions. The reason is often obscure. In one study, the most common associated diseases (collectively 60% of total cases) included cholecystitis, cardiac disease (only 50% having overt congestive failure), acute or chronic infection, GI tract disease (mostly ulcerative or inflammatory) and cancer.

Obstructive jaundice may be extrahepatic or intrahepatic in origin. The classic example is extrahepatic common bile duct obstruction from stone or carcinoma. Here, one expects an increase in serum bilirubin mostly due to the direct-acting fractions, since conjugated bilirubin cannot escape into the small intestine and backs up, regurgitating into the bloodstream. After a time, however, some of the conjugated bilirubin breaks down in the plasma to the unconjugated form, so that there may be a sort of false increase of the indirect fraction producing a less clear-cut direct-to-indirect ratio. Also, after a prolonged period of cholestasis, there often is some degree of secondary liver damage, which may tend to obscure results. In jaundice due to liver cell damage, such as is found in hepatitis and often in decompensated (considerably active) cirrhosis, both direct and indirect bilirubin are elevated in varying proportions. The indirect may be increased because of inability of the damaged cells to conjugate normal amounts of unconjugated serum bilirubin. The direct fraction increase usually results from intrahepatic cholestasis secondary to bile sinusoid blockage by damaged hepatic cells. Jaundice due to carcinoma may be caused by extrahepatic direct biliary obstruction or secondary to intrahepatic blockage of small biliary ducts by expanding tumor masses. Drug toxicity jaundice is due to hypersensitivity reactions to certain drugs, notably Thorazine, causing intrahepatic jaundice of a type that simulates extrahepatic obstruction.

In patients with considerable jaundice in whom liver function or other tests do not show a clearcut pattern to determine cause, a steroid test may be of value in differentiating hepatocellular damage (due to viral hepatitis, cholangitis or active cirrhosis) from extrahepatic obstruction. Prednisone (10 mg every 6 hours) is given for 5 days, after baseline bilirubin values are obtained. The anti-inflammatory effect of adrenocorticosteroids will usually demonstrate acute hepatocellular damage by a decrease in total bilirubin values of more than 50% in less than 5 days. In extrahepatic obstruction due to a tumor or intrahepatic obstruction due to drugs, no significant (or less than 50%) decrease occurs in total bilirubin. The results in cases of obstructing common bile duct stones are variable, because in some cases the obstruction may be due to edema around a stone, which will be relieved by steroids. As in similar nonspecific tests, occasional false positives and negatives occur.

Urine Bilirubin and Urobilinogen

These tests follow much the same pattern as direct and indirect bilirubin. After bile reaches the duodenum, intestinal bacteria convert most of the bilirubin to urobilinogen. Much urobilinogen is lost in the feces, but part is absorbed into the bloodstream. Once in the blood, most of the urobilinogen goes through the liver and is extracted by hepatic cells. Thence, it is excreted in the bile and once again reaches the duodenum. Not all the blood-borne urobilinogen reaches the liver; some is removed by the kidneys and excreted in urine. A positive 1:20 dilution is the maximum normal quantity (see p. 116).

Direct-acting (conjugated) bilirubin will also be partially excreted by the kidney if the serum level of conjugated bilirubin is elevated. Indirect (unconjugated) bilirubin apparently cannot pass the glomerular filter, so it does not appear in urine. However, when serum indirect bilirubin is high, more conjugated bilirubin is produced and excreted into the bile; consequently, more urobilinogen is produced in the intestine. A fraction of this gets back into the blood stream and thence into the urine, so that increased urine urobilinogen is found when increased indirect bilirubin is present. When increased serum indirect bilirubin is due only to increased RBC destruction, the serum direct-acting (conjugated) bilirubin is close to normal, because the liver excretes most of what it produces into the bile ducts. Since the serum direct-acting bilirubin is normal, the urine does not contain increased direct-acting bilirubin in jaundice due to hemolytic anemia.

When complete biliary obstruction occurs, no bile can reach the duodenum and no urobilinogen can be formed. The stool normally gets its color from bilirubin breakdown pigments, so that in complete obstruction the stools lose their color and become gray-white (so-called clay-color). The conjugated bilirubin backs up (regurgitates) into the bloodstream, and tests for urine direct-acting bilirubin give positive results. In cases of severe hepatocellular damage, urobilinogen is formed and absorbed into the bloodstream, but the damaged liver cells cannot extract it adequately, and thus increased amounts get into the urine. In addition, there may be direct-acting bilirubin in the urine secondary to leakage back into the blood from damaged liver cells, as described earlier. Incidentally, urine bilirubin is often called bile, which is technically incorrect, since direct-acting bilirubin is only one component of bile. However, custom and convenience make the term widely used.

Alkaline Phosphatase
Much is still unknown regarding mechanisms of formation and excretion of alkaline phosphatase, an enzyme produced mainly in liver and bone. Apparently formation is relatively small in the normal liver, and the compound is excreted into the bile by a different mechanism than that of bilirubin excretion. The great usefulness of the alkaline phosphatase test in liver disease is its unusual sensitivity to partial or mild degrees of biliary obstruction, either extrahepatic or intrahepatic. Under such circumstances, the alkaline phosphatase may be elevated with a normal serum bilirubin. In mild cases of acute liver cell damage there may be little, if any, alkaline phosphatase elevation. When a phase of temporary intrahepatic obstruction exists in acute liver cell damage, alkaline phosphatase is usually elevated, but promptly decreases once the acute episode is finished, whereas serum bilirubin often is still climbing. In cirrhosis, the alkaline phosphatase is variable, depending on degree of decompensation and obstruction. Inactive mild or moderate cirrhosis and uncomplicated fatty liver usually do not result in elevation, and active cirrhosis may or may not cause increased values. Alkaline phosphatase is one of the best indications of liver

space-occupying lesions, whether carcinoma or infection — it may be elevated in these cases when all other tests are negative. The reason is not always clear.

Since osteoblasts in bone produce large amounts of alkaline phosphatase, greatly increased osteoblastic activity hinders usefulness of alkaline phosphatase as a liver function test. Paget's disease, hyperparathyroidism, rickets and osteomalacia, and osteoblastic metastatic carcinoma to bone all give consistently elevated values. In a patient with jaundice, one can surmise that at least a portion of an alkaline phosphatase elevation is due to liver disease. When doubt exists as to the origin of alkaline phosphatase increase, several alternatives are available. One possibility is use of another enzyme that provides similar information but is more specific for liver origin. Enzymes that have been widely used for this purpose are leucine aminopeptidase (LAP, p. 449), 5'-nucleotidase (5-NT, p. 449) and gamma-glutamyl transpeptidase (GGTP, p. 211). Of these, LAP was the first to be introduced, but it is significantly less sensitive than alkaline phosphatase. The methodology of 5-NT is probably a little too difficult for reliable results in the average laboratory; according to at least one report, about 10% of patients with bone disease may display slight elevation. The GGTP has equal or greater sensitivity to alkaline phosphatase in obstructive liver disease and greater sensitivity in hepatocellular damage. Various reports in the literature state that GGTP is not elevated in bone disease. However, some data in these reports suggest that GGTP may occasionally display mild elevation in bone disease. Another method for differentiating tissue origin of alkaline phosphatase is isoenzyme separation of specific bone and liver fractions by the use of heat, chemical or electrophoretic techniques. Of these, electrophoresis is more difficult but probably more reliable.

Serum Glutamic-Oxaloacetic Transaminase, Serum Glutamic-Pyruvic Transaminase, Lactic Dehydrogenase

Aspartate transaminase (formerly serum glutamic-oxaloacetic transaminase, GOT or SGOT) is an enzyme found in several organs, but especially in heart and liver tissues. In cases of acute cellular destruction in either organ, the enzyme is released into the bloodstream from damaged cells. Elevated values usually appear 8 hours after injury. If the original episode is not continued or repeated, serum levels reach a peak in 24–36 hours and then fall to normal (usually in 4–6 days). In mild injury, serum levels may be only transiently and minimally elevated or may even remain within normal limits. In acute hepatitis, SGOT usually is elevated according to the severity and extent of hepatocellular damage and the particular time the test was drawn. In the acute phase, values are often over 10 times normal. However, later the values fall toward normal, so that a test drawn in the subsiding phase may show moderate or possibly only mild abnormality. In extrahepatic obstruction there is no elevation unless secondary parenchymal acute damage is present; when elevations occur, they are usually only mild to moderate (less than 10 times normal values). In cirrhosis, SGOT may or may not be abnormal, depending on the degree of hepatic decompensation or cell necrosis taking place. Elevation of SGOT is generally mild to moderate in these cases (less than 10 times normal). Usually, but not always, only active cirrhosis shows significant abnormalities. The same is true in fatty liver. In alcoholic patients in delirium tremens, SGOT is usually elevated, even without demonstrable liver damage. In liver passive congestion there may be variable degrees of SGOT elevation if the episode is severe and acute; since congestive heart failure with secondary liver passive congestion is common in heart disease, this makes it difficult to interpret whether SGOT elevation is due only to liver congestion or to a possible myocardial infarct. In metastatic carcinoma, up to half the cases show abnormality, but generally only if metastases are extensive and usually with only mild or moderate elevation.

Serum alanine transaminase (formerly serum glutamic-pyruvic transaminase, SGPT) is an enzyme found mostly, although not exclusively, in liver. In liver disease SGPT is elevated under roughly the same circumstances as SGOT, but seems less sensitive, apparently requiring somewhat more extensive or severe acute parenchymal damage to give abnormal values. An advantage of SGPT is that it is relatively specific for liver cell damage, although slight elevations in myocardial infarct have occasionally been reported. The SGPT level usually returns to normal ranges before the SGOT.

Lactic dehydrogenase (LDH) is found in most of the same tissues as SGOT and is elevated in many of the same conditions. For some reason, acute liver damage does not ordinarily release much LDH, so that LDH is a relatively insensitive indicator of acute hepatocellular destruction, usually not rising over twice normal, even in hepatitis. One exception is infectious mononucleosis, which frequently does cause both SGOT and LDH elevation. Nevertheless, in some cases of passive congestion from heart failure or in an occasional case of viral hepatitis, LDH can rise to levels several times normal, so that LDH values have not been very reliable in differentiating cardiac from hepatic damage. LDH enzyme fractionation (p. 224) may help solve this problem. LDH can often rise to levels higher than twice normal in metastatic carcinoma to the liver, and it is thus valuable as an addition to the usual tests for metastasis, especially when jaundice is present. It is interesting that LDH becomes elevated in a significant number of patients with various malignancies, even without liver metastases.

The LDH "liver" isoenzyme (slow-moving fraction, fraction #5) is more sensitive than total LDH to hepatocellular injury, roughly equal to SGOT, as well as being more specific.

Gamma-Glutamyl Transpeptidase

This enzyme is found primarily in liver and kidney, with a smaller amount in heart muscle. Gamma-glutamyl transpeptidase (GGTP) may be elevated in a wide variety of hepatic diseases, although in no case with 100% sensitivity. Some reports have indicated increased detection of hepatic metastases compared to other enzymes, although at least one investigator found little difference from results with alkaline phosphatase. In general, the majority of reports claim somewhat increased sensitivity over standard enzymes used to characterize hepatic function, both in acute hepatocellular damage and in obstruction. Certain drugs that affect liver cell microsomes, such as diphenylhydantoin (Dilantin) and phenobarbital, may produce GGTP elevation. Elevations also occur with some frequency in diabetes, various neurologic and brain disorders and alcoholism. In bone disease GGTP is usually normal, in contrast to alkaline phosphatase; however, some reports indicate that slight increase may, in fact, occur in some patients with bone abnormality. There has been a great deal of interest in the GGTP elevation found in alcoholism. Alcohol may produce GGTP elevation without massive intake, without light-microscope evidence of hepatocellular damage and without abnormality of other enzymes. In summary, GGTP is relatively (but not entirely) specific for liver disease compared to alkaline phosphatase, is very sensitive to a wide variety of hepatic abnormalities, and is especially sensitive to the hepatic effects of alcohol.

Prothrombin Time

In certain situations prothrombin time (PT) can be a useful liver test. The liver synthesizes prothrombin but apparently needs vitamin K to do so. Vitamin K is a fat-soluble vitamin, present in most adequate diets, which is also synthesized by intestinal bacteria; in either case, it is absorbed from the small bowel in combination with dietary fat molecules. Consequently, interference with vitamin K metabolism can take place either from deficiency due to diet or destruction of intestinal bacteria, defective intestinal absorption due to lack of bile salts or through primary small bowel malabsorption, or inadequate utilization secondary to destruction of liver parenchyma. Normally, the body has considerable tissue stores of vitamin K, so that it usually takes several weeks to get significant prothrombin deficiency on the basis of inadequate vitamin K alone. The usual cause of prothrombin difficulties is liver disease. The main point to remember is that it takes very severe liver disease, more often chronic but sometimes acute, before prothrombin levels become significantly abnormal. In the usual case of viral hepatitis, the PT is either normal or only slightly increased. In massive hepatocellular necrosis the PT may be significantly elevated, but it seems to take a few days to occur. In mild or moderate degrees of cirrhosis there is usually little change. In severe end-stage cirrhosis the PT is often elevated and usually does not give much response to vitamin K therapy. In metastatic carcinoma PT is usually normal, except with biliary tract obstruction.

Bromsulphalein

The dye bromsulphalein (BSP) is metabolized and excreted by hepatic parenchymal cells in a manner very similar to bilirubin. Injection of a standard dose (calculated from patient blood volume as estimated by patient weight) and determination of percent disappearance from serum at a standard time interval provides one estimate of overall liver cell function. The BSP test gives abnormal results more frequently than other biochemical tests in "inactive" cirrhosis (no active hepatic cell injury or inflammation) and also in primary or metastatic tumor within the liver. Nevertheless, use of BSP is being discouraged by many authorities and in many cases it is being replaced by indocyanine green (Cardio-Green) because of patient reactions to BSP that, though rare, may be severe or even fatal. Other considerations include: (1) the test seldom provides information that is not obtainable in other ways; (2) the test shows only nonspecific abnormality in a wide variety of liver conditions that include any cause of jaundice; and (3) false results are often obtained when opiates or gallbladder x-ray contrast media are present in the blood or when a patient is obese (p. 451).

Serum Proteins

Albumin is chiefly synthesized in the liver, so that most acute or chronic destructive liver diseases of at least moderate severity show decreased serum albumin on electrophoresis. In addition, there may be other changes. In cirrhosis of moderate to severe degree, there is a decreased albumin and usually a diffuse gamma globulin elevation, sometimes fairly marked. Far-advanced cirrhosis sometimes has a characteristic pattern with a gamma globulin configuration that even includes the beta range (so-called slurring into the beta). However, a considerable number show only the gamma range elevation, and a few have normal gamma levels. Hepatitis may also have moderate elevation of the gamma globulins. Biliary obstruction eventually causes elevated beta globulins, since beta globulins carry cholesterol.

Blood Ammonia

One function of the liver is the synthesis of urea from various sources of ammonia, most of which comes from protein-splitting bacteria in the GI tract. In cirrhosis, there is extensive liver cell destruction and fibrous tissue replacement of areas between nodules or irregularly regenerating liver cells. This architectural distortion also distorts the hepatic venous blood supply and leads to shunting into the systemic venous system often manifested by esophageal varices. Thus, two conditions should exist for normal liver breakdown of ammonia: (1) enough functioning liver cells must be present and (2) enough ammonia must reach these liver cells. With normal hepatic blood flow, blood ammonia elevation occurs only in extremely severe liver decompensation. With altered blood flow in cirrhosis, less severe decompensation is needed to produce elevated blood ammonia. Nevertheless, the blood ammonia is not directly dependent on the severity of cirrhosis but only on the presence of hepatic failure.

Hepatic failure produces a syndrome known as prehepatic coma (hepatic encephalopathy), which progresses to actual hepatic coma. Clinical symptoms of prehepatic coma include mental disturbances of various types, characteristic changes in the electroencephalogram, and a peculiar flapping intention tremor of the distal extremities. However, each element of this triad may be produced by other causes, and one or more may be lacking in some patients. The ensuing hepatic coma may also be simulated in the hyponatremia or hypokalemia that cirrhotic patients often manifest, or in gastrointestinal bleeding, among other causes. Blood ammonia shows the best correlation with hepatic encephalopathy or coma of any current laboratory test. However, blood ammonia is not elevated in all of these patients, so that a normal blood ammonia does not rule out the diagnosis. Arterial ammonia levels are slightly more reliable than venous ones. The blood ammonia has been proposed as an aid in the differential diagnosis of massive upper gastrointestinal bleeding, since elevated values would mean severe liver disease and thus suggest esophageal varices as the cause of the bleeding. However, since cirrhotics may also have acute gastritis or peptic ulcer, this use of the blood ammonia has not been widely accepted. At present, the blood ammonia is mainly utilized as an aid in diagnosis of hepatic encephalopathy or coma, since elevated values would suggest liver failure as the cause of the symptoms. Otherwise, ammonia is not a useful liver function test, since elevations usually do not occur until hepatic failure.

Liver Scan

If a radioactive colloidal preparation is injected intravenously, it is picked up by the reticuloendothelial system. The Kupffer cells of the liver take up most of the radioactive material in normal circumstances, with a small amount being picked up by spleen and bone marrow. If a sensitive radioactive counting device is placed over the liver, a sort of photograph can be obtained of the distribution of radioactivity. A similar procedure can be done with thyroid and kidney, using radioactive material that these organs normally take up (such as iodine in the case of the thyroid). Certain diseases may be suggested on liver scan if the proper circumstances are present.

1. Space-occupying lesions, either tumorous or inflammatory, often show as discrete filling defects if they are over 2 cm in size.

2. Cirrhosis has a characteristic although nonspecific appearance, but has to be well established, and best results are obtained in far-advanced cases.

3. Fatty liver has irregular isotope distribution like cirrhosis, but only if severe.

4. Liver scanning may be useful to differentiate abdominal masses from an enlarged liver.

Undoubtedly, more sensitive equipment will become available and, perhaps, better radioactive isotopes. At present, useful as the liver scan may be, it is often difficult to distinguish between cirrhosis, fatty liver, and disseminated metastatic carcinoma with nodules less than 2 cm in diameter. Liver scan is reported to detect metastatic carcinoma in 70–85% of patients tested (literature range 57–97%), and to suggest a false positive diagnosis in 5–10% of patients without cancer. The majority of these false positive studies are in patients with cirrhosis.

Liver Biopsy

This procedure has been greatly simplified, and its morbidity and mortality markedly reduced, by the introduction of small-caliber biopsy needles, such as the Menghini. Nevertheless, there is a small but definite risk. Contraindications to biopsy include a PT near the anticoagulant range or a platelet count under 50,000/cu mm. Liver biopsy is especially useful in the following circumstances:

1. To differentiate between cirrhosis, hepatitis, and extrahepatic obstruction, when the clinical picture or laboratory values are confusing or atypical. In classic cases, there usually is no need for biopsy, although some believe that a tissue diagnosis is worth the risk.

2. To prove the diagnosis of metastatic or primary hepatic carcinoma in a patient who would otherwise be operable or who does not have a known primary lesion. (In a patient with an inoperable known primary lesion, such a procedure would be academic.)

3. In hepatomegaly of unknown origin whose etiology cannot be determined otherwise.

4. In a relatively few selected patients who have systemic diseases affecting the liver, such as miliary tuberculosis, in whom the diagnosis cannot be established by other means.

A discussion of liver biopsy should be concluded with a few words of caution. Two disadvantages are soon recognized by anyone who deals with a large number of liver specimens. First, the procedure is a needle biopsy, and this means a very small fragment of tissue, often partially destroyed, taken in a random sample manner from a large organ. Localized disease is easily missed. Second, many diseases produce nonspecific changes that may be spotty, may be healing, or may be minimal. Even with an autopsy specimen it may be difficult to put a definite label on many situations, including the etiology of many cases of cirrhosis. The pathologist should be furnished with the pertinent history, physical findings and laboratory data; sometimes these have as much value for interpretation of the microscopic findings as the histologic changes themselves. In summary, liver biopsy is often indicated in difficult cases, but do not expect it to be infallible or even invariably helpful.

Computerized Axial Tomography and Ultrasound

Computerized axial tomography (CAT), if available, can aid in liver disease detection. From preliminary reports, CAT has approximately the same detection rate as liver scan for space-occupying lesions. Cysts can frequently be distinguished from solid lesions. In common bile duct obstruction, a dilated biliary tree can be visualized in most patients, suggesting that the obstruction is extrahepatic. Gallstones may be outlined in some cases. B-mode ultrasound is capable of delineating a dilated biliary tract, reportedly in 80% or more cases. Intrahepatic mass lesions can also be seen, but with more difficulty than with liver scan or CAT. Ultrasound can differentiate between cystic and solid lesions, in most cases.

Fetoprotein Test

Fetal liver produces an $alpha_1$ globulin called alphafetoprotein (AFP), which becomes the dominant fetal serum protein in the 1st trimester, reaching a peak at 12 weeks, then declining to 1% of the peak at birth. By 1 year of age, a much greater decrease has occurred. Hepatomas were found to produce a similar protein; therefore a test for hepatoma could be devised using antibodies against AFP antigen. Original techniques, such as immunodiffusion, were relatively insensitive, and could not detect normal quantities of fetoprotein in adult serum. Extensive studies using immunodiffusion in several countries revealed that 30–40% of hepatoma patients who were white had positive tests, while the rate among Chinese and blacks was 60–75%. Men seemed to have a higher positive rate than women. Besides hepatoma, embryonal cell carcinoma and teratomas of the testes had an appreciable positivity rate. Reports of "false positive" results with other conditions included several in cases of gastric carcinoma with liver metastases and a few in cases of pregnancy in the 2d trimester. Subsequently, when much more sensitive radioimmunoassay techniques were devised, small quantities of AFP were detected in normal adult individuals. Radioimmunoassay has increased the abnormality rate in hepatoma somewhat, especially in white patients, while elevations accompanying other conditions are also more frequent. For example, according to one report, AFP was increased in approximately 75% of hepatoma cases, 75% of embryonal carcinomas or teratomas of the testes, 20% of pancreatic or gastric carcinomas, and 5% of colon and lung carcinomas. Others have found occasional elevation in patients with viral hepatitis, in some patients with active cirrhosis, and in a scattering of patients with other conditions. Therefore, sensitivity and, to an even greater degree, specificity depend on the assay technique used.

LABORATORY FINDINGS IN COMMON LIVER DISEASES

Having discussed various individual liver function tests, it may be useful to summarize the typical laboratory abnormalities associated with certain common liver diseases.

Acute Viral Hepatitis

After an incubation period, acute viral hepatitis most often begins with some combination of gastrointestinal symptoms, fever, chills, and malaise, lasting 4–7 days. During this phase there is no clinical jaundice. Leukopenia with a relative lymphocytosis is common, and there may be a few atypical lymphocytes. Hemoglobin and platelet counts usually are normal. Liver function tests reflect acute hepatocellular damage, with SGOT and SGPT levels usually over 10 times normal. The alkaline phosphatase frequently is elevated, but usually less than 3 times normal. In the last 1–2 days of this period, urine tests often are positive for bile, even without icterus, and sometimes even with the serum bilirubin within normal range. Serum bilirubin values begin climbing toward the end of this initial phase. The next development is visible jaundice; during this period, clinical symptoms tend to subside. The serum bilirubin continues to rise for a time, then slowly falls. Both direct and indirect fractions are increased. Alkaline phosphatase often begins to fall shortly after clinical icterus begins. A convalescent phase eventually ensues, with return of all tests to normal, beginning with the alkaline phosphatase and ending with Hanger's test (cephalin-cholesterol flocculation test) (p. 448) and BSP. Some patients continue to manifest a low-grade hepatitis (chronic persistent or chronic active), reflected by variable and intermittent SGOT abnormalities (usually mild or moderate in degree) with or without alkaline phosphatase elevation. Some patients never develop jaundice during viral hepatitis; this is known as anicteric hepatitis. In such situations, function tests reveal mild-to-moderate acute hepatocellular damage, with minimal obstructive component. The etiologic agents and serologic tests are discussed in Chapter 16.

Biliary Obstruction

Obstruction may be complete or incomplete, extrahepatic or intrahepatic. Extrahepatic obstruction is most often produced by gallstones in the common bile duct or by carcinoma of the head of the pancreas. Intrahepatic obstruction is most often found in the obstructive phase of acute hepatocellular damage, as seen in "active" cirrhosis or infectious hepatitis, or by liver reaction to certain drugs, such as chlorpromazine (Thorazine). Serum bilirubin becomes markedly elevated, with the direct-acting fraction predominating. Usually, but not always, complete extrahepatic obstruction has a more marked total bilirubin elevation with a greater proportion of the direct-acting fraction than does acute hepatocellular necrosis, in which the direct and indirect fractions are often nearly equal. As time goes on, the serum bilirubin in extrahepatic obstruction may not have a marked direct-indirect fraction disproportion. Drug-induced jaundice mimics extrahepatic obstruction closely in all respects. Alkaline phosphatase is usually over 3 times normal in biliary obstruction. In the early phase of complete extrahepatic obstruction SGOT is normal but later may become abnormal when prolonged obstruction creates liver cell damage. This contrasts to the marked elevations in viral hepatitis. The most common diagnostic problems involve differentiating extrahepatic obstruction from drug jaundice, some cases of severe active cirrhosis and occasional cases of subsiding hepatitis. If the PT time is markedly prolonged, a good response to parenteral vitamin K would suggest extrahepatic obstruction. Percutaneous transhepatic cholangiography (p. 221), ultrasound or CAT scan may help differentiate extrahepatic from intrahepatic obstruction by demonstrating a dilated biliary duct system. If these modalities are not available, the steroid test may be of help. It usually is not possible to differentiate extrahepatic obstruction from drug jaundice by chemical tests. Liver biopsy often cannot demonstrate the etiology of obstruction, and is mainly useful to rule out certain of the intrahepatic etiologies, such as cirrhosis or hepatitis.

Fatty Liver

Fatty liver is a common cause for hepatomegaly of unknown etiology. In uncomplicated fatty liver, function tests are variable. There may be no abnormality at all. However, 75% reportedly have an abnormal BSP, the degree of abnormality being variable. Alkaline phosphatase may be elevated in nearly 48%, usually less than twice normal. Elevated SGOT is found in 40% of patients, usually less than 5 times normal, and more often with severe degrees of fatty metamorphosis. Serum bilirubin may be raised in 35% of patients, but most have minimal abnormality, usually less than twice normal and without jaundice. However, severe fatty liver may present clinically with jaundice, but this is very uncommon.

Cirrhosis

A wide spectrum of test results is exhibited by cirrhosis, depending on whether the disease is active or inactive and on degree of hepatocellular destruction. With inactive cirrhosis, the most frequent abnormality is found in the BSP. Early cases may not show any abnormal tests, or may have an elevated BSP. In more advanced cases, the BSP usually is abnormal to a varying degree. In moderate degrees of inactive cirrhosis there may, in addition, be minimal or mild abnormalities in the SGOT, alkaline phosphatase and serum bilirubin, although no definite pattern can be stated. In advanced cases the PT begins to rise and mild abnormalities in other liver function tests become more frequent.

In "active" cirrhosis (florid cirrhosis or alcoholic hepatitis), liver function tests show evidence of mild-to-moderate acute hepatocellular damage. Serum bilirubin may be normal or elevated; if elevated, usually only to a mild extent, but occasionally to a severe degree. Alkaline phosphatase is often less than 3 times normal, although occasionally it may be higher, and SGOT usually is less than 10 times normal. Active cirrhosis may have a clinical and chemical pattern simulating either the minimal changes of advanced fatty liver, the moderate abnormalities of subacute hepatitis or the picture of obstruction with secondary liver damage. A history of chronic alcoholism and physical findings of spider angiomata and splenomegaly would help point toward cirrhosis. Liver biopsy is the best diagnostic test.

In childhood cirrhosis, the possibility of Wilson's disease (p. 419) should be considered. Primary biliary cirrhosis would be likely in a 30–50-year-old female with pruritus, slow onset of jaundice, protracted clinical course, liver biopsy showing bile duct destruction and abnormal antimitochondrial antibody test (p. 450).

Metastatic Carcinoma

A clinical picture compatible with obstructive jaundice, active cirrhosis or hepatomegaly of unknown origin may be produced by metastatic carcinoma, or the carcinoma may be completely occult. The liver is a frequent target for metastases, some of the most common primary sites being lung, breast, prostate and both the upper and lower gastrointestinal tract. Earlier reports frequently stated that metastases to a cirrhotic liver were rare, but later studies dispute this. Depending on the number, size and location of tumor deposits, the patient may or may not develop jaundice; some may do so even without much involvement. In carcinoma of the head of the pancreas, obstruction of the common bile duct may occur relatively early with onset of a typical picture of posthepatic obstruction. About 25% of patients with metastatic carcinoma to the liver become clinically jaundiced, and about the same number have elevated bilirubin (most often, the direct-acting fraction) without evident jaundice. By far the most frequently noted abnormality is hepatic enlargement. A significant minority may have physical findings compatible with portal hypertension or cirrhosis.

In many cases of metastatic carcinoma to the liver the patient is not jaundiced. Alkaline phosphatase is very often elevated in these circumstances; and this may be true, although not always, even when only a relatively few nodules are present. Therefore, the typical pattern for metastatic carcinoma to the liver is a normal bilirubin with elevated alkaline phosphatase. If the serum bilirubin is elevated, the "typical" metastatic pattern becomes much less frequent, or is obscured, and a significant minority develop abnormal enzyme tests indicative of acute hepatocellular damage. Diagnosis, therefore, is much more difficult in the presence of jaundice, since these tests are often elevated (at least temporarily) from any of a great variety of etiologies. As mentioned previously, a liver scan is very useful, and LDH may be of some further help. Liver biopsy may be indicated, depending on the circumstances.

To conclude liver function tests, perhaps some comments are indicated on the use of these procedures. Some doctors order every test available and keep repeating them all, even those which give essentially the same information. For example, the SGPT is ordered with the SGOT because SGPT is more specific for liver disease. After the first results, it is usually sufficient to follow only one of these enzymes. The same is true of alkaline phosphatase and its substitutes (GGTP, LAP, 5-NT; p. 449). Whichever enzyme is used, if the result is normal, this suggests that bone rather than liver is the source of increased alkaline phosphatase, and the alkaline phosphatase alone can be followed without repeating the other enzyme. If SGOT level suggests severe acute hepatocellular damage or if signs of obvious liver disease, such as jaundice, are present, it would be useless to assay one of these other enzymes since all of them are likely to be elevated, regardless of bone contribution to alkaline phosphatase. Therefore, rather than enzyme differentiation, many prefer alkaline phosphatase isoenzyme fractionation, which has the added benefit that concurrent elevation of both bone and liver fractions can be demonstrated. For this, isoenzyme electrophoresis is more reliable.

Serum cholesterol is not a very helpful liver function test, since the PT gives essentially the same information and is technically more easy and reliable. Urine bile is not necessary if the serum direct-acting bilirubin value is known. Serum protein electrophoresis is valuable mainly in helping pick up some cases of cirrhosis. Liver scan is most helpful in showing metastatic carcinoma. Liver biopsy can frequently provide a definitive answer, thereby shortening the patient's stay in the hospital and making lengthy repetition of lab tests unnecessary. The earlier a biopsy is obtained, the more chance one has to see clear-cut diagnostic changes. If, for some reason, a liver biopsy is thought to be contraindicated, and if the serum bilirubin is more than twice normal limits, ultrasound, CAT scanning, percutaneous transhepatic cholangiography or possibly the steroid test may be helpful in differentiating intrahepatic from extrahepatic obstruction.

Liver function tests should be selected to fit the clinical situation. Therefore, one suggestion for a good initial liver test "profile" might include bilirubin (total and direct), SGOT, alkaline phosphatase, and PT. The SGOT should demonstrate the presence of acute hepatocellular injury; the alkaline phosphatase, obstruction and also many cases of space-occupying lesions; and the PT, if abnormal, suggests a serious degree of hepatic damage. Of course, to interpret these tests, one must know what conditions (for example, cardiac failure with liver congestion) could affect each of these tests, must have other clinical information, and must be prepared to repeat certain of the procedures in 3–4 days to establish a pattern. The clinical circumstances dictate to some extent the choice of tests in any situation. If hepatitis is suspected, an SGOT level contributes the most toward establishing the diagnosis. In possible cirrhosis without jaundice, the SGOT and PT are useful. (The LDH and liver scan also may be helpful, since metastatic carcinoma may closely mimic cirrhosis.) If all tests are normal and cirrhosis is strongly suggested, a BSP may be indicated. In possible metastatic carcinoma, alkaline phosphatase and liver scan are the best tests. Other tests may be indicated in special circumstances. Liver biopsy may be necessary in any difficult case as the only way to prove a diagnosis. There are too many exceptions to any of the so-called diagnostic or typical liver function test patterns.

EXTRAHEPATIC BILIARY TRACT

The major subdivisions of the biliary tract are the intrahepatic bile ducts, the common bile duct and the gallbladder. The major diseases of the biliary system are gallbladder infection (cholecystitis, acute or chronic), gallbladder stones and obstruction to the common bile duct by stones or tumor. Obstruction to intrahepatic bile channels can occur as a result of acute hepatocellular damage, but this aspect was noted in the discussion of liver function tests and will not be included here.

Acute cholecystitis usually presents with upper abdominal pain, most often accompanied by fever and a leukocytosis. Occasionally, difficulty in diagnosis may be produced by a right lower lobe pneumonia or peptic ulcer, and cholecystitis occasionally results in ST and T-wave electrocardiographic changes that might point toward myocardial disease. Acute cholecystitis is very frequently associated with gallbladder calculi, usually in the cystic duct. Some degree of increased bilirubin is found in 25–30% of patients, and some studies report as high an incidence as 50%. Bilirubinemia may occur even in patients without stones. Acute cholecystitis without stones is said to be most common in elderly persons. SGOT is said to be elevated in nearly 75% of cholecystitis patients; this is more likely if jaundice is present. In one study, about 20% had SGOT levels more than 6 times normal, and 6% more than 10 times normal. Of these, some had jaundice and some did not. About 20% of cholelithiasis patients are reported to have common duct stones. About 40% of the patients with common duct stones do not become jaundiced. Common duct stones usually occur in association with gallbladder calculi, but occasionally may be present alone. Cholecystitis patients sometimes develop elevated serum amylase, usually less than 2 times normal limits. About 15% of patients are said to have some degree of concurrent acute pancreatitis.

In uncomplicated obstructive jaundice due to common duct stones or tumor, SGOT and LDH are usually normal. Nevertheless, in some instances SGOT may become elevated very early (sometimes to more than 10 times normal) in the absence of demonstrable hepatocellular damage. The striking SGOT elevation may lead to a misdiagnosis of hepatitis. Several reports indicate that LDH was also considerably elevated in these patients, usually 5 times the upper limits of normal. Since LDH is usually less than twice normal in viral hepatitis (although occasional exceptions occur), higher LDH values point toward the "atypical obstruction" enzyme pattern. Both SGOT and LDH values may fall steadily after 2–3 days.

Radiologic Procedures

Diagnosis of stones in the gallbladder or common bile duct rests mainly with the radiologist. On plain films of the abdomen 20–25% of gallbladder stones are said to be visible. Oral cholecystography consists of oral administration of a radiopaque contrast medium that is absorbed by intestinal mucosa and secreted by liver cells into the bile. When bile enters the common duct, it takes a certain amount of pressure to force open the ampulla of Vater. During the time this pressure is building up, bile enters the cystic duct into the gallbladder, where water is reabsorbed, concentrating the bile. This process allows concentration of the contrast medium as well as the bile and, therefore, outlines the interior of the gallbladder as well as delineates any stones of sufficient size. An average of 70% of those with gallbladder calculi may be identified by oral cholecystography. Repeat examination (using a double dose of contrast medium or alternative techniques) is necessary if the original study does not show any gallbladder function. In most of the remaining patients with gallbladder calculi, oral cholecystography reveals a poorly functioning or a nonfunctioning gallbladder. Less than 5% of patients with gallbladder stones are said to have a completely normal oral cholecystogram. (Over 50% of patients with cholecystitis and gallbladder tumor have abnormal oral cholecystograms.)

There are certain limitations to the oral method. Although false negative examinations (gallbladder calculi and a normal test) are relatively few, false positive results (nonfunctioning gallbladder but no gallbladder disease) have been reported in some studies in more than 10% of cases. In addition, neither oral cholecystography nor plain films of the abdomen are very useful in detecting stones in the common bile duct. Visualization of the common bile duct by the oral method is frequently poor, whether stones are present or not.

Intravenous cholecystography supplements the oral procedure in some respects. Nearly 50% of common duct stones may be identified. Intravenous injection of the contrast medium is frequently able to outline the common duct and major intrahepatic bile ducts.

Limitations of the intravenous technique include poor reliability in demonstrating gallbladder calculi, since there are an appreciable number of both false positive and false negative results. There also is a considerable incidence of patient reaction to the contrast medium, although newer techniques (drip infusion) have markedly reduced the danger of reaction.

A limitation to both the oral and the intravenous procedure is the fact that both depend on a patent intrahepatic and extrahepatic biliary system. If the serum bilirubin is over 2 mg/100 ml (and the increase is not due to hemolytic anemia), neither oral nor intravenous cholangiography is usually satisfactory.

When jaundice is present, it is sometimes possible to do percutaneous transhepatic cholangiography. This consists of inserting a cannula into one of the intrahepatic bile ducts through a biopsy needle and injecting the contrast medium directly into the duct. This procedure outlines the biliary duct system and is, therefore, useful in confirming the presence of extrahepatic obstruction in a patient with jaundice. The technique is not easy, and it requires considerable experience; more than 25% of attempts fail. There is a definite risk of producing bile peritonitis, which occasionally has been fatal. Preparation for surgical intervention should be made in advance in case this complication does develop.

B-mode ultrasound can visualize dilated hepatic bile ducts in about 80% of patients with extrahepatic biliary tract obstruction and thus may be useful to help differentiate intrahepatic from extrahepatic obstruction. CAT scan may provide the same information.

REFERENCES

Adams, J. T., et al.: Serum glutamic oxalacetic transaminase activity in cholecystitis, Surgery 68:492, 1970.

Bessman, S. P.: Blood Ammonia, in Sobotka, H., and Stewart, C. P. (ed.): *Advances in Clinical Chemistry* (New York: Academic Press, Inc., 1959), vol. 2.

Betro, M. G., et al.: Gamma-glutamyl transpeptidase in diseases of the liver and bone, Am. J. Clin. Pathol. 60:672, 1973.

Blahd, W. H. (ed.): *Nuclear Medicine* (2d ed.; New York: McGraw-Hill Book Company, Inc., 1971).

Bradus, S., et al.: Hepatic function and serum enzyme levels in association with fatty metamorphosis of the liver, Am. J. Med. Sci. 246:35, 1963.

Breen, K. J., and Schenker, S.: Liver function tests, CRC Crit. Rev. Clin. Lab. Sci. 2: 573, 1971.

Buonocore, E.: Transhepatic percutaneous cholangiography, Radiol. Clin. North Am. 14:527, 1976.

Cooley, R. N.: Diagnostic accuracy of radiologic studies of the biliary tract, small intestine, and colon, Am. J. Med. Sci. 246:610, 1963.

Enquist, I. F., et al.: Validity of the bromsulphalein test in patients with acute severe upper gastrointestinal hemorrhage, Am. J. Surg. 107:306, 1964.

Feizi, T.: Immunoglobulins in chronic liver disease, Gut 9:193, 1968.

Felix, E. L., et al.: The value of the liver scan in preoperative screening of patients with malignancies, Cancer 38:1137, 1976.

Fenster, F., and Klatskin, G.: Manifestations of metastatic tumors of the liver, Am. J. Med. 31:238, 1961.

Frank, B. B., and Raffensperger, E. C.: Hepatic granulomata, Arch. Intern. Med. 115:223, 1965.

Gabuzda, G. J.: Hepatic Coma: Clinical Considerations, Pathogenesis, and Management, in Dock, W., and Snapper, I. (eds.): *Advances in Internal Medicine* (Chicago: Year Book Medical Publishers, Inc., 1962), vol. 11.

Ginsberg, A. L.: Very high levels of SGOT and LDH in patients with extrahepatic biliary tract obstruction, Am. J. Digest. Dis. 15:803, 1970.

Gregory, P. B., and Cooney, D. P.: Misleading SGOT (aspartate aminotransferase) values in obstructive jaundice due to pancreatic carcinoma, Am. J. Dig. Dis. 21:509, 1976.

Leevy, C. M.: Fatty liver: A study of 270 patients with biopsy proven fatty liver and a review of the literature, Medicine 41:249, 1962.

Levine, R. A., and Klatskin, G.: Unconjugated hyperbilirubinemia in the absence of overt hemolysis, Am. J. Med. 36:541, 1964.

Leyton, B., et al.: Correlation of ultrasound and colloid scintiscan studies of the normal and diseased liver, J. Nucl. Med. 14:27, 1973.

Mehlman, D. J., et al.: Serum alpha-fetoglobulin with gastric and prostatic carcinoma, N. Engl. J. Med. 285:1060, 1971.

Oxley, D. K.: Nuclear diagnosis of disseminated cancer of the breast, Am. J. Clin. Pathol. 64:780, 1975.

Reaves, L. E., III: Syndromes of constitutional hyperbilirubinemia, Postgrad. Med. 39:270, 1966.

Schiff, L. (ed.): *Diseases of the Liver* (3d ed.; Philadelphia: J. B. Lippincott Company, 1969).

Shehadi, W. H.: Radiologic examination of the biliary tract: Plain film of the abdomen; oral cholecystography, Radiol. Clin. North Am. 4:463, 1966.

Sherlock, S.: Chronic active hepatitis, Postgrad. Med. 50:206, 1971.

Spellberg, M. A.: Intrahepatic cholestasis vs. posthepatic jaundice: Methods of diagnosis, Med. Clin. North Am. 48:53, 1964.

Steigmann, F., and Shah, M. N.: Fatty liver with jaundice: A diagnostic enigma with surgical implications, Am. J. Gastroenterol. 54:126, 1970.

Waldmann, T. A., and McIntire, K. R.: The use of a radioimmunoassay for alpha-fetoprotein in the diagnosis of malignancy, Cancer 34:1510, 1974.

Wise, R. E.: Current concepts of intravenous cholangiography, Radiol. Clin. North Am. 4:521, 1966.

Zawadzki, Z., and Kraj, M. A.: Alpha-fetoprotein in hepatocellular disease and neoplastic disorders, Am. J. Gastroenterol. 61:45, 1974.

Zieve, L., et al.: Normal and abnormal variations and clinical significance of the one-minute and total serum bilirubin determinations, J. Lab. Clin. Med. 38:446, 1951.

Zimmerman, H. J., and Seeff, L. B.: Enzymes in Hepatic Disease, in Coodley, E. L. (ed.): *Diagnostic Enzymology* (Philadelphia: Lea & Febiger, 1970), p. 1.

20 / Cardiac, Pulmonary and Miscellaneous Diagnostic Procedures

MYOCARDIAL INFARCTION

CLINICAL SIGNS AND SYMPTOMS are extremely important in both suspicion and diagnosis. The type of pain with its distribution and response to nitroglycerin may be very characteristic. A history may show predisposing factors, previous anginal pain or symptoms of heart failure. Even when diagnosis is virtually certain on clinical grounds alone, the physician often will want laboratory confirmation, and this becomes more important when symptoms are atypical or minimal. An ECG is the most useful direct test available. Approximately 50% of myocardial infarctions show unequivocal changes on the first ECG. Another 30% have abnormalities compatible with, but not diagnostic of, infarction, often obscured by certain major conduction irregularities, such as bundle branch block, or previous digitalis therapy. About 20% do not show significant changes, and this occasionally happens even in otherwise characteristic cases. Laboratory tests cannot directly show infarction, but certain values are regularly elevated in this condition and may give a pattern that is helpful when combined with the clinical picture. In classic cases a polymorphonuclear leukocytosis begins between 12 and 24 hours after onset of symptoms, usually in the range of 10,000–20,000/cu mm. It generally lasts between 1 and 2 weeks, depending on the extent of tissue necrosis. Leukocytosis is accompanied by increased temperature of moderate degree and increased erythrocyte sedimentation rate (ESR). The ESR abnormality persists longer than leukocytosis, remaining elevated sometimes as long as 3–4 weeks.

Enzyme Indicators

SERUM ASPARTATE TRANSAMINASE (AST OR SGOT).—Certain enzymes are present in cardiac muscle and are released when tissue necrosis occurs. Aspartate (glutamic-oxaloacetic) transaminase becomes elevated between 8 and 12 hours after infarction, reaches a peak between 24 and 48 hours and falls to normal within 3–8 days. The SGOT blood levels have a very rough correlation with the extent of infarct, and may be only transiently and minimally abnormal. The SGOT levels may be elevated due to acute damage to parenchymal cells of other organs. Elevation is common in liver cell necrosis (p. 210), happens often with sufficient skeletal muscle

223

damage (including trauma or extensive surgical damage) and is found fairly frequently in acute pancreatitis. In some of these situations, myocardial infarct may have to be considered in differential diagnosis of symptoms. Chronic hypokalemia may elevate SGOT (and creatine phosphokinase).

Conditions other than those just mentioned may elevate SGOT. Morphine or meperidine (Demerol) may temporarily raise SGOT. Elevations have also been reported in occasional cases of warfarin (Coumadin) anticoagulant therapy and with large doses of salicylates.

LACTIC DEHYDROGENASE (LDH). — Between 24 and 48 hours postinfarction, LDH becomes elevated, reaches a peak between 48 and 72 hours, and slowly falls to normal between 5 and 10 days. Thus, LDH tends to parallel SGOT at about double the time interval. LDH is more sensitive than SGOT and is reported to be elevated even in small infarcts that showed no SGOT abnormality. When LDH values are quoted, total serum LDH is meant.

In acute liver cell damage, total LDH is not as sensitive as SGOT. In acute or chronic passive congestion of the liver, LDH is most often normal or only minimally elevated, although occasionally substantial elevations do occur. Since LDH fraction 1 is contained in RBC as well as cardiac muscle, LDH is greatly influenced by accidental hemolysis in serum, and thus must be collected and transported with care. Heart valve prostheses may produce enough low-grade hemolysis to affect LDH, and LDH is also abnormal in many patients with megaloblastic and moderate or severe hemolytic anemias. Skeletal muscle contains LDH, so that total LDH (or even hydroxybutyric acid dehydrogenase) values are not reliable in the first week after extensive surgery. Finally, LDH may be elevated in 60–80% of those with pulmonary embolism (reports vary from 30% to 100%), in some cases of malignant neoplasms and leukemia and in some patients with uremia.

Lactic dehydrogenase is actually a group of enzymes. The individual enzymes (isoenzymes) that make up total LDH have different concentrations in different tissues. Therefore, the tissue responsible for elevated total LDH may often be identified by fractionation (separation) and measurement of individual isoenzymes. In addition, since the population normal range for total LDH is rather wide, abnormal elevation of one isoenzyme may occur without lifting total LDH out of the total LDH normal range.

Five main fractions (isoenzymes) of LDH are measured. Using the standard international nomenclature (early U.S. investigators used opposite terminology), fraction 1 is found mainly in RBC and in heart and kidney tissues; fraction 3 in lung tissue; and fraction 5 mainly in liver tissue. Skeletal muscle has significant representation in all fractions, although there is relatively more fraction 5. Various methods of isoenzyme separation are available; the two most commonly used are heat and electrophoresis. Heating to 60° C for 30 minutes destroys most activity except for fractions 1 and 2, the heat-stable fractions. Using electrophoresis, the fast-moving fractions are 1 and 2 (heart), while the slowest-migrating fraction is 5 (liver). Electrophoresis has the advantage that one can see the relative contributions of all five fractions.

The relative specificity of LDH isoenzymes is very useful because of the large number of diseases that affect standard "heart" enzyme tests. For example, one study of patients in hemorrhagic shock with no evidence of heart disease found elevated SGOT in 70%, LDH in 52% and SGPT in 37%. LDH enzyme fractionation offers a way to diagnose myocardial infarction when liver damage is suspected of contributing to total LDH increase. In liver damage without myocardial infarct, fraction 1 is normal and most of the increase is due to fraction 5. If myocardial infarct and liver damage coexist, fractions 1 and 5 are both elevated.

There are several characteristic LDH isoenzyme patterns illustrated and described in Figure 20–1. However, not all patients with the diseases listed necessarily have the "appropriate" isoenzyme configuration; the frequency with which the pattern occurs depends on the particular disease and the circumstances. For example, the characteristic abnormality in pulmonary embolization is a fraction 3 increase, but embolization may actually produce increase in any of the fractions or may be associated with a normal pattern. Multiorgan disease may produce combinations of the various patterns. In shock the various fractions tend to move toward equal height; in malignancy, although all components may be elevated, the midzone or the 4 and 5 fractions tend to be accentuated.

The LDH isoenzymes may help evaluate postsurgical chest pain. Skeletal muscle contains both fraction 1 and fraction 5, so that total LDH, HBD or fraction 1 elevations are not reliable during the first week after extensive

Fig 20–1.—Representative LDH isoenzyme patterns with most frequent etiologies. **A,** normal. **B,** fraction *1* increased with *1* becoming greater than *2:* acute myocardial infarct; artifactual hemolysis; hemolytic or megaloblastic anemia; renal cortex infarct. **C,** fraction *5* increased: acute hepatocellular damage (hepatitis, passive congestion, active cirrhosis); muscle crush injury. **D,** fraction *3* increased: pulmonary embolization; lymphoproliferative disorders; acute pancreatitis. **E,** midzone fractions unequally elevated: tumor. **F,** all fractions elevated, tending toward equal height: shock.

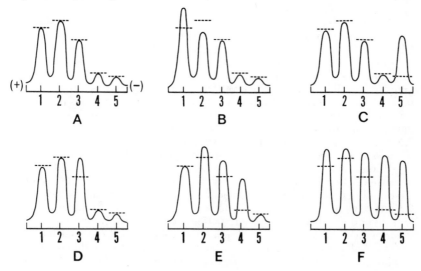

surgery. However, a normal LDH-1/LDH-2 ratio in samples obtained 24–48 hours after onset of symptoms would be considerable evidence against myocardial infarct. Creatine phosphokinase (CPK) isoenzymes, if available, would be of even greater assistance in the first 24 hours.

Most LDH fractions are stable for several days at refrigerator temperature. LDH-5 rapidly decreases if the specimen is frozen.

HYDROXYBUTYRIC ACID DEHYDROGENASE (HBD).—This has been used as a substitute for LDH fast-moving (heart) isoenzyme measurement. Actually, HBD is total LDH that is forced to act on an alphaketobutyric acid substrate instead of pyruvic or lactic acid. Under these conditions, the fast-moving LDH fractions show relatively greater activity than the slow-moving fraction, so that HBD therefore indirectly measures fast-moving fraction 1 (heart) activity. However, if fraction 5 (liver) is elevated sufficiently, it will also produce measurable HBD effect, so that HBD is not as specific as electrophoresis or heat fractionation in separating heart from liver isoenzymes. Nevertheless, since HBD assay is easier to perform (and therefore cheaper) than LDH isoenzymes, some follow the practice of obtaining a more specific isoenzyme method if in doubt about LDH heart vs liver contribution. Once the "heart" fraction is proved elevated, they follow subsequent activity levels with HBD.

CREATINE PHOSPHOKINASE (CPK).—Available as an aid in diagnosis of cardiac and skeletal muscle lesions, CPK is being advocated as a substitute for SGOT in heart disease. Creatine phosphokinase is found only in heart muscle, skeletal muscle and brain. Use of CPK in primary diseases of skeletal muscle is discussed elsewhere (p. 418). In myocardial infarction CPK behaves like SGOT. However, acute liver cell damage (which frequently causes an abnormal SGOT) has no effect on CPK. This is an advantage, since the situation often arises in which an elevated SGOT (or LDH) might be due to severe hepatic passive congestion from heart failure rather than from fresh myocardial infarction.

While CPK is present in brain tissue as well as muscle, reports differ to some extent as to the effect of central nervous system disease on serum CPK levels. According to one report, CPK may be elevated in a wide variety of conditions that affect the brain, including bacterial meningitis, encephalitis, cerebrovascular accident, hepatic coma, uremic coma and grand-mal epileptic attacks. Elevation is not always present; even when present, the degree of elevation varies considerably. Elevations have been reported in some patients in acute phases of certain psychiatric diseases, notably schizophrenia; the cause is not known.

Since CPK is frequently utilized to differentiate acute cardiac and hepatic disease, it is worth noting that hepatic coma and delirium tremens, two conditions associated with liver damage, may induce elevated CPK values because of effects on tissue other than that of the liver. Thus, CPK is often abnormal in delirium tremens, presumably due to muscular exertion. Elevations have also been reported (for reasons unknown) in many patients with hypothyroidism and in some patients with tachyarrhythmias (mostly ventricular) and chronic hypokalemia. Elevation of CPK is associated with effects of alcohol on muscle. For example, 24–48 hours following heavy drinking episodes, CPK levels become abnormal in the majority of patients, as well as in most patients with delirium tremens. Levels of CPK are said to be normal in chronic alcoholics without heavy intake.

After intramuscular injection, CPK is frequently elevated. Since therapeutic injections are common, this probably constitutes the most frequent cause of CPK elevation. Specimens must be drawn before injection or at least within 1 hour after injection. Trauma to muscle makes CPK unreliable for a few days postoperatively.

Normal CPK values for black males are double those for white males; values for black and white females are nearly equal.

Isoenzymes of CPK are now becoming available. There are three major categories: CPK-BB (CPK-1), found in brain and lung; CPK-MM (CPK-3), found in skeletal muscle; and the hybrid CPK-MB (CPK-2), found in cardiac muscle. Isoenzymes offer a reliable way to detect myocardial damage without regard to skeletal muscle contribution to CPK values. The CPK-MB level begins to rise 3–6 hours after onset of infarct, reaches a peak in 12–24 hours, and returns to normal in 48–72 hours (sometimes earlier). There is a rough correlation between the size of the infarct and the degree of elevation. Since small infarcts may not elevate the MB fraction dramatically, it is important to time specimen collection so as not to miss the peak. Some recommend 4 specimens, 1 every 6 hours after onset of symptoms, although 3 specimens, 1 every 8 hours, seems a more reasonable compromise.

There is some dispute as to whether ischemia without actual infarct will elevate either total CPK or CPK-MB. The controversy revolves around the fact that currently there is no way to rule out the possibility that a small infarct may have occurred in a patient who clinically is thought to have only ischemia.

In equivocal cases it is helpful to obtain LDH isoenzyme determinations as well as CPK-MB, both to enhance diagnostic specificity and because specimens for CPK may have been obtained too late to detect elevation. If the 3 CPK isoenzyme samples are obtained 1 every 8 hours and LDH isoenzymes are performed at 24 and 48 hours, nearly all infarcts should be documented. Of course, if one of the CPK-MB determinations is strongly positive, it might not be necessary to obtain further samples.

Although CPK-MB is found mainly in cardiac muscle, much smaller amounts are located in skeletal muscle. Skeletal muscle contains two types of muscle fibers, so-called type I, which contains only CPK-MM, and type II, which contains CPK-MB in addition to CPK-MM. Type II comprises 40% of the fibers in such muscles as the quadriceps. In Duchenne's muscular dystrophy, especially in the earlier stages, the amount of CPK-MB may be increased, presumably due to skeletal muscle type II involvement, with CPK-MM increased to a much greater degree. An increase in CPK-MB may also occur in some patients with gangrene or severe ischemia of the extremities. In addition, patients with acute myositis of various types, idiopathic myoglobinemia, Reye's syndrome and Rocky Mountain spotted fever frequently display some degree of CPK-MB elevation.

In patients undergoing defibrillation or cardiac resuscitation, CPK-MB value is usually normal unless actual myocardial injury (such as contusion) takes place. At least one report indicates that the CPK-MB value is normal in most patients with myocarditis, pericarditis and subacute bacterial endocarditis, even when LDH isoenzymes display a "cardiac" pattern. Coronary angiography likewise is associated with normal MB values. In open-heart surgery, such as coronary artery revascularization, appearance of CPK-MB isoenzyme elevation raises the question of myocardial infarct, even though operative manipulation of the heart takes place. Nearly 15% of such patients (ranging from 1–37%) have displayed MB elevation just prior to operation. Others have MB increase during institution of cardiopulmonary bypass or anesthesia induction before actual cardiac surgery begins.

Elevation of the CPK-BB value is not common. It is occasionally elevated after pulmonary embolization, and one report indicated that it may occasionally be increased in some patients who undergo cardiopulmonary resuscitation. In brain disorders, where one theoretically would expect release of CPK-BB, the actual isoenzyme detected in serum is usually CPK-MM. In some patients, an unusually accentuated albumin may be mistaken for CPK-BB using electrophoresis. Total CPK elevation in myxedema is due to the MM fraction.

The Heart Scan

Heart scanning can now be performed in two ways. Scan for acute myocardial infarction is done with technetium pyrophosphate or certain other radiopharmaceuticals. These agents localize in acutely damaged myocardium, producing a focal area of increased radioactivity. The scan is not reliable less than 24 hours after onset of infarct, and returns to normal by 6–7 days after infarct. Best results are obtained with transmural infarcts and with locations in the anterior and lateral walls of the left ventricle. Subendocardial infarcts, especially when small, are much more likely to be missed. Another consideration is necessity to transport the patient to the scanner, unless the institution is one of the few that can provide a portable unit. Combined use of CPK and LDH isoenzymes has lessened scan necessity in diagnosis. Heart scanning may, however, assist in the diagnosis of acute myocardial infarct that occurs during or after cardiac surgery, when enzyme or isoenzyme diagnosis is not reliable. Some additional areas of difficulty in myocardial scanning include the fact that size of the scan abnormality cannot at present be reliably correlated to infarct size, Ventricular aneurysms may concentrate the phosphate radiopharmaceuticals in a manner suggesting infarct, and this unexplained capability may persist for years.

Heart scanning can also be done by using radioactive elements, such as potassium, rubidium and thallium, that localize in viable myocardium. Scars and infarcts are seen as areas without uptake. Areas of ischemia (if sufficiently large) also may be detected by scanning before and after exercise.

PERICARDIAL EFFUSION

Pericardial effusion may be a consideration in differential diagnosis of an enlarged heart on chest x-ray. Two techniques are available to demonstrate increased pericardial fluid: (1) the radioisotope heart (or cardiac blood pool) scan and (2) ultrasound (echosonography). The first involves placing a radioisotope compound into the bloodstream, where it mixes with blood inside the heart. Scanning this region provides a picture of the interior dimensions of the heart as outlined by the intracardiac blood pool; this can be compared to the x-ray cardiac silhouette or (depending on technique) to adjacent lung and liver blood pools. Pericardial effusion separates the heart pool from the x-ray heart border or from adjacent structures. Effusion over 200 ml can be detected with reasonable efficiency. Ultrasound is even more sensitive in detecting effusion, although a B-mode or M-mode detector is needed.

PULMONARY EMBOLISM

Pulmonary emboli are often difficult either to diagnose or to confirm. Sudden dyspnea is the most common symptom, but clinically there may be any combination of chest pain, dyspnea and possibly hemoptysis. Diseases that must be also considered are myocardial infarction and pneumonia. Pulmonary embolism is often associated with chronic congestive heart failure, cor pulmonale, postoperative complications of major surgery, and fractures of the pelvis or lower extremities – all situations in which myocardial infarct itself is more likely. The classic x-ray findings of a wedge-shaped lung shadow are often absent or late in developing, because not all cases of embolism develop actual pulmonary infarction, even when the embolus is large.

Laboratory tests in pulmonary embolism have not been very helpful. Initial reports of a characteristic test triad (elevated bilirubin and LDH with normal SGOT) proved disappointing, because only 20–25% of patients display this combination. Reports that LDH is elevated in 80% of patients are probably optimistic. In addition, LDH may be elevated in myocardial infarction or liver passive congestion, conditions which could mimic or be associated with embolism. Theoretically, LDH isoenzyme fractionation should help, since the classic isoenzyme pattern of pulmonary embolism is a fraction 3 increase. Unfortunately, this technique also has proved disappointing, since a variety of patterns have been found in embolization, and fraction 3 may be normal. Total CPK initially was advocated to differentiate embolization from myocardial infarct, but reports indicate that total CPK may become elevated in some patients with embolism. The CPK isoenzymes, however, are reliable in confirming myocardial infarct; and a normal CPK-MB plus normal LDH isoenzyme fraction 1 and 2 ratio (obtained at proper times) is also reliable in ruling out myocardial infarct.

The Lung Scan

The most useful screening procedure for pulmonary embolism is the lung scan. Serum albumin is tagged with a radioisotope and the tagged albumin molecules are treated in such a way as to cause aggregation into larger molecular groups (50–100 μ). This material is injected into a vein, passes through the right side of the heart, and is sent into the pulmonary artery. The molecules then are trapped in small arterioles of the pulmonary artery circulation, so that a radiation detector scan of the lungs shows a diffuse radioactive uptake throughout both lungs from these trapped radioactive molecules. A scan is a visual chart of the radioactivity counts over a specified area received by the radiation detector. The isotope solution is too dilute to cause any difficulty by its partial occlusion of the pulmonary circulation; only a small percentage of the arterioles are affected, and the albumin is metabolized in 3–4 hours. If a part of the pulmonary artery circulation is already occluded by a thrombus, the isotope does not reach that part of the lung, and the portion of lung affected does not show any uptake on the scan (positive scan).

The lung scan becomes "positive" immediately after total occlusion of the pulmonary artery or any branches of the pulmonary artery that are of significant size. There does not have to be actual pulmonary infarction, since the scan results do not depend on tissue necrosis, only on mechanical vessel occlusion. However, in conditions that temporarily or permanently occlude or cut down lung vascularity there will be varying degrees of "positivity" on lung scan; these include cysts, abscesses, many cases of carcinoma, scars and a considerable number of pneumonias, especially when necrotizing. However, many of these conditions may be at least tentatively ruled out by comparison of the scan results with a chest x-ray. A chest x-ray should therefore be obtained with the lung scan.

Asthma in the acute phase may also produce focal perfusion defects due to bronchial obstruction; these disappear after treatment and therefore could mimic emboli. Congestive heart failure or pulmonary edema frequently cause multiple perfusion abnormalities on scan; this is a major problem in the elderly, since dyspnea is one of the symptoms associated with embolization. Emphysema may produce quite striking scan defects, even when chest x-ray is normal. The findings may simulate embolization or may be a source of confusion when emphysema and emboli coexist. Emphysema abnormality can be differentiated from that of embolization by a follow-up lung scan after 6–8 days. Defects due to emphysema persist unaltered, whereas those from emboli tend to change configuration. The repeat study could be performed earlier, but with increased risk of insufficient time lapse to permit diagnostic changes.

The lung scan (like the chest x-ray) is nonspecific; i.e., a variety of conditions produce abnormality. Certain findings increase the probability of embolization. Serial studies provide the best information. In some cases, a xenon ventilation study (p. 454) may help differentiate emboli from other etiologies of perfusion defect; but when congestive failure is present, when the defect is small and when embolization is superimposed on severe emphysema, xenon may not be reliable. Pulmonary artery angiography provides a more definitive answer than the lung scan, but it is a relatively complicated invasive procedure, entails some risk, and may miss small peripheral clots. The lung scan, therefore, is more useful than angiography as a screening procedure. A normal lung scan effectively rules out pulmonary embolization. A minimum of four views (anterior, posterior and both lateral projections) must be performed to constitute an adequate perfusion lung scan study.

SARCOIDOSIS

This disease, of as yet unknown etiology, is manifested by noncaseating granulomatous lesions in many organ systems, most commonly in lungs and thoracic lymph nodes. The disease is much more common in blacks. Laboratory studies may suggest or support the diagnosis. Anemia is not frequent but appears in about 5% of cases. Splenomegaly is present in 10-30%. Leukopenia is found in approximately 30%. Eosinophilia is reported in 10-60%, averaging 25% of cases. Thrombocytopenia is very uncommon, reported in less than 2% of several large series. Serum protein abnormalities are common, with hyperglobulinemia in nearly 50% and frequently decreased albumin. Hypercalcemia is reported in about 20%, although some authors give higher figures. Alkaline phosphatase is elevated in nearly 35%, which probably reflects either liver or bone involvement. The two major diagnostic procedures available are the Kveim skin test and biopsy.

The Kveim test consists of intradermal inoculation of an antigen composed of human sarcoidal tissue. A positive reaction is given by development of a papule in 4-6 weeks which, on biopsy, yields the typical noncaseating granulomas of sarcoidosis. The test is highly reliable, with less than 3% false positives. The main difficulty is inadequate supplies of sufficiently potent antigen. For this reason, few laboratories are equipped to do the Kveim test. Between 40% and 80% of cases give positive results, depending on the particular lot of antigen and the duration of disease. In chronic sarcoidosis (more than 6 months after onset of illness), the patient is less likely to exhibit a positive Kveim test. Steroid treatment depresses the Kveim reaction, and may produce a negative test. The value of the Kveim test is especially great when no enlarged lymph nodes are available for biopsy, when granulomas obtained from biopsy are nonspecific, or when diagnosis on an outpatient basis is necessary. A recent report has challenged the specificity of the Kveim test, suggesting that a positive test is related more to chronic lymphadenopathy than to any specific disease.

Biopsy is the most widely used means for diagnosis at present. Peripheral lymph nodes are involved in 60-95% of cases, although often they are small. The liver is said to show involvement in 75% of cases, although it is palpable in 20% or less. Difficulties with biopsy come primarily from the fact that the granuloma of sarcoidosis, although characteristic, is nonspecific. Other diseases that may sometimes or often give a similar histologic pattern are early miliary tuberculosis, histoplasmosis, some fungal diseases, some pneumoconioses, and the so-called pseudosarcoid reaction sometimes found in lymph nodes draining areas of carcinoma.

ERYTHROCYTE SEDIMENTATION RATE

This procedure consists of filling a calibrated tube of standard diameter with anticoagulated whole blood and measuring the rate of RBC sedimentation during a specified period, usually 1 hour. When the RBC settle toward the bottom of the tube, they leave an increasingly large zone of clear plasma, which is the area measured. Many diseases cause abnormally great red cell sedimentation (rate of fall in the tube system). These include acute and chronic infection, tissue necrosis and infarction, well-established malignancy, rheumatoid-collagen diseases, abnormal serum proteins and certain physiologic stress situations, such as pregnancy. Most of the sedimentation effect seems due to alterations in plasma proteins, mainly fibrinogen and globulins. The erythrocyte sedimentation rate (ESR) has two main uses: (1) as a means of following the activity or clinical course of certain diseases, such as acute rheumatic fever or acute glomerulonephritis, and (2) to demonstrate or confirm the presence of occult organic disease, either when the patient has symptoms but no definite physical or laboratory evidence of organic disease or in some cases when the patient is completely asymptomatic.

The ESR has three main limitations: (1) it is a very nonspecific test, (2) it is sometimes normal in diseases where usually it is abnormal and (3) technical factors may considerably influence the results. The tubes must be absolutely vertical; even small degrees of tilt have great effect on degree of sedimentation. Most types of anemia will falsely increase the ESR as performed by the Wintrobe method using oxalate anticoagulant; the Westergren method, using citrate or EDTA, is not affected. The Wintrobe method may be "corrected" for anemia, but this is not accurate. On the other hand, sickle cell anemia and polycythemia falsely decrease the ESR. Normal values (at least for the Westergren method) usually quoted for the ESR may be too low in persons over age 40 and definitely are too low in those over age 60. After age 60, at least 10 mm/hour should be added to normal values.

FAT EMBOLIZATION

A syndrome most often associated with severe bone trauma, fat embolization may also occur in fatty liver, diabetes and other conditions. Symptoms may be immediate or delayed. If immediate, shock is frequent. Delayed symptoms occur 2–3 days after injury, and pulmonary or cerebral manifestations are most prominent. Frequent signs are fever, tachycardia, tachypnea, upper body petechiae (50% of patients), and decreased hemoglobin. Laboratory diagnosis includes urine examination for free fat (special technique, p. 127), which is positive in 50% of cases during the first 3 days, and serum lipase, which is elevated in nearly 50% of patients from, roughly, day 3 to 7. Fat in sputum is unreliable; it gives many false positives and negatives. Chest x-rays sometimes demonstrate diffuse tiny infiltrates, sometimes coalescing, described in the literature as having a "snowstorm" appearance. Some patients develop a laboratory picture suggestive of disseminated intravascular coagulation. A recent report has indicated that diagnosis by cryostat frozen section of peripheral blood clot is sensitive and specific, but adequate confirmation of this is not yet available.

SELECTED TESTS OF INTEREST IN PEDIATRICS

NEONATAL IGM LEVELS.—Maternal IgG (immunoglobulin-G, p. 245) can cross the placenta, but not IgA or IgM. Chronic infections involving the fetus, such as congenital syphilis, toxoplasmosis, rubella and cytomegalic inclusion disease, lead to IgM production by the fetus. Increased IgM levels in cord blood at birth or in neonatal blood during the first few days of life suggest chronic intrauterine infection. Infection near term or subsequent to birth results in IgM increase beginning 6–7 days postpartum.

Unfortunately, there are pitfalls when interpreting such data. Many cord blood samples become contaminated with maternal blood, thus falsely raising IgM values. Normal values are controversial; 20 mg/100 ml is the most widely accepted upper limit. Various techniques have different reliabilities and sensitivities. Finally, some investigators state that fewer than 40% of rubella or cytomegalovirus infections cause elevated IgM before birth.

AGAMMAGLOBULINEMIA.—This condition may lead to frequent infections. Electrophoresis displays decreased gamma globulin, which can be confirmed by quantitative immunoglobulin technique.

NITROBLUE TETRAZOLIUM TEST.—Chronic granulomatous disease of childhood is a rare, sex-linked disorder of WBC manifested by repeated infections and ending in death before puberty. Polymorphonuclear leukocytes are able to attack high-virulence organisms, such as streptococci and staphylococci, but are unable to destroy those of lower virulence, such as the gram-negative rods. The nitroblue tetrazolium test is negative. Some normal granulocytes are able to reduce this substance to a dark blue color, but those in patients with chronic granulomatous disease are unable to do so. The nitroblue tetrazolium test has also been reported to separate persons with bacterial infection from persons with leukocytosis of other etiologies (p. 445). It has been advocated as a screening test for infection when the WBC count is normal and as a means to differentiate bacterial and viral infection in febrile patients. There is a great divergence of opinion in the literature on the merits of this procedure, apportioned about equally between those who find it useful and those who feel that it is not reliable because of unacceptable degrees of overlap between patients in various diagnostic categories. Many modifications of the original technique have been proposed, which add to the confusion.

SERUM FETOPROTEIN.—This test has been discussed elsewhere as a screening test for hepatoma (p. 215). Some reports indicate that fetoprotein tends to be elevated in acute hepatitis of infancy but not in biliary atresia, thus providing another aid in differentiating these two causes of neonatal jaundice.

Fetoprotein in amniotic fluid has proved useful in antenatal detection of open neural tube defects (spina bifida, anencephaly, p. 376).

PORPHYRIAS

In these related diseases the main similarity is the abnormal secretion of substances that are precursors of the porphyrin compound heme (of hemoglobin). The known pathways of porphyrin synthesis begin with glycine and succinate, which are combined to eventually form a compound known as delta aminolevulinic acid (ALA). This goes on to produce a substance known as porphobilinogen, composed of a single pyrrole ring. From there, four of these rings are joined to form the tetrapyrrole compound proporphyrinogen; this is the precursor of protoporphyrin, which in turn is the precursor of heme (Fig 20–2). The tetrapyrrole compounds exist in 8 isomers, depending on where certain side groups are located. The only iso-

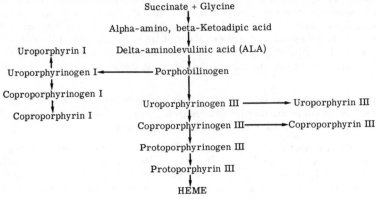

Fig 20–2.—Porphyrin synthesis.

meric forms that are clinically important are I and III. Normally, very small amounts of proporphyrin degradation products appear in the feces or in the urine; these are called coproporphyrins or uroporphyrins. (Their names refer to where they were first discovered, but both may appear in either urine or feces.)

The porphyrias have been classified in several ways, none of which is entirely satisfactory. The most common system includes erythropoietic porphyria (congenital porphyria), hereditary hepatic porphyria, cutanea tarda and toxic porphyria. Erythropoietic porphyria is a rare congenital disease characterized clinically by skin photosensitivity, pink discoloration of the teeth, and sometimes mild hemolytic anemia. Uroporphyrin and coproporphyrin I are excreted and are the only abnormal chemical findings.

Hereditary hepatic porphyria may be subdivided into three types; acute intermittant porphyria (AIP; Swedish genetic porphyria); variegate porphyria (VP; South African genetic porphyria); and hereditary coproporphyria (HC). In addition to episodes of acute porphyria, skin lesions (often due to photosensitivity) are present in VP and HC. The skin manifestations resemble those of cutanea tarda, and some of these patients were probably included in the cutanea tarda group in previous classifications. All three subdivisions manifest increase in the enzyme ALA-synthetase, which produces ALA from its precursors. However, AIP is characterized by decrease of 50% or more in the enzyme uroporphyrinogen-I-synthetase, which produces uroporphyrinogen I from porphobilinogen; VP and HC are said to have normal levels of this enzyme. Assay for uroporphyrinogen-I-synthetase is reported to provide a means of detecting AIP in the nonsymptomatic phase. The procedure is available in only a few reference laboratories.

Acute episodes of hereditary hepatic porphyria are manifested clinically by intermittent attacks of colicky abdominal pain. This is often accompanied by a leukocytosis and thus can mimic a variety of diseases, such as appendicitis and pancreatitis. In addition, severe constipation and episodes of abnormal mental behavior may occur. These attacks may be precipitated by barbiturates. (Other drugs have occasionally been incriminated.) In these acute episodes, an almost pathognomonic finding is the presence of porphobilinogen in the urine. Urinary uro- and coproporphyrins are relatively normal in many cases of acute porphyria when urine is freshly voided. Porphyrinogens may be increased; these compounds and porphobilinogen may break down to porphyrins. If this occurs, uroporphyrin type III and coproporphyrin type III are produced, but are not diagnostic, since they may be increased in other conditions. A compound called Waldenström's porphyrin — a complex of uroporphyrin type I and III — may also be present. Porphobilinogen is nearly always present during one of the clinical attacks, but the duration of excretion is highly variable. It may occasionally disappear if not searched for initially. Between attacks, some patients excrete porphobilinogen and others do not. Urine ALA is usually increased during acute attacks but not as markedly as porphobilinogen. During remission, ALA also may become normal.

Porphobilinogen is usually detected by color reaction with Ehrlich's reagent and confirmed by demonstrating that the color is not removed by chloroform (Watson-Schwartz test). Since false positive results may occur, it is essential to further confirm a positive test by butanol (butyl alcohol) extraction. Porphobilinogen will not be extracted by butanol, whereas butanol will remove most of the other Ehrlich-positive, chloroform-negative substances. A positive finding in the porphobilinogen test is the key to diagnosis of symptomatic acute porphyria; analysis and quantitation of urinary porphyrins or ALA are useful only if the Watson-Schwartz test results are equivocal. Glucose administration may considerably decrease porphobilinogen excretion.

Some investigators prefer the Hoesch test rather than the modified Watson-Schwartz procedure. The Hoesch test also uses Ehrlich's reagent but is less complicated and is said to be more specific for porphobilinogen (although the possibility of drug-induced false reactions has not been adequately investigated).

Some feel that a positive finding for porphobilinogen should be confirmed by quantitative chemical techniques (available in reference laboratories) due to experience with false positive Watson-Schwartz test results in various laboratories.

Cutanea tarda is a chronic type of porphyria. There usually is some degree of photosensitivity, but it does not develop until after puberty. There often is some degree of liver disease. These patients excrete abnormal amounts of uroporphyrin and coproporphyrin III.

Toxic porphyria may be produced by a variety of chemicals, but the most common is lead. Lead poisoning produces abnormal coproporphyrin III excretion but not uroporphyrin III. ALA is also excreted.

TESTS FOR ALLERGY

The atopic diseases were originally defined as sensitization based on hereditary predisposition (thus differentiating from nonaffected persons exposed to the same commonly found antigens), characterized by immediate urticarial skin reaction to offending antigen and by the Prausnitz-Küstner reaction. Prausnitz and Küstner demonstrated in 1921 that serum from a sensitized person, when injected into the skin of a nonsensitized person, would produce a cutaneous reaction when challenged by appropriate antigen (cutaneous passive transfer). The serum factor responsible was known as reagin (skin-sensitizing antibody). In 1966, reagin was found to be immunoglobulin E (IgE, p. 245), which has been shown to trigger immediate local hypersensitivity reactions by causing release of histamines and vasoactive substances from mast cells, which, in turn, produce local anaphylaxis in skin or mucous membranes. The IgE system thus mediates so-called atopic dermatitis, allergic rhinitis and many cases of asthma. Allergens may come from the environment (pollens, foods, allergenic dust, molds), from certain chronic infections (fungus, parasites), from medications (penicillin) or from industrial sources (cosmetics, chemicals). Sometimes there is a strong hereditary component; sometimes none is discernible. Discovery that IgE is the key substance in these reactions has led to measurement of serum IgE levels as a test for presence of atopic allergy sensitization.

Serum IgE level can be measured by radioimmunodiffusion or other techniques and has been useful in diagnosis of certain conditions, such as aspergillus-associated asthma (p. 172). Measurement of IgE is also being employed to investigate etiology of asthma and atopic dermatitis. The current system is called the radioallergosorbent test (RAST). Specific antigen is bound to a carrier substance and allowed to react with specific IgE antibody. The amount of IgE antibody bound is estimated by adding radioactive anti-IgE antibody and quantitating the amount of labeled anti-IgE attached to the IgE-antigen complex. The type of antigen, the degree and duration of stimulation and current exposure to antigen all influence IgE levels to any particular antigen at any point in time. Studies thus far indicate that RAST has an 80–85% correlation with results of skin testing using the subcutaneous injection method (range 60–100%, depending on the investigator and the antigen used). It seems a little less sensitive than the intradermal skin test method, but some claim that it predicts the results of therapy better, i.e., is possibly more specific. Since only a limited number of antigens are available for use in the RAST system, each antigen to be tested for must be listed by the physician. Some advise obtaining a serum total IgE assay in addition to RAST; if the RAST panel is negative and serum IgE is high, this suggests allergy to antigens not included in the RAST panel. Total serum IgE can be normal, however, even if one or more antigens on the RAST panel are positive. There is some cross reaction between certain antigens in the RAST system. The RAST profile is more expensive than skin testing with the same antigens.

REFERENCES

Ahmad, M., et al.: Limited diagnostic specificity of technetium-99m stannous pyrophosphate myocardial imaging in acute myocardial infarction, Am. J. Cardiol 39: 50, 1977.

Alford, C. A.: Immunoglobulin determinations in the diagnosis of fetal infection, Pediatr. Clin. North Am. 18:99, 1971.

Allen, J. C.: Recurrent infections in man associated with immunologic or phagocythe deficiencies, Postgrad. Med. 50:88, 1971.

Berg, T., and Johansson, S. G. O.: Allergy diagnosis with the radioallergosorbant test, Int. Arch. Allergy Appl. Immunol. 40:770, 1971.

Berger, R. L., et al.: Diagnosis and management of massive pulmonary embolism, Surg. Clin. North Am. 48:311, 1968.

Bernstein, I. L.: Experiences with RAST in the Diagnosis and Management of Inhalant Allergy, In Evans, R. (ed.): *Advances in the Diagnosis of Allergy: RAST* (Miami: Symposia Specialists, 1975).

Coleman, R. E., et al.: Improved detection of myocardial infarction with technetium-99m stannous pyrophosphate and serum MB creatine phosphokinase, Am. J. Cardiol. 37:732, 1976.

Czucs, M. M., Jr.: Diagnostic sensitivity of laboratory findings in acute pulmonary embolization, Ann. Intern. Med. 74:161, 1971.

Ehsani, A., et al.: Effects of electrical countershock on serum creatine phosphokinase (CPK) isoenzyme activity, Am. J. Cardiol. 37:12, 1976.

Emerson, P. M., and Wilkinson, J. H.: Lactate dehydrogenase in the diagnosis and assessment of response to treatment of megaloblastic anaemia, Brit. J. Haematol. 12:678, 1966.

Eshchar, J., and Zimmerman, H. J.: Creatine phosphokinase in disease, Am. J. Med. Sci. 253:272, 1967.

Evarts, C. M.: The fat embolization syndrome: A review, Surg. Clin. North Am. 50:493, 1970.

Fleisher, G. A., et al.: Serum creatine kinase, lactic dehydrogenase, and glutamic-oxaloacetic transaminase in thyroid disease and pregnancy, Mayo Clin. Proc. 40:300, 1965.

Galen, R. S.: The enzyme diagnosis of myocardial infarction, Hum. Pathol. 6:141, 1975.

Gilbertsen, V. A.: Erythrocyte sedimentation rates in older patients, Postgrad. Med. 38:A-44, 1965.

Hauman, A., et al.: Cryostat test for fat embolism, Lab. Med. 2:37, 1971.

Israel, H. L.: Diagnosis of sarcoidosis, Ann. Intern. Med. 68:1323, 1968.

Israel, H. L., and Goldstein, R. A.: Relation of Kveim-antigen reaction to lymphadenopathy, N. Engl. J. Med. 284:345, 1971.

Itano, M.: The detection of CPK_1 (BB) in serum, Am. J. Clin. Pathol. 65:351, 1976.

Kottinen, A., et al.: Serum enzymes and isoenzymes: extrapulmonary sources in acute pulmonary embolization, Arch. Intern. Med. 133:243, 1974.

Lafair, J. S., and Myerson, R. M.: Alcoholic myopathy, Arch. Intern. Med. 122:417, 1968.

Light, R. W., and Bell, W. R.: LDH and fibrinogen-fibrin degradation products in pulmonary embolism, Arch. Intern. Med. 133:372, 1974.

Mayock, R. L., et al.: Manifestations of sarcoidosis, Am. J. Med. 35:67, 1963.

Meltzer, H. Y.: Creatine kinase and aldolase in serum: Abnormality common to acute psychoses, Science 159:1368, 1968.

Meyer, U. A., et al.: Intermittent acute porphyria—demonstration of a genetic defect in porphobilinogen metabolism, N. Engl. J. Med. 286:1277, 1972.

Nathan, L. E., et al.: Application of an automated determination of isoenzyme-5 of lactate dehydrogenase to the diagnosis of hepatic disease, Clin. Chem. 19:1036, 1973.

Pitt, B., and Strauss, H. W.: Myocardial imaging in the non-invasive evaluation of patients with suspected ischemic heart disease, Am. J. Cardiol. 37:797, 1976.

Platt, M. R., et al.: Technetium stannous pyrophosphate myocardial scintigrams in recognition of myocardial infarction in patients undergoing coronary artery revascularization, Ann. Thorac. Surg. 21:311, 1976.

Pollack, A.: Diagnosing porphyria. Why aren't labs interested? Lab. Management 14(10):24, 1976.

Quinn, J. L., III: The lung: The challenge of nuclear medicine, Am. J. Roentgenol. 105:251, 1969.

Roberts, R., and Sobel, B. E.: CPK isoenzymes in evaluation of myocardial ischemic injury, Hosp. Practice 11:55, 1976.

238   CLINICAL LABORATORY MEDICINE

Roberts, R., and Sobel, B. E.: Elevated plasma MB creatine phosphokinase activity. A specific marker for myocardial infarction in perioperative patients, Arch. Intern. Med. 136:421, 1976.

Russell, S. M., et al.: Ischemic rhabdomyolysis and creatine phosphokinase isoenzymes: a diagnostic pitfall, J.A.M.A. 235:632, 1976.

Sax, S. M., et al.: Atypical increase in serum creatine kinase activity in hospital patients, Clin. Chem. 22:87, 1976.

Schlegel, R. J.: Chronic granulomatous disease 1974, J.A.M.A. 231:615, 1975.

Schrader, W. H.: Erythrocyte sedimentation rate, Postgrad. Med. 34:A-42, 1963.

Sinnott, J. L.: The laboratory investigation of the porphyrin disorders: A review, Med. Lab. Sci. 33:133, 1976.

Tschudy, D. P., et al.: Acute intermittent porphyria: Clinical and selected research aspects, Ann. Intern. Med. 83:851, 1975.

Tysinger, D. S.: Pulmonary function testing for the general hospital and physician, J. Med. Assoc. State Ala. 39:658, 756, 834, 922, 1113, 1970; 40:33, 106, 1970.

Wackers, F. J. T., et al.: Value and limitations of thallium-201 scintigraphy in the acute phase of myocardial infarct, N. Engl. J. Med. 295:1, 1976.

Weidner, W., et al.: Roentgen techniques in the diagnosis of pulmonary thromboembolism, Am. J. Roentgenol. 100:397, 1967.

Weinsaft, P. P., and Haltaufderhyde, V.: Erythrocyte sedimentation rate in the aged, J. Am. Geriatr. Soc. 13:738, 1965.

Windhorst, D. B.: Functional Defects of Neutrophils, in Stollerman, G. H., et al. (eds.): *Advances in Internal Medicine* (Chicago: Year Book Medical Publishers, Inc., 1970), vol. 16, p. 329.

21 / Serum Proteins

ALBUMIN AND GLOBULIN, both free and combined with other substances containing lipid or carbohydrate, make up the serum proteins. Normal total protein concentration is 6.5–8 gm/100 ml. Normal globulin range is 1–3 gm and that of albumin 4–6 gm. Plasma contains fibrinogen in addition to the ordinary serum proteins. The globulin molecule is approximately 2½ times as large as that of albumin, although quantitatively albumin is normally 2–3 times the level of globulin. Albumin seems most concerned with maintaining the serum oncotic pressure, where its osmotic influence is about 4 times that of globulin. The globulins, on the other hand, seem to have more varied assignments and form the main transport system for many substances, as well as having an active role themselves in certain immunologic mechanisms.

Most serum albumin seems produced by the liver. The origin of various globulins is not well understood, although some, if not all, are apparently synthesized by the reticuloendothelial system. Both of these protein categories can be elevated and depressed in various conditions.

SERUM PROTEIN FRACTIONS

METHODS OF FRACTIONATION. — There are four widely used procedures for fractionating the serum proteins. "Salting-out" by differential chemical solubility will yield rough separation into albumin and globulin. Cohn has devised a more complicated chemical fractionation method by which certain parts of the protein spectrum may be separated from one another as a large-scale industrial-type procedure. The ultracentrifuge has recently been used to study some of the subgroups of the globulins. This is possible because the sedimentation rate at high speeds depends on the molecular size and shape, the type of solvent used to suspend the protein and the force of centrifugation. The velocity of any particular class of globulins under standard conditions depends primarily on molecular size and is known as the Svedberg number; the most common classes of globulins are designated as 7S, 19S or 22S. Electrophoresis can also be used; current standard methods include filter paper, cellulose acetate film, agarose and polyacrylamide gel as a migrating field. In clinical medicine, electrophoretic techniques are becoming routine and will form the backbone of this discussion. The albumin to globulin (A/G) ratio is usually done by a chemical method and should be discarded, since electrophoresis will not only give the same information but also pinpoint the areas where serum protein

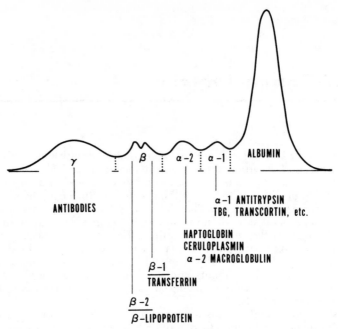

Fig 21–1. — Some important components of serum protein fractions.

shifts take place, which sometimes have as much diagnostic importance as the shifts themselves.

Different methods give slightly different values for various protein fractions. For example, serum albumin by electrophoresis may be about 0.5 gm/100 ml less than by the usual chemical method. This is fortunately not often very important. Also, the laboratory must rigidly standardize its electrophoretic technique, since variations in electric current, buffer solution and other technical aspects will give different results. That is why normal values should be prepared by the individual laboratory for its own particular procedure.

Serum protein electrophoresis ordinarily will display bands corresponding to albumin, alpha₁ and alpha₂ globulins, beta globulins, and gamma globulins. According to the quantitation or density of these bands, a special instrument will translate this into a linear pattern, which is a rough visual approximation of the amount of substance present. The main problem with this method is the difficulty in separating some of the serum components. It has been found that by using potato starch in a gel-like state, the separation of some of these fractions will be sharper; this is especially true in some of the abnormal hemoglobins. Polyacrylamide gel has also been used. However, these procedures are technically somewhat more difficult than the other techniques, and filter paper and cellulose acetate remain the routine clinical laboratory methods of choice. With filter paper or cellulose acetate,

alpha$_2$ migrates faster toward the anode than beta; with starch or polyacrylamide gel, the reverse occurs.

Serum Albumin

Elevation of serum albumin is very unusual other than in dehydration.
Most changes involve diminution, although the normal range is somewhat
large, and small decreases are thus lost without previous knowledge of the
individual patient's normal levels. In pregnancy, albumin decreases progressively until delivery and does not return to normal until about 8 weeks
postpartum. In infants, adult levels are reached at about 1 year of age.
Thereafter, serum proteins are relatively stable except for a gradual decrease after age 70. Malnutrition leads to decreased albumin, presumably
from lack of essential amino acids, but also possibly from impaired liver
manufacture and unknown causes. Impaired synthesis may itself be a
cause of decreased albumin, since it is found in most forms of clinical liver
disease. In chronic cachectic or wasting diseases, such as tuberculosis or
carcinoma, the albumin is often decreased, but it is not clear whether this
is due to impaired synthesis or to other factors. Chronic infections seem to
have much the same effect as the cachectic diseases.

Serum albumin may be directly lost from the bloodstream by hemorrhage, burns, exudates or leakage into the gastrointestinal tract in various
malabsorption diseases. In many acute illnesses or injuries, the albumin is
quickly decreased. This might be thought of as a response to stress and
seems to have a different mechanism from hypoalbuminemia found in
malnutrition or simple loss of protein. This will be discussed further. Finally, there may be a genetic cause, such as familial idiopathic dysproteinemia, in which the albumin is greatly decreased while all the globulin
fractions are elevated and seem to take over most of the functions of albumin. In nephrosis there is a marked decrease in serum albumin secondary
to direct loss in the urine.

Alpha$_1$ Globulins

Alpha$_1$ globulin is increased in pregnancy and by estrogen administration and occasionally by neoplasia, tissue necrosis and infection. Alpha$_1$
globulin is absent or nearly so in alpha$_1$ antitrypsin deficiency, a hereditary
disorder that predisposes to development of emphysema. Serum protein
electrophoresis detects homozygous disease but frequently displays a
normal alpha$_1$ peak in those who are heterozygous. Immunoassay is needed to detect heterozygotes or confirm electrophoretic findings (p. 423).

Alpha$_2$ Globulins

Alpha$_2$ globulins as a group are seldom depressed; diminution of one
component is usually masked in the normal range. Haptoglobin is decreased in hemolytic anemia and severe liver disease, ceruloplasmin in
Wilson's disease. On the other hand, a considerable number of diseases
may cause an increase. An increase in the alpha$_2$ globulin is coupled with a
decrease in albumin in various stress situations. They may include acute
infections, injury, trauma, burns, extensive neoplasia or certain chronic illnesses in the active stage, such as rheumatic fever or rheumatoid arthritis.
This is also found in acute myocardial infarct and similar conditions in

which tissue necrosis takes place. Haptoglobin elevation is found in most of the conditions just mentioned. In similar but more chronic illnesses albumin may be decreased or may be normal; the alpha$_2$ globulin may be slightly or moderately elevated, and the gamma globulin is increased. There are certain other diseases that often show alpha$_2$ increase. In the nephrotic syndrome there is classically a marked alpha$_2$ peak, which may sometimes be joined by a beta globulin elevation. In addition, there is, of course, greatly decreased albumin. In hyperthyroidism, far-advanced diabetes and adrenal insufficiency there is reportedly a slightly to moderately elevated alpha$_2$ in some cases.

Beta Globulins

A decrease in the beta globulins is not very common. Transferrin is frequently decreased in protein malnutrition. The beta globulins may be increased in many conditions. An increase in transferrin produced by chronic iron deficiency anemia and by pregnancy in the 3d trimester leads to a beta increase of varying degree that occasionally has a homogeneous spikelike configuration simulating a monoclonal peak. In patients in whom serum cholesterol is elevated, the beta globulins are also likely to be increased; this includes hypothyroidism, biliary cirrhosis, nephrosis and some cases of diabetes. In liver disease in general, there is some variability. Beta globulin is usually, but not always, elevated in obstructive jaundice; it may be found elevated to some extent in many cases of hepatitis, but not as often as in obstructive jaundice. It is often elevated in cirrhosis; when so, it is often joined to the gamma globulin and occasionally does not even appear as a separate peak. This will be discussed later. Finally, beta elevations may occasionally be seen in certain other diseases, including malignant hypertension, Cushing's disease, periarteritis nodosa and sometimes carcinoma. These changes are probably due to increase in complement. Hemolysis may produce an artifactual needle-like spike in the beta or pregamma area. A double peak in the beta area is frequently observed when the cellulose acetate method is used. Electrophoresis on polyacrylamide gel produces reversal of the alpha$_2$ and beta area positions compared to paper or cellulose acetate electrophoresis (i.e., the beta area on paper becomes alpha$_2$ on polyacrylamide gel).

Gamma Globulins

Gamma globulins exhibit a wide variety of changes. They are decreased in hypo- and agammaglobulinemia, which may be either primary or secondary. The secondary type sometimes may be found with long-term steroid treatment, the nephrotic syndrome, occasionally in overwhelming infection, and relatively often with chronic lymphocytic leukemia, lymphosarcoma, or multiple myeloma.

Many diseases cause increase in gamma globulin. Almost all types of infections are followed by increased gamma globulin, although the increase may not be sufficient to cause abnormal changes on paper electrophoresis, especially if the infection is mild or acute. Chronic infections characteristically show electrophoretic gamma increase, especially tuberculosis. Collagen diseases, including rheumatoid arthritis and lupus erythematosus, often cause considerably elevated values, and this may be true also in many hypersensitivity diseases. Sarcoidosis, syphilis and lymphogranuloma venereum are other well-known etiologies. Gamma globulin is frequently increased in Hodgkin's disease, malignant lymphoma, and chronic lymphocytic leukemia. Multiple myeloma and certain uncommon diseases characteristically show a marked increase of a special homogeneous spike-like pattern, and this will be discussed later. A final general category for gamma increase is the group of liver diseases. In hepatitis, there is classically a relatively mild separate increase in both beta and gamma globulins with a decrease of albumin, but this does not always occur. In cirrhosis, there is characteristically a marked increase in gamma globulin. The most suggestive pattern is a combination of beta and gamma without the usual separation between the two. However, in most cases, one merely sees an ordinary gamma globulin elevation; of considerable degree in some, slight in others and no gamma elevation in about 10%. In obstructive jaundice, one often sees an increase in alpha$_2$, beta and gamma, all three, to varying degree.

Typical Electrophoretic Patterns

By way of summary, several typical electrophoretic patterns will be presented with diseases in which they will most commonly be found (Fig 21 – 2). It must be strongly emphasized that these patterns are by no means pathognomonic of any one disease or groups of diseases, that they will sometimes not occur in a disease in which they should be present and that there will be considerable variation in the shape and height of the electrophoretic peaks in individual patients, which may obscure the pattern. In other words, the patterns are simply intended as a rule of thumb.

The first of these patterns presents what is called the acute stress, or acute reaction, pattern and consists of a decreased albumin and elevated alpha$_2$ globulin. This is found in acute infections in the early stages; some cases of myocardial infarct and tissue necrosis; some cases of severe burns, surgery, and other stress situations; and in some of the rheumatoid diseases with acute onset. The second pattern consists of a slightly or moderately decreased albumin, a slightly or moderately elevated gamma globulin and a slightly elevated or normal alpha$_2$. This is the chronic inflammatory pattern and is found in chronic infections of various types, cirrhosis and rheumatoid-collagen diseases. There may, of course, be various stages of transition between this chronic pattern and the previously described acute one. Next is the so-called nephrotic type, in which one sees a greatly decreased albumin and a considerably increased alpha$_2$ with or without an increase in beta. This differs from the acute stress pattern in that the alpha$_2$ elevation of the nephrotic syndrome is usually either slightly or moderately greater than that seen in acute stress, while the albumin fraction in the nephrotic syndrome has a definitely greater decrease (sometimes to extremely low levels) than the albumin values of the acute stress pattern.

Fourth is the frequently found pattern in far-advanced cirrhosis consisting of a decreased albumin with moderately or considerably increased gamma globulin and variable degrees of incorporation of the beta into the gamma. The more pronounced the "slurring" becomes, the more suggestive for cirrhosis. However, complete incorporation of the beta into the gamma is actually uncommon, and this is only one of several patterns that

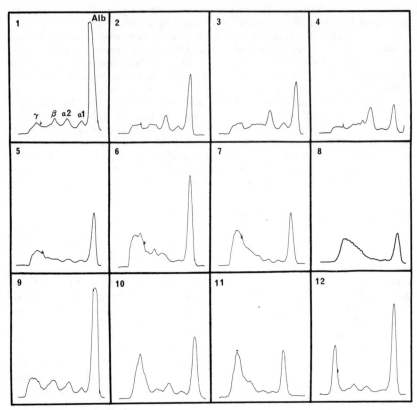

Fig 21–2.—Typical serum protein electrophoretic patterns. **1,** normal (*arrow near gamma region indicates serum application point*); **2,** acute stress pattern; **3,** acute stress or nephrotic syndrome; **4,** nephrotic syndrome; **5,** chronic inflammation (mild to moderate), cirrhosis; **6,** cirrhosis, granulomatous diseases, rheumatoid-collagen group; **7,** suggestive of cirrhosis, but could be found in the granulomatous diseases or the rheumatoid-collagen group; **8,** characteristic pattern of cirrhosis; **9,** slight nonspecific elevation of gamma, possibly also beta globulin fraction (? chronic disease); **10,** same as **6,** configuration of gamma peak superficially mimics myeloma, but is more broad-based; **11,** same interpretation as **10;** **12,** myeloma, Waldenström's, idiopathic or secondary monoclonal gammopathy.

may be found in cirrhosis. The fifth pattern consists of a greatly increased, but diffuse, gamma globulin, with or without a small but independent beta increase and a moderately decreased albumin. This is most often found in some cases of cirrhosis; in granulomatous diseases, such as sarcoidosis or far-advanced pulmonary tuberculosis; in subacute bacterial endocarditis; and in certain of the collagen diseases such as lupus or periarteritis.

Finally, there is a so-called monoclonal gammopathy spike (m-protein and paraprotein are synonyms). This is located in the gamma area (much less frequently in the beta and rarely in the alpha$_2$) and consists of a high, relatively thin spike configuration that is more homogeneous and needle-shaped than the other gamma or beta elevations discussed earlier. The majority of persons with the monoclonal spike on serum electrophoresis have myeloma. However, a sizable minority do not, and these are divided among Waldenström's macroglobulinemia, secondary paraproteinemia and idiopathic monoclonal gammopathy.

Certain conditions may produce globulin peaks that simulate monoclonal configuration; alpha$_2$ in nephrotic syndrome or with elevated haptoglobin; beta due to pregnancy in the 3d trimester, elevated transferrin, presence of serum free hemoglobin or contamination by fibrinogen; and gamma in rare patients with severe chronic disease.

Immunoglobulins

Gamma globulins (called immunoglobulins in current immunologic terminology) are not a homogeneous group. There are three main subdivisions: IgG (immunoglobulin G), which migrates in the gamma region on electrophoresis; IgA, which migrates in the pregamma or the area between gamma and beta; and IgM, which migrates in the prebeta or beta (Fig 21–3). There are two additional groups called IgD and IgE. IgG comprises about 75% of serum immunoglobulins and has a normal 7S molecular weight. IgG immunoglobulins constitute the majority of the antibodies, especially the warm-temperature incomplete type. IgM accounts for 5–7% of total immunoglobulins, and is a macroglobulin (19S) group. It includes cold agglutinins, ABO blood group isoagglutinins, and rheumatoid factor. IgA constitutes about 15% of immunoglobulins. Although most are 7S, some molecules are larger. It is found primarily in secretions, such as saliva, tears, gastrointestinal secretions from stomach and accessory organs and those from the respiratory tract. IgD is a normal 7S molecule that makes up less than 1% of the immunoglobulins; its function is not known. IgE also has a 7S weight and less than 1% frequency. It seems involved with certain allergic conditions, especially atopic (skin sensitivity) disorders, and is associated with reaginic antibody.

The normal immunoglobulin molecule is composed of two heavy chains (each chain of 50,000 molecular weight) and two light chains (each of 20,000 molecular weight) connected by disulfide bridges. IgM is a pentomeric arrangement of five complete immunoglobulin units.

Fig 21–3.—Diagrammatic relationship of immunoglobulins to the standard cellulose acetate serum protein electrophoretic pattern.

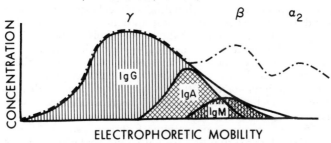

TABLE 21-1.—IMMUNOGLOBULIN
NOMENCLATURE

CURRENT TERMINOLOGY	SYNONYMS
IgG	γ (gamma) G
	γ_2
	7S γ
IgA	γA
	γ_1A
	β_2A
IgM	γM
	γ_1M
	β_2M
	19S γ

MULTIPLE MYELOMA

Multiple myeloma is a malignancy of plasma cells involving bone marrow that frequently produces multisystem disease. Patients are usually more than 40 years old, with the highest incidence occurring in age group 50–60. The plasma cells infiltrate bone marrow at some time during the course of the disease, but this ordinarily does not result in peripheral blood plasmacytosis. Bone marrow aspiration usually is suggestive of myeloma by the time symptoms develop, but sometimes may take longer to become diagnostic. There usually are over 20% plasma cells in the myeloma bone marrow. If less than this, many have to be immature if a diagnosis is to be possible, because other diseases can sometimes give up to 20% marrow plasma cells of the mature type. Anemia is found in 60–80% of patients (or more, depending on the stage of the disease). It is generally moderate in degree (although sometimes severe) and of normocytic-normochromic type. Total WBC count is usually normal, with leukopenia reported in 15–20% of cases. Thrombocytopenia may be found in approximately 10% of patients. Red cell rouleaux formation in peripheral blood smears is common and often provides a clue to the diagnosis. The ESR is usually moderately to markedly elevated. By far the most common symptom in myeloma is bone pain, most often in the spine. X-rays display abnormality in 80–85% of patients. The most typical finding is the "punched-out" osteolytic lesion, most commonly in skull, vertebral spine and pelvis. Between 6% and 25% demonstrate diffuse osteoporosis as the only abnormality; the rest display various combinations of focal osteolytic lesions, osteoporosis and pathologic fractures. Results of bone scan are not as frequently abnormal in myeloma as in metastatic tumor involving bone. The alkaline phosphatase value tends to be normal, except when fractures develop. Hypercalcemia occurs in 20–35% of myeloma patients. Cryoglobulins are found in approximately 5%, and amyloid in 5–10%. Azotemia is frequent, especially in the later stages of the disease. Many patients develop a tendency toward infection, and this may be the reason they are seen by the physician.

About 75–80% of myeloma patients feature plasma cell secretion of abnormal monoclonal serum protein with a molecular weight (160,000 or

7S) typical of a normal complete immunoglobulin molecule. Of all patients with monoclonal protein, about two thirds have myeloma. In those myeloma patients with normal weight serum monoclonal protein, roughly 70% can be categorized as IgG, about 25% as IgA and fewer than 2% as IgD or IgE.

In addition to normal weight serum monoclonal protein many patients excrete an abnormal, incomplete, low molecular weight protein, known as Bence Jones protein. Bence Jones protein is composed only of immunoglobulin light chains and therefore has a low molecular weight (40,000 or 3.5S). Unlike normal weight monoclonal proteins, it is able to pass the glomerular filter into the urine. In most cases it is cleared rapidly from plasma; therefore, even when Bence Jones proteinuria is marked, this substance usually is not demonstrable in serum by ordinary electrophoretic techniques and frequently not even by immunoelectrophoresis. About 70–80% of myeloma patients produce Bence Jones; 50–60% have a normal weight serum monoclonal protein in addition to urine Bence Jones, and about 20% (literature range 10–26%) reveal Bence Jones in urine as the only protein abnormality ("light chain" myeloma). Light chain myeloma is frequently associated with hypogammaglobulinemia on standard serum protein electrophoresis. Clinically, there tends to be somewhat greater incidence of azotemia, hypercalcemia and lytic bone lesions than seen in ordinary myeloma.

The classic method of detecting Bence Jones is by a carefully done heat coagulability test, where it appears on heating to 60° C and disappears on boiling, only to reappear if the urine is cooled. As mentioned earlier (p. 110), with a few exceptions Bence Jones gives a positive sulfosalicylic acid test for urine protein, but dipsticks frequently give negative results. It has been found that since various technical problems and human factors make the heat method unreliable, urine electrophoresis is the best method for demonstrating Bence Jones. In urine, it appears as a single homogeneous spike similar to that of monoclonal protein in serum. The normal weight monoclonal serum proteins of myeloma do not appear in the urine. In many cases it is necessary to concentrate the urine (50–100 times) to detect small quantities of Bence Jones protein.

Whereas light chain myeloma involves selective production of the light chain fragment of immunoglobulin molecules, there is a rare condition known as Franklin's disease (heavy chain disease) characterized by selective production of the heavy chain fragment. The clinical picture is most often similar to that of malignant lymphoma. Bone marrow aspiration findings are variable, and lymph node biopsy may suggest lymphoma or contain a mixed cell infiltrate.

OTHER MONOCLONAL GAMMOPATHIES

Waldenström's (Primary) Macroglobulinemia

This is a lymphoproliferative disorder characterized by monoclonal IgM (molecular weight 1,000,000 or 19S) production, with classic clinical features of lymphadenopathy, hepatosplenomegaly, anemia, hyperglobulinemia with rouleaux formation and the hyperviscosity syndrome. From 10% to 30% of Waldenström patients (literature range 0–60%) excrete

Bence Jones protein in the urine. Although typical findings are a mixture of mature lymphocytes and plasmacytoid lymphocytes, in some cases the histologic picture on biopsy is suggestive of a diffuse type of lymphocytic lymphoma. Bone marrow aspiration may yield normal findings, nonspecific lymphoid infiltration or lymphoma-like infiltrate. On skeletal x-ray, "punched-out" osteolytic lesions of the type seen in myeloma are usually absent. The hyperviscosity syndrome consists of shortness of breath, various neurologic abnormalities and visual difficulty with "sausage-shaped" segmentation of retinal veins. Serum viscosity (as measured by the Ostwald viscosimeter or other methods) is increased. In some patients the disease could be interpreted as malignant lymphoma or lymphocytic leukemia with IgM production; in a few instances, plasma cells predominate, and osteolytic bone lesions are present that would be compatible with an IgM myeloma. Since plasma cells are derived from lymphocytes, many are inclined to view these disorders as a spectrum. However, since clinicians usually insist on a specific diagnosis, the "intermediate" forms create a problem.

Idiopathic Monoclonal Gammopathy

Idiopathic monoclonal gammopathy is defined as monoclonal protein in the absence of disease known to be associated with it. True incidence is hard to define, since patients with nonneoplastic "secondary" paraproteinemia were frequently not segregated from paraproteinemia without other disease in many reports in the literature. Nonneoplastic monoclonal gammopathy apparently is more common with advanced age. Some investigators found incidence between 0.3% and 3.0% in populations tested, with the higher rates in the elderly. There is disagreement about whether overt myeloma will develop if followed long enough, although it is reported in some cases.

Secondary Monoclonal Gammopathy

This may be further subdivided into those associated with neoplasia and those associated with nonneoplastic disorders. In the neoplasm group monoclonal proteins are most often found with malignant lymphoma and chronic lymphocytic leukemia. Among carcinomas, those of the rectosigmoid are most frequent, followed by prostate, breast and lung. Incidence in one large cancer hospital ranged from 0.2% in the fourth decade to 5.7% in the ninth. In three large series of patients with monoclonal gammopathy, 6–8% of cases were associated with lymphoma or lymphocytic leukemia and 4–8% with other types of neoplasms. Nonneoplastic diseases that have been associated with monoclonal proteins are many and varied, but the greatest number appear in the rheumatoid-collagen-autoimmune group, cirrhosis, chronic infection (particularly tuberculosis, biliary tract, urinary tract and lung), Gaucher's disease, osteitis deformans (Paget's disease of bone) and sarcoidosis. Most of these conditions are ordinarily associated with polyclonal hyperglobulinemia rather than monoclonal. Incidence of nonneoplastic monoclonal protein in the three series mentioned varied from 4% to 10%. Monoclonal protein type in the secondary paraproteinemias may be IgG, IgA or IgM. Occasional patients in either the neoplastic or nonneoplastic group excrete urine Bence Jones protein, usually in small amount. In some cases the heat test is falsely positive due to an increase in normal light chains associated with polyclonal gammopathy.

Diagnostic Techniques

In many instances the diagnosis of myeloma or Waldenström's macroglobulinemia can be made by serum protein electrophoresis and bone marrow aspiration; in those patients without a monoclonal-type serum peak, urine electrophoresis on a concentrated specimen would be essential. In problem cases, it is necessary to resort to serum and urine immunoelectrophoresis. Many authorities advocate immunoelectrophoresis in all patients since this is the only way to classify monoclonal immunoglobulin disorders with certainty. (Even subgrouping of IgG and IgA is now possible.) Although subclassification of myeloma into immunoglobulin categories at present has more academic than practical application from the standpoint of therapy, such classification may become important in the future and, in any event, provides additional confirmation of the diagnosis. About 1–2% of myeloma patients fail to secrete abnormal proteins in either serum or urine that are detectable even by immunoelectrophoresis ("nonsecretory" myeloma).

Immunoelectrophoresis consists of three steps: (1) The unknown (patient's) serum is subjected to ordinary electrophoresis in a substance such as agar gel; this separates the immunoglobulins from one another to some extent. (2) Antiserum against a specific type of human globulin (or a polyvalent antiserum against several types) is added to a trench cut near the electrophoretic bands, and the immunoglobulins and anti-immunoglobulin antibodies diffuse toward each other. (3) The areas of reaction be-

Fig 21–4.—Procedure for immunoelectrophoresis (modified from Terry and Fahey). **Step 1,** electrophoresis of human serum globulins on agar gel. **Step 2,** addition of antihuman globulin antibody mixture to a nearby trough, and diffusion of the separated globulin fractions and the antibody mixture components toward each other. **Step 3,** formation of precipitin lines at interaction of globulin fractions and specific antibodies to these fractions from the antiglobulin antibody mixture. The globulin fractions have different rates of diffusion and thus produce precipitin lines in different areas.

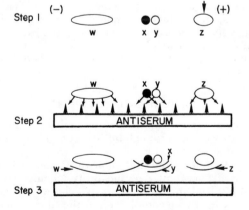

tween the patient's immunoglobulin fractions and their corresponding antibodies form visual precipitin lines (Fig 21 – 4). The combination of electrophoresis and agar diffusion antigen-antibody reaction produces better separation of the immunoglobulin components and demonstrates abnormal quantities of any type present. Immunoelectrophoresis is currently most useful in differentiating macroglobulinemia from other types of monoclonal gammopathy. If the monoclonal peak is shown to be IgM, this is evidence against myeloma, since only a few cases of IgM myeloma have been reported. On the other hand, if the peak is not IgM, this rules out Waldenström's macroglobulinemia. The idiopathic or secondary paraproteinemias can be either IgG, IgA or IgM.

Immunoelectrophoresis for light chains is also useful. Normally there are two types of light chains, known as kappa and lambda, present in serum, with about twice as much kappa produced as lambda. Malignant monoclonal gammopathies, such as myeloma or Waldenström's, usually have an abnormal predominance of either kappa or lambda, with the other markedly decreased or absent. Interestingly, although kappa myeloma is about twice as common as lambda myeloma in most of the myeloma immunoglobulin categories, IgD myeloma is predominantly a lambda type. Commercial companies have had problems in producing consistently good antisera to kappa and lambda light chains. Controls must be run with every lot of antiserum to guard against false results.

Occasionally, there may be other types of abnormal serum proteins in myeloma, Waldenström's macroglobulinemia, malignancy, and some of the other diseases, such as lupus. Among these are cryoglobulins. These are abnormal globulins that have the interesting property of coagulating when cooled to certain temperatures. They are not generally demonstrable as distinct peaks on paper electrophoresis, but are incorporated into areas occupied by other globulins.

There are screening tests for both cryoglobulins and macroglobulins. The cryocrit is essentially a cold precipitation test for cryoglobulins adapted to yield a rough quantitative result. Serum of the patient is placed in the icebox overnight, then centrifuged in a Wintrobe hematocrit tube. Normally, less than 2% of precipitate will be found. To test for cryofibrinogen, heparinized plasma is used for the same procedure. Macroglobulins are screened by the Sia test, which is actually a test for euglobulin. The procedure consists very simply of adding a drop of the patient's serum to distilled water. Most of the macroglobulins are insoluble in water, so that the formation of a precipitate suggests the presence of macroglobulins. The test is not very reliable.

SERUM COMPLEMENT

Serum complement is an important immunologic enzyme system that makes up about 10% of the serum globulins. Complement has many activities, some of which are undoubtedly still unknown; most attention has been focused on its role in the immunologic system, where effects have been demonstrated on vascular permeability, chemotaxis, phagocytosis, immune adherence and immune cell lysis. The most famous laboratory procedure directly involving complement is the complement fixation (CF) test method. There are 9 major components, ranging from alpha to gamma in electrophoretic mobility. There are also inhibitors of some of these components. Nomenclature in this system has been confusing because numbers assigned to the components are not in the same order as the order in which the components are activated in a complement activation sequence and also because subcomponents exist in some of the components. Total complement is abbreviated C; the major components are numbered C1 through C9. (Some use the symbol C' instead of C.) Component C1 has three subcomponents: C1q, C1r and C1s. Component C3 has also been called beta-1C.

The most common congenital disease associated with complement is hereditary angioedema. This is due to absence of C1 inhibitor, and the diagnosis is established by assay of C1 (C1 esterase) inhibitor. In some cases C1 inhibitor is present but nonfunctional. If immunologic methods are used for assay, this would lead to apparent normal results. Since C1, when activated, will split C2 and C4, lack of C1 inhibitor will lead to decreased C2 and C4 in appropriate test settings, so that a functional decrease in C1 esterase inhibitor can be inferred even if immunologic C1 assays provide normal results.

Acquired complement abnormalities are much more common than congenital ones. Total complement is temporarily elevated following onset of various acute or chronic inflammatory diseases or acute tissue damage, although type B viral hepatitis is associated with decreased complement. Most of the clinical conditions in which complement measurement is useful are associated with decreased levels. Both total complement (C) and C3 are usually reduced in active poststreptococcal glomerulonephritis, lupus nephritis and acute renal transplant rejection. Both may be decreased in systemic lupus erythematosus (SLE) without clinical nephritis, although the classic pattern in SLE without nephritis is for total complement to be decreased and C3 to be normal. Gram-negative septicemia may result in decreased C3 levels while C1 levels are normal. Component C3 is unstable and may decrease significantly in blood or serum that stands more than 1 or 2 hours at room temperature.

LIPOPROTEINS

Thus far, discussion has concerned the serum proteins in general. There is a special category known as lipoproteins that are combinations of various lipids with the plasma proteins. Lipids, in general, are insoluble in water and most biologic fluids, and depend for transport on binding to various plasma proteins. Unesterified fatty acids make up about 5% of the blood lipid, are mostly carried by serum albumin and seem to provide a readily available and excellent source of energy when carbohydrate is deficient. The other blood lipids are bound to globulin in various proportions and are known as lipoproteins. The lowest density lipoproteins are also those of the largest molecular size and are known as chylomicrons. These are composed mainly of triglycerides with a thin covering of protein and are the particles that are initially formed after intestinal fat absorption and that give postprandial plasma its characteristic milky appearance. The chylomicrons are eventually broken down enzymatically into unesterified fat-

TABLE 21-2.—MAJOR LIPOPROTEIN SUBGROUPS

LIPID-PROTEIN FRACTIONS	ULTRACENTRIFUGE S_f	ULTRACENTRIFUGE SPECIFIC GRAVITY	ELECTROPHORESIS	COMPOSITION
Chylomicrons	400–40,000	—	Neutral fat zone (point of application)	About 80% triglycerides
Very low-density (beta) lipoproteins	20–400	Less than 1.006	Prebeta	About half triglycerides, half cholesterol and phospholipid
Low-density (beta) lipoproteins	10–20 0–10	1.006–1.019 1.019–1.063	Beta Beta	About half cholesterol, rest predominantly phospholipid and protein
High-density (alpha) lipoproteins	—	Over 1.063	Alpha	About half protein, rest predominantly cholesterol and phospholipid
Albumin-unesterified fatty acids	—	—	—	—

ty acids and other lipid fractions. One subgroup is composed predominantly of triglyceride and has a very low density. There is a class of intermediate although still relatively low-density lipoproteins that are bound to beta globulins and are composed predominantly of cholesterol with smaller amounts of phospholipids and triglycerides. These are known as low-density beta lipoproteins. The highest density molecules are also the smallest. These are bound to the alpha$_1$ globulin and are composed predominantly of protein with smaller amounts of cholesterol, phospholipids and triglycerides. They are alpha or high-density lipoproteins. Serum lipids may be determined chemically or by electrophoresis. On electrophoresis the results usually are reported in terms of immobile lipid, prebeta, beta and alpha lipoprotein. This corresponds to chylomicrons, very low-density, low-density and high-density lipoproteins, respectively (Table 21 – 2).

There has been much recent interest in the significance of the lipoproteins in atherosclerosis. Large numbers of studies have been carried out, various populations have been examined, various diets have been tried and endless pages of statistics have been published. There is general but not unanimous agreement that when beta lipoproteins are elevated, there may be an increased tendency toward atherosclerosis and, therefore, of myocardial infarct. In addition, many believe that serum triglyceride elevation has an equal significance. Since beta lipoproteins are the main carriers of serum cholesterol, the majority of investigators believe (without unanimous agreement) that the serum cholesterol can be used as an indirect measure of beta lipoprotein and, therefore, as one parameter of increased atherogenic risk. Decreased high density (alpha) lipoprotein has been reported to increase risk of coronary atherosclerosis. Finally, some lab aspects must be considered:

1. Cholesterol levels have been shown to deviate 10% from mean values during any 24-hour period and show differences of 5 – 50 mg/100 ml in day-to-day variation. Some individuals display even greater changes.

2. It has also been found that there is a well-documented tendency by the serum lipids, especially cholesterol, to fluctuate considerably for as much as 2 months after myocardial infarct. Therefore, values taken soon after a myocardial infarct may not be representative of the patient's usual levels.

3. The normal values quoted vary considerably from one population to the next, depending on diet, heredity, age, sex and even types of occupa-

TABLE 21 – 3. – LIPID NORMAL VALUES

AGE	TOTAL CHOLESTEROL (MG/100 ML)	TRIGLYCERIDES (MG/100 ML)
1 – 19	120 – 230	10 – 140
20 – 29	120 – 240	10 – 140
30 – 39	140 – 270	10 – 150
40 – 49	150 – 310	10 – 160
50 – 59	160 – 330	10 – 190

CLASSIFICATION OF LIPOPROTEINEMIAS

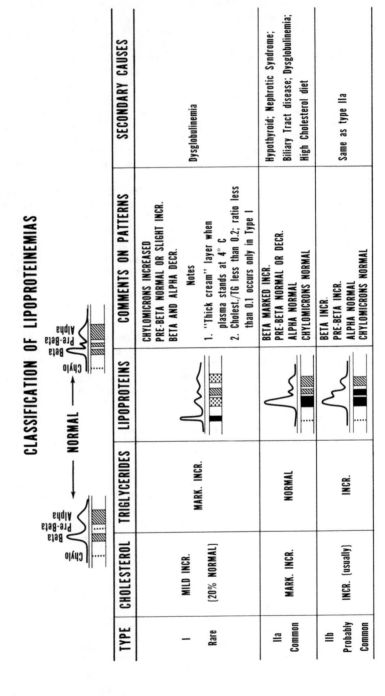

TYPE	CHOLESTEROL	TRIGLYCERIDES	LIPOPROTEINS	COMMENTS ON PATTERNS	SECONDARY CAUSES
I Rare	MILD INCR. (20% NORMAL)	MARK. INCR.		CHYLOMICRONS INCREASED PRE-BETA NORMAL OR SLIGHT INCR. BETA AND ALPHA DECR. Notes 1. "Thick cream" layer when plasma stands at 4° C 2. Cholest./TG less than 0.2; ratio less than 0.1 occurs only in Type I	Dysglobulinemia
IIa Common	MARK. INCR.	NORMAL		BETA MARKED INCR. PRE-BETA NORMAL OR DECR. ALPHA NORMAL CHYLOMICRONS NORMAL	Hypothyroid; Nephrotic Syndrome; Biliary Tract disease; Dysglobulinemia; High Cholesterol diet
IIb Probably Common	INCR. (usually)	INCR.		BETA INCR. PRE-BETA INCR. ALPHA NORMAL CHYLOMICRONS NORMAL	Same as type IIa

Type	Frequency			Pattern	Notes	Associated Conditions
III	Uncommon	INCR. (20% NORMAL)	INCR. (10% NORMAL)	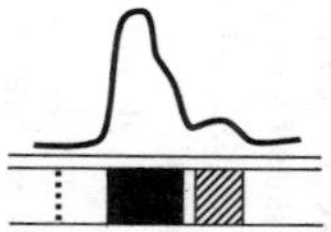	BETA INCR. ("BROAD BETA" IN 2/3 CASES) PRE-BETA NORMAL OR MILD INCR. ALPHA NORMAL CHYLOMICRONS NORMAL — Notes: Need ultracentrifugation for diagnosis (Demonstration of "floating beta")	Diabetes Mellitus; Hepatic Disease
IV	Most Common	NORMAL (20% INCR.)	INCR.	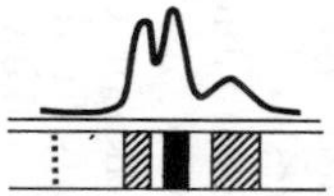	PRE-BETA MOD. OR MARK. INCR. BETA AND ALPHA NORMAL OR MILD DECR. CHYLOMICRONS NORMAL — Notes: Sometimes called "Carbohydrate-induced hyperlipemia"	Hypothyroid; Nephrotic Syndrome; Pregnancy; Estrogen; Diabetes Mellitus; Pancreatitis; Dysglobulinemia
V	Uncommon	INCR. (40% NORMAL)	INCR.	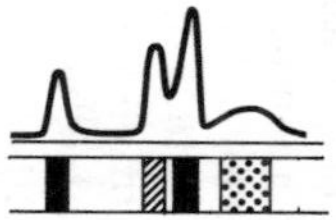	PRE-BETA INCR. BETA AND ALPHA DECR. CHYLOMICRONS INCR. — Notes: 1. "Thick cream" layer 2. Cholest./TG ratio usually above 0.15 when plasma stands at 4° C.	Pancreatitis; Alcoholism; Diabetes Mellitus

Fig 21–5. — Classification of lipoproteinemias.

tion where stress is a factor. For example, normal values for an average American population (Table 21–3) are considerably higher than those for an average Japanese group. Normal values for total cholesterol, which are probably near the true normal range, are 150–250 mg/100 ml; those for average American populations are 150–300 mg/100 ml.

Finally, the technical aspects of lipid and cholesterol determination are very important. Many methods for cholesterol determination are in use, and surveys have shown disturbingly great fluctuation among values of different laboratories using different methods or even the same method. Accuracy for serum cholesterol has been relatively poor, except under rigid quality control programs and with certain standard methods, and sometimes not even then. If one is to rely on cholesterol values, he should know the laboratory to which he sends patients and find out how they run their controls and what variation they expect from duplicate samples. Triglyceride values have been shown in laboratory surveys to be generally even less reproducible than cholesterol values. It becomes even more necessary to send triglycerides to a reliable laboratory. Therefore, diet or other treatment may be given credit for moderate decreases in cholesterol, whereas in reality it may be due to physiologic or laboratory variability. Other diseases that characteristically cause high cholesterol are idiopathic hypercholesterolemia, biliary cirrhosis, hypothyroidism and the nephrotic syndrome.

The lipoprotein disease classification (Fig 21–5) proposed by Frederickson's group is now becoming standard.

Tests useful in establishing and categorizing lipoprotein disease include inspection of serum (after it has been kept overnight at ice-box temperature), cholesterol, triglyceride, lipoprotein electrophoresis and ultracentrifugation. Visual inspection, cholesterol and triglyceride are the most important; they serve as screening procedures and in many cases as diagnostic tests. Normal values for all three are reasonable evidence (although not completely so) against serious lipoprotein disease (Table 21–4).

If visual inspection discloses a creamlike precipitate of chylomicrons, normal cholesterol and triglycerides signify Frederickson type I, whereas elevation of either points toward type V. Likewise, if serum has normal chylomicron content, elevation of cholesterol with normal triglyceride is type II, whereas the opposite means type IV. If both cholesterol and tri-

TABLE 21–4.–PROBABILITY OF DETECTING HYPER-
LIPOPROTEINEMIA BY LIPID ANALYSIS ALONE

	PERCENTAGE DETECTABLE BY LIPID CONCENTRATION		
TYPE	ABNORMAL CHOLESTEROL	ABNORMAL TRIGLYCERIDE	ABNORMAL CHOLESTEROL OR TRIGLYCERIDE
I	80	100	100
II	89	24	92
III	82	91	91
IV	22	100	100
V	61	100	100

From Frederickson, D. S., et al.: The Typing of Hyperlipoproteinemia: A Progress Report (1968), in Holmes, W. L., et al. (eds.): *Drugs Affecting Lipid Metabolism* (New York: Plenum Press, 1969).

glyceride are significantly abnormal, this may be type II or type III. Type II has recently been subdivided into IIa and IIb. IIa has increased beta and cholesterol but normal prebeta and triglyceride. Type IIb has elevated cholesterol, triglyceride, beta, and prebeta. Type III is uncommon; it is similar to IIb in that both cholesterol and triglyceride are elevated, but it frequently has a slightly different electrophoretic pattern (broad beta) and always has a peculiar "floating beta" component (a beta-mobility protein which floats at 1.006 density instead of 1.013), which can only be demonstrated by ultracentrifugation. Types II and IV constitute the majority of lipoproteinemias; V is less common, and I and III are uncommon.

Type IV is probably more common than II. Most type IV patients have the acquired form. Type II is more frequently congenital than type IV; however, the majority of type II patients have the acquired form, the most common etiology being a high cholesterol diet.

Some specimens from patients with types IIb, III, or IV may be somewhat cloudy or faintly milky in appearance; this must be differentiated from the thicker, creamlike precipitate of increased chylomicrons.

Lipoprotein electrophoresis is not absolutely necessary to phenotype most patients; however, it is useful in some cases to confirm the diagnosis, to help separate types IIa, IIb, III and some cases of IV, and to quantitate the alpha (HDL) fraction. In classic cases, type III displays a "broad beta" band that obliterates the normal valley between beta and prebeta peaks. Definitive diagnosis of type III must be done by ultracentrifugation.

Certain considerations affect interpretation of these lab results. Patients should be on a normal diet for several days previous to testing and must be fasting for at least 10 hours. If a test cannot be done the same day, the serum must be refrigerated but not frozen; freezing alters prebeta and chylomicron fractions, although cholesterol and triglyceride determinations can be done. Certain lipoprotein types can be caused by specific diseases; in such a case, treatment must be directed primarily toward the etiologic disease. Normal range for cholesterol and triglyceride is age-related. Although there is no agreement as to what values are truly normal, Table 21–3 lists normal ranges according to Frederickson. Because of laboratory technical limitations, one must be cautious in attributing significance to borderline results.

On electrophoresis, occasional persons display increased prebeta but normal triglyceride levels. If lab error is ruled out, these patients may have a congenital variant called "Lp system" or "sinking prebeta." This is not thought to have any clinical significance.

Plasma or serum may be used for lipoprotein analysis. Plasma collected with EDTA is preferred if the specimen cannot be tested the same day.

Two rare diseases display characteristic lipoprotein electrophoresis patterns. Tangier disease has no alpha peak. Bassen-Kornzweig syndrome (associated with "pin-cushion" RBC, called acanthocytes, and neurologic abnormalities) lacks a beta peak.

REFERENCES

Alper, C. A., and Rosen, F. S.: Clinical Application of Complement Assays, in Stollerman, G. H. (ed.): *Advances in Internal Medicine* (Chicago: Year Book Medical Publishers, Inc., 1975), vol. 20, p. 61.

Azar, H. A., et al.: "Nonsecretory" plasma cell myeloma, Am. J. Clin. Pathol. 58:618, 1972.

Beaumont, J. L., et al.: Classification of hyperlipidaemias and hyperlipoproteinaemias, Bull. WHO 43:891, 1970.

Berman, H. H.: Waldenström's macroglobulinemia with lytic osseous lesions and plasma-cell morphology, Am. J. Clin. Pathol. 63:397, 1975.

Bernier, G. M.: Adult hypogammaglobulinemia, Am. J. Med. 36:618, 1964.

Bistrian, B. R.: Protein status of general surgical patients, J.A.M.A. 230:858, 1974.

Bloch, K. J., et al.: Gamma heavy chain disease—an expanding clinical and laboratory spectrum, Am. J. Med. 55:61, 1973.

Burgert, W., Jr.: Alpha-1 antitrypsin deficiency, Postgrad. Med. 47:63, 1970.

Cannon, D. C.: Immunoglobulin analysis in clinical diagnosis. 1. Quantitative methods, Postgrad. Med. 46:55, 1969.

Castelli, W. P., and Moran, R. F.: Lipid studies for assessing the risk of cardiovascular disease and hyperlipidemia, Hum. Pathol. 2:153, 1971.

Castelli, W. P., et al.: HDL cholesterol and other lipids in coronary heart disease, Circulation 55:767, 1977.

Deegan, M. J.: Bence Jones protein: nature, metabolism, detection, and significance, Ann. Clin. Lab. Sci. 6:38, 1976.

Delaney, W. E.: Identification and quantitation of immunoglobulins, Ann. Clin. Lab. Sci. 2:75, 1972.

Fahey, J. L., et al.: Serum hyperviscosity syndrome, J.A.M.A. 192:120, 1965.

Fahey, J. L., et al.: Plasma cell myeloma with D-myeloma protein (IgD myeloma), Am. J. Med. 45:373, 1968.

Fessel, W. J., et al.: What is the albumin level? Arch. Intern. Med. 114:547, 1964.

French, A. B.: Protein-losing gastroenteropathies, Am. J. Dig. Dis. 16:661, 1971.

Harkness, D. R.: Structure and function of immunoglobulins, Postgrad. Med. 48:64, 1970.

Korngold, L.: Plasma Proteins: Methods in Study and Changes in Diseases, in Stefanini, M. (ed.): Advances in Clinical Pathology (New York: Grune & Stratton, Inc., 1966), vol. 1, p. 340.

Kyle, R. A.: Multiple myeloma: review of 869 cases, Mayo Clin. Proc. 50:29, 1975.

Kyle, R. A., and Bayrd, E. D.: "Benign" monoclonal gammopathy: A potentially malignant condition? Am. J. Med. 40:426, 1966.

Kyle, R. A., et al.: Diagnosis of syndromes associated with hyperglobulinemia, Med. Clin. North Am. 54:917, 1970.

Law, D. K., et al.: The effects of protein caloric malnutrition on immune competence of the surgical patient, Surg. Gynecol. Obstet. 139:257, 1974.

Leonardy, J. G.: Serum protein electrophoresis in office practice, South. Med. J. 64:129, 1971.

Levy, R. I.: Prominent prebeta lipoprotein band and normal plasma triglyceride level: Normal variant, J.A.M.A. 226:574, 1973.

Lipo, J. F., and Preston, J. A.: Lipoprotein phenotyping, CRC Crit. Rev. Clin. Lab. Sci. 2:461, 1971.

Maldonado, J. E., et al.: Pathophysiology of the monoclonal gammopathies, Postgrad. Med. 53:102, 1973.

Martin, N. H.: The immunoglobulins: A review, J. Clin. Pathol. 22:117, 1969.

Mattioli, C., and Tomasi, T. B., Jr.: Human Serum Immunoglobulins, in Dowling, H. F. (ed.): Disease-a-Month (Chicago: Year Book Medical Publishers, Inc., April 1970).

Michaux, J., and Heremans, J. F.: Thirty cases of monoclonal immunoglobulin disorders other than myeloma or macroglobulinemia, Am. J. Med. 46:562, 1969.

Migliore, P. J., and Alexanian, R.: Monoclonal gammopathy in human neoplasia, Cancer, 21:1127, 1968.

Osserman, E. F., and Takatsuki, K.: Plasma cell myeloma: Gamma globulin synthesis and structure, Medicine 42:357, 1963.

Perry, M. C., and Kyle, R. A.: The clinical significance of Bence Jones proteinuria, Mayo Clin. Proc. 50:234, 1975.

Pruzansky, W., and Ogryzlo, M. A.: Changing pattern of diseases associated with M components, Med. Clin. North Am. 56:371, 1972.

Ravel, R.: Serum protein electrophoresis in cirrhosis, Am. J. Gastroenterol. 52:509, 1969.

Ritzmann, S. E., and Levin, W. C.: Cryopathies: A review, Arch. Intern. Med. 107: 754, 1961.

Rothschild, M. A.: Serum albumin, Am. J. Dig. Dis. 14:711, 1969.

Sharp, H. L.: Alpha-1 antitrypsin deficiency, Hosp. Practice 6:83, 1971.

Spiro, R. G.: Glycoproteins: Structure, metabolism, and biology, N. Engl. J. Med. 269:566, 616, 1963.

Stone, M. J., and Frenkel, E. P.: The clinical spectrum of light chain myeloma, Am. J. Med. 58:601, 1975.

Tullis, J. L., et al.: Albumin, J.A.M.A. 237:355, 1977.

Williams, R. C., Jr., et al.: Studies of "benign" serum M-components, Am. J. Med. Sci. 257:275, 1969.

Zawadzki, Z. A., and Edwards, G. A.: Dysimmunoglobulinemia in the absence of clinical features of multiple myeloma and macroglobulinemia, Am. J. Med. 42:67, 1967.

Zawadzki, Z. A., and Edwards, G. A.: Pseudoparaproteinemia due to hypertransferrinemia, Am. J. Clin. Pathol. 54:802, 1970.

Zawadzki, Z. A., and Edwards, G. A.: Dysimmunoglobulinemia associated with hepatobiliary disorders, Am. J. Med. 48:196, 1970.

22 / Bone and Joint Disorders

RHEUMATOID DISEASES

THE RELATIONSHIP between the rheumatoid diseases and those of the so-called collagen-vascular group is both close and uncertain. Many of the clinical symptoms found classically in one disease or syndrome may be found in another; the difference is on emphasis of certain aspects over others. This similarity extends to laboratory tests and makes it even more difficult to separate borderline or problem cases into one clear-cut group or the other. Until the exact etiology of each disease is known, things are likely to continue in this fashion. It may be that a common mechanism is operating, which affects different target organs or tissues in different people. This would help to explain the spectrum of clinical and laboratory findings that become evident in large series of cases. Fortunately, most patients can be assigned to satisfactory categories using available clinical and laboratory data.

Rheumatoid Arthritis

Rheumatoid arthritis (RA) is a chronic systemic disease whose most prominent symptoms occur in joints. The small joints of the hands and feet, especially the proximal interphalangeal joints, are usually affected at some time, as are various larger joints of the extremities. Involvement tends to be a slow migratory process, which may be symmetrical.

In active RA, hemoglobin concentration may be normal or mildly decreased. Uric acid is normal. Serologic tests are the usual method of laboratory diagnosis unless joint aspiration is performed. Rheumatoid arthritis and related diseases are associated with production of several globulins, both IgG and IgM, called rheumatoid factors, of which the most important is an IgM macroglobulin. This has the ability to combine in vitro with normal gamma globulin. Complement is fixed during the reaction. Therefore, various types of serologic tests may be set up using this basic reaction, differing mainly in the type of indicator system used to visually demonstrate results. The original method was known as the Rose-Waaler, or sheep cell agglutination test, using antisheep RBC antibodies to combine with sheep RBC, then allowing the rheumatoid factor in the patient's serum to combine with the antibody gamma globulin coating the sheep cells. Clumping of RBC indicated a positive result. It was found subsequently that synthetic particles such as latex could be coated with gamma globulin and the coated particles clumped by rheumatoid factor, thus giving a flocculation test. Just as happened with the serologic test for syphilis (p. 385), many combinations of ingredients have been tried, with resulting variations in sensitivity and specificity—too many to discuss individually. However, one must make a distinction between tube tests and rapid slide tests, since the slide tests in general have a slightly greater sensitivity but correspondingly less specificity. They should be used mainly for screening purposes. Some false positive results can be eliminated by heat-inactivating patient serum at 56° C for 30 minutes.

The latex fixation tube test for RA, known also as the Plotz-Singer latex test, today is the most widely used and standard method. The average sensitivity in well-established clinical cases of adult RA is about 76% (range 53–94%). Normal controls average about 1% positive. For comparison, a widely used commercial latex slide test (Hyland "RA-test") averages about 89% positive in known adult RA patients, but reportedly averages about 10% positive in normal controls. Besides a certain small percentage of Plotz-Singer false positives in apparently normal persons, certain diseases give a significantly high number of reactions in a manner analogous to the "biologic false positive" of syphilis serology. These include collagen diseases, sarcoidosis, syphilis, various liver diseases, including cirrhosis and hepatitis, certain more rare diseases and possibly even old age. The incidence of these reactions for the conditions mentioned is 10–40%; the incidence is highest in the collagen-vascular group (p. 484).

Juvenile Rheumatoid Arthritis and Rheumatoid Arthritis Variants

Juvenile rheumatoid arthritis (Still's disease) is usually considered to be part of rheumatoid arthritis, since about half of these children display similar clinical symptoms. Although incidence of positive RA latex tests is only 5–40%, it is known that even in patients with onset in adult years, there is correlation both with duration and activity (but not severity) of the disease; most patients with positive test results have active symptoms more than 6 months. Nevertheless, in about half of the juvenile patients, there is sufficient clinical difference from adult RA to question whether this "atypical" subgroup is the same disease. In particular, sacroiliitis and cervical spine involvement occur in many of these patients. The sacroiliitis is frequently accompanied by iritis or anterior uveitis. About 10% of the patients develop spondylitis. Incidence of the HL-A B-27 antigen (p. 89) is over 50% in patients with atypical rheumatoid disease, whereas B-27 is not a feature of adult RA and is found in fewer than 20% of patients whose symptoms are more typical of adult RA.

So-called rheumatoid arthritis variants include rheumatoid-like joint inflammation that differs from classic RA in various respects (similar to those noted in the juvenile RA atypical subgroup) and that occurs in association with another recognized disease. Other RA variants are ankylosing spondylitis (Marie-Strümpell disease), arthritis associated with Reiter's syndrome and psoriasis, and enteropathic arthritis (*Yersinia enterocolitica* enteritis, ulcerative colitis and Crohn's disease). Peripheral joint involvement may resemble classic RA or may be atypical. Tests for RA are positive in 5–15% of patients or even more, depending on the investigator and the method used. However, if patient serum is heat-inactivated and a latex tube test is used, results in these diseases are most often reported as positive in less than 5%. Ankylosing spondylitis, Reiter's syndrome and *Yersi-*

nia enteritis have a close association with HL-A B-27 antigen. In the others, if sacroiliitis or spondylitis are present, the association is frequent; if not, B-27 incidence is much lower.

COLLAGEN-VASCULAR DISEASES

Collagen-vascular diseases are an ill-defined collection of syndromes that have certain points of similarity, among which the most striking are fibrinoid necrosis of collagenous tissue and involvement of various subdivisions of arteries by an inflammatory process. Some diseases emphasize one of these aspects and some the other. The main connection between these often quite dissimilar syndromes is the probability that their basic etiology is some manifestation of a disorder involving immunologic hypersensitivity. Since the three most common diseases in this group are disseminated lupus erythematosus, polyarteritis nodosa and scleroderma, these three will be discussed briefly from the laboratory point of view.

Lupus Erythematosus

Lupus erythematosus features various combinations of facial skin rash, arthritis, nephritis, systemic symptoms such as fever and malaise, and inflammation of serous membranes such as the pericardium. The disease is by far most common in women, predominantly young or middle-aged adults. Hepatomegaly is found in about 30% of patients, splenomegaly in nearly 20% and adenopathy in nearly 50%. There is anemia in up to 80% of patients, mostly of moderate degree, but severe and hemolytic in rare cases. The WBC count is classically slightly to moderately lower than normal, but not always. Thrombocytopenia is present in a large minority of cases. There are often one or more manifestations of abnormal plasma proteins; these may include cold-precipitable cryoglobulins, circulating anticoagulants, autoantibodies, elevated gamma globulins, false positive rheumatoid arthritis and syphilis serologic reactions and certain even rarer phenomena.

LE CELL PREPARATION. — The most useful test in lupus, and the one usually required for definitive diagnosis, is the lupus erythematosus (LE) cell preparation. This test depends on the fact that antibodies against various nuclear constituents that are produced in lupus react with nuclei of damaged cells, either tissue cells or white blood cells. The nuclear material is converted to a homogeneous amorphous mass that stains basophilic with Wright's stain. This mass is then phagocytized by polymorphonuclear neutrophlis; these neutrophils containing the hematoxylin (blue staining) bodies in their cytoplasm are the so-called LE cells. These LE cells are considered by many to be specific for lupus erythematosus with one exception, a syndrome identical to ordinary lupus, which is produced by hypersensitivity to the drug hydralazine (Apresoline). Nevertheless, one report indicates that for patients taking more than 1.5 gm of procainamide per day, LE cell preparations will be positive in 50% of cases and will show antinuclear antibodies in 75%. Others believe that LE cells are not diagnostic of lupus, but only strongly suggestive. It is true that LE cells have been reported in certain other drug sensitivity cases, but some believe these were not true LE cells. Certain patients with chronic active hepatitis have occasionally demonstrated LE cells, but the possibility that these patients may in addition have had subclinical lupus never has been completely ruled out. This has been made into a syndrome called "lupoid hepatitis," although some of these patients had cirrhosis rather than chronic hepatitis. The syndrome is not universally accepted. Cases also are reported from time to time when patients with classic rheumatoid arthritis or one of the other collagen diseases produce a few LE cells. In rheumatoid arthritis, some investigators report an incidence of 15–20%. Again, in some of these patients, it is almost a matter of philosophy whether the diagnosis is rheumatoid arthritis with LE cells or lupus with predominantly rheumatoid-type symptoms. Finally, artifacts may be confused with true LE cells. To be definitive, the basophilic hematoxylin body must be completely amorphous, without any remaining nuclear structure whatever. In many situations, one finds examples of neutrophils with phagocytized nuclear material that still retains some identity as a nucleus, such as residual chromatin pattern. These are not true LE cells; they are called "tart cells." Increased numbers of these may be seen in lupus, but they do not have any diagnostic significance. Also confused by inexperienced persons are neutrophils with ingested RBC.

Different methods may be used for LE cell preparations. Their common denominator is some way to traumatize a number of the WBC. After this, there is an incubation period while the nuclei of the damaged cells are converted to hematoxylin bodies and then ingested by some of the living neutrophils. The preparation is centrifuged, and smears of the neutrophil layer are made. After Wright's stain, the smears are searched for LE cells. When hematoxylin bodies are formed, groups of neutrophils sometimes are found surrounding one of the bodies preparatory to one neutrophil phagocytizing it. These groupings are called rosettes and are considered by some investigators as equal in importance to true LE cells; others insist on finding classic LE cells for definite diagnosis. It must be emphasized that the LE phenomenon is often intermittent, sometimes present for varying periods and sometimes absent. There is some correlation to the activity of the disease, but not entirely. It is possible (although not usual) for LE cell preparations to give positive results one day and not the next, and sometimes several preparations done the same day may have both positive and negative results. This seems due to the nature of the disease, the strictly empirical nature of the test and, to some extent, the technical aspects of the test itself. Adrenocortical steroid treatment often suppresses LE cell production.

Fluorescent antinuclear antibody test.—The antinuclear factor responsible for the LE cell phenomenon is not the only autoantibody or "factor" demonstrable in systemic lupus. A wide variety of such factors has been demonstrated, reactive against either nuclear or cytoplasmic constituents with varying degrees of tissue and cellular constituent specificity. Fluorescent tests for antinuclear antibodies(ANA) have been devised, using a variety of methods to obtain suitable nuclei. Most of these tests have positive results in over 95% of lupus patients, while LE cell preparation has positive results in 60–80% of patients, depending on several factors such as duration, activity and severity of disease (p. 485). The LE preparation is currently still the most specific test for systemic lupus erythematosus, although there is some dispute as to how specific it actually is. Nevertheless, the high sensitivity of the fluorescent antinuclear antibody test makes it much more efficient for screening than the LE preparation. If the fluorescent ANA test is negative, chances of a positive LE preparation are very low. Since any test has the possibility of technical error, a negative ANA in a patient with high probability of lupus should be repeated.

The fluorescent ANA test is a nonspecific reaction. Assays for specific varieties of antinuclear antibodies have been developed. The most important antinuclear antibodies currently tested for act against native (double-stranded) deoxyribonucleic acid (DNA), single-stranded DNA, DNA-histone complex (sNP), acidic nuclear proteins (Sm), and nucleolar ribonucleic acid (RNA). A commercial radioimmunoassay kit is available to test for anti-native DNA, which is present in 70–90% of systemic lupus erythematosus (SLE) patients. (Range in the literature is 64–100%, probably influenced by differing methodologies and patient group characteristics.) There is some evidence that active SLE is more likely to display abnormality than inactive disease, although anti-native DNA may be absent even in active SLE. Some data indicate that high titers of anti-native DNA correlate closely with positive results in LE preparations, whereas normal or mildly elevated anti-native DNA titers can be found either with positive or negative LE preparations. The percentage of abnormal anti-native DNA results found in other rheumatoid-collagen diseases has varied widely among investigators, from less than 5% to 25–50%. The majority have found very few positive anti-native DNA results in rheumatoid arthritis and have reported less than 20% positive anti-native DNA results in other connective tissue diseases and allied conditions such as Sjögren's syndrome. This has led to claims that the test for anti-native DNA is highly specific for SLE and that it provides an indication of disease activity. Data available to date only partially substantiate these claims.

Commercial companies have marketed 2-minute slide latex agglutination tests for SLE based on latex particles coated with DNA. The two tests available so far have substantial differences in sensitivity, but both demonstrate fewer positive results in SLE than the LE preparation.

Polyarteritis Nodosa

Polyarteritis nodosa features inflammation of small and medium-sized arteries. Single organs or multiple systems may be involved, although usually the lungs are spared. The kidney is the organ that most frequently shows abnormalities, with hematuria the main sign. Hypertension is fairly common. Laboratory studies usually show a moderate leukocytosis with neutrophilic increase and immaturity of the ordinary type seen with infections. Mild anemia is also common. There often is an increase in serum gamma globulin. The main diagnostic procedure is biopsy. The most common type is muscle biopsy, and the usual region is the gastrocnemius because it is easy to reach. However, if biopsy is done, it should be from some muscle with a painful area if any are present; random samples give poor results. The biopsy should be generous, since the lesions of polyarteritis lie in small arteries. The incidence of positive single muscle biopsies in fairly definite cases of polyarteritis ranges from 20 to 40%; obviously, it will be on the lower side in mild or questionable cases. Another difficulty is that occasionally patients with classic RA may have arteritis nearly identical to polyarteritis. Lupus patients also may have arteritis, but the lesions tend to be in arterioles. Other more rare syndromes of the collagen-vascular group may create histologic difficulty. Therefore, the clinical picture has as much importance as the biopsy report.

Scleroderma

Scleroderma (progressive systemic sclerosis) leads to progressive dense connective tissue replacement of certain areas that normally contain only small amounts of loose collagen. These include the dermis of the skin, the submucosa of the esophagus or other parts of the gastrointestinal tract, and the heart. The lungs frequently develop a slowly progressive type of diffuse fibrosis, radiologically most prominent in the lung bases. In addition, the kidneys are often affected by a somewhat different histologic process, similar to malignant hypertension. The disease is most common in middle-aged women. Clinically, the skin changes produce tautness and lack of elasticity; this most often occurs in the hand and is often accompanied by Raynaud's phenomenon. Esophageal involvement leads to dysphagia, while small bowel changes may produce localized dilatation. Laboratory tests usually show the hemoglobin to be normal. There may be an increased erythrocyte sedimentation rate, and there may be associated hypergammaglobulinemia of a diffuse type, although this is not a constant feature. Scleroderma produces a relatively high incidence of positive rheumatoid factor tests and also of biologic false positive syphilis serologies. Diagnosis usually can be made clinically but may be suggested by barium swallow esophageal x-rays in patients who have esophageal symptoms. Biopsy of an affected skin area is the procedure of choice if the diagnosis cannot be made clinically.

ACUTE RHEUMATIC FEVER

Acute rheumatic fever (ARF) is a disease that has a specific etiologic agent and yet demonstrates some similarity with the rheumatoid-collagen-vascular group. The etiologic agent is the beta hemolytic Lancefield group A streptococcus. Apparent hypersensitivity or other effect of this organism causes connective tissue changes manifested by focal necrosis of collagen and the development of peculiar aggregates of histiocytes, "Aschoff bodies." Symptoms of ARF include fever, a migratory type of polyarthritis, and frequent development of cardiac damage manifested either by symptoms or only by electrocardiographic changes. Diagnosis or confirmation of diagnosis often rests on appropriate laboratory tests. Throat culture should be attempted; the finding of beta hemolytic streptococci, Lancefield group A, would be a strong point in favor of the diagnosis if the clinical picture is highly suggestive. However, throat cultures often show negative results. Blood culture findings are almost always negative. Beta streptococci produce an enzyme known as streptolysin-O. About 7–10 days after infection, antibodies to this material begin to appear. Highest incidence of positive results is during the third week after onset of ARF. At this time, 90–95% abnormal results are obtained; thereafter, the antibody titer drops steadily. At the end of 2 months only 70–75% are positive; at 6 months, 35%; at 12 months, 20%. Therefore, since the streptococcus most often cannot be isolated, antistreptolysin titers of over 200 Todd units may be helpful evidence of a recent infection. However, this does not actually prove that the disease in question is ARF or that the streptococcal infection that produced the antibodies was recent enough to cause the present symptoms. Commercial tests that detect several other antistreptococcal antibodies in addition to antistreptolysin, such as anti-ADNase, may be more sensitive for screening than antistreptolysin alone. The erythrocyte sedimentation rate (ESR) is usually elevated during the clinical course of ARF and is a useful indication of current activity of the disease. However, the ESR is very nonspecific and only indicates an active inflammatory process somewhere in the body. In a minority of ARF patients, peculiar subcutaneous nodules develop, most often near the elbows. These are composed of focal collagen necrosis surrounded by palisading of histiocytes. In some cases, therefore, biopsy of these nodules may help confirm the diagnosis of ARF. However, biopsy is not usually done if other methods make the diagnosis reasonably certain. Also, the nodules are histologically similar to those of rheumatoid arthritis. During the acute phase of the disease there usually is a moderate leukocytosis, and most often there is a mild to moderate anemia.

OTHER JOINT DISEASES

Gout

Gout usually involves single specific joints, usually including some of the small joints of the extremities (typically the metatarsal-phalangeal joint of the great toe). The disease is most common in males. Acute attacks are frequently accompanied by fever and leukocytosis. Renal impairment due to uric acid deposition is fairly common late in the course of untreated patients. Patients with gout usually have an elevated serum uric acid level and respond specifically to colchicine.

Although elevation of uric acid is characteristic of gout, more uric acid elevations are due to other diseases than to gout. Perhaps the most frequent etiology in hospitalized patients is chronic renal disease with azotemia. Other conditions frequently associated with increased uric acid levels include tumors of blood cells (leukemia, polycythemia vera and other myeloproliferative diseases), especially during treatment; therapy with thiazide diuretics, and eclampsia.

Synovial fluid aspirated from an acutely inflamed joint reveals needle-shaped crystals of sodium monophosphate within neutrophils or lying free. These may be seen with the ordinary microscope but are best visualized using compensated polarized light. With the color compensator, urate crystals exhibit negative birefringence (yellow against a red background with the axis of the crystal parallel to the axis of the compensator). When injected into a joint some steroids form needle-like crystals, which may mimic nonpolarized uric acid crystals.

Pseudogout

Pseudogout clinically resembles gout to some degree but tends to affect large joints such as the knee rather than small peripheral joints. Joint x-rays indicate some differences from classic gout but are frequently not a sufficient basis for diagnosis. Synovial fluid examination discloses calcium pyrophosphate crystals, either within neutrophil cytoplasm or extracellular. These appear as short needles or short rods, but sometimes compensated polarized light (imparting a positive birefringence, blue on red background) is necessary for reliable differentiation from uric acid.

Septic Arthritis

Septic arthritis is diagnosed by direct aspiration and culture of the synovial fluid.

SYNOVIAL FLUID ANALYSIS

When synovial fluid is aspirated, 1 ml or more should be placed in a sterile tube for possible culture and a similar quantity into a heparinized tube for cell count. The remainder can be used for other procedures. A cell count is performed from anticoagulated fluid using 0.9% saline as the WBC pipette diluent (the usual diluent, Turk's solution, contains acetic acid, which coagulates synovial fluid mucin).

MUCIN CLOT. — The Ropes test for mucin clot is performed by adding a few drops of aspirate to 10 – 20 ml of 5% acetic acid in a small beaker. After waiting 1 minute, the beaker is shaken. A well-formed clot remains compact; a poor clot is friable and shreds apart easily. In general, noninflammatory arthritides form a good clot. In noninfectious inflammation, the clot may be good to poor, while that associated with acute bacterial infection is poor.

VISCOSITY (STRING SIGN). — Aspirate is allowed to drip slowly from the end of a needle. The length of the strand formed by each drop before it separates is the endpoint. In normal fluid and in noninflammatory arthritides the strands string out more than 3 cm. In acute inflammatory conditions fluids drip with little, if any, stringing.

SYNOVIAL FLUID GLUCOSE. — Synovial fluid glucose is usually within 10 mg/100 ml of serum glucose and always within 20 mg/100 ml. A blood specimen for glucose should be obtained as close as possible to the joint aspiration. The patient should have fasted at least 6 – 8 hours to achieve baseline values and to compensate for delay in glucose level equilibration between blood and synovial fluid. In degenerative arthritis, synovial fluid glucose level usually is normal. In acute infectious arthritis, there is a mild to moderate decrease (10 – 50 mg/100 ml decrease from serum levels), and in infectious arthritis, there is a marked decrease (usually more than 50 mg/100 ml decrease from serum levels).

OTHER EXAMINATIONS. — Other examinations include a serologic test for rheumatoid arthritis. The RA tests on synovial fluid occasionally show positive results before serum tests. In SLE, LE cells frequently form in synovial fluid and can be demonstrated on the same Wright's stained smear used for differential cell count. In arthritis of Reiter's syndrome, synovial fluid total hemolytic complement (C') is considerably elevated. In addition,

TABLE 22-1.—CLASSIC SYNOVIAL FLUID FINDINGS

	VISCOSITY	CELL COUNT, CU MM	PMN, %	GLUCOSE LEVEL	MUCIN CLOT	MISCELLANEOUS PROCEDURES
Normal	High	0–600	25	Normal	Good	—
Traumatic arthritis	High	5,000 Many RBC	50	Normal	Good	—
Osteoarthritis	High	2,000	25	Normal	Good	Cartilage fragments
Acute rheumatic fever	Low	2,000–10,000	50	Occasional decrease	Good or poor	—
Systemic lupus erythematosus	High	5,000	25	Normal	Good	LE cell preparations
Rheumatoid arthritis	Low	5,000–60,000	50	Usually decreases	Poor	RA tests
Gout (acute episode)	Low	5,000–60,000	50	Sometimes decreases	Poor	Urate crystals
Septic arthritis	Low	Over 50,000	90	Marked decrease	Poor	Culture

large macrophages that ingest neutrophils and various granules are said to be characteristic, although they may appear in any of the RA variants and occasionally in other conditions.

Typical synovial fluid findings are summarized in Table 22 – 1.

JOINT SCANNING

Besides synovial fluid examination, joint scanning is a procedure that may offer useful information. For screening purposes, the scan could be performed with one of the isotope-labeled phosphate compounds used for bone scanning. These scans display abnormality in most joints that have a significant degree of inflammation, even when subclinical. Joint scanning permits a reasonably accurate assessment of the number, location and degree of activity of involved joints and offers an objective (although only semiquantitative) method for evaluating results of therapy. Although fairly sensitive, the phosphate agents are not ideal for joint scanning, since increased concentration denotes increased activity of bone osteoblasts in response to adjacent synovial abnormality rather than a primary synovial reaction. Other etiologies for osteoblastic stimulation, such as osteochondritis dissecans, traumatic joint disease, active osteoarthritis, healing fractures and the later stages of aseptic necrosis, may all produce abnormal bone scan images, which sometimes are hard to differentiate from arthritis. In such cases other compounds may be employed, including technetium pertechnetate or labeled albumin. These tend to remain in blood vessels, thereby indicating regions of increased vascularity or hyperemia, such as the synovial membrane when involved in active arthritis. These compounds are a little less sensitive than the phosphates but are more specific for synovial disease.

BONE SCANNING

Certain disorders affecting bone have been discussed elsewhere (hyperparathyroidism, p. 376; metastatic tumor in bone, p. 401). The commonest diagnostic problems involve fractures, osteomyelitis and metastatic tumor. The nonradiologic procedures most frequently used in bone disease are serum alkaline phosphatase (p. 210) and bone scanning.

Strontium-85 was the first agent to be widely used in bone scanning. Its relatively high patient radiation dose and the problems with excretion by the colon led to replacement by fluorine-18, which in turn has been superseded by the technetium-labeled phosphates. Bone scan abnormality is due to increased osteoblastic activity, whether neoplastic, reactive, reparative or metabolic. Local hyperemia is also a factor.

Bone scan provides important information in the evaluation of trauma and unexplained pain in areas where an occult fracture is a possibility. Whereas some fractures are immediately evident on x-ray, in many cases the fracture line cannot be seen, especially in the spine, ribs, face and smaller bones of the extremities. The radiologist is then forced to look for secondary changes produced by healing, which will not become evident before 10 – 14 days and in some cases may never be detectable. On bone scan, many fracture sites become abnormal within 3 days after trauma; and the great majority, in 5 days. Once evident, the abnormality persists for a variable amount of time, the average being approximately 2 years. A fracture site revealed on x-ray but not on scan at least 7 days after trauma usually represents an old, healed injury. Severe osteoporosis or severe malnutrition retard osseous reaction and may result in an equivocal or falsely negative scan. As noted previously, various types of joint disease can be visualized on the bone scan and may on occasion present problems in differentiation of the disease from possible fracture in the neighborhood of the joint.

Osteomyelitis is another disease in which bone scan may be invaluable. X-ray changes do not usually appear before 10–14 days after onset and may be delayed further or be difficult to interpret. Bone scan becomes abnormal days or weeks before x-rays. Although the exact time after onset necessary for most patients to display abnormality is not as clearly defined in osteomyelitis as in fracture, the literature seems to suggest 5–7 days. If bone scan is negative and osteomyelitis is strongly suspected, a gallium scan (p. 164) may be helpful, or the bone scan may be repeated after several days. Certain conditions resemble osteomyelitis clinically and to some degree on scan. These include cellulitis, arthritis and focal bone necrosis or infarct. Patients already receiving steroid or antibiotic therapy before onset of osteomyelitis may display changes in normal bone response. These changes can affect the bone scan latent period or the image characteristics.

Metastatic tumor detection is the reason for the majority of current bone scan requests. All malignancies capable of metastasis may reach bone. Some of these, including prostate, breast, lung, kidney, urinary bladder, thyroid and possibly malignant lymphoma, are more likely to do so than other tumors (p. 493). Tumor-related bone scanning is indicated in several situations: (1) to establish operability of the neoplasms just mentioned before embarking on extensive curative surgery (with the exception of thyroid and low-grade urothelial malignancies), (2) to follow results of therapy, (3) to investigate unexplained symptoms that may be due to occult tumor and (4) to investigate pain that may originate in bone. Until bone scanning became available, skeletal x-ray survey was the mainstay of diagnosis. Numerous comparisons have shown that bone scanning detects 15–40% more bone metastases (literature range 7–57%) than x-ray. This difference is related to osteoblastic reaction induced by the tumor, which may occur even when the lesion is osteolytic on x-ray. On the other hand, about 5% of metastases are seen on x-ray but not on scan (literature range 3–8%); these are usually "pure" osteolytic lesions. The implication of these figures is that bone scan is sufficient for routine detection of metastases in the major bone-seeking tumors and that x-ray should be reserved for specific anatomical areas in which the scan is equivocal or the etiology of a scan abnormality is in doubt. X-ray would also be useful when there is strong suspicion of bone malignancy yet the scan is negative, when the scan is normal in areas of bone pain and to help differentiate metastasis from focal severe osteoarthritis.

Bone scanning does have disadvantages—especially the fact that it is a nonspecific technique. The variety of conditions that may produce abnormal bone scans include fractures (even those of long duration), osteomyelitis, active osteoarthritis, joint synovial inflammation, areas of bone necrosis or infarct, myositis ossificans, renal osteodystrophy, Paget's disease of bone, certain benign bone tumors such as fibrous dysplasia and osteoid osteoma, and various artifacts such as ossification centers in the sternum or costochondral junction calcification. On the other hand, when tumor produces widespread bone marrow invasion, the spine or other bones may sometimes display a homogeneous appearance on scan that may be misinterpreted as normal unless certain other findings are taken into account. As a general rule, the greater the number of focal asymmetric lesions on bone scan, the more metastatic tumor should be suspected. Healing fractures (which actually may have occurred at different times) and Paget's disease create the most interpretive difficulty. Some institutions routinely scan only the spine, pelvis and ribs instead of the total body. A question may arise about the probability of metastases elsewhere. One large study encompassing a wide variety of tumors indicates that the incidence of solitary uptake (other areas negative) in the skull is about 4%; in the extremities as a unit, about 9%; in the humerus, about 1%; in the femur, 5%; in the tibia or fibula, 2%, and elsewhere in the extremities, quite rare.

REFERENCES

Alarcon-Segovia, D., et al.: Significance of the lupus erythematosus phenomenon in older women with chronic hepatic disease, Mayo Clin. Proc. 40:193, 1965.

Aprill, C. N., et al.: Pheripheral joint imaging: Variations in normal children, J. Nucl. Med. 13:367, 1972.

Bardana, E. J., and Pirofsky, B.: Recent advances in the immunopathogenesis of systemic lupus erythematosis, West. J. Med. 122:130, 1975.

Bendersky, G.: Etiology of hyperuricemia, Ann. Clin. Lab. Sci. 5:456, 1975.

Bianchi, F. A., and Keech, M. K.: Comparison of two slide tests in rheumatoid arthritis, J.A.M.A. 185:318, 1963.

Brewer, E. J., Jr., et al.: Criteria for the classification of juvenile rheumatoid arthritis, Bull. Rheum. Dis. 23:712, 1972–73 series.

Calabro, J. J.: The three faces of juvenile rheumatoid arthritis, Hosp. Practice 9:61, 1974.

Caplan, H. I.: The use of latex fixation tests in non-rheumatic states, Ann. Intern. Med. 59:449, 1963.

Cheng, C. T., and Persellin, R. H.: Interference by C1q in slide latex tests for rheumatoid factor, Ann. Intern. Med. 75:683, 1971.

deShazo, R. D.: The spectrum of systemic vasculitis, Postgrad. Med. 58:78, 1975.

Ehrlich, G.: Intermittent and periodic rheumatic syndromes, Bull. Rheum. Dis. 24:746, 1973–74 series.

Feinstein, A. R.: The natural histories of acute rheumatic fever, Bull. Rheum. Dis. 17:423, 1966.

Fernandez-Madrid, F., and Mattioli, M.: Antinuclear antibodies (ANA): Immunological and clinical significance, Semin. Arthritis Rheum. 6:83, 1976.

Gelfand, M. J., and Silberstein, E. B.: Radionuclide imaging: Use in diagnosis of osteomyelitis in children, J.A.M.A. 237:245, 1977.

Goldgraber, M. B., and Kirsner, J. B.: Scleroderma of the gastrointestinal tract: A review, A. M. A. Arch. Pathol. 64:255, 1957.

Good, A. E.: Reiter's disease, Postgrad. Med. 61:153, 1977.

Gray, R. L., and Gottlieb, N. L.: The HL-A B-27 histocompatibility antigen in rheumatoid arthritis variants, J. Florida M. A. 63:339, 1976.

Hall, A. P.: Serologic tests in rheumatoid arthritis, Med. Clin. North Am. 45:1181, 1961.

Handmaker, H., and Leonards, R.: The bone scan in inflammatory osseous disease, Semin. Nucl. Med. 6:95, 1976.

Hoffbauer, F. W.: Lupoid hepatitis, Postgrad. Med. 38:376, 1965.

Hoffer, P. B., and Gevant, H. K.: Radionuclide joint imaging, Semin. Nucl. Med. 6: 121, 1976.

Hollander, J. E. (ed.): *Arthritis* (7th ed.; Philadelphia: Lea & Febiger, 1966).

Kitridou, R. C.: Synovianalysis, Am. Fam. Physician 5:101, 1972.

Marty, R., et al.: Bone trauma and related benign disease: Assessment by bone scanning, Semin. Nucl. Med. 6:107, 1976.

Nakamura, R. M.: Diagnostic laboratory tests for systemic lupus erythematosis and related disorders, Lab. Med. 6(6):11, 1975.

Neustadt, D. H.: Ankylosing spondylitis, Postgrad. Med. 61:124, 1977.

Notman, D. D., et al.: Profiles of antinuclear antibodies in systemic rheumatic diseases, Ann. Intern. Med. 83:464, 1975.

O'Duffy, J. D.: Psoriatic arthritis, Postgrad. Med. 61:165, 1977.

Osmond, J. D., et al.: Accuracy of ^{99m}Tc-diphosphonate bone scans and roentgenograms in the detection of prostate, breast, and lung carcinoma metastases, Am. J. Roentgenol. Radium Ther. Nucl. Med. 125:972, 1975.

Palumbo, P. J., et al.: Musculoskeletal manifestations of inflammatory bowel disease, Mayo Clin. Proc. 48:411, 1973.

Ramer, S., and Bluestone, R.: Colitic arthropathies, Postgrad. Med. 61:141, 1977.

Rosenthall, L.: ^{99m}Tc-phosphate complex joint imaging, Appl. Radiol. Nucl. Med. 5: 179, 1976.

Rosenthall, L., and Kaye, M.: Technetium-99m-pyrophosphate kinetics and imaging in metabolic bone disease, J. Nucl. Med. 16:33, 1975.

Rosenthall, L., et al.: Observation on the use of ^{99m}Tc-phosphate imaging on peripheral bone trauma, Radiology 119:637, 1976.

Rothfield, N. F.: The role of antinuclear reactions in the diagnosis of systemic lupus erythematosus: A study of 53 cases, Arthritis Rheum. 4:223, 1961.

Rothfield, N. F.: Serologic tests in rheumatic diseases, Postgrad. Med. 45:116, 1969.

Schaller, J.: Juvenile rheumatoid arthritis, Postgrad. Med. 61:117, 1977.

Singer, J. M.: The latex fixation test in rheumaticoid diseases: A review, Am. J. Med. 31:766, 1961.

Smith, D. M.: Common adult osteopenic states: Osteoporosis and osteomalacia, Am. Fam. Physician 14:160, 1976.

Smith, L. H., and Riggs, B. L.: Clinical and laboratory considerations in metabolic bone disease, Ann. Clin. Lab. Sci. 5:252, 1975.

Stevens, M. B., et al.: The clinical significance of extracellular material (ECM) in LE-cell preparations, N. Engl. J. Med. 268:976, 1963.

Tofe, A. J., et al.: Correlation of neoplasms with incidence and localization of skeletal metastases: An analysis of 1,355 diphosphonate bone scans, J. Nucl. Med. 16: 986, 1976.

Tofe, A. J., et al.: Incidence of solitary skull and extremity involvement in whole-body scintigrams, J. Nucl. Med. 17:755, 1976.

Vaughn, J. H.: Rheumatologic disorders due to immune complexes, Postgrad. Med. 54:129, 1973.

Weitzman, R. J., and Walker, S. E.: The L.E. cell test revisited, Lab. Med. 7(6):23, 1976.

23 / Acid-Base and pH

FLUID AND ELECTROLYTE PROBLEMS are common in hospitalized patients. In general, most of these situations are produced secondary to other disease processes or as undesirable side effects of therapy. In addition, a few diseases characteristically lead to certain electrolyte alterations that are important for diagnosis and treatment.

Fluid and electrolytes in one form or another make up nearly all of the human body. It is useful to think of these constituents as though they were contained in three separate compartments among which are variable degrees of communication: individual cells, containing intracellular fluid; vascular channels, containing blood or lymph; and the extracellular nonvascular tissue components, the interstitial fluid. Shifts of fluid and electrolytes between and within these compartments take place continually as the various activities concerned with hemostasis, cell metabolism and organ function go on. These changes can to some degree be monitored clinically by their effects on certain measurable parameters, including the pH and concentration of certain ions (electrolytes) in a fairly accessible substance, the blood. This chapter covers blood pH and its disturbances, and the next chapter takes up certain electrolyte and fluid disorders.

BLOOD pH: THE BICARBONATE-CARBONIC ACID SYSTEM

Blood pH comes from the French words *puissance hydrogen,* meaning the strength or power of hydrogen. The hydrogen ion concentration of blood expressed in terms of gram molecular weights of hydrogen per liter (mols/L) is so much less than 1 (for example, 0.0000001) that it is easier to communicate this information in terms of logarithms (thus the previous example becoming 1×10^{-7}). The symbol pH simplifies this even more, because pH is defined as the negative logarithm of the hydrogen ion concentration (in the preceding example, 1×10^{-7} becomes 10^{-7} which then becomes 7.0). In this way, a relatively simple scale is substituted for very cumbersome tiny numbers. In the pH scale, therefore, a change of 1.0 pH unit means a tenfold change in hydrogen ion concentration (7.0 to 6.0 means 10^{-7} to 10^{-6} mols/L.).

The normal pH of arterial blood is 7.4, with a normal range between 7.36 and 7.44. It seems that blood pH must be maintained within relatively narrow limits, because pH outside the range 6.8 to 7.8 is incompatible with life. Therefore, hydrogen ion content is regulated by a series of buffer substances. A buffer is a substance that can bind hydrogen ions to a certain extent without developing marked change in pH. Among substances which act as buffers are hemoglobin, plasma protein, phosphates, and the bicarbonate-carbonic acid system. Bicarbonate is by far the body's most important buffer substance; it is present in large quantities and can be controlled by the lungs and kidneys.

A brief review of the bicarbonate-carbonic acid system recalls that CO_2 in aqueous solutions exists in potential equilibrium with carbonic acid ($CO_2 + H_2O \rightleftharpoons H_2CO_3$). The enzyme carbonic anhydrase catalyzes this reaction toward attainment of equilibrium; otherwise, the rate of reaction would be minimal. Carbon dioxide is produced by cellular metabolism and released into the bloodstream. There, most of it diffuses into the RBC where carbonic anhydrase catalyzes its hydration to carbonic acid (H_2CO_3). Carbonic acid readily dissociates into hydrogen ions (H^+) and bicarbonate ions (HCO_3^-). Eventually, only a small amount of dissolved CO_2 and a much smaller amount of undissociated H_2CO_3 remain in the plasma. Therefore, the great bulk of the original CO_2 (amounting to 75%) is carried in the blood as bicarbonate, with only about 5% still in solution (as dissolved CO_2 or undissociated H_2CO_3) and about 20% coupled with hemoglobin as a carbamino compound or, to a much lesser extent, with other buffers, such as plasma proteins.

This situation can best be visualized by means of the Henderson-Hasselbalch equation. This states that $pH = pK + \log \dfrac{base}{acid}$, where pK is the dissociation constant (ability to release hydrogen ions) of the particular acid chosen, such as H_2CO_3. The derivation of this equation will be disregarded to concentrate on the clinically useful parts, the relationship of pH, base and acid. If the bicarbonate-acid system is to be interpreted by means of the Henderson-Hasselbalch equation, then $\dfrac{base}{acid} = \dfrac{HCO_3^-}{H_2CO_3}$ since bicarbonate is the base and carbonic acid is the acid. Actually, most of the so-called carbonic acid represented in the equation is dissolved CO_2, which is present in plasma in an amount greater than 100 times the quantity of undissociated H_2CO_3. Therefore, the formula should really be $\dfrac{HCO_3^-}{H_2CO_3 + CO_2}$, but it is customary to let H_2CO_3 stand for the entire denominator. The next step is to note from the Henderson-Hasselbalch equation that pH is proportional ($\cong$) to $\dfrac{base}{acid}$. This means that in the bicarbonate-carbonic acid system, $pH \cong \dfrac{HCO_3^-}{H_2CO_3}$.

The kidney is the main regulator of HCO_3^- manufacture (the numerator of the equation) and the lungs primarily control CO_2 excretion (the denominator).

The kidney has several means of excreting hydrogen ions. One is the conversion of monohydrogen phosphate to dihydrogen phosphate (HPO_4^{2-} to $H_2PO_4^-$). Another is the formation of ammonia (NH_3) in renal tubule cells by deamination of certain amino acids, such as glutamine. Ammonia then diffuses into the urine, where it combines with H^+ to form ammonium ion (NH_4^+). A third mechanism is the one with which there is most concern now, the production of HCO_3^- in the renal tubule cells. These cells possess carbonic anhydrase, which catalyzes the formation of H_2CO_3 from CO_2. The H_2CO_3 dissociates, leaving HCO_3^- and H^+. The H^+ is excreted in the urine by the phosphate or ammonium pathways or combined with some other anion. The HCO_3^- goes into the bloodstream where it forms part of the pH buffer system, as was already mentioned. Not only does HCO_3^- assist in buffering H^+ within body fluids, but HCO_3^- filtered at the glomerulus into the urine can itself combine with urinary H^+ (produced by the renal tubule cells from the H_2CO_3 cycle and excreted into the urine).

The lungs, on the other hand, take H_2CO_3, change it to CO_2 and water with the aid of carbonic anhydrase and blow off the CO_2. In this process, a mechanism for excreting H^+ exists, because the HCO_3^- in the plasma can combine with free H^+ to form H_2CO_3, which can then be eliminated from the lungs in the form of CO_2, as was just described. This process can probably handle excretion of most normal and mildly abnormal H^+ quantities. However, when large excesses of free H^+ are present in body fluids, the kidney plays a major role, because not only is H^+ excreted directly in the urine, but HCO_3^- is formed, which helps buffer additional amounts of H^+ in the plasma.

Going back to the Henderson-Hasselbalch equation, which is now modified to indicate that pH is proportional ($\cong$) to $\dfrac{HCO_3^-}{H_2CO_3}$, it is easy to see that variations in either the numerator or denominator will change pH. If HCO_3^- is increased without corresponding increase in H_2CO_3, the ratio will be increased and the pH will rise. Conversely, if something happens to increase H_2CO_3 or dissolved CO_2, the denominator will be increased, the ratio will be decreased, the pH will fall and so on. Clinically, an increase in normal plasma pH is called alkalosis and a decrease is called acidosis. The normal ratio of HCO_3^- to H_2CO_3 is 20:1.

LABORATORY DETERMINATIONS OF pH and CO_2

Next will be described the laboratory tests used in pH problems, which, incidentally, are often called acid-base because of the importance of bicarbonate and carbonic acid changes involved.

CARBON DIOXIDE COMBINING POWER. — Venous blood is drawn aerobically with an ordinary syringe and the serum is removed after clotting and centrifugation. The CO_2 tension of this serum is then equilibrated to normal alveolar levels of 40 mm Hg by simply having the technician blow his own alveolar air into the specimen through a tube arrangement. This maneuver adjusts the amount of dissolved CO_2 to the normal amounts found in normal arterial blood. HCO_3^- of the serum is then converted to CO_2 by acid hydrolysis in a vacuum and the released gas is measured. The released CO_2 thus consists of the dissolved CO_2 of the specimen already present plus the converted HCO_3^- (and thus the denominator plus the numerator of the Henderson-Hasselbalch equation). Subtraction of the known amount of dissolved CO_2 and H_2CO_3 in normal blood from this measurement gives what is essentially a value for serum HCO_3^- alone (the so-called combining power since HCO_3^- combines with H^+). The inaccuracy that may be caused by these manipulations should be obvious.

CARBON DIOXIDE CONTENT.—Total CO_2 content is determined from heparinized arterial or venous blood drawn anaerobically. This may be done in a vacuum tube or a syringe that is quickly capped. (Mineral oil is not satisfactory for sealing.) The blood is centrifuged and the plasma removed. At this point, all the CO_2 present is still at the same CO_2 tension or partial pressure of dissolved gas that the patient possessed. Next, the plasma is analyzed for CO_2 in a method which converts HCO_3^- and H_2CO_3 to the gas form. Thus, CO_2 content measures the sum of HCO_3^-, H_2CO_3 and dissolved CO_2. Since the amount of dissolved CO_2 and H_2CO_3 in blood is very small, normal values for CO_2 content are quite close to those of the CO_2 combining power (which measures only HCO_3^-). Since the specimen has been drawn and processed with little or no contact with the outside air, the result is obviously more accurate than that obtained from the CO_2 combining power.

SERUM BICARBONATE.—Serum is obtained from blood drawn aerobically and assayed for HCO_3^- without equilibration. This technique is used for most automated CO_2 equipment and even in many laboratories using manual methods. This is even less accurate than CO_2 combining power. The serum is frequently exposed to air for relatively long periods of time. Only large changes in CO_2 or HCO_3^- will be detected.

PCO_2.—A fourth method is one popularized by Astrup. This is based on the fact that most of the denominator of the Henderson-Hasselbalch equation is dissolved CO_2, since the partial pressure of CO_2 (the PCO_2) of the specimen is proportional to the amount of dissolved CO_2, the PCO_2 is therefore proportional to the denominator of the Henderson-Hasselbalch equation and may be used as a measure of the denominator. In practice, a small amount of whole blood (plasma can be used), collected anaerobically, is analyzed for PCO_2, using a CO_2 electrode. The HCO_3^- may then be calculated (from the Henderson-Hasselbalch equation), or the PCO_2 value itself may be used in conjunction with pH to differentiate acid-base abnormalities. PCO_2 by electrode is without question the method of choice for acid-base problems. pH is usually measured at the same time on the same specimen.

pH MEASUREMENT.—pH has been quite a problem so far as laboratory technique is concerned. Most instruments measure the difference in electric charge between two electrodes placed into the unknown solution, which in this case is plasma or whole blood. Unfortunately, the pH changes of blood are relatively very small, so that the instrument must be very sensitive. The more sensitive it is made, the more difficult to gain stability and reliability of results, since only a small error in the equipment may show up as a significant pH change. More recently, better machines have been put on the market and direct pH reading is now a routine part of blood gas measurement. On the technical side, it should be noted that at room temperature, plasma pH decreases at the rate of about 0.015 pH unit every half hour. Unless measurement is done within ½ hour after drawing, the blood should be refrigerated; it can then be kept up to 4 hours. Venous specimens are nearly as accurate as arterial blood for pH if blood is drawn before the tourniquet is released and the patient's hand or arm is kept without motion after tourniquet application. Room air contact must be avoided.

CLINICAL DISTURBANCES OF pH

With this background, one may proceed to the various clinical disturbances of pH. These have been classically known as the state of acidosis when pH is decreased toward the acid side of normal, and alkalosis when pH is elevated toward the alkaline side of normal. Acidosis, in turn, is usually subdivided into metabolic and respiratory etiology, and the same for alkalosis.

METABOLIC ACIDOSIS.—This type of acidosis may have at least three main causes.

Acid-Gaining Acidosis.—Hydrogen ions not included in the CO_2 system are added to the blood. The common situations are:

1. *Direct administration*—such as treatment with ammonium chloride, or the late effects of salicylate poisoning. Ammonium chloride (NH_4Cl) releases H^+ ions and Cl^- ions as the liver utilizes this compound for NH_3 in order to synthesize urea. Aspirin is acetylsalicylic acid, which in large quantities will eventually add enough H^+ ions to cause acidosis, even though in the early stages there is respiratory alkalosis (to be discussed later).

2. *Excess metabolic acid formation*—found in diabetic ketoacidosis, starvation, or severe dehydration. These conditions cause utilization of body protein and fat for energy instead of carbohydrate, with production of ketone bodies and various metabolic acids.

The results of acid-gaining acidosis are a decrease in free HCO_3^- which is used up trying to buffer the excess H^+. Thus, the numerator of the Henderson-Hasselbalch equation is decreased, the normal 20:1 ratio is decreased and the pH is, therefore, decreased. The CO_2 content (or CO_2 combining power) is also decreased because the bicarbonate, which it measures, has been decreased as a primary response to the addition of excess acid.

Base-Losing Acidosis.—This situation is caused by severe intestinal diarrhea, especially if prolonged or in children. Diseases such as cholera or possibly ulcerative colitis or severe dysentery might do this. The mechanism is direct loss of HCO_3^- from the lumen of the small intestine. Normally, HCO_3^- is secreted into the small intestine, so that the contents of the small intestine are alkaline in contrast to the acidity of the stomach. Most of the HCO_3^- is reabsorbed; however, prolonged diarrhea or similar conditions could mechanically prevent intestinal reabsorption enough to cause significant HCO_3^- loss in the feces. In addition, the H^+ ions that were released from H_2CO_3 in the formation of HCO_3^- by carbonic anhydrase are still present in the bloodstream and help decrease pH. However, the primary cause is the direct loss of HCO_3^-; the numerator of the Henderson-Hasselbalch equation is decreased, the 20:1 ratio is decreased and the pH is decreased. Naturally, the CO_2 content is also decreased.

Renal Acidosis. — This occurs in kidney failure that produces the clinical syndrome of uremia. As mentioned previously, the kidney has the major responsibility for excreting large excesses of H^+. In uremia, H^+ from metabolic acids that normally would be excreted this way are retained in the bloodstream due to loss of renal tubular function. As in acid-gaining acidosis, the excess H^+ must be buffered; therefore, part of the available body fluid HCO_3^- is used up. This decreases the numerator of the Henderson-Hasselbalch equation, decreases the normal 20:1 ratio and therefore decreases pH. Again, the CO_2 content is decreased.

RESPIRATORY ACIDOSIS. — The second major category of acidosis is that called respiratory acidosis. This may be due to any condition that causes pulmonary CO_2 retention. These include the respiratory muscle paralysis of polio, the respiratory brain center depression sometimes seen in encephalitis or with large doses of such drugs as morphine, primary lung disease (such as pulmonary fibrosis or severe emphysema) that destroys oxygen-exchange ability and sometimes heart diseases (such as chronic congestive heart failure). The basic problem here is H_2CO_3 excess, produced by the CO_2 retention. Thus, the denominator of the Henderson-Hasselbalch equation is increased, the normal 20:1 ratio is decreased and the pH is decreased. The CO_2 content is sometimes normal but is usually increased, because of kidney attempts to handle the excess CO_2 by forming more HCO_3^- and excreting more H^+ ions.

METABOLIC ALKALOSIS. — Alkalosis may also be divided into metabolic and respiratory types. In metabolic alkalosis, there are three relatively common situations which should be discussed.

Alkali Administration. — Usually in this situation sodium bicarbonate is taken in large quantities for the treatment of peptic ulcer symptoms. In this case, excess HCO_3^- is absorbed above the amount needed to neutralize stomach hydrochloric acid (HCl). The numerator of the Henderson-Hasselbalch equation is increased, the normal 20:1 ratio is increased, and the pH therefore rises. Content of CO_2 will naturally also rise because of the additional HCO_3^-. Lactate, citrate or acetate in sufficient quantities may also produce alkalosis, since they are metabolized to HCO_3^-.

Acid-Losing Alkalosis. — This most frequently results from severe or protracted vomiting, such as may occur with pyloric stenosis. Gastric HCl is lost in vomiting. This was originally produced by conversion of H_2CO_3 to HCO_3^- and H^+, mediated by carbonic anhydrase of the gastric mucosa. The HCO_3^- is kept in the bloodstream, but the H^+ are secreted into the gastric lumen as HCl. When HCl is lost through vomiting, the H^+ are continually being lost, causing the CO_2 content to be increased, because the HCO_3^- released when HCl is produced is still in the bloodstream and increases when HCl is being formed at an increased rate. Therefore, the 20:1 ratio is increased and the pH is increased. Since H_2CO_3 is decreased as it is being continually used to produce more HCl, the lungs tend to retain CO_2 to compensate. Therefore, PCO_2 may actually increase, although not enough to prevent increase of the 20:1 ratio.

Hypokalemic Alkalosis.—This is most commonly due to excess potassium ion (K^+) loss by the kidney, such as might happen with overuse of certain diuretics that cause K^+ as well as sodium ion (Na^+) loss. Normally, most body K^+ is intracellular, whereas the majority of Na^+ and H^+ are extracellular. When excess K^+ is lost in the urine, intracellular K^+ diffuses out of the cells to replace some of that being lost from plasma; Na^+ and H^+ move into the cells to replace the K^+ that has moved out. Thus, H^+ are lost from extracellular fluid and plasma. A second mechanism depends on the fact that sodium is reabsorbed from the urine into the renal distal tubule cells by an active transport mechanism. This transport mechanism involves excretion of H^+ and K^+ into the urine to replace the reabsorbed Na^+. In this exchange (or transport) system H^+ and K^+ compete with each other. Therefore, if an intracellular deficit of K^+ exists (in the tubule cells), more H^+ are excreted into the urine to allow the reabsorption of the same quantity of sodium. The result of renal H^+ loss and extracellular fluid H^+ loss is an acid-losing type of alkalosis. Therefore, more H^+ are manufactured by the kidney from H_2CO_3 in order to replace lost extracellular H^+; more HCO_3^- ions are thereby formed, and the numerator of the Henderson-Hasselbalch equation is increased. The denominator is eventually increased if the lungs attempt to compensate by increasing CO_2 retention by slower breathing. However, respiratory compensation is frequently minimal or insignificant in hypokalemic alkalosis, so that the P_{CO_2} frequently remains normal. Also, the urine pH is decreased because of the excess H^+ being excreted in the urine. This is the opposite of what one would ordinarily expect, because, in acidosis, the kidney usually attempts to compensate by excreting more H^+ (acid urine), whereas in alkalosis it would normally try to conserve H^+ and thus produce a urine of higher pH (alkaline urine).

RESPIRATORY ALKALOSIS.—The other major subdivision of alkalosis is that of respiratory alkalosis, which occurs when the respiratory mechanism blows off more CO_2 than normally, due to respiratory center stimulation from some cause. The main conditions in which this happens are the so-called hyperventilation syndrome, caused by hysteria or anxiety; high fever, and direct stimulation of the respiratory center by drugs. Overdose of aspirin can cause this in the early stages, although later, after more of the aspirin is absorbed, a metabolic acidosis develops. In hyperventilation, from whatever cause, respirations are increased and deeper, blowing off more CO_2. This creates a H_2CO_3 deficit since it is being used up to replenish CO_2 by the lung carbonic anhydrase enzymes. Therefore, the denominator of the Henderson-Hasselbalch equation is decreased, the 20:1 ratio is increased and plasma pH increases. Carbon dioxide content will decrease, because when H_2CO_3 is lost due to formation of CO_2 in the lungs, HCO_3^- is converted to H_2CO_3 in the kidney to compensate secondarily for or replace the decreasing plasma carbonic acid.

To summarize plasma pH problems: In metabolic acidosis there is eventual HCO_3^- deficit leading to decreased plasma pH and decreased CO_2 content (or CO_2 combining power). In respiratory acidosis there is primary H_2CO_3 excess, which causes decreased plasma pH, but the CO_2 content is increased due to renal attempts at compensation. In metabolic alkalosis there is eventual bicarbonate excess leading to increased plasma pH and increased CO_2 content. In respiratory alkalosis there is primary carbonic acid deficit, which causes increased plasma pH, but the CO_2 content is decreased due to renal attempts at compensation. The urine pH usually reflects the status of the plasma pH except in hypokalemic alkalosis, where there is acid urine pH despite plasma alkalosis.

As noted, CO_2 content or combining capacity essentially constitutes the numerator of the Henderson-Hasselbalch equation. The PCO_2 is essentially a measurement of the equation denominator, and can be used in conjunction with pH to indicate acid-base changes. This is the system popularized by Astrup and Siggaard-Andersen. The PCO_2 follows the same direction as the CO_2 content in classic acid-base syndromes. In metabolic acidosis, the PCO_2 is decreased, because acids other than H_2CO_3 accumulate, and CO_2 is blown off by the lungs in attempts to decrease body fluid acidity. In metabolic alkalosis, the PCO_2 is increased if the lungs compensate by hypoventilation; in mild or acute cases, PCO_2 may remain normal. In respiratory alkalosis, the PCO_2 is decreased, because increased ventilation blows off more CO_2. In respiratory acidosis, the PCO_2 is increased because of CO_2 retention due to decreased ventilation.

Interpretation of pH Data

Acid-base data interpretation has always been one of the least understood areas of medicine. Use of the Henderson-Hasselbalch equation makes it simple, in classic noncorrected cases. The equation numerator (HCO_3^- or CO_2 content) and denominator (PCO_2) usually follow each other; as one increases or decreases, so does the other, and therefore, the direction of change for one can be predicted from the behavior of the other. The pH follows the same direction of abnormality as PCO_2 and CO_2 content in metabolic acidosis or alkalosis; it goes in the opposite direction in cases of respiratory acidosis or alkalosis. Therefore, if pH is known and either HCO_3^- or PCO_2 is known, it can be surmised whether the disorder is respiratory or metabolic in origin. Normal values for PCO_2 are 35 – 45 mm Hg and for CO_2 content 20 – 30 mEq/L. In metabolic acid-base disorders, the numerator (HCO_3^-) of the Henderson-Hasselbalch equation is primarily affected, while the denominator (PCO_2) attempts to compensate by means of regulating the breathing rate. In respiratory acid-base disorders, the denominator (PCO_2) is primarily affected while the numerator (HCO_3^-) attempts to compensate by kidney action.

The above explanations refer to uncomplicated noncorrected cases with attempts at compensation. Since attempts at compensation may, for some reason, not be adequate, or even may be impossible, changes in the compensatory component may not be as marked as the primary change or may even be confined to population normal range. This is more likely to occur in metabolic alkalosis, especially the hypokalemic type. On the other hand, compensatory changes may substantially succeed in correcting pH to normal range. Finally, attempts at therapy or the presence of one physiologic abnormality superimposed on a disease with others may complicate matters.

Two other concepts that form an integral part of the Astrup system should be defined. The term "buffer base" refers to all substances in the buffering system of whole blood which are able to bind excess H^+. Bicarbonate forms slightly over half of total buffer base; hemoglobin makes up about one third of total buffer base, consisting of three quarters of the non-bicarbonate buffer system. Normal buffer base values for any patient are therefore calculated on the basis of the actual hemoglobin concentration as well as normal figures for pH and HCO_3^-. The term "base excess" refers to any difference in the measured total quantity of blood buffer base from the patient's calculated normal value. Thus, an increase in total buffer base (such as an increase in HCO_3^-) is considered a "positive" base excess; a decrease in total buffer base from calculated normal (such as a decrease in HCO_3^-) is considered a "negative" base excess.

In many cases involving acid-base disturbances, the diagnosis is obvious, and the only reason for obtaining CO_2 studies is to gauge the severity of the disorder. Determination of pH would not be needed. This would be the situation in diabetic acidosis, for example. However, in other patients, the underlying disorder is not obvious; there may be intervening attempts at therapy, or compensatory mechanisms may obscure a classic picture. In these cases, pH measurement is essential to interpret values of P_{CO_2} or CO_2 content. The problem is one of diagnosis rather than simple estimation of severity.

REFERENCES

Albert, M. S.: Acid-base disorders in pediatrics, Pediatr. Clin. North Am. 23:639, 1976.

Blumentals, A. S. (ed.): Symposium on acid-base balance, Arch. Intern. Med. 116: 647–742, 1965.

Davis, R. P.: Logland: A Gibbsian view of acid-base balance, Am. J. Med. 42:159, 1967.

Elkinton, J. R.: Renal acidosis: Diagnosis and treatment, Med. Clin. North Am. 47: 935, 1963.

Felig, P.: Diabetic ketoacidosis, N. Engl. J. Med. 290:1360, 1974.

Filley, G. F.: *Acid-Base and Blood Gas Regulation* (Philadelphia: Lea & Febiger, 1971).

Kassirer, J. P.: Serious acid-base disorders, N. Engl. J. Med. 291:773, 1974.

McCurdy, D. K.: Mixed metabolic and respiratory acid-base disturbances: Diagnosis and treatment, Chest 62 [Suppl]:35S–44S, 1972.

Nahas, G. G. (ed.): Current concepts of acid-base measurement, Ann. NY Acad. Sci. 133:1–274, 1966.

Simmons, D. H., and Shkolnick, S.: Acid-base alterations in pulmonary disease, Dis. Chest 45:175, 1964.

Still, G., and Rodman, T.: The measurement of the content of carbon dioxide in plasma, Am. J. Clin. Pathol. 38:435, 1962.

Weisberg, H. F.: A better understanding of anion-cation ("acid-base") balance, S. Clin. North Am. 39:1, 1959.

Weisberg, H. F.: pH of venous blood (Questions and Answers), J.A.M.A. 194:688, 1965.

Weisberg, H. F.: Antics with "acid-base" semantics, Lab. Med. 3:11, 1972.

Winters, R. W., et al.: *Acid-Base Physiology in Medicine: A Self-Instruction Program* (Westlake, OH: The London Company, 1967).

24 / Serum Electrolytes

CHAPTER 23 discussed pH and its clinical variations. The present chapter will attempt to cover the most frequent conditions associated with abnormalities of the major body electrolytes: sodium, potassium and chloride.

Before going further, a clear distinction must be made between total body electrolyte concentration and serum concentration. Total body concentration of any electrolyte such as sodium includes an intravascular component (comprising the concentration of the electrolyte within serum and within RBC), an interstitial fluid component and an intracellular component. Since most ions are diffusible to variable degrees among each of the three compartments, the serum concentration often does reflect the concentration in other fluid compartments. However, since the concentration of various electrolytes (such as sodium and potassium) differs in cells and extracellular fluid, in many situations the serum concentration does not accurately reflect intracellular electrolyte conditions. Furthermore, the serum electrolyte concentration depends on the amount of water present (plasma volume). A normal quantity of a particular electrolyte such as sodium may appear to have a low serum value if it is diluted by an excess of water. Likewise, an actual electrolyte deficit may show normal serum values if the plasma volume is decreased by excess water loss. Therefore, the serum levels of any electrolyte may or may not reflect the total body concentration, depending on the situation. Unfortunately, serum levels are the only electrolyte measurement that is readily available. A knowledge of what happens to total body levels as well as serum levels is essential to understand problems in certain situations.

SERUM SODIUM ABNORMALITIES

The most frequent electrolyte abnormalities, from both clinical situations and abnormal laboratory values, are found with sodium. This is true because sodium is the most important cation of the body, both from a quantitative standpoint and from its influence on maintaining electrical neutrality. The most common causes of low or high serum sodium values are enumerated in Table 24-1. Some of the situations and the mechanisms involved require further explanation.

In protracted and severe vomiting, such as occurs with pyloric obstruction or stenosis, gastric fluid is lost in large amounts and a hypochloremic (acid-losing) alkalosis develops, as described in Chapter 23. Serum sodium values are usually within normal range, since gastric contents have a relatively low sodium content. Occasional patients may even show hypernatre-

TABLE 24-1.—CLINICAL SITUATIONS FREQUENTLY
ASSOCIATED WITH SERUM SODIUM ABNORMALITIES

Hyponatremia
1. Sodium and water depletion (deficit hyponatremia)
   a) Loss of GI secretions with replacement of fluid but not electrolytes
      (1) Vomiting
      (2) Diarrhea
      (3) Tube drainage
   b) Loss from skin with replacement of fluids but not electrolytes
      (1) Excessive sweating
      (2) Extensive burns
   c) Loss from kidney
      (1) Diuretics (mercurial, chlorothiazide)
      (2) Chronic renal insufficiency (uremia) with acidosis
   d) Metabolic loss
      (1) Starvation with acidosis
      (2) Diabetic acidosis
   e) Endocrine loss
      (1) Addison's disease (or sudden withdrawal of long-term steroid therapy)
   f) Iatrogenic loss from serous cavities
      (1) Paracentesis or thoracentesis
2. Excessive water (dilution hyponatremia)
   a) Congestive heart failure
   b) Cirrhosis
   c) Acute or chronic renal insufficiency (oliguria)
   d) Excessive water administration
   e) Diabetic acidosis (therapy without adequate sodium replacement)
3. Intracellular loss (tired cell syndrome)
   a) Cachexia and severe malnutrition
   b) Cirrhosis
   c) Carcinomatosis
Hypernatremia
Dehydration is the most frequent overall clinical finding in hypernatremia.
1. Deficient water intake (either orally or intravenously)
2. Excess water output (excess sweating, diabetes insipidus)
3. Occasional cases of severe protracted vomiting or diarrhea
4. Some cases of cerebral disease with ADH control loss

mia if fluid loss exceeds loss of electrolytes. Despite normal serum levels, total body sodium is somewhat depleted, so replacement therapy should also include some sodium. Serum potassium values are most often low, due to direct loss and to alkalosis that develops when so much hydrochloric acid (HCl) is lost. Similar findings are produced by continuous gastric tube suction if continued over 24 hours.

In severe or long-standing diarrhea, the most common acid-base abnormality is a base-losing acidosis. Serum sodium, chloride and potassium values are most often normal, despite considerable depletion of total body stores of these electrolytes, especially of potassium. The normal serum findings are explained by the marked loss of water characteristic of diarrhea. The diarrhea seen in sprue differs somewhat from the electrolyte pattern of diarrhea from other causes in that hypokalemia is a somewhat more frequent finding. Regardless of the serum values, known deficits of water and electrolytes must be cautiously replaced.

Diabetic acidosis and its treatment provide very interesting electrolyte problems. Lack of insulin causes metabolism of protein and fat to provide energy that normally is available from carbohydrates. Ketone bodies and other metabolic acids accumulate; the blood sugar level is also elevated, and both sugar and ketones are excreted in the urine. Glycosuria produces an osmotic diuresis; a certain amount of serum sodium is lost with the sugar and water, and other sodium ions accompany the strongly acid ketone anions.

The effects of diuresis, as well as of accompanying electrolyte loss, are manifested by severe dehydration. The serum sodium and chloride levels are often low in untreated diabetic acidosis, although (because of water loss) less often they may be within normal range. The serum potassium level is usually normal. Nevertheless, even with normal serum levels, considerable total body deficits exist for all these electrolytes. The treatment for severe diabetic acidosis is insulin and large amounts of intravenous fluids. Sodium and chloride usually are given with the fluid to replace their deficits. After insulin administration, potassium ions tend to move into body cells, being no longer needed to combine with ketone acid anions. Also, potassium is apparently taken into liver cells when glycogen is formed from plasma glucose under the influence of insulin. In most patients, the serum potassium level falls to nearly half admission values after 3–4 hours of fluid and insulin therapy (if adequate urine output is present), due to continued urinary potassium loss, shifts into body cells and rehydration. After this time, potassium supplements should be added to the other treatment.

Sweat consists of water with a small but significant sodium chloride content. In extensive sweating, especially in a patient with fever, large amounts of water are lost. In addition, enough sodium and chloride loss occurs to produce total body deficits, sometimes of surprising degree. However, because of even more severe water deficit, the serum electrolyte values are normal or elevated.

In extensive burns, plasma and extracellular fluid leak into the damaged area in large quantities. If the affected area is extensive, hemoconcentration becomes noticeable and enough plasma may be withdrawn from the circulating blood volume to bring the patient close to or into shock. Plasma electrolytes accompany this loss from the circulation. The serum sodium level may be normal or decreased. If the patient is supported over the initial reaction period, fluid will begin to return to the circulation after about 48 hours. Therefore, after this time, fluid and electrolyte requirements should be much less, so as not to overload the circulation. Silver nitrate treatment for extensive burns may itself cause clinically significant hyponatremia (due to electrolyte diffusion into the hypotonic silver nitrate solution).

Role of Kidney in Electrolyte Physiology

Thus far, electrolyte disturbances have been relatively straightforward. In other common or well-recognized syndromes, abnormality is closely tied to the role of the kidney in water and electrolyte physiology. A brief résumé of current information on this subject may be helpful in understanding clinical situations discussed later.

Formation of urine begins with the glomerular filtrate, which is similar to plasma, except that plasma proteins are too large to pass the glomerular capillary membrane. In the *proximal convoluted tubules,* about 85% of filtered sodium is actively reabsorbed by the tubule cells. The exchange mechanism is thought to be located at the tubule cell border along the side opposite from the tubule lumen; sodium is thus actively pumped out of the tubule cell into the renal interstitial fluid. Sodium from the urine passively diffuses into the tubule cell to replace that which is pumped out. Chloride and water passively accompany sodium from the urine into the cell and from thence into the interstitial fluid. Most of the filtered potassium is also reabsorbed, probably by passive diffusion. At this time, some hydrogen ion (H^+) is actively secreted by tubule cells into the urine, but not to the extent that occurs farther down the nephron (electrolyte pathways and mechanisms are substantially less well known for the proximal tubules than for the distal tubules).

In the *ascending (thick) loop of Henle,* sodium is still actively reabsorbed, except that the tubule cells are now impermeable to water. Therefore, since water cannot accompany reabsorbed sodium and remains behind in the urine, the urine at this point becomes relatively hypotonic (the excess of water over what would have been present had water reabsorption continued is sometimes called "free water," and purely from a theoretical point of view is sometimes spoken of as though it were a separate entity, almost free from sodium and other ions).

In the *distal convoluted tubules,* three processes go on. (1) Sodium ions continue to be actively reabsorbed (in addition to the sodium pump located at the interstitial side of the cell, which is pushing sodium out into the interstitial fluid, another transport mechanism on the tubule lumen border now begins actively to extract sodium from the urine into the tubule cells). Intracellular hydrogen and potassium ions are actively excreted by the tubule cells into the urine in exchange for urinary sodium. There is competition between hydrogen and potassium for the same exchange pathway. However, since hydrogen ions are normally present in much greater quantities than potassium, most of the ions excreted into the urine are hydrogen. (2) The urinary acidification mechanisms other than bicarbonate reabsorption ($NaHPO_4$ and NH_3) are operable here. (3) Distal tubule cells are able to allow reabsorption of water in a selective fashion. Permeability of the distal tubule cell to water is altered by a mechanism under the influence of antidiuretic hormone (ADH). There is a limit in possible quantity of water reabsorbed, because reabsorption is passive; ADH simply acts on cell membrane permeability, controlling the ease of diffusion. Therefore, only "free water" (the theoretical excess of hypotonic water from isotonic urine) is actually reabsorbed.

In the *collecting tubules,* the tubular membrane is likewise under the control of ADH. Therefore, any "free water" not reabsorbed in the distal convoluted tubules plus water that constitutes actual urine could theoretically be passively reabsorbed here. However, three factors act to control the actual quantity reabsorbed: first, the state of hydration of the tubule cells and renal medulla in general, which determines the osmotic gradient toward which any reabsorbed water must travel; second, the total water reabsorption capacity of the collecting tubules, which is limited to about 5% of normal glomerular filtrate, and third, the amount of "free water" reabsorbed in the distal convoluted tubules, which helps determine the total quantity of water reaching the collecting tubules.

Whether collecting tubule reabsorption capacity will be exceeded and, if so, to what degree, is naturally dependent on the total quantity of water available. The amount of water reabsorbed compared to degree of dilution (hypotonicity) of urine reaching the collecting tubules determines the degree of final urine concentration.

Effect of Adrenal Cortex Dysfunction

Certain adrenal cortex hormones control sodium retention and potassium excretion. Aldosterone is the most powerful, but cortisone and hydrocortisone do have some effect. In *Addison's disease* there exists a state of adrenocortical insufficiency, so that normal sodium-retaining influences on the kidney are lacking. Usually there is enough just barely to maintain sodium balance; however, when placed under stress of any type, the remaining adrenal cortex cells cannot give a normal hormone response and prevent development of a critical situation. The so-called crisis of Addison's disease is simply the result of overwhelming fluid and salt loss from the kidneys, and responds to replacement. Serum sodium and chloride levels are low, serum potassium is usually high normal or elevated and the patient is markedly dehydrated. The CO_2 content (or combining power) may be normal or may be slightly decreased due to the mild acidosis that accompanies severe dehydration. In the syndrome *primary aldosteronism* there is oversecretion of aldosterone leading to sodium retention and, therefore, potassium loss. The serum potassium value is low and the serum sodium is often mildly elevated, although a substantial minority of patients have serum sodium values within normal range. For some reason, the low potassium levels do not seem to cause symptoms as severe as those in other, more acute types of hypokalemia, and the main clinical symptom of this disease is hypertension. Sodium retention usually is not sufficient to produce edema. In *Cushing's syndrome* there is overproduction of hydrocortisone, which in some cases may lead to hypokalemia and/or hypernatremia. If this occurs, however, it usually is mild, and the patient does not have clinical symptoms directly referable to serum electrolyte abnormalities. Hypertension is fairly common in Cushing's syndrome.

Dilutional Syndromes

In cirrhosis, hyponatremia and hypokalemia are frequent, separately or concurrently. There are a variety of etiologies: ascitic fluid sequestration; attempts at diuresis, often superimposed on poor diet or sodium restriction; paracentesis therapy, and hemodilution. Electrolyte abnormalities are more likely to appear when ascites is present, and to become most severe if azotemia complicates liver disease. Hemodilution is a frequent finding in cirrhosis, especially with ascites; this may be due to increased activity of aldosterone, which is normally deactivated in the liver, or sometimes is attributable to "inappropriate" secretion of ADH.

Congestive heart failure is frequently associated with hyponatremia (and, much less frequently, hypokalemia). The most frequent cause of hyponatremia is overtreatment with diuretic therapy, usually in the presence of dietary sodium restriction. However, sometimes the hyponatremia may be dilutional, due to retention of water as glomerular filtration rate is decreased by heart failure or by "inappropriate" secretion of ADH. If hypokalemia is present, it usually is a side effect of diuretics.

Iatrogenic electrolyte disturbances most often result in decreased concentration of one or more serum electrolyte values. This may be due to treatment administered by a physician, or to conscious or unconscious attempts at therapy by the patient or relatives. For example, marked sweating leads to thirst; ingestion of large quantities of water alone would dilute body fluid sodium, already depleted, even further. A baby with diarrhea may be treated at home with water or sugar water; this replaces water without adequate replacement of electrolytes and has the same dilutional effect as in the preceding example. On the other hand, the infant may be given boiled skimmed milk or soup, which are high-sodium preparations; the result may be hypernatremia if fluid intake is not adequate. On the physician's side, the effects of excessive diuretic therapy have been mentioned. Probably even more common is dilutional hyponatremia induced by intravenous infusion of electrolyte-free solutions such as 5% dextrose in water. Superimposed on inadequate oral intake or previous deficits, this may have a dilutional effect. If renal water excretion is impaired, normal maintenance fluid quantities may lead to dilution, whereas excessive infusions may produce actual water intoxication or pulmonary edema. There may also be problems when excessive losses of fluid or various electrolytes occur for any reason and replacement therapy is attempted but either is not adequate or is excessive. The net result of any of the situations mentioned is a fluid and/or electrolyte problem, which must be carefully and logically reasoned out, beginning from the primary deficit (the etiology of which may still be active) and proceeding through subsequent events. Adequate records of fluid and electrolyte administration are valuable in solving the problem.

Recognition of dilutional syndromes is often difficult. Three laboratory procedures may be of help. The first is a plasma volume determination, most often done using albumin tagged with ^{131}I (RISA). The second is a serum water determination. Serum water value elevation in the presence of normal plasma protein levels is good evidence in favor of a dilutional syndrome. Measurement of substances that are relatively constant in blood, such as hemoglobin, total protein or creatinine, may be useful to indicate hemodilution or concentration. These are most helpful when previous baseline values exist. An obvious drawback is that values for any serum constituent may change due to disease rather than from water shifts.

Speaking of iatrogenic dilutional syndromes, it should be mentioned that the normal physiologic response to surgery is that of moderate fluid and electrolyte retention. In the first 24 hours after surgery there tends to be decreased urine output, with fluid and electrolytes remaining in the body that would normally be excreted. Because of this, care should be taken not to overload the circulation with too much intravenous fluid on the first postoperative day. Incidentally, in certain patients such as those undergoing extensive surgical procedures and those admitted originally for other problems, it is often useful to have preoperative serum electrolyte values so that subsequent electrolyte problems can be better evaluated.

Inappropriate Antidiuretic Hormone Secretion

Antidiuretic hormone (ADH) has been mentioned as one regulator of plasma volume, via its action on renal distal tubule water reabsorption. It is produced by the posterior pituitary under control of the hypothalamus. Several factors influence ADH production: blood osmotic changes (concentration and dilution, acting on osmoreceptors in the hypothalamus), blood volume changes, certain neural influences such as pain and certain drugs, such as morphine and alcohol. Lack or insufficient production of ADH leads to the syndrome known as diabetes insipidus. Water cannot be retained normally by the kidney; a continual diuresis of dilute urine is produced, and marked dehydration results. Pitressin given parenterally corrects the defect. Another syndrome involving ADH is now being well recognized, although it is not frequent. This is so-called inappropriate secretion of ADH, or "inappropriate ADH" (IADH). Basically, this syndrome results from water retention by ADH in situations in which one would not expect ADH to be secreted. The criteria for IADH syndrome include hyponatremia with serum hypo-osmolality; continued renal excretion of sodium despite hyponatremia; urine osmolality that shows a significant degree of concentration (instead of the maximally dilute urine one would expect), and no evidence of blood volume depletion. In other words, ADH is secreted despite hemodilution and/or decreased serum osmolality. The reason for increased sodium excretion is not definitely known; it is thought that increase of interstitial fluid volume by water retention may lead to suppression of sodium reabsorption (in order not to reabsorb even more water). Blood volume often is in normal range (since sodium is not retained), and there usually is no edema (since interstitial fluid expansion usually is only moderate).

In diagnosing IADH a problem may arise concerning what urine osmolality value qualifies as a significant degree of concentration. If the serum and urine specimens are obtained "together" and if the serum demonstrates significant hyponatremia and hypo-osmolality, a urine osmolality value greater than that of the serum specimen would be considered more concentrated than usual. However, in some cases of IADH the urine does not necessarily have to possess higher osmolality than the serum if it can be demonstrated that water retention is taking place despite a hypotonic plasma. Also, since some patients with IADH may have low urine sodium levels due to low body intake of sodium, the diagnosis of IADH may be assisted by administering a test dose of sodium. In IADH, infusion of saline does not correct the hyponatremia; most of the sodium will appear in the urine as long as the patient does not restrict fluids (fluid restriction will cause sodium retention in IADH). Water restriction is the treatment of choice.

This syndrome in its classic form has been reported mainly in some cases of intracranial injury or cerebral infection, and in a few patients with bronchogenic carcinoma (especially the undifferentiated "oat cell" type).

There are, however, somewhat more frequent situations that have many features of IADH without its classic syndrome. The dilutional hyponatremia of cirrhosis and congestive heart failure may sometimes be of this type, although usually other mechanisms can better account for hyponatremia, such as overuse of diuretics. However, in some cases, IADH seems to contribute; these patients differ from those with the classic IADH syndrome in that edema is often present, and the urine contains very little sodium. In other words, the main feature is water retention with dilutional hyponatremia. This has been called the "refractory dilutional syndrome"; treatment with sodium can be dangerous; therapy consists of water restriction.

Tired Cell Syndrome

Another syndrome involving hyponatremia is without any really good explanation, although here again IADH may contribute in part. These persons have a chronic wasting illness such as carcinomatosis, chronic malnutrition or simple old age. Serum sodium levels are mildly or moderately decreased. As a rule, these persons do not have symptoms from their hyponatremia and seem to have physiologically adjusted to the lower serum level. Treatment with salt does not raise the serum values. Apparently the only cure is to improve the patient's state of nutrition, especially his body protein, which takes considerable time and difficulty. This situation has been called the "tired cell syndrome."

Laboratory Investigation of Hyponatremia

Laboratory tests frequently cannot provide a clear-cut etiology for hyponatremia. Urine sodium determination helps detect hyponatremia owing to renal salt loss, whether from intrinsic kidney disease or from diuretics (if the effect of diuretic therapy on the kidney is still present). These patients should have urine sodium concentrations over 20 mEq/L. "Simultaneous" serum and urine osmolalities can segregate those with IADH syndrome. If the patient has hyponatremia and low urine sodium, and in addition displays clinical edema, hemodilution is the most probable diagnosis. Laboratory indicators for hemodilution are noted on page 287, but provide best information if the episode of hyponatremia is acute and if the test had been done prior to onset of hyponatremia so that the normal state for the measurement would be available for comparison. Subject to this drawback, measurement of hematocrit (or hemoglobin) and total protein may be useful. Hematocrit and total protein which are elevated from previous values in the presence of hyponatremia suggest sodium depletion. Hyponatremia plus hematocrit and total protein which are decreased from previous values is more suggestive of hemodilution. In this situation, decrease in plasma proteins is not as reliable as hematocrit, due to the frequency of albumin decrease in many severe illnesses. In the case of decreased hematocrit, occult bleeding must be ruled out. Serum water determination (p. 456) is another possible aid if plasma proteins are not altered by disease. Increase of hematocrit and plasma proteins, especially when accompanied by hypernatremia, suggests water deficit. Plasma volume determination (p. 104) is the most accurate way to prove dilution or dehydration, but may not be available.

SERUM POTASSIUM ABNORMALITIES

The situation with abnormal potassium values is in many respects comparable to that of sodium (Table 24–2). Some of these situations are also tied to sodium and were discussed earlier. These include diabetic acidosis with treatment, adrenal diseases such as primary aldosteronism and Addison's disease, certain cardiac problems and the effect of diuretics, particularly the chlorothiazide group. Hypokalemia is frequent in cirrhosis. There are, likewise, similarities in that dilution with potassium-free fluids such as glucose water or saline may lead to potassium deficit. Besides the effect of outright dilution, there is in addition an element of continued renal loss. The kidney is apparently set up best to conserve sodium and to excrete potassium (since one way to conserve sodium is to excrete potassium ions in exchange), so that when normal intake of potassium stops, it takes time for the kidney to adjust and stop losing normal amounts of potassium ions. In the meantime, a deficit may be created. The potentiality for gastrointestinal hypokalemia should be mentioned again. Although potassium is present in GI tract secretions only in relatively small amounts, with continued loss of these secretions the body will eventually lose enough potassium to require replacement. This is especially true in diarrhea.

Hypokalemia has a close relationship to alkalosis. Increased plasma pH (alkalosis) results from decreased extracellular fluid H^+ concentration; the extracellular fluid deficit draws hydrogen from body cells, leading to decreased intracellular concentration and therefore less H^+ available in renal tubule cells for exchange with urinary sodium. This means increased potassium excretion in exchange for urinary sodium, and eventual hypokalemia. Besides being produced by alkalosis, hypokalemia can itself lead to alkalosis—or, at least, a tendency toward alkalosis. Hypokalemia results from depletion of intracellular potassium (the largest body store of potassium). Hydrogen ion diffuses into body cells to replace partially the intracellular cation deficit caused by potassium deficiency; this tends to deplete extracellular fluid hydrogen levels. In addition, more hydrogen is excreted into the urine in exchange for sodium, since the potassium that normally would participate in this exchange is no longer available. Both mechanisms tend eventually to deplete extracellular fluid hydrogen. As noted in

TABLE 24-2.—CLINICAL SITUATIONS COMMONLY
ASSOCIATED WITH SERUM POTASSIUM ABNORMALITIES

Hypokalemia
1. Inadequate intake (cachexia or severe illness of any type)
2. Intravenous infusion of potassium-free fluids
3. Protracted vomiting
4. Renal loss (primary aldosteronism; diuretics)
5. Treatment of diabetic acidosis without potassium supplements
6. Treatment with large doses of ACTH or cortisone
7. Cirrhosis

Hyperkalemia
1. Renal failure with oliguria ("renal shutdown")

Chapter 23, in alkalosis due to hypokalemia an acid urine is produced, contrary to the usual situation in alkalosis. This incongruity is due to the intracellular acidosis that results from hypokalemia.

High potassium values are found in relatively few diseases. Of these, the only common situation is renal shutdown with failure to produce adequate urine quantities and therefore inability to excrete enough potassium.

Serum calcium is an important body electrolyte that is covered further in Chapter 30. A list of the most common diseases associated with disorders of calcium metabolism has been included there, along with typical laboratory findings.

CLINICAL AND LABORATORY FINDINGS IN ELECTROLYTE IMBALANCE

Before concluding this material, it might be useful to describe some of the clinical symptoms of electrolyte imbalance. Interestingly enough, they are very similar for low sodium, low potassium and high potassium. They include muscle weakness, nausea, anorexia and mental changes, which usually tend toward drowsiness and lethargy. The ECG in hypokalemia is very characteristic, and with serum values below 3.0 mEq/L usually shows depression of the S-T segment and flattening or actual inversion of the T wave. In hyperkalemia the opposite happens; the T wave becomes high and peaked; this usually begins with serum potassium values over 7.0 mEq/L (normal values being 4.0 – 5.5 mEq/L). One final note on hypokalemia — potassium antagonizes the action of digitalis, and hypokalemia may allow digitalis toxicity with doses that would ordinarily be nontoxic. Conversely, very high concentrations of potassium are toxic to the heart, so that intravenous infusions should never give more than 20.0 mEq/hour even with good renal function.

In the clinical laboratory, the four commonly used "electrolyte" determinations include serum sodium, chloride, CO_2 and potassium. Serum chlorides have not been specifically mentioned because, in general, they follow the serum sodium (except in a few situations such as the hyperchloremic alkalosis of vomiting). Usually it is sufficient to get all four of these test results initially and after that to follow only the important ones, namely sodium and potassium. If the initial CO_2 is normal (or close to it), there usually is no need to keep reordering it unless something specific is in mind. Serum chloride levels, as mentioned, usually parallel the sodium levels and are useful mainly as a rough check on the sodium values. Therefore, chlorides also can generally be omitted or only spot-checked after the initial values are received. It usually is not necessary to get repeat determinations on chloride or CO_2 except in special circumstances or when the initial CO_2 is markedly abnormal.

SERUM AND URINE OSMOLALITY. — This may assist in diagnosis of certain fluid and electrolyte problems. Osmolality (p. 134) is the measurement of the number of osmotically active particles in a solution. It is determined by the degree of induced freezing point change in a special machine. Units are milliosmoles (mOsm) per liter of water. Therefore, osmolality depends not only on the quantity of solute particles but also on the quantity of water in which they are dissolved. Sodium is by far the major constituent of serum osmolality. Plasma proteins have little osmotic activity and are essentially noncontributory to serum osmolality. Serum (or plasma) osmolality may be estimated from the formula $mOsm = (1.86 \times sodium) + \dfrac{BS}{18} + \dfrac{BUN}{2.8} + 5$, with blood sugar (BS) and blood urea nitrogen (BUN) in mg/100 ml and Na (sodium) in mEq/L. A quick approximation is $2Na + \dfrac{BS}{20} + \dfrac{BUN}{3}$. Normal adult range is 275–300 mOsm. The ratio of serum sodium concentration to serum osmolality (Na/Osm) is normally 0.43–0.50.

Decreased serum osmolality is almost always caused by hyponatremia. Therefore, low serum sodium levels are most often accompanied by low osmolality in dilution syndromes, salt (without water) depletion and the tired cell syndrome. Some patients lose salt and water concurrently; some of the extracellular water loss is replaced from intracellular water, with the final result being a relative sodium deficit. The effect of serum sodium dilution on serum osmolality may be counterbalanced to some degree by the presence of dehydration. In hyponatremia without coincident increase in the other solutes, the Na/Osm ratio is said to be normal (i.e., there is a decrease both in sodium and osmolality). An appreciable minority of patients with hyponatremia have osmolality in the normal range. Some of these patients may be dehydrated; others may have cardiac, renal or hepatic disease. These diseases characteristically reduce the Na/Osm ratio, this being partially attributed to the effects of increased blood sugar, urea or unknown metabolic substances. Especially in uremia, osmolality changes cannot always be accounted for by effects of BUN alone. Patients in shock may develop disproportionately elevated measured osmolality compared to calculated osmolality; again, this points toward circulating metabolic products. Besides elevating osmolality, these substances displace a certain amount of sodium from serum, thus lowering sodium levels. One milliequivalent of sodium will be displaced by each 35 mg/100 ml blood sugar or each 5 mg/100 ml BUN increase over normal limits. Elevated serum lipids will also displace sodium, but without elevating osmolality.

Increased osmolality may be produced by water deficit (dehydration), sodium overload, hyperglycemia, uremia, unknown metabolic products, or various drugs or chemicals, especially ethyl alcohol. The difference between calculated and measured osmolality gives a clue to the presence of unusual solutes. Many substances do not affect osmolality; those which do are potentially dialyzable. Osmolality is one of the criteria for diagnosis of hyperosmolar nonketotic acidosis and of the IADH syndrome. Renal dialysis units may determine osmolality of the dialysis bath solution to help verify that electrolyte composition is within acceptable limits.

REFERENCES

Agarwal, B. N. and Agarwal, P.: Magnesium deficiency in clinical medicine: A review, J. Am. Med. Wom. Assoc. 31:72, 1976.

Boyd, D. R., and Baker, R. J.: Osmometry: A new bedside laboratory aid for the management of surgical patients, Surg. Clin. North Am. 51:241, 1971.

Butcher, H. R., Jr.: The pathophysiology of sodium depletion in man, Surg. Clin. North Am. 45:345, 1965.

Emmett, M., and Narins, R. G.: Clinical use of the anion gap, Medicine 56:38, 1977.

Epstein, F. H., et al.: Cerebral hyponatremia, N. Engl. J. Med. 265:513, 1961.

Finkel, R. M.: Hyponatremia, Med. Clin. North Am. 56:645, 1972.

Goldberger, E.: *A Primer of Water, Electrolyte, and Acid-Base Syndromes* (3d ed.; Philadelphia: Lea & Febiger, 1965).

Leaf, A.: The clinical and physiologic significance of the serum sodium concentration, N. Engl. J. Med. 267:24, 77, 1962.

Lindeman, R. D.: Hypokalemia: Causes, consequences, and correction, Am. J. Med. Sci. 272:5, 1976.

Lindeman, R. D., and Papper, S.: Therapy of fluid and electrolyte disorders, Ann. Intern. Med. 82:64, 1975.

Lobdell, D. H.: Freezing-point osmometry – Simple and valuable procedure, Lab. Med. 1:43, 1970.

Mansberger, A. R., et al.: Refractometry and osmometry in clinical surgery, Ann. Surg. 169:672, 1969.

Martin, H. E., et al.: Fluid and electrolyte therapy of severe diabetic acidosis and ketosis, Am. J. Med. 24:376, 1958.

Mena, I.: The role of manganese in human disease, Ann. Clin. Lab. Sci. 4:487, 1974.

Mendoza, S. A.: Syndrome of inappropriate antidiuretic hormone secretion (SIADH), Pediatr. Clin. North Am. 23:681, 1976.

Parenteral water and electrolyte solutions, Med. Lett. Drugs Ther. 12:77, 1970.

Randall, H. T.: Fluid, electrolyte, and acid-base balance, Surg. Clin. North Am. 56:1019, 1976.

Scheiner, E., et al.: Water and electrolyte disturbances in cancer patients, Med. Clin. North Am. 50:711, 1966.

Sunderman, F. W., Jr.: Current status of zinc deficiency in the pathogenesis of neurological, dermatological and musculoskeletal disorders, Ann. Clin. Lab. Sci. 5:132, 1975.

Takasu, T., et al.: Hyponatremia in congestive heart failure, Ann. Intern. Med. 55:368, 1961.

Whang, R.: Hyperkalemia: Diagnosis and treatment, Am. J. Med. Sci. 272:19, 1976.

25 / Diagnosis of Malabsorption

THE FUNCTION OF THE GASTROINTESTINAL TRACT is to perform certain mechanical and enzymatic procedures on food and then to absorb necessary constituents into the bloodstream and excrete the remainder. When the usual dietary constituents are not absorbed normally, symptoms may develop that form part of the syndrome known as malabsorption (Table 25–1). There are three basic types of malabsorption. The first concerns the interruption of one of the stages in fat absorption (indicated in Table 25–1 by I, II and III); this primarily concerns fat absorption and also those substances dependent on the presence of lipid. Another broad category is intrinsic defect of the small bowel mucosa, listed in the classification as IV, A–D. This type shows interference with not only fat and fat-soluble substances but also carbohydrates and many other materials. The third category is represented by IV, E and also by the deficiency disease called pernicious anemia. In these cases, lack of one specific substance normally produced by the gastrointestinal tract leads to malabsorption of other substances dependent on this substance for absorption.

CLINICAL AND LABORATORY FINDINGS

Steatorrhea, meaning the appearance of excess quantities of fat in the stool, is a frequent manifestation of most of the malabsorption syndromes from most causes. Many patients with steatorrhea also have diarrhea, but the two are not synonymous; a patient can have steatorrhea without diarrhea. In children, the principal diseases associated with steatorrhea and malabsorption are celiac disease and cystic fibrosis of the pancreas. In adults, the most common causes are tropical sprue, nontropical sprue (the adult form of celiac disease) and pancreatic insufficiency. The clinical picture is roughly similar for all these diseases, but varies according to cause, severity and duration. The most common chief complaints of severe malabsorption, in general, are diarrhea and weakness, weight loss and mild functional gastrointestinal complaints (anorexia, nausea, mild abdominal pain). Physical findings and laboratory results tend to differ with the various etiologies. In severe cases of sprue tetany, bone pain, tongue surface atrophy and even bleeding may be found. Physical examination may show abdominal distention and also peripheral edema in nearly half the patients. In pancreatic insufficiency, physical examination may be normal or show malnutrition. Neurologic symptoms are found with moderate frequency in pernicious anemia, but may be present with other etiologies. Laboratory findings vary according to severity and etiology, but in

TABLE 25-1.—CLASSIFICATION OF MALABSORPTIVE
DISORDERS (WITH COMMENTS ON OCCURRENCE AND
ASSOCIATED ABNORMALITIES)

I. Inadequate mixing of food with bile salts and lipase. Mild chemical
steatorrhea common, but clinical steatorrhea uncommon. Actual diarrhea
uncommon. Anemia in approximately 15–35%; most often iron deficiency,
rarely megaloblastic
  A. Pyloroplasty
  B. Subtotal and total gastrectomy (occasional megaloblastic anemias reported)
  C. Gastrojejunostomy
II. Inadequate lipolysis—lack of lipase or normal stimulation of pancreatic
secretion. Steatorrhea only in far-advanced pancreatic destruction, and
diarrhea even less often
  A. Cystic fibrosis of the pancreas
  B. Chronic pancreatitis
  C. Cancer of the pancreas or ampulla of Vater
  D. Pancreatic fistula
  E. Severe protein deficiency
  F. Vagus nerve section
III. Inadequate emulsification of fat—lack of bile salts. Clinical steatorrhea
uncommon, sometimes occurs in very severe cases. Usually no diarrhea
  A. Obstructive jaundice
  B. Severe liver disease
IV. Primary absorptive defect—small bowel
  A. Inadequate length of normal absorptive surface. Unusual complication of
surgery
    1. Surgical resection
    2. Internal fistula
    3. Gastroileostomy
  B. Obstruction of mesenteric lymphatics (rare)
    1. Lymphoma
    2. Hodgkin's disease
    3. Carcinoma
    4. Whipple's disease
    5. Intestinal tuberculosis
  C. Inadequate absorptive surface due to extensive mucosal disease. Except
for *Giardia* infection and regional enteritis, most of these diseases are
uncommon. Steatorrhea only if there is extensive bowel involvement
    1. Inflammatory
      a) Tuberculosis
      b) Regional enteritis or enterocolitis (diarrhea very common)
      c) *Giardia lamblia* infection (diarrhea common; malabsorption rare)
    2. Neoplastic
    3. Amyloid disease
    4. Scleroderma
    5. Pseudomembranous enterocolitis (diarrhea frequent)
    6. Radiation injury
    7. Pneumatosis cystoides intestinalis
  D. Biochemical dysfunction of mucosal cells
    1. "Gluten-induced" (steatorrhea and diarrhea very common)
      a) Celiac disease (childhood)
      b) Nontropical sprue (adult)

(table continued)

TABLE 25-1.—*Continued*

    2. Enzymatic defect

        a) Disaccharide malabsorption (diarrhea frequent symptom)

        b) Pernicious anemia (deficiency of "gastric" intrinsic factor)

    3. Cause unknown. Uncommon except for tropical sprue (which is common only in the tropics)

        a) Tropical sprue (diarrhea and steatorrhea common)

        b) Severe starvation

        c) Diabetic visceral neuropathy

        d) Endocrine and metabolic disorder (e.g., hypothyroidism)

        e) Zollinger-Ellison syndrome (diarrhea common; steatorrhea may be present)

        f) Miscellaneous

  E. Malabsorption associated with altered bacterial flora (diarrhea fairly common)

    1. Small intestinal blind loops, diverticula, anastomoses (rare)

    2. Drug (oral antibiotic) administration (infrequent but not rare)

---

sprue most often include one or more of the following: anemia, steatorrhea, hypoproteinemia, hypocalcemia and hypoprothrombinemia. In pancreatic insufficiency, the main abnormalities are steatorrhea and decreased carbohydrate tolerance (sometimes overt diabetes). In pernicious anemia the patient has only anemia without diarrhea, steatorrhea or the other test abnormalities. The majority of stomach operations do not cause diarrhea or abnormalities of fat absorption.

Steatorrhea is due to excess excretion of fat in the stools from inability to absorb lipids. Anemia is most often macrocytic, but sometimes is caused by iron deficiency or is a mixed type due to various degrees of deficiency of folic acid, vitamin B_{12} and iron. Calcium may be deficient because of gastrointestinal loss due to diarrhea. Prothrombin formation by the liver is often impaired in various degrees because of lack of vitamin K. This is a fat-soluble vitamin that is produced by bacteria in the small bowel. Long-term oral antibiotics may reduce the bacterial flora by killing these bacteria and thus interfere with vitamin K formation; inability to absorb fat will secondarily prevent vitamin K and vitamin A, which are dependent on fat solubility for intestinal absorption, from entering the bloodstream. Malnutrition resulting from lack of fat and carbohydrate absorption leads to hypoproteinemia, mainly secondary to lack of normal production of albumin by the liver. This also contributes to the peripheral edema that many patients show.

Generally speaking, the patients usually present in one of two ways. In the first group the major finding on admission is anemia, and once malabsorption is suspected, either by the finding of megaloblastic bone marrow changes or by other symptoms or signs suggestive of malabsorption, the problem becomes one of differentiating between pernicious anemia and other types of malabsorption. In the second group, the patient presents with one or more clinical symptoms of malabsorption, either mild or marked in severity; the diagnosis has to be firmly established and the etiology investigated. There are several basic tests for malabsorption which, if used intelligently, usually can lead to the diagnosis and in some cases to the cause.

FECAL FAT. — *Qualitative fecal fat* may be stained by Sudan III dye, whereby neutral fat will appear as bright orange droplets. The fatty acids normally do not stain. These fatty acids and the original neutral fat may then be converted to stainable fatty acids by heat and acid hydrolysis. The preparation is then stained and examined a second time to determine if the droplets are increased from the first examination. The reliability of this type of procedure is debated in the literature, but it seems fairly accurate if the technician is experienced. Naturally, there will be difficulty in distinguishing normal results from only low-grade degrees of steatorrhea. It is possible to get some idea of etiology by estimating the amount of neutral fat vs fatty acid; lack of fatty acid suggests pancreatic disease.

The basic diagnostic test for presence of steatorrhea is *quantitative fecal fat*. Stool collections are taken over a minimum of 3 full days. The patient should be on a diet containing approximately 50 – 150 gm fat a day (average 100 gm) beginning 2 days before the test collection. It is necessary to make sure that the patient is actually eating enough of this diet to take in at least 50 gm of fat a day; it is also obviously important to make sure that all the stools are collected and the patient is not incontinent of feces. If the patient has constipation, which some do have, it may be necessary to use a bedtime laxative. Normal diet results in an average excretion of less than 7 gm fat/24 hours; 5–7 gm/24 hours is equivocal, since many patients with minimal steatorrhea and a small but significant percentage of normal persons fall into this range. Finally, it should be noted that some patients with partial or complete malabsorption syndromes may have normal fecal fat excretion. This seems most common in tropical sprue.

PLASMA CAROTENE. — Carotene is the fat-soluble precursor of vitamin A and is adequately present in most normal diets that contain green or yellow vegetables. Normal values are considered 70–300 μg/100 ml; 30–70 μg/100 ml are usually considered moderately decreased levels, and less than 30 μg/100 ml means severe depletion. Other causes of low plasma carotene, besides malabsorption, are poor diet, severe liver disease and high fever. There is considerable overlap between carotene values in malabsorption and in normal control patients, but this usually is over the 30-μg level. However, this test is valuable mostly as a screening procedure.

X-RAY EXAMINATION. — A "small bowel series" is done by letting barium pass into the small intestine. There are several changes in the normal radiologic appearance of the small bowel that are suggestive of malabsorption. These changes appear in 70–90% of patients, depending on the severity of disease, the etiology and the particular investigator. The radiologic literature agrees that many chronic diseases, especially when associated with fever and cachexia, may cause an interference with digestion of such severity as to produce a pattern that may be confused with sprue. Secondary malabsorption cannot be distinguished from primary unless it is due to certain rare causes such as tumor. The so-called diagnostic patterns of sprue are thus characteristic of, but not specific for, primary small intestine absorption, and are not present in probably 20% of the patients.

RADIOISOTOPE TECHNIQUES. — To test for fat malabsorption, a neutral fat named triolein combining glycerol and fatty acid has been tagged with ^{131}I. It is also possible to tag a simple fatty acid such as oleic acid with ^{131}I. This radioactive fat can be administered in several ways, usually as a capsule or as part of a fatty meal. After a certain period, a specimen of blood can be drawn and measured for radioactivity. The stool also can be measured for radioactivity, with either procedure giving an idea of how much fat was either absorbed or rejected by the intestinal mucosa. In malabsorption due to pancreatic disease, radioactive fatty acid (oleic acid) is absorbed normally, but not radioactive neutral fat (triolein). In primary small bowel malabsorption, both types of fat show abnormal absorption. There have been many reports on this subject. The main problem with the test is a technical one, and this concerns the way the radioactive fat is administered. Apparently results differ quite markedly according to whether the radiosotope is given as a capsule or as an integral part of a fatty meal, and even the type of fatty vehicle has some influence on absorption. This test is promising but is not yet standardized. At present, it is probably better to avoid using radioactive fat techniques, since the same information generally can be obtained in other ways and the accuracy of these procedures is open to considerable question.

SCHILLING TEST. — Pernicious anemia is an interesting disease in which a combination of specific (anatomical) lesions and factor deficiency lead to a characteristic clinical picture. This has been discussed more fully in Chapter 2. Briefly, pernicious anemia patients have atrophic gastritis, a complete lack of gastric hydrochloric acid (anacidity, p. 303) and a partial or complete deficiency of so-called intrinsic factor. This is produced by the stomach and is necessary for the absorption of vitamin B_{12}, which normally takes place in the ileum. Laboratory findings vary according to the duration and severity of the disease, but classically consist of a macrocytic anemia in which the average red cell size is slightly larger than normal; a megaloblastic bone marrow in which the normal red cell series is distorted into a peculiar appearance that is characteristic and is called megaloblastic change, and often by secondary abnormality in the white cells and platelets leading to low blood levels (leukopenia and thrombocytopenia) and mature neutrophil hypersegmentation. In true pernicious anemia, oral administration of usual dietary amounts of vitamin B_{12} ($1-2$ μg/day) will have no measurable effect on the clinical course or the hematologic picture. A few patients will respond to a dose of as little as 5 μg and nearly all to 100 μg, presumably by the effect of mass action on the small intestine mucosa despite intrinsic factor deficiency.

The Schilling test consists of oral administration of 0.5 μg of vitamin B_{12}, that has been tagged with radioactive cobalt. At the same time, 1,000 μg of nonisotopic vitamin B_{12} is given intramuscularly to saturate tissue-binding sites and to allow a portion of any labeled B_{12} absorbed from the intestine to be excreted or flushed out into the urine. In the normal person, approximately 33% of the absorbed radioactive B_{12} will thus appear in the urine and the total normal 24-hour urinary excretion is $8-40\%$ of the original oral dose. Since poor renal function may delay excretion, a 48-hour collection may be necessary if the blood urea nitrogen (BUN) is elevated. Normal

48-hour values are the same as those for 24 hours. In classic pernicious anemia, the Schilling test will have a positive result, i.e., less than 8% urinary excretion of the radioisotope for 24 hours, if no intrinsic factor has been given with the test dose. The test is then completely repeated after 3 days, using adequate amounts of intrinsic factor. It will then show normal values, since the added intrinsic factor will now allow normal vitamin B_{12} absorption.

The Schilling test, with and without intrinsic factor, is extremely helpful in distinguishing pernicious anemia from various other malabsorption syndromes, which may show part or all of the classic pernicious anemia clinical and laboratory findings. A considerable number of patients with sprue and a few with some of the other malabsorption diseases may have positive Schilling test results without intrinsic factor, but B_{12} malabsorption will not be corrected by the addition of intrinsic factor. This differential procedure is especially helpful because other laboratory tests may be confusing. For example, some patients with primary malabsorption may fail to have steatorrhea, and some may have anacidity, especially in the older age groups. In fact, about 30% of normal patients over age 70 apparently do not produce hydrochloric acid. Finally, occasional patients with classic pernicious anemia also show the impaired absorptive function test results that one would expect in other malabsorption syndromes. The Schilling test can thus be very helpful and, incidentally, can be done even if the patient already has been started on treatment, as long as intrinsic factor is not being given.

One additional caution: some pernicious anemia patients may exhibit abnormal Schilling test results with added intrinsic factor, but then revert to a typical normal absorption response with intrinsic factor after treatment with parenteral vitamin B_{12}.

False positive tests (false low values) may be produced by incomplete urine collection (normal output is greater than 600 ml/24 hours and usually is over 800 ml). Measurement of urine creatinine excretion is also helpful as a check on complete collection. Some laboratories routinely collect two consecutive 24-hour urine specimens, since the initial 24-hour collection may be incomplete, and vitamin B_{12} excretion during the second 24 hours may be sufficient to bring total 48-hour excretion to normal range. A second nonisotopic vitamin B_{12} injection is administered 24 hours after the first, since this has been shown to increase B_{12} excretion during the second 24 hours. If the first 24-hour excretion gives normal results, the second can be discontinued. False normal results are much less of a problem than false positive, but may be caused by fecal contamination of the urine.

If a bone marrow aspiration to document megaloblastic change is contemplated, it should be performed before the Schilling test. The nonisotopic B_{12} parenteral "flushing dose" will quickly convert the megaloblastic changes to normal.

D-XYLOSE TEST.—Besides quantitative (fecal) fat studies, the most important test for malabsorption is the D-xylose test. Rather than a screening test for malabsorption per se, it is a test that identifies the sprue-type diseases and differentiates them from other malabsorption etiologies. Originally, an oral glucose tolerance test was used in malabsorption, since it was found that most patients with sprue showed a flat curve. However, some patients with obvious malabsorption had a normal curve, and it was also found in several large series that up to 20% of normal patients had a so-called flat curve, so this test was abandoned. D-Xylose is a pentose isomer that is absorbed in much the same manner as glucose from the jejunum. The standard test dose is 25 gm D-xylose in 250 ml water, followed by another 250 ml water. The patient is fasted overnight, since xylose absorption is delayed by other food. After the test dose, the patient is kept at bed rest for 5 hours without food. The normal person's peak blood levels are reached in approximately 2 hours and fall to fasting levels in approximately 5 hours. Xylose is excreted mostly in the urine with approximately 80–95% of the excretion in the first 5 hours and the remainder in 24 hours. Side effects of the oral xylose are mild diarrhea and abdominal discomfort in a small number of patients. Normal values for (2-hour) blood xylose levels are over 25 mg/100 ml; 20–25 mg/100 ml is equivocal, and less than 20 mg/100 ml is strongly suggestive of malabsorption. The 5-hour urine xylose normal values are greater than 5 gm; 4–5 gm is equivocal, and less than 4 gm is suggestive of malabsorption. Values for 24-hour urine collection are normally greater than 5 gm. It is obviously very important to make sure that the urine collection is complete and that there is no fecal contamination of the urine. A catheter may have to be used if the patient is incontinent of urine or if there is a question of fecal contamination, but catheterization should be avoided if at all possible. Two main physiologic circumstances may affect the 5-hour urinary excretion—renal insufficiency and advanced age. It was found that there may be abnormally low 5-hour urine excretion of xylose in persons over age 65. However, one study claims that the 24-hour urine collection is normal in these patients unless actual malabsorption is present. If the serum creatinine level is borderline or elevated, the 5-hour urine xylose excretion is also likely to be abnormally low, and again the 24-hour urine may be useful. In these cases, however, the 2-hour blood levels may help, for they should be normal and are not affected by the two conditions mentioned. Otherwise, the 5-hour urine excretion is more reliable than the blood levels, which tend to fluctuate.

The xylose test may be helpful in differential diagnosis and etiology of malabsorption. Most patients with cystic fibrosis and pancreatic insufficiency are said to have normal urine xylose values. This is also true of most patients with liver disease. Patients with classic pernicious anemia have normal xylose test results, although it must be remembered that many of these patients are aged and may have low urine results from this cause. In megaloblastic anemia of pregnancy some patients have abnormal xylose test results, although probably the majority show normal values. A minor percentage of patients with partial gastrectomy are reported to have abnormal urine values. Patients with functional diarrhea and duodenal ulcer have normal results.

In malabsorption diseases, there is excellent D-xylose correlation with proved sprue and celiac disease. The urine results are more often clearcut than the blood levels. There is no correlation with the amount of steatorrhea present. Patients with regional enteritis involving extensive areas of the jejunum may have abnormal results, while normal results are associated with this disease when it is localized to the ileum. Patients with Whipple's disease and multiple jejunal diverticula may also have abnormal results. Finally, in certain diseases other than malabsorption, for some reason patients sometimes have abnormal urinary xylose excretion. Myxedema shows this quite often. There are reports that this may also occur in diabetic neuropathic diarrhea, rheumatoid arthritis, acute or chronic alcoholism and occasionally in severe congestive heart failure. Ascites is reported to produce abnormal urine excretion with normal plasma levels. Although probably not common in the diseases just mentioned, abnormal results still occur often enough that one must be aware of this fact.

SMALL INTESTINE BIOPSY.—It has been demonstrated that in classic sprue, both tropical and nontropical, the mucosa of the small intestine shows characteristic histologic abnormalities. Instead of the normal monotonous fingerlike villous pattern, the villi are thickened and blunted with flattening of the cuboidal epithelium, and may eventually fuse and often disappear altogether. Depending on the degree of change in the villi, biopsies may show moderate or severe changes. These same changes to a much lesser degree may be found in many of the other conditions causing malabsorption, including even subtotal gastrectomy. However, these usually are not of the severity seen in sprue and generally can be differentiated by the clinical history or other findings. Other causes of malabsorption, such as Whipple's disease, which characteristically shows many para-aminosalicylic acid (PAS)-positive macrophages in the mucosa, may be detected on biopsy.

COMMENT.—This chapter has considered certain tests for intestinal malabsorption. In my opinion, the most useful tests in initial screening for malabsorption syndromes are the D-xylose, plasma carotene and qualitative fecal fat. (Some institutions do not do the plasma carotene, however.) If all of these have normal results, chances of demonstrating steatorrhea by other means are very low. If one or all are abnormal, it may be necessary to do a quantitative fecal fat study. X-ray studies may show compatible abnormalities and may also reveal some of the secondary causes of steatorrhea. A careful history, physical examination and appropriate laboratory studies usually can rule out many of the causes of malabsorption, including most of those in categories I–III in Table 25–1. Jejunal biopsy may occasionally be necessary, but the diagnosis usually can be made by routine methods. In patients over age 60 it might be useful to obtain both a 5-hour and 24-hour D-xylose urine collection, with the 5-hour value added to the next 19 hours to give the total 24-hour figure. If pernicious anemia is suspected, a Schilling test without intrinsic factor is needed. If the Schilling test without intrinsic factor has abnormal results, it is followed by a Schilling test with intrinsic factor. A bone marrow test to demonstrate megaloblastic change and a gastric analysis for anacidity are highly desirable.

REFERENCES

Adlersberg, D., et al.: The roentgenologic appearance of the small intestine in sprue, Gastroenterology 26:548, 1954.

Collins, J. R.: Small intestinal mucosal damage with villous atrophy: A review of the literature, Am. J. Clin. Pathol. 44:36, 1965.

Etheridge, C. L.: Protein-losing enteropathy, Med. Clin. North Am. 48:75, 1964.

Gardner, F. H.: Hematologic aspects of sprue, Am. J. Clin. Nutr. 8:179, 1960.

Gordon, R. S., et al.: Protein-Losing Gastroenteropathy, in Dowling, H. F. (ed.): *Disease-a-Month* (Chicago: Year Book Medical Publishers, Inc., August 1966).

Herbert, V.: Detection of malabsorption of vitamin B_{12} due to gastric or intestinal dysfunction, Semin. Nucl. Med. 2:220, 1972.

Jeffries, G. H., et al.: Malabsorption, Gastroenterology 46:434, 1964.

Joske, R. A., and Curnow, D. H.: The D-xylose absorption test, Australas. Ann. Med. 11:4, 1962.

Katz, A. J., and Falchuk, Z. M.: Current concepts in gluten-sensitive enteropathy (Celiac sprue), Pediatr. Clin. North Am. 22:767, 1975.

Longstreth, G. F., and Newcomer, A. D.: Drug-induced malabsorption, Mayo Clin. Proc. 50:284, 1975.

McIntire, P. A.: Use of radioisotope techniques in the clinical evaluation of patients with megaloblastic anemia, Semin. Nucl. Med. 5:79, 1975.

Moore, J. G.: Simple fecal tests of absorption: A prospective study and critique, Am. J. Dig. Dis. 16:97, 1971.

Rogers, A. I.: Steatorrhea, Postgrad. Med. 50:123, 1971.

Rogers, A. I., and Rothman, S. L.: Blind loop syndrome, Postgrad. Med. 55:99, 1974.

Ruffin, J. M., and Roufail, W. M.: Whipple's disease: Evolution of current concepts, Am. J. Dig. Dis. 11:580, 1966.

Shiner, M.: Problems in interpretation of intestinal mucosal biopsies, J.A.M.A. 188:165, 1964.

Stenman, U. H.: False-positive tests for intrinsic-factor antibody, Lancet 2:428, 1976.

Stranchen, J. A.: An augmented Schilling test in the diagnosis of pernicious anaemia, Lancet 2:545, 1976.

Summerskill, W. H. J., and Moertel, C. G.: Malabsorption syndrome associated with anicteric liver diseases, Gastroenterology 42:380, 1962.

Texter, E. C., et al.: Laboratory procedures in the diagnosis of malabsorption, Med. Clin. North Am. 48:117, 1964.

Thaysen, E. H., and Mullertz, S.: The D-xylose absorption tolerance test, Acta Med. Scand. 171:521, 1962.

Waldmann, T. A.: Protein-losing enteropathy and kinetic studies of plasma protein metabolism, Semin. Nucl. Med. 2:251, 1972.

Wenger, J.: Blood carotene in steatorrhea and the malabsorption syndrome, Am. J. Med. 22:373, 1957.

Wilson, F. A., and Dietschy, J. M.: Differential diagnostic approach to clinical problems of malabsorption, Gastroenterology 61:911, 1971.

Wollaeger, E. E., and Scudamore, H. H.: Spectrum of diseases causing steatorrhea, Arch. Intern. Med. 113:819, 1964.

26 / Gastrointestinal Function

GASTRIC ANALYSIS

GASTRIC ANALYSIS has two main uses: to determine gastric acidity and to obtain material for exfoliative cytology. We shall discuss only the first here.

When gastric aspiration is performed to determine gastric acidity, the usual purpose is either to determine degree of acid production in persons with ulcer or ulcer symptoms or to determine if the stomach is capable of producing acid as part of a workup for pernicious anemia. Since passing the large-caliber tube needed is not met with enthusiasm by the patient, it is important that the physician understand what information can be obtained and be certain that this information is really necessary.

One problem in evaluating gastric acid secretion data from the literature is the term "achlorhydria," which is often used as a synonym for "anacidity." The classic method of gastric analysis involved titration with 0.1 N sodium hydroxide to the end point of Topfer's reagent (pH 2.9–4.0); this represented "free' hydrochloric acid (HCl). Next the specimen was titrated to the end point of phenolphthalein (pH 8.3–10.0); this represented "total" acid. The difference was said to represent "combined acid," thought to be protein-bound and weak organic acids, but probably including small amounts of HCl. Achlorhydria technically is defined as absence of *free* acid (pH will not drop below 3.5 on stimulation) but not necessarily complete lack of *all* acid. True anacidity is absence of all acid, now defined as a pH that does not fall below 6.0 or decrease more than 1 pH unit after maximum stimulation. Therefore, achlorhydria is not the same as anacidity, but nevertheless the two terms are often used interchangeably.

Gastric acidity used to be reported in degrees or units; this is the same as milliequivalents per liter. Most authorities today recommend timed collection and report values obtained in milliequivalents per hour, i.e., secretion rate instead of concentration. A 1-hour basal specimen is collected; normal values are not uniform, but seem most often to be quoted as 1–6 mEq/hour. Histamine, betazole (Histalog) or pentagastrin is then administered, and four 30-minute consecutive specimens are collected. Maximum acid output (MAO) is the sum of all four 30-minute collections. Acidity used to be measured by titration with chemical indicators but is now frequently obtained with a pH electrode.

Proper placement of the gastric tube is critical; many recommend assistance by fluoroscopy.

A method of tubeless gastric analysis called Diagnex Blue is available. A blue dye is coupled to a cation exchange resin. Free HCl in the stomach replaces the indicator dye, which is absorbed and then excreted in the urine. Presence of dye in the urine thus indicates gastric acid secretion. Oral caffeine rather than parenteral histamine is used to stimulate acid production. This is a useful test in workup of a patient for pernicious anemia, since only a urine specimen is required rather than gastric aspiration. The degree of acid secretion is not relevant, only whether any acid is being produced. However, the test is useful only if acid production is demonstrated, since about 50% of those showing no free acid by the Diagnex caffeine stimulation procedure will have acid production induced by histamine. If the Diagnex Blue test does indicate gastric acid, however, there obviously is no need for histamine administration.

Gastric aspiration to determine gastric acidity is useful in the following circumstances.

Diagnosis of Pernicious Anemia. — Presence of acid secretion rules out pernicious anemia. Complete lack of acid secretion after maximum stimulation is consistent with pernicious anemia, but may occur in up to 30% of persons over age 70 and occasionally in presumably normal younger persons. If basal secretion fails to demonstrate acid, stimulation is necessary. Alcohol or caffeine has been used, but if demonstrable acid production does not occur, histamine, betazole (Histalog) or pentagastrin is necessary. Of these, histamine has the most side effects and pentagastrin the least. Anacidity rather than achlorhydria is the classic gastric analysis finding in pernicious anemia, but as noted previously, the older term "achlorhydria" is still being used with the same meaning as "anacidity."

Diagnosis of Gastric Cancer. — Given a known gastric lesion, anacidity after maximum stimulation is strong evidence against peptic ulcer. However, only about 20% of gastric carcinoma is associated with complete anacidity, so gastroenterologists tend to rely more on gastroscopy than gastric analysis.

Diagnosis of Zollinger-Ellison Syndrome. — These patients have a gastrin-producing tumor, usually in the pancreas (p. 398), and typically demonstrate a high basal acid secretion with minimal change after stimulation. Specifically, gastric analysis is strongly suggestive when the basal output is 15 mEq/hour or the ratio of basal to maximum output is 0.6 or greater (i.e., basal level is 60% or more of MAO value after maximum stimulation). Some would consider basal levels of 10 mEq/hour and a basal-MAO ratio greater than 0.4 as evidence suggesting a need for further workup so as not to miss a gastrin-producing tumor. In one report, 70% of Zollinger-Ellison patients had basal acid output of over 15 mEq/hour as opposed to 10% of duodenal ulcer patients; 80% displayed a basal-MAO ratio of 0.6 as compared to 2% of duodenal ulcer patients. The best diagnostic procedure is serum gastrin assay (p. 398).

Diagnosis of Marginal Ulcer. — After partial gastric resection with gastro-jejunostomy (Billroth II procedure or variant), abdominal pain or GI bleeding may raise the question of ulcer in the jejunum near the anastomosis. A MAO value greater than 25 mEq/hour is strongly suggestive of marginal ulcer; one less than 15 mEq/hour is evidence against the diagnosis.

Differentiation of Gastric from Duodenal Ulcer. — Duodenal ulcer patients as a group tend to have gastric acid hypersecretion, while gastric ulcer patients most often have normal or even low rates. Patients with gastric ulcer usually have MAO values less than 40 mEq/hour. About 25–50% of duodenal ulcer patients display MAO greater than 40 mEq/hour. Conversely, very low acid secretion rates are evidence against duodenal ulcer. Basal secretion greater than 10 mEq/hour is evidence against gastric ulcer.

Determining Type and Extent of Gastric Resection. — Knowing the amount of acid is sometimes helpful in the surgical treatment of duodenal ulcer. Some surgeons prefer to do a hemigastrectomy (removal of half the stomach) rather than a subtotal gastrectomy (two-thirds resection) because postoperative complications are fewer in the former. If the patient is a hypersecretor, the surgeon may add vagotomy to a hemigastrectomy, or he may perform a subtotal resection to reduce HCl-producing cells or lessen stimulation of those that remain.

Evaluation of Vagotomy Status. — Patients undergoing a surgical procedure that includes bilateral vagotomy may later experience symptoms that might be due to recurrent ulcer, or manifest a proved recurrent ulcer. The question then arises whether vagotomy is complete. The Hollander test employs insulin hypoglycemia (20 units regular insulin or 0.1 units/kg) to stimulate gastric acid secretion through intact vagal nerve fibers. Although disagreement exists on what values are considered normal, the majority employ: (1) basal acid output less than 2 mEq/hour; (2) for postinsulin values, either total acid output less than 2 mEq/hour in any 1-hour period, or increase in acid concentration of less than 20 mEq/L in 2 hours. Most agree that a "positive" response means incomplete vagal section. Interpretation of the "negative" response (failure to secrete sufficient acid under stimulus of hypoglycemia) is more controversial. Antrectomy or partial gastrectomy removes HCl-secreting cells, and a "negative" response thus could be due either to vagal section or to intact vagus but insufficient total gastric HCl secretory activity.

DIFFERENTIAL TESTS IN DIARRHEA

As mentioned previously, besides anemia, chronic diarrhea is a prominent symptom of the various malabsorption diseases and may be the chief complaint. There are many conditions that cause a chronic diarrhea, which must be differentiated from the relatively common types that last only a few days and usually respond to ordinary treatment. Diarrhea in infants will not be specifically discussed, since this is a special problem peculiar to that age group.

In all age groups with long-term or chronic diarrhea, a stool should be obtained for culture to rule out the presence of *Salmonella* or *Shigella* bacteria. A stool should also be obtained for ova and parasites, with special emphasis on the possibility of amoebas being present. One of the malabsorption syndromes may be causing the diarrhea, either in children or in young and middle-aged adults; in children, this would be due to either cystic fibrosis of the pancreas or celiac disease. In an adult, the various forms of sprue and, more rarely, some of the secondary malabsorption causes might be considered. In children and young and middle-aged adults, ulcerative colitis is a possibility, especially if there is blood in the stools. This would call for a sigmoidoscopic examination. In adults over age 40, carcinoma of the colon has been found to cause diarrhea in a significant proportion of cases. A barium enema and sigmoidoscopic examination are necessary. In the aged, in addition to carcinoma, fecal impaction is a frequent cause of diarrhea, and this usually can be determined easily by ordinary rectal examination. In many cases, no organic etiology for persistent diarrhea can be found. This situation is often called "functional diarrhea" and is attributed to psychiatric causes. The organic diseases listed here must be ruled out before deciding that a patient has a psychosomatic disorder.

OTHER PROCEDURES IN GASTROINTESTINAL DISEASE

The most frequent major diseases affecting the gastrointestinal tract may be divided into benign and malignant and localized into upper GI (stomach and duodenum) and lower GI (colon). The major benign disease of the upper GI tract area is peptic ulcer; those of the lower GI are diverticulosis and mucosal polyp. The malignant disease usually affecting either area is the same—adenocarcinoma. As a general rule, GI carcinoma is not common under age 40 (although it can occur), and increases steadily in probability after that age (many other types of cancer do likewise). The major clinical symptom of peptic ulcer is epigastric pain that classically occurs between meals and is relieved by food or antacids. Patients with gastric carcinoma may have similar pain, nonspecific pain or simple gastric discomfort. The major symptom of colon carcinoma is change in bowel habits, either toward chronic diarrhea or constipation. However, either upper or lower GI carcinoma may be relatively asymptomatic until very late.

Laboratory tests for these GI lesions may be divided into three categories: screening tests, x-ray and direct visualization techniques.

SCREENING TESTS.—The most useful screening test is examination of the feces for blood. Usually this blood is occult (not grossly visible); sometimes it is grossly visible; if from the upper GI tract, it is often black ("tarry"), while lower GI bleeding may still show unchanged blood and color the stool red. Anemia of the chronic iron deficiency type is often present, although not always, and sometimes may be severe. Occult blood in the feces can be demonstrated by simple chemical tests for hemoglobin. All are based on peroxidase activity of hemoglobin, which is detected when it catalyzes the oxidation of a color reagent by a peroxide reagent. The most popular tests have included benzidine, guaiac (as powder, tablet or impregnated filter paper) and orthotolidin. Many studies have been done evaluating one or more of these methods. Results have often been conflicting and, at times, completely contradictory. Nevertheless, some consensus emerges. Benzidine is the most sensitive of the reagents but yields a great number of false positive results. It is currently not available in the United States. Orthotolidin most commonly in the form of a tablet called Hematest, has intermediate sensitivity, consistently detecting 10–15 ml blood placed in the stomach experimentally. False positive results (on unrestricted diet) were most often reported to be 20–30%. Guaiac in powder form provided surprisingly divergent results for different investigators, but the majority reported a lesser degree of sensitivity than with Hematest. A guaiac-impregnated filter paper kit named Hemoccult has been available since 1966. This is said to be approximately 25% as sensitive as guaiac powder or orthotolidin. Limits of consistent detection are apparently about 15–25 ml blood placed in the stomach. On an unrestricted diet, false positive results ranged 1–12%, most being trace or weak reactions. This seems to be the current method of choice, although more evaluations would be desirable.

Certain precautions have been emphasized to minimize false positive reactions and increase detection of true lesions:

1. The patient should be on a meat-free high-residue diet, beginning at least 24 hours prior to collection of the stool. Eliminating meat decreases weak false positive reactions. Some advocate boiling a fecal suspension to destroy plant peroxidases. The high-residue component increases detection of significant lesions. If patients must be screened on an unrestricted diet, possibly someone who manifests a weakly positive result could be restudied on a restricted diet.

2. At least 3 stool specimens should be collected, with tests performed on at least 2 areas from each. This is due to intermittent bleeding from some lesions.

3. Stool specimens should be tested within 48 hours after collection. Conversion of positive to negative results or vice versa has been reported after storage, although data is conflicting. One report indicates that large doses of vitamin C may produce false negative results.

Besides ulcer, polyp or malignancy, other serious GI diseases such as ulcerative colitis, regional enteritis and diverticulitis may give guaiac-positive stools.

Gastric analysis may be helpful in screening peptic ulcer from cancer of the stomach, as mentioned earlier. Low free acid or anacidity (with histamine) is suspicious for cancer if a stomach lesion is known to be present.

X-RAYS.—X-ray procedures include upper GI series for stomach and duodenum, and barium enema for the colon. In the upper GI series, the patient swallows a barium mixture, and a series of x-ray films shows this radiopaque material filling the stomach and duodenum. Barium enema means barium washed into the colon through a tube, after all feces are eliminated by laxatives and regular enemas. The major cause of poor barium enema studies is inadequate colon preparation. If feces remain in the colon after preparation for this procedure, obviously the barium cannot fill these areas, and small lesions may be missed.

DIRECT VISUALIZATION.—Direct visualization techniques include gastroscopy for stomach and proctoscopy and sigmoidoscopy for rectal and sigmoid colon lesions. Biopsy and specimens for cytology (Papanicolaou smears) can be obtained at the same time. Simple rectal examination allows many rectal and prostate cancers to be detected by the doctor's finger. For this reason, rectal examination is always included as a part of any good physical examination.

In summary, rectal examination and stool tests for occult blood are the best simple screening procedures for GI tumors. If these are positive, or arouse strong clinical suspicion, one can proceed to x-ray studies of the area indicated. When possible, direct visualization techniques are extremely helpful. Fiberoptic colonoscopy can detect lesions throughout the colon.

PANCREATIC FUNCTION

The pancreas is an important gastrointestinal accessory organ and may be involved in disease from both its exocrine and endocrine aspects. Pancreatic enzymes consist mainly of starch-digesting amylase, fat-digesting lipase and protein-digesting trypsin, as well as bicarbonate and certain other substances. These are secreted through the pancreatic duct, which enters the duodenum close by the common bile duct. Intrinsic diseases of the pancreatic parenchyma or obstruction of the pancreatic duct by tumor and by disease in surrounding areas such as the ampulla of Vater may cause diminution or complete absence of pancreatic secretions and secondarily lead to symptoms from lack of these important digestive enzymes. The diseases of the endocrine system that involve the islands of Langerhans in the pancreas will be discussed in the next chapter.

The most important parenchymal diseases are acute and chronic pancreatitis and carcinoma of the pancreas. Classic acute pancreatitis is manifested by sudden onset of severe epigastric pain that may radiate elsewhere, often to the back. There may be nausea and vomiting. If severe, there may be abdominal distention, rigidity of the abdomen and shock. In severe and classic disease, the diagnosis is frequently obvious; unfortunately, various symptoms found in acute pancreatitis regardless of severity may occur in other diseases. In disease of mild or moderate degree, or in patients with a chronic low-grade or intermittent type of pancreatitis, symptoms may be vague or atypical. The most common diseases that clinically are confused with acute (or sometimes chronic) pancreatitis are perforated peptic ulcer, biliary tract inflammation or stones, intestinal infarction and intra-abdominal hemorrhage. Myocardial infarct may sometimes enter the differential diagnosis since the pain may occasionally radiate to the upper abdomen; in addition, the SGOT may be elevated in more than half of acute pancreatitis patients.

Laboratory findings in acute pancreatitis vary according to the severity of the disease. In severe disease there may be a moderate leukocytosis with a shift to the left. Moderate hyperglycemia may be present, and in very severe disease outright diabetes may develop. There may be a mild jaundice, probably due to edema around the ampulla of Vater. Serum calcium may be decreased, sometimes to quite low values. This decrease usually appears 3–14 days after onset of symptoms, most frequently on the 4th or 5th day. It is attributed to the liberation of pancreatic lipase into the peritoneal cavity, with resulting digestion of fat and the combination of fatty acids with calcium, which we see grossly as fat necrosis. Again, in very severe disease there may be hemorrhagic phenomena due either to release of proteolytic enzymes such as trypsin into the blood, or release of blood into the abdominal cavity from a hemorrhagic pancreas.

Diagnostic Tests

AMYLASE. — In acute pancreatitis, the most important laboratory test is the measurement of alpha amylase. Alpha amylase actually has several components (isoenzymes), some derived from the pancreas and some from salivary glands. Clearance from serum takes place in about 2 hours; a significant portion is via the kidney by glomerular filtration and the remainder (some data indicate over 50%) by other pathways. Serum levels will become abnormal between 2 and 12 hours after onset in up to 80% of patients and within 24 hours in up to 90%. Thereafter there is a relatively early return to normal, in most patients reaching a peak by 24 hours and returning to normal in 48 – 72 hours. In some patients the serum amylase will remain elevated longer due to continued pancreatic cell destruction, but in a fair number it will not. In certain situations there may be falsely low or normal serum amylase levels. The administration of glucose will cause a decrease in serum amylase, so that one should wait at least 1 hour and preferably 2 after the patient has eaten to get a serum amylase measurement. One should realize that values taken during intravenous fluid therapy containing glucose may be unreliable. In massive hemorrhagic pancreatic necrosis there may not be any serum amylase elevation at all because no functioning cells are left to produce it. Pancreatic destruction of this degree is uncommon, however.

A list of the more important etiologies for elevated serum amylase include:

1. Primary acute or chronic relapsing pancreatitis: idiopathic, traumatic or associated with alcohol, viral hepatitis or hyperparathyroidism

2. Hyperamylasemia associated with biliary tract disease: cholecystitis, biliary tract lithiasis, tumor or spasm of the sphincter of Oddi produced by morphine and Demerol or following biliary tract cannulation

3. Hyperamylasemia associated with nonbiliary acute intra-abdominal disease: perforated or nonperforated peptic ulcer, peritonitis, intra-abdominal hemorrhage, intestinal obstruction or infarct, recent abdominal surgery

4. Nonpancreatic or non-alpha amylase: acute salivary gland disease or macroamylasia

5. Miscellaneous: renal failure, diabetic ketoacidosis, pregnancy, cerebral trauma, extensive burns, drug hypersensitivity (thiazides, ethacrynic acid, oral contraceptives, tetracyclines) and cholecystography using radiopaque dyes (approximately 72 hours in some cases)

In some instances of biliary tract disease there is probably a retrograde secondary pancreatitis; in others, release of amylase into the circulation when pancreatic duct obstruction takes place; still others have no convincing anatomical explanation. Likewise, in some cases of acute nonbiliary tract intra-abdominal disease there is a surface chemical pancreatitis; when intestinal obstruction or infarction occurs, there may be escape of intraluminal enzyme, but in other instances no definite cause is found.

Urine amylase determination may also be helpful, especially when serum amylase is normal or equivocally elevated. Urine amylase usually rises within 24 hours after the serum amylase and as a rule remains abnormal for 7 – 10 days after the serum concentration returns to normal. Various investigators have used 1-, 2- and 24-hour collection periods with roughly equal success. The shorter collections have to be very accurately timed, while the 24-hour specimen may involve problems in complete collection. It is important to have the results reported as units per hour. Frequently the values are reported as units/100 ml, which is inaccurate because it is influenced by fluctuating urine volumes. One drawback of both serum and urine amylase is their relation to renal function. When renal function is sufficiently diminished to produce serum BUN elevation, amylase excretion also diminishes, leading to mild· or moderate elevation in serum amylase and decrease in urine amylase.

Because renal excretion of amylase depends on adequate renal function, amylase urinary excretion correlates with creatinine clearance (p. 131). In acute pancreatitis, however, there seems to be increased clearance of amylase compared to creatinine. The amylase to creatinine clearance ratio (A/CCR) is based on this observation. This procedure involves "simultaneous" collection of one serum and one urine specimen and does not require a timed or complete urine collection. The A/CCR becomes abnormal 1–2 days subsequent to the serum amylase but remains abnormal for 7–10 days, slightly longer than urine amylase. This is said to be an excellent diagnostic procedure in acute pancreatitis, more specific and sensitive than serum amylase and with fewer technical drawbacks than urine amylase. Many of the etiologies for hyperamylasemia that do not evoke a secondary pancreatitis have normal A/CCR values. The exact degree of specificity is not yet established; reports have appeared that A/CCR may be elevated in some cases of diabetic ketoacidosis and burns. Behavior in renal failure is variable. In mild azotemia, the A/CCR may be normal, but in more severe azotemia or in uremia sufficient to require dialysis, it may be elevated. In addition, different investigators have adapted different ratio numbers as upper limits of normal, and there have been suggestions that the particular amylase method used will influence results. More data is needed before final conclusions about A/CCR can be made.

Chronic pancreatitis and its resulting pancreatic insufficiency may often be very difficult to diagnose. This depends again on the degree of pancreatic destruction and whether it occurs acutely or in a low-grade fashion. The serum amylase in chronic pancreatitis is still important, although much more unreliable than in acute disease. In about half the patients it is within normal range. Repeated determinations are necessary at intervals of perhaps 3 days. Moreover, the values may be borderline or only slightly elevated, leading to confusion with the other causes of elevated amylase mentioned previously. In this situation, the urine amylase or the A/CCR ratio is the most helpful test.

LIPASE. — Serum lipase is considered more specific for pancreatic damage than amylase. Lipase levels rise slightly later than serum amylase, although usually within 24 hours, and tend to remain abnormal longer, in most instances returning to normal in 7–10 days. Urine lipase is not currently used. Although the traditional viewpoint was that serum lipase was elevated less frequently than serum amylase in pancreatitis, some recent work employing newer analytic methods has disputed this.

OTHER TESTS. — Amylase isoenzyme fractionation by electrophoresis (or other methods) is becoming available. Results to date show several isoenzymes of both pancreatic and salivary type. In clinical acute pancreatitis, reports indicate that the expected increase in pancreatic-type isoenzymes is observed. In hyperamylasemia without clinical pancreatitis, some patients exhibit increased pancreatic-type isoenzymes and some, increased salivary type. These techniques are not yet widely available, and more data are needed.

Macroamylase is a macromolecular complex that contains alpha amylase bound to other molecules. Macroamylase in serum (macroamylasemia) reacts in chemical tests for amylase to produce apparent elevated serum amylase, although macroamylasemia may occur without exceeding serum amylase normal limits. Macroamylase does not pass the glomerular filter, so elevated serum amylase with reduced A/CCR is suggestive of macroamylasemia. Since occasional patients with elevated serum amylase due to salivary-type amylase may have reduced A/CCR, however, macroamylase should be confirmed by special techniques such as selective chromatography.

CHRONIC PANCREATITIS. — Chronic pancreatic insufficiency may occur as a result of pancreatitis or hemochromatosis in adults and in the disease known as cystic fibrosis of the pancreas in children. The diagnosis may be quite difficult, since the disease either represents an end-stage phenomenon with no acute process going on, or else may take place slowly and subclinically over a long period. The classic case of chronic pancreatitis consists of diabetes, pancreatic calcification on x-ray and steatorrhea. The diagnosis of diabetes will be discussed in the next chapter. Steatorrhea may be demonstrated by quantitative fecal fat studies, as described in Chapter 25. Either of these parameters may be normal or borderline in many patients.

It may be desirable to attempt to assess pancreatic function by several methods. One of these is the measure of pancreatic trypsin excreted in the stools. A diluted portion of stool is placed on a photographic film, and the presence of trypsin is indicated by digestion of the gelatin covering of the film. However, this test is inaccurate because proteolytic bacteria exist in the colon and may themselves digest the gelatin. The stool may be examined directly and useful information obtained. Theoretically, in pancreatic insufficiency, there should be a large amount of neutral fat and very little fatty acid. However, a variable amount of fatty acid may in reality be present because some of the colon bacteria apparently are able to convert neutral fat to fatty acid. In the presence of demonstrable steatorrhea, a normal D-xylose test result is usually found in pancreatic insufficiency or cystic fibrosis. Reports have appeared advocating measurement of serum amylase after injection of the pancreatic-stimulating hormone secretin. There is still controversy over the usefulness of this procedure. Also possible is direct measurement of pancreatic fluid constituents after secretin stimulation by means of duodenal tube drainage. This technique would have to be done by an experienced gastroenterologist and is not widely available.

Pancreas scanning using selenomethionine (^{75}Se), an amino acid analogue, is helpful in certain situations. To produce worthwhile results, a stationary imaging device such as the Anger scintillation camera must be used. The patient fasts overnight, and the scan is begun shortly after a high-protein meal to stimulate the organ. Under these conditions, a normal scan is effective in ruling out serious pancreatic disease. Abnormal scans may be produced by a variety of conditions, including nonfasting, active peptic ulcer, gastric surgery or vagotomy, chronic pancreatitis, pancreatic tumor and malnutrition. Usual degrees of acute pancreatitis tend to produce abnormal scan image. Islet cell tumors are usually too small to be demonstrated, and most often exist with a normal scan.

Computerized axial tomography (CAT) and B-mode ultrasound are probably more useful than current methods of pancreas scanning. Both can detect abnormality in approximately 80% of patients, but are able to demonstrate focal or generalized gland enlargement; therefore an abnormal study has fewer possible etiologies. However, it is frequently difficult to differentiate between acute pancreatitis and tumor. It seems that CAT is easier to perform and interpret than ultrasound. Ultrasound (and, to a lesser extent, CAT) cannot always visualize the normal pancreas.

Cystic Fibrosis

Finally, a few words should be said about the diagnosis of cystic fibrosis of the pancreas. This classically occurs in children, but may not be manifested until adolescence or even occasionally in adults. It is a hereditary disease carried by a recessive gene. The disease affects the mucous glands of the body, but for some reason seems to affect those of the pancreas more than any others. The pancreatic secretions become thickened and eventually block the pancreatic acini, leading to secondary atrophy of the pancreatic cells. The same process may be found elsewhere, as in the lungs, where inspissated secretions may lead to recurrent bronchopneumonia, and in the liver, where thickened bile may lead to plugging of the small ducts and to a secondary cirrhosis in very severe disease. These patients usually do not have a watery type of diarrhea, but this is not always easy to ascertain by the history. The diagnosis is made because the sweat glands of the body are also involved in the disease. Although these patients excrete normal *volumes* of sweat, the sodium and chloride *concentration* of the sweat is abnormal in that much higher values of these electrolytes are lost. Cystic fibrosis and its diagnosis are discussed in Chapter 33.

Cystic fibrosis in children should be differentiated from so-called celiac disease. Celiac disease is basically the childhood form of the nontropical sprue seen in adults, both of which in many cases seem due to hypersensitivity to a substance known as gluten. This substance is found in wheat, oats and barley, and causes both histologic changes and clinical symptoms that are indistinguishable from those of tropical sprue, which is not influenced by gluten. These patients have normal sweat electrolytes, often will respond to a gluten-free diet and behave like ordinary patients with the malabsorption syndrome.

REFERENCES

Ambromovage, A. M., et al.: The twenty-four hour excretion of amylase and lipase in the urine, Ann. Surg. 167:539, 1968.
Anderson, M. C.: Review of pancreatic disease, Surgery 66:434, 1969.
Banks, P. A.: Acute pancreatitis, Gastroenterology 61:382, 1971.

Colcher, H.: Guidelines for fiberoptic examination in upper gastrointestinal bleeding, Adv. Intern. Med. 20:399, 1975.

Cooley, R. W.: The diagnostic accuracy of radiologic studies of the biliary tract, small intestine, and colon, Am. J. Med. Sci. 246:610, 1963.

Czerniak, P., et al: Usefulness of radionuclides in evaluation of stomach disorders, Semin. Nucl. Med. 2:288, 1972.

Danovitch, S. H.: Clinical usefulness of gastric secretory studies, Geriatrics 28:119, 1973.

Friedman, B. L.: Radionuclide determination of gastrointestinal blood loss, Semin. Nucl. Med. 2:265, 1972.

Gambill, E. E., and Mason, H. L.: One-hour value for urinary amylase in 96 patients with pancreatitis: Comparative diagnostic value of tests of urinary and serum amylase and serum lipase, J.A.M.A. 186:24, 1963.

Ginsberg, A. L.: Alterations in immunologic mechanisms in diseases of the gastrointestinal tract, Am. J. Dig. Dis. 16:61, 1971.

Goldberg, J. M.: Diagnostic use of pancreatic lipase determination by radial enzyme diffusion, and design of a routine pancreatic profile, Clin. Chem. 22:638, 1976.

Gorden, H. E., et al.: Diagnosis and management of gastrointestinal bleeding, Ann. Intern. Med. 71:993, 1969.

Greegor, D. H.: Detection of silent colon cancer in routine examination, CA 19:330, 1969.

Helfat, A., et al.: Re prevalence of macroamylasemia: Further study, Am. J. Gastroenterol. 62:54, 1974.

Katz, D., et al.: Sources of bleeding in upper gastrointestinal hemorrhage: A re-evaluation, Am. J. Dig. Dis. 9:447, 1964.

Legaz, M. E., and Kenny, M. A.: Electrophoretic amylase fractionation as an aid in diagnosis of pancreatic disease, Clin. Chem. 22:57, 1976.

Lifton, L. J., et al.: Amylase vs. lipase in the diagnosis of acute pancreatitis. Clin. Chem. 20:880, 1974.

Morris, D. W., et al.: Reliability of chemical tests for fecal occult blood in hospitalized patients, Am. J. Dig. Dis. 21:845, 1976.

Morrisey, R., et al.: The nature and significance of hyperamylasemia following operation. Ann. Surg. 180:67, 1974.

Ostrow, J. D., et al.: Sensitivity and reproducibility of chemical tests for fecal occult blood with an emphasis on false-positive reactions, Am. J. Dig. Dis. 18:930, 1973.

Piper, D. W., et al.: The assessment of gastric secretion in man, M. J. Aust. 57:549, 1970.

Rogers, A.: Immunoglobulins and the gastrointestinal tract, Postgrad. Med. 48:75, 1970.

Ruzicka, F. F., and Rossi, P.: Normal vascular anatomy of the abdominal viscera, Radiol. Clin. North Am. 8:3, 1970.

Salt, W. B., Jr., and Schanker, S.: Amylase, its clinical significance: A review of the literature, Medicine 55:269, 1976.

Schiffer, C. F., et al.: Amylase/creatinine clearance fraction in patients on chronic hemodialysis, Ann. Intern. Med. 86:65, 1977.

Schindler, R.: Critical evaluation of biopsy techniques for the diagnosis of gastritides, Am. J. Dig. Dis. 7:167, 1962.

Sparberg, M., and Kirsner, J. B.: Gastric secretory activity with reference to HCl, Arch. Intern. Med. 114:508, 1964.

Steigmann, F., and Hyman, S.: Acute gastrointestinal bleeding, Postgrad. Med. 41:252, 1967.

Stein, A. M.: Macroamylasemia, Postgrad. Med. 55:103, 1974.

Stoehlein, J. R., et al.: Hemoccult detection of fecal occult blood quantitated by radioassay, Am. J. Dig. Dis. 21:841, 1976.

Toffler, A. H., and Spiro, H. M.: Shock or coma as the predominant manifestation of painless acute pancreatitis, Ann. Intern. Med. 57:655, 1962.

Van Goidsenhoven, G. E., et al.: Pancreatic function in cirrhosis of the liver, Am. J. Dig. Dis. 8:160, 1963.

Wiggans, G., et al.: Computerized axial tomography for diagnosis of pancreatic cancer, Lancet 2:233, 1976.

Williams, L. F.: Gastrointestinal hemorrhage as a postoperative phenomenon, Am. J. Surg. 116:375, 1968.

Winauer, S. J.: Fecal occult blood testing, Am. J. Dig. Dis. 21:885, 1976.

27 / Tests for Diabetes and Hypoglycemia

DIABETES

BESIDES EXOCRINE DIGESTIVE ENZYMES secreted into the duodenum, the pancreas has endocrine functions centered in the islands of Langerhans. Their location is primarily in the tail and body of the pancreas; their hormones are glucagon and insulin, and their secretion is directly into the bloodstream. True diabetes mellitus results from hypofunction of the pancreatic islands of Langerhans, specifically the islet beta cells that produce insulin. This may be idiopathic or secondary to pancreatic involvement by carcinoma, pancreatitis or hemochromatosis. The idiopathic type is by far the most common. Its clinical features will not be discussed except to point out that there are two general categories of diabetics—those whose disease begins relatively early in life and is more severe, who require insulin for management and show severe insulin deficiency on assay, and a second group whose disease begins in late middle age or afterward, is less severe and can be treated with small doses of insulin or with oral medication, and who show some degree of insulin production.

Most laboratory tests for diabetes attempt to reflect pancreatic islet hypofunction, qualitative or quantitative, by measuring insulin production. Direct insulin assay was once technically too difficult for any but a few research laboratories. Therefore, emphasis in clinical medicine has been on indirect methods, whose end point usually demonstrates the action of insulin on a relatively accessible and measurable substance, the blood sugar. This necessity for indirect measurement of insulin makes certain flaws inherent in all laboratory procedures based on blood sugar determination. These problems derive from any technique that attempts to assay one substance by monitoring its action on another. Ideally, one should measure a substrate that is specific for the reaction or enzyme in question under test conditions that eliminate the effects on utilization by any other factors. The blood sugar level does not meet any of these criteria.

The blood sugar level depends primarily on the liver, which exerts its effect on blood glucose homeostasis via its reversible conversion of glucose to glycogen as well as gluconeogenesis from fat and protein. Next most important is tissue utilization of glucose, which is mediated by pancreatic insulin but is affected by many factors in addition to insulin.

The actual mechanisms involved in the regulation of blood sugar levels are complex, and in many cases only partially understood. Insulin is

315

thought to act primarily on tissues at the cellular level, but its mode of action still has not been definitively established. The most accepted current theory involves alteration of cell membrane permeability to glucose. Others have suggested some influence on the hexokinase enzyme system that mediates the conversion of glucose to glucose-6-phosphate; also, there is some evidence that insulin enhances glycogen, protein and fat synthesis. In addition, insulin may have a direct effect on the liver, possibly by suppressing glucose formation from glycogen (glycogenolysis).

The liver is affected by at least three important hormones: epinephrine, glucagon and hydrocortisone (cortisol). Epinephrine from the adrenal medulla stimulates breakdown of glycogen to glucose, apparently by converting inactive hepatic cell phosphorylase to active phosphorylase, which mediates the conversion of glycogen to glucose-1-phosphate. In addition, there is evidence that gluconeogenesis from lactate is enhanced via the enzyme adenosine 3, 5-monophosphate. Glucagon is a hormone that is produced by the pancreatic alpha cells and released by the stimulus of hypoglycemia. It is thought to act on the liver in a manner similar to epinephrine. Hydrocortisone (cortisol), cortisone and similar 11-oxygenated adrenocorticosteroids also influence the liver, but in a different manner. One fairly well documented pathway is enhancement of glycogen synthesis from amino acids. This increases the carbohydrate reserve available to augment blood sugar levels; thus, steroids like cortisol essentially stimulate gluconeogenesis. In addition, cortisol deficiency leads to anorexia and also causes impairment of carbohydrate absorption from the small intestine.

Methods of Blood Glucose Determination

The technique of blood sugar determination must be considered because different methods vary in specificity and sensitivity to glucose. The blood specimen itself is important; for each hour of standing at room temperature glucose values of whole blood decrease 10 mg/100 ml unless a preservative is added. Fluoride is considered the best preservative at present. Plasma or serum are more stable than whole blood; if serum can be removed from the cells before 2 hours, serum glucose values remain stable up to 24 hours at room temperature (some authors report occasional decreases). Refrigeration assists this preservation. Serum or plasma values are 10–15% higher than those of whole blood. This is important, because normal values quoted in the literature are mostly those from whole blood, while most present-day automated equipment uses serum. Venous blood is customarily used for glucose measurement; capillary (arterial) blood produces values that are approximately 30 mg/100 ml higher but may vary considerably, with sometimes as much as 100 mg/100 ml difference. This venous-capillary divergence is said to be negligible when the patient is fasting.

A considerable number of methods for blood glucose determination are widely used. These may be conveniently categorized as nonspecific reducing substance methods producing results significantly above true glucose values (Folin-Wu manual method and neocuproine SMA 12/60 automated method); methods that are not entirely specific for glucose but that yield results fairly close to true glucose (Somogyi-Nelson, orthotoluidine, ferricyanide), and true glucose (glucose oxidase and hexokinase). There are certain technical differences and interference by certain medications or metabolic substances that account for nonuniformity of laboratory methodology and that in some instances may affect interpretation (p. 487). Normal values mentioned in this chapter are for serum and for true glucose (unless otherwise specified).

A more recent test for blood glucose is a rapid semiquantitative paper dipstick method named Dextrostix. A portion of the paper strip is impregnated with glucose oxidase, an enzyme specific for glucose, plus a color reagent. One drop of whole blood is used; the color that develops is compared to a reference color chart. Evaluations of this test to date provide a consensus that, with experience, values between 40 and 130 mg/100 ml usually agree within at least ± 30−40% with values obtained from standard methods. Persons without much familiarity with the technique may obtain more erratic results. Dextrostix tends to underestimate to varying degrees any concentration of glucose over approximately 130 mg/100 ml. The method has been found useful to differentiate between hypoglycemia and hyperglycemia, and to provide a gross approximation of diabetic blood sugar control for outpatients. Additional considerations are possible differences between capillary (fingerstick) blood and venous blood values, alluded to previously; also, the fact that fluoride blood preservatives will inactivate the glucose oxidase enzyme.

The diagnosis of diabetes is made by demonstrating abnormally increased blood sugar under certain controlled conditions. If insulin deficiency is large, carbohydrate homeostatic mechanisms are unable to compensate and the fasting blood sugar levels are consistently elevated. If insulin deficiency is smaller, abnormality is noted only when an unusually heavy carbohydrate load is placed on the system. In uncompensated insulin deficiency, a fasting blood sugar (FBS) reveals abnormality; in equivocal cases or in compensated insulin deficiency, a variety of carbohydrate tolerance test procedures are available to unmask the defect. To use and interpret these procedures, the various factors involved must be thoroughly understood.

Glucose Tolerance Test: Standardization of Procedure

Glucose tolerance tests (GTT) are provocative tests in which a relatively large dose of glucose challenges the body homeostatic mechanisms. All other variables being normal, it is assumed that the subsequent rise and fall of the blood sugar is due mainly to production of insulin in response to hyperglycemia, and that the degree of insulin response is mirrored in the behavior of the blood glucose. Failure to realize that this assumption is predicated on all other variables being normal explains a good deal of the confusion that exists in the literature and in clinical practice.

The most important factor in the GTT is the need for careful standardization of the test procedure. Without these precautions any type of glucose tolerance test yields such varied results that an abnormal response cannot be interpreted. *Previous carbohydrate intake* is very important. If diet has been low in both calories and carbohydrates for as little as 3 days preceding the test, glucose tolerance may be diminished temporarily and the GTT may shift more or less toward diabetic levels. This has been especially true in starvation, but the situation does not have to be this extreme. Even a normal caloric diet that is low in carbohydrates may influence the GTT. A preparatory diet has been recommended that includes approximately 300 gm carbohydrates/day for 3 days preceding the test, although others believe that 100 gm for each of the 3 days is sufficient. The average American diet contains approximately 100–150 gm carbohydrates; it is obviously necessary in any case to be sure the patient actually eats at least 100 gm a day for 3 days. *Inactivity* has been reported as a significant influence on the GTT, also toward the diabetic side. One study found almost 50% more diabetic GTT response in bedridden patients compared to ambulatory patients otherwise identical in most other respects. There is a well-recognized trend toward decreasing carbohydrate tolerance with *advanced age*. Although the degree of abnormality is not enough to affect fasting sugar normal range, glucose tolerance upper limits increase about 1 mg/100 ml/year beyond age 50. There are three schools of thought as to the interpretation of this fact. One group feels that effects of aging either unmask latent diabetes or represent true diabetes due to impairment of islet cell function in a manner analogous to subclinical renal function decrease through arteriosclerosis. Another group applies arbitrary correction formulas to decrease the number of abnormalities to a predetermined figure based on estimates of diabetes incidence in the given population. The most widely accepted viewpoint regards these changes as physiologic rather than pathologic; and, to avoid labeling these persons diabetic, it extends the upper limits of normal by adding 1 mg/100 ml to each GTT value for each year over age 50. Fasting values are not affected. The effect of *obesity* is not certain. Some believe that obesity per se has little influence on the GTT. Others believe that obesity decreases carbohydrate tolerance; they have found significant differences after weight reduction, at least in obese mild diabetics. *Fever* tends to produce a diabetic-type GTT response; this is true regardless of the etiology, but more so with infections. *Diurnal variation* in glucose tolerance has been reported, with significantly decreased carbohydrate tolerance during the afternoon in many persons whose GTT curves were normal in the morning. This suggests that tests for diabetes should be done in the morning.

The Oral Glucose Tolerance Test

The oral dose of glucose has been fairly well standardized at 100 gm dextrose. Some have used as little as 50 gm with equally good results. This is administered as a 50% solution or dissolved in 300–500 ml water, in either case flavored by some substance such as lemon juice. The dose may be calculated from body weight.

Blood specimens are taken fasting, then ½ hour, 1, 2 and 3 hours after dextrose ingestion. Fajans and Conn advocate an additional specimen at 1½ hours. After ingestion and a lag period, the blood sugar curve rises sharply to a peak, usually in 15–60 minutes. In one study, 76% had maximal values at ½ hour, 17% at 1 hour. The curve then falls steadily but more slowly, reaching normal levels at 2 hours. These may be fasting values or simply within normal blood sugar ranges.

Occasionally, after the fasting level is reached, there may follow a transient dip below the fasting level, usually not great, then a return to fasting values. This relative hypoglycemic phase of the curve (when present) is thought to be due to a lag in the ability of the liver to change from converting glucose to glycogen (in response to previous hyperglycemia) to its other activity of supplying glucose from glycogen. In some cases, residual insulin may also be a factor. This "hypoglycemic" phase, if present, is generally between the 2d and 4th hours. Several reports indicate that so-called terminal hypoglycemia, which is a somewhat exaggerated form of this phenomenon, occurs in a fairly large number of patients with GTT indicative of mild diabetes. They believe that an abnormally marked hypoglycemic dip often appears in mild diabetics 3–5 hours after meals or a test dose of carbohydrates, and may be one of the earliest clinical manifestations of the disease.

Criteria for interpretation of the oral GTT have varied widely. This situation is brought about because of the absence of a sharp division between diabetics and nondiabetics, variations in methodology and variations in adjustment for the many conditions that may affect the GTT quite apart from diabetes mellitus; some of these factors have been mentioned previously, and others will be discussed later. The criteria of Fajans and Conn are probably the most widely accepted (other reasonably established criteria are listed on page 483). Normal oral GTT values (mg/100 ml true glucose) include:

TIME	SERUM (MG/100 ML)	WHOLE BLOOD (MG/100 ML)
Fasting	70–110	60–100
1 hour	< 185	< 160
(1½ hours)	(< 160)	(< 145)
2 hours	< 140	< 120

Note: Add 1 mg/100 ml/year over age 50 to each nonfasting value.

For the diagnosis of diabetes mellitus, at least two of these figures must be abnormal (assuming all other factors that could influence the GTT are eliminated). If only one single value on the curve is abnormal, it is considered suspicious, but not diagnostic, of diabetes. Other authorities suggest slightly different criteria (p. 483). Taking a representative sample of the literature, normal values for (whole blood) FBS range from 100 to 120 mg/100 ml; 1-hour levels, from 150 to 170 mg/100 ml; and 2-hour values from "FBS" to 120 mg/100 ml. Nevertheless, the criteria of Fajans and Conn correlate well enough with the clinical course of diabetes to have thus far warranted acceptance in the interest of diagnostic uniformity.

Screening Tests for Diabetes

Screening tests for diabetes attempt to circumvent the multiple blood sugar determinations required for the GTT. The FBS and the 2-hour postprandial (2-hour pc) blood sugar level have been widely used. Since these methods constitute, in essence, isolated segments of the GTT, interpretation of their results must take several problems into consideration in addition to those inherent in the GTT.

An abnormality in the FBS, for example, raises the question of whether a full GTT is needed for confirmation of diabetes. Most authors believe that *if the FBS is elevated, there is no need to do the full glucose tolerance test.* Whatever the etiology for the abnormal FBS, the GTT will also be abnormal; since it is known in advance that the GTT will be abnormal, no further information will be gained from performing the GTT. Most also agree that a normal FBS is not reliable in screening for diabetes. In one study, 63% of those with diabetic GTT had normal FBS; and others have had similar experiences, although perhaps with less striking figures.

Most investigators believe that of all the GTT values and criteria, the 2-hour level is the most crucial. The 2-hour value alone has therefore been proposed as a screening test. This recommendation is based on the fact that the helpfulness of blood sugar levels prior to the 2-hour time point is open to some question. Fajans and Conn state that "the diagnosis of diabetes mellitus cannot be made with confidence on the basis of an abnormal elevation of blood sugar level at ½ or 1 hour if it is accompanied by a normal 2-hour blood sugar level in the GTT." The main reason for this lies in the effect of gastric emptying on glucose absorption. It has been fairly well proved that normal gastric emptying does not deliver a saturation dose. Therefore, slow gastric emptying tends to produce a low or "flat" GTT. On the other hand, either unusually swift gastric transit or delivery of a normal total quantity of glucose to the small intestine within a markedly shortened time span results in abnormally high amounts of glucose absorbed during the initial phases of the tolerance test. Since homeostatic mechanisms are not instantaneous, the peak values of the tolerance curve reach abnormally high figures before the hyperglycemia is brought under control. An extreme example of this situation occurs in the "dumping syndrome" produced by gastrojejunostomy.

If previous time interval specimens are considered unreliable, the question then is justified as to whether the 2-hour value alone is sufficient. In many cases, if the 2-hour level is definitely abnormal, a full GTT would not add any useful information, although an FBS would provide some further indication of the severity of derangement in carbohydrate homeostasis. If the 2-hour level is equivocal (140 mg/100 ml ± 10 mg/100 ml), a GTT should be done, since abnormalities in other areas of the curve would give added support to the suspicion of diabetes. This assumes also that nonpancreatic diabetogenic influences are ruled out. There are several provisos to this situation that must be kept in mind. If the 2-hour postprandial specimen follows an ordinary meal rather than being part of a standard tolerance test, the problem of adequate carbohydrate preparation may obscure results as well as possible variations in the amount and type of sugar ingested. Also, Fajans and Conn, as well as others, report one variation of the normal oral GTT that drops relatively swiftly to normal at approximately 1½ hours and then rebounds above 140 mg/100 ml by 2 hours. In one report this phenomenon occurred in as many as 5–10% of patients. This is the basis for the suggested inclusion of a 1 ½-hour specimen into the oral GTT procedure. Finally, Fajans and Conn call attention to their follow-up data on persons with normal 2-hour values but abnormal or borderline levels elsewhere in the GTT curve. Subsequent retesting over periods of years frequently revealed progression to a degree of carbohydrate impairment diagnostic of diabetes. With these limitations, the 2-hour postprandial blood sugar is a very useful screening test. It is definitely more sensitive than the FBS, and its specificity could be increased by utilizing the standard carbohydrate preparation and a standard oral glucose test dose.

Glucose Tolerance in Other Diseases

Besides the intrinsic and extrinsic factors that modify response to the oral glucose tolerance test procedure, other diseases besides diabetes mellitus regularly produce diabetic-type GTT patterns or curves. Among these are adrenal, thyroid and pituitary hormone abnormalities that influence liver or tissue response to blood glucose levels. *Cushing's syndrome* results from hypersecretion of hydrocortisone. Since this hormone stimulates gluconeogenesis, among its other actions, 70–80% of these patients exhibit decreased carbohydrate tolerance, while 25% of those with Cushing's syndrome demonstrate overt diabetes. *Pheochromocytomas* of the adrenal medulla (or elsewhere) have been reported to produce hyperglycemia in nearly 60% of the affected patients, and glucosuria in a lesser number. These tumors produce norepinephrine or epinephrine, either continually or intermittently. The diabetogenic effects of epinephrine were mentioned earlier, and it has been noted that those pheochromocytomas that secrete norepinephrine rather than epinephrine are not associated with abnormalities of carbohydrate metabolism. *Primary aldosteronism* leads to the overproduction of aldosterone, the chief electrolyte-regulating adrenocortical hormone. This increases renal tubular excretion of potassium and retention of sodium. Patients with primary aldosteronism frequently may develop decreased carbohydrate tolerance. According to Conn, this is most likely due to potassium depletion,which in some manner adversely affects the ability of pancreatic beta cells to respond normally to a hyperglycemic stimulus. Parenthetically, there may be some analogy in the reports that *chlorothiazide diuretics* may cause added decrease in carbohydrate tolerance in diabetics, thus acting as diabetogenic agents. Some say no such effect exists in normal persons, but others maintain that it does in a few. Chlorothiazide often leads to potassium depletion as a side effect; indeed, one report indicates that potassium supplements will reverse the diabetogenic effect. However, other mechanisms have been postulated.

Thyroid hormone has several effects on carbohydrate metabolism. First, thyroxine acts in some way on small intestine mucosal cells to increase hexose sugar absorption. In the liver, thyroxine causes increased gluconeogenesis from protein and increased breakdown of glycogen to glucose. The metabolic rate of peripheral tissues is increased, resulting in an increased rate of glucose utilization. Peripheral tissue glycogen is depleted. Nevertheless, the effect of *hyperthyroidism* on the GTT is variable. Apparently the characteristic hyperthyroid curve is one that peaks unusually high, sometimes with glucosuria, but which returns to normal ranges by 2 hours. However, in one extensive survey, as many as 7% were reported to have diabetic curves and another 2% had actual diabetes mellitus. Surprisingly, the type of curve found in any individual patient was without relation to the severity of the hyperthyroidism. In *myxedema*, a "flat" oral GTT (defined as a peak rise of less than 25 mg/100 ml above FBS) is common. However, in hypothyroidism a normal or even a diabetic-type curve may be found, since absorption defects vary in degree and are counterpoised against decreased tissue metabolism.

Hyperpituitarism, especially acromegaly, may produce a diabetic or pseudodiabetic GTT. Growth hormone (somatotropin) is thought to have its own ability to stimulate gluconeogenesis. Actually, the influence of the pituitary on carbohydrate metabolism has been mainly studied in conditions of pituitary hypofunction; in hypopituitarism, a defect in gluconeogenesis was found that was due to a combination of thyroid and adrenocorticosteroid deficiency rather than to deficiency of either agent alone.

In *acute pancreatitis,* perhaps 25–50% of patients may have transient hyperglycemia. In chronic pancreatitis, abnormal glucose tolerance or outright diabetes mellitus is extremely common.

A variety of nonendocrine disorders may produce diabetogenic effects on carbohydrate tolerance. *Chronic renal disease with azotemia* frequently demonstrates a diabetic curve of varying degree, sometimes even to the point of fasting hyperglycemia. The reason is not definitely known. It is said that the tolbutamide test (discussed in Chapter 35) is normal in nondiabetics with azotemia. Hyperglycemia with or without glucosuria occurs from time to time in patients with *cerebral lesions.* These may include tumors, skull fracture, cerebral infarction, intracerebral hemorrhage and encephalitis. The mechanism is not known, but experimental evidence suggests some type of center with regulatory influence on glucose metabolism located in the medulla and the hypothalamus, and perhaps elsewhere. Similar reasoning applies to the transient hyperglycemia, sometimes accompanied by glucosuria, seen in *severe carbon monoxide poisoning.* This is said to appear in 50% of these patients, and seems to be due to a direct toxic effect on the cerebral centers responsible for carbohydrate metabolism. One subgroup of *lipoproteinemia* (p. 254) is also said to frequently elicit some degree of decreased carbohydrate tolerance, which sometimes may include fasting hyperglycemia.

Malignancies of varying types are reported to produce decreased carbohydrate tolerance in varying numbers of patients, but the true incidence and the mechanism involved are difficult to ascertain due to the presence of other diabetogenic factors such as fever, cachexia, liver dysfunction and inactivity.

Liver disease often affects the oral GTT; this is not surprising in view of the importance of the liver in carbohydrate homeostasis. Abnormality is most often seen in cirrhosis; the degree of abnormality has a general (although not exact) correlation with degree of liver damage. In well-established cirrhosis, the 2-hour postprandial blood sugar is usually abnormal. The FBS is variable, but is most often normal. Fatty liver may produce GTT abnormality similar to that of cirrhosis. In infectious hepatitis there is less abnormality than in cirrhosis; results become normal during convalescence and may be normal throughout in mild disease.

Myocardial infarction has been shown to precipitate temporary hyperglycemia, glucosuria or decreased carbohydrate tolerance. In one representative study, 75% had abnormal GTT during the acute phase of infarction, with 50% of these being frankly diabetic curves; follow-up showed that about a third of the abnormal curves persisted. Besides the well-known increased incidence of atherosclerosis (predisposing to infarction) in overt or latent diabetics, emotional factors in a stress situation and hypotension or hepatic passive congestion with liver damage may be contributory. *Emotional hyperglycemia* is considered a well-established entity and probably is secondary to epinephrine effect.

Oral glucose tolerance tests in *pregnancy* are the subject of dispute. Some investigators believe that the oral GTT in gravid women does not differ from that of nulliparas, and thus any abnormalities in the curve are suspicious of latent diabetes. Others believe that pregnancy itself, especially in the last trimester, tends to exert a definite diabetogenic influence. This view is reinforced by observations that various *synthetic estrogen-progesterone combinations used for contraception* often mimic the diabetogenic effects of pregnancy. This may occur in 18–46% of patients, and, as in pregnancy, the FBS is most often normal. The exact mechanism is not clear; some offer an explanation of altered intestinal absorption.

Salicylate overdose in children frequently produces a clinical situation that closely resembles diabetic acidosis. Salicylate in large quantities has a toxic effect on the liver, leading to decreased glycogen formation and to increased breakdown of glycogen to glucose. Therefore, there may develop a mild to moderate elevation in blood sugar, accompanied by ketonuria. Plasma ketone tests may even be positive, although usually only to mild degree. Salicylic acid metabolites give positive results in tests for reducing substances such as Clinitest (p. 110), so that such tests falsely suggest glucosuria. In addition, salicylate stimulates the central nervous system respiratory center in the early phases of overdose, so that increased respiration may suggest the Kussmaul breathing of diabetic acidosis. The CO_2 content (or combining power) is decreased. Later on, a metabolic acidosis develops.

Differentiation from diabetic acidosis can be accomplished by simple tests for salicylate in plasma or urine. A dipstick test called Phenistix (p. 117) is very useful for screening purposes. A positive plasma Phenistix reaction for salicylate is good evidence of salicylate poisoning. A positive result in urine is not conclusive, since in urine the procedure will detect nontoxic levels of salicylate, but a negative urine result would be strong evidence against the diagnosis. Definitive chemical quantitative or semi-quantitative tests for blood salicylate levels are available. It is important to ask about a history of medication given to the patient or the possibility of accidental ingestion in children with suspicious clinical symptoms.

Salicylate intoxication is not frequent in adults. When it occurs, there is much less tendency toward development of a pseudodiabetic acidosis syndrome. In fact, in adults, salicylate in nontoxic dose occasionally produces hypoglycemia, which tends to occur 2–4 hours postprandially.

Dilantin is reported to decrease glucose tolerance; and overdose occasionally produces a type of nonketotic hyperglycemic coma.

Controversy on Clinical Relevance of the Oral Tolerance Test

Complete discussion of the oral GTT must include reference to other studies that attack the clinical usefulness of the procedure. These comprise reports of large series of normal persons showing up to 20% "flat" GTT results, studies that showed different curves in repeat determinations after time lapse and others in which various types of curves were obtained on repeated tests in the same individual. Some investigators feel there is inadequate evidence that GTT abnormality actually indicates true diabetes mellitus (at least, with the normal values customarily used), since many persons with abnormal GTT fail to progress to clinical diabetes and the population incidence of diabetes is far short of that predicted by GTT screening. Therefore, sensitivity, specificity, reproducibility and clinical relevance have all been challenged, even under standardized test conditions. Nevertheless, at present the oral GTT is still the standard parameter of carbohydrate tolerance and the laboratory basis for the diagnosis of diabetes mellitus.

Intravenous Glucose Tolerance Test

This test was devised to eliminate some of the objections to the oral GTT. Standard procedure for the intravenous test (IV-GTT) is as follows: The patient has a 3-day high-carbohydrate preparatory diet. After an FBS is obtained, a standard solution of 50% glucose is injected intravenously over a 3–4-minute period. Blood samples are obtained at ½, 1, 2 and 3 hours, although it would seem more informative to omit the ½-hour specimen and substitute a 1½-hour sample. The curve reaches a peak immediately after injection (300–400 mg/100 ml, accompanied by glucosuria), then falls steadily but not linearly toward fasting levels. Criteria for interpretation are not uniform. However, most believe that a normal response is indicated by return to fasting levels by 1–1¼ hours. The height of the curve has no significance. Most agree that the IV-GTT is adequately reproducible. In diabetes, fasting levels are not reached in 2 hours and often not even by 3. The curve in liver disease is most characteristically said to return to normal between 1¼ and 2 hours; however, some patients with cirrhosis have a diabetic-type curve. Many of the same factors that produce a diabetogenic effect on the oral GTT do likewise to the intravenous procedure; these include carbohydrate deprivation, inactivity, old age, fever, uremia, stress, neoplasms and the various steroid-producing endocrine diseases. There are, however, several differences from the oral GTT. Alimentary problems are eliminated. The IV-GTT is said to be normal in pregnancy, also in hyperthyroidism, although one report found occasional abnormality in thyrotoxicosis. The IV-GTT is conceded to be somewhat less sensitive than the oral procedure, although, as just noted, a little more specific.

Cortisone Glucose Tolerance Test

Fajans and Conn attempted to improve the sensitivity of the oral GTT. They found that the addition of adrenocortical steroids to the procedure magnified slight degrees of defective carbohydrate tolerance and produced an increased number of abnormal curves in a group of patients with a history or genetic background strongly predisposing toward diabetes. For example, of 17 persons with "suspicious" oral GTT, 88% had positive cortisone glucose tolerance test (C-GTT). Follow-ups tended to substantiate the test results, since Fajans and Conn report that 25% of those with positive C-GTT and normal oral GTT developed outright diabetes and 10% probable diabetes. The procedure for the C-GTT is as follows: After standard 3-day carbohydrate diet, oral cortisone acetate is given at specified intervals; then the standard oral GTT is run. Normal values are approximately 20 mg/100 ml above those of the standard oral GTT. The 2-hour value is the most crucial, just as in the standard GTT. Several reports have subsequently agreed with these findings regarding sensitivity and specificity. Others have not been enthusiastic. However, Fajans and Conn correctly point out that several misconceptions about C-GTT exist. The test does not disclose genetic susceptibility to diabetes, only a certain degree of decreased carbohydrate tolerance. The test and interpretation must be done as originally described, and, if comparison with standard oral GTT results is desired, the criteria of Fajans and Conn for the oral GTT must also be used. These authors further maintain that obesity per se does not seem to influence either the standard or C-GTT, although obesity in diabetics further decreased carbohydrate tolerance. Old age, inadequate carbohydrate diet and most other diabetogenic factors that influence the standard oral GTT do likewise to the C-GTT. Cortisone priming seems to increase greatly the number of abnormal GTTs in pregnancy, and apparently the significance of this is not yet established. At present, the C-GTT is recommended by its originators mainly as a research tool; its usefulness lies in demonstrating probable diabetes in some persons with only minimally decreased carbohydrate tolerance.

Plasma (or Serum) Insulin Assay

Insulin was the first substance used successfully in radioisotope immunoassay, and it is now available in most sizable reference laboratories. In general, juvenile diabetics have low fasting insulin levels, and an oral GTT using insulin determinations will usually produce a flat curve. Mild diabetics possess normal fasting insulin levels and display a GTT curve that has a delayed rise, either to normal height or to a point moderately above normal; in either case the curve thereafter falls in a normal fashion. Decreased tolerance due to many other causes produces similar curves; an insulin GTT has not been more efficient in uncovering subclinical diabetes than blood sugar GTT. Some maintain that the ratio of insulin values to glucose values obtained on the same specimen during the oral GTT is more reliable than insulin values alone. At any rate, most investigators feel that, at present, plasma insulin levels should not be used for diagnosis of diabetes mellitus.

Plasma anticoagulated with EDTA is reported to produce values equal to serum, but heparin is said to be associated with values greater than serum.

Patients being treated with insulin develop anti-insulin antibodies after approximately 6 weeks. These antibodies interfere with insulin RIA measurement by competing with insulin antibodies used in the test. Whether values will be falsely increased or decreased will depend on the method used. Endogenous antibodies will not interfere with tolerance tests, since their quantity remains unchanged throughout the test; only the baseline value is affected.

Classification of Diabetes

A new classification of diabetes has been proposed and is gaining considerable acceptance. This is partially based on the various laboratory tests discussed. The categories are:

1. Prediabetes: all laboratory tests normal; genetic predisposition.

2. Subclinical diabetes: cortisone GTT abnormal; oral GTT normal.

3. Latent (chemical) diabetes: oral GTT abnormal; FBS normal or abnormal; no clinical symptoms.

4. Overt diabetes: FBS abnormal; clinical diabetes.

Glucosuria

Besides measurement of blood glucose or carbohydrate tolerance, certain other procedures are widely used or proposed for the detection of diabetes mellitus. The appearance of glucose in the urine has long been utilized both for detection and as a parameter of treatment. As a clue to diagnosis, urine sugar depends on hyperglycemia that exceeds the renal tubular threshold for glucose. This is usually quoted as 170 mg/100 ml (Somogyi whole blood values) for venous blood. Of some interest regarding the threshold concept in diabetics is evidence that some diabetics possess either low thresholds or, especially in the elderly, unusually high ones (up to 300 mg/100 ml). It has also been shown that arterial blood glucose levels are much better correlated with glucosuria than venous ones. Nevertheless, routine urine testing provides a method for practical continuous outpatient monitoring of therapy and for the prevention of ketoacidosis. This aspect provides another argument for more routine use of the full GTT, since glucosuria can be correlated with degree of hyperglycemia. Incidentally, many diabetic patients and many of those involved in mass surveys take their urine sugar test before breakfast, which actually is the least likely time to produce glucosuria.

The problem of causes of hyperglycemia not due to diabetes mellitus was discussed earlier. Renal threshold assumes importance in another way because of the condition known as renal glucosuria. This may be congenital or acquired; the acquired type may be idiopathic or secondary to certain diseases such as the Fanconi syndrome, acute tubular necrosis or renal rickets. In all types there is glucosuria at lower blood sugar levels than normal. Some report that a significant number of those with the nonfamilial idiopathic variety of renal glucosuria eventually develop overt diabetes mellitus, although others do not agree.

Glucosuria of pregnancy occurs in the last trimester. Reported incidence depends on the sensitivity of the testing methods used, ranging from 5% to 35% or even 70%. The etiology seems to be a combination of increased glomerular filtration rate and temporarily decreased renal threshold. Lactosuria is even more common. Glucosuria without hyperglycemia occurs in 20% of patients with lead poisoning. This is due to a direct toxic effect on the renal tubule cells. Glucosuria of a transient nature has been reported in 24% of normal newborn infants. A study utilizing paper chromatography revealed galactosuria, usually in amounts too small for detection by routine techniques, to be even more common.

Mentioned here only for the sake of completeness are the two main types of urine sugar tests: the copper sulfate tests for reducing substances, and the glucose oxidase enzyme papers. The merits, drawbacks and technical aspects of these tests, as well as a general discussion of glucosuria, are included in Chapter 12.

Diagnosis of Diabetic Coma

Diabetic coma may occur without a history of diabetes or in circumstances where history is not available. Other major etiologies of coma have to be considered, including insulin hypoglycemia, meningitis or cerebrovascular accident, shock, uremia and barbiturate overdose. Diabetic coma yields a clearcut, fast diagnosis by means of a plasma acetone test. Anticoagulated blood is obtained; a portion is centrifuged for 2 to 3 minutes, and the plasma is tested for acetone. Diabetic acidosis severe enough to produce coma will be definitely positive (except for the rare cases of lactic acidosis or hyperosmolar coma [p. 458]). The other etiologies for coma will be negative, since they rarely produce the degree of acidosis found in diabetic coma. The findings of urinary glucose and acetone strongly suggest diabetes, but may occur in other conditions. Such findings would not entirely rule out insulin overdose (always a consideration in a known diabetic), since the urine could have been produced before the overdose. This would be unlikely, however, if urinary acetone were strongly positive. An elevated blood sugar also is strong evidence of diabetic coma, especially in marked degrees of elevation. Other conditions that might combine coma with hyperglycemia (cerebrovascular accident, acute myocardial infarction) have only mild or moderate hyperglycemia in those instances where hyperglycemia is produced. Besides blood sugar determination, a simple empirical test to rule out hypoglycemia is to inject some glucose solution intravenously. Cerebral damage is investigated by cerebrospinal fluid examination. Uremia is determined by means of the blood urea nitrogen, although other etiologies of coma besides primary renal disease may have an elevated BUN. Drug ingestion is established by careful history, analysis of stomach contents and identification of the drug in blood samples (one anticoagulated and one clotted specimen are preferred). Shock is diagnosed on the basis of blood pressure; further laboratory investigation depends on the probable etiology.

HYPOGLYCEMIA

Whereas diabetes is caused by insulin deficiency, a syndrome is produced by insulin excess. The best-known cause is functioning islet cell tumor (insulinoma), usually adenoma, but occasionally carcinoma. In these patients, symptoms are most often precipitated by fasting. The first effects are vague malaise and apathy, followed by hypoglycemia signs. These include nausea, weakness, nervousness, tachycardia and sweating. If hypoglycemia is allowed to continue, fainting or even coma will follow, often with convulsions. Sometimes central nervous system symptoms predominate; these are identical to those of central nervous system hypoxia and produce bizarre behavior and blurring of consciousness. Differential diagnosis includes alcoholism, uremia, hyperventilation, barbiturate overdose and diabetic coma. Hypoglycemia may be produced by other causes; the most important of these is *functional hypoglycemia*. This condition is fairly common, and differs from organic hypoglycemia in that attacks are brought on by intake of carbohydrates. It represents an abnormal response of the pancreas to only moderately increased carbohydrate loads, resulting in oversecretion of insulin by the pancreas and the development of temporary hypoglycemia 1–3 hours later when the initial blood sugar elevation is eliminated and some of the excess insulin is still present. The initial blood sugar elevation is no greater than that of a normal person. Somewhat different conditions are found in certain postgastrectomy patients, where gastric emptying is swift and complete so that ingested carbohydrates are suddenly dumped into the duodenum, resulting in abnormally high blood sugar levels and temporary hypoglycemia after hastily produced insulin has overcome the initial hyperglycemia. This is called the dumping syndrome or alimentary hypoglycemia. The initial blood sugar elevation is definitely greater than that of a normal person.

Diagnostic Procedures

Diagnosis of islet cell tumor is important, since the condition is surgically correctable but accurate diagnosis is a necessity to avoid unnecessary operation. The basic criterion is Whipple's triad, which consists of:

1. attacks of central nervous system or hypoglycemia symptoms while fasting

2. an FBS of 10 mg/100 ml or more below FBS normal lower limits at some time

3. Relief of symptoms by glucose

The diagnosis may have to be confirmed by some other method. Several procedures are available that serve as screening or confirmatory tests.

ORAL 5-HOUR GLUCOSE TOLERANCE TEST.—The patient fasts for 8–12 hours, unless symptoms are brought on sooner. The standard oral GTT procedure is then carried out, but with hourly blood samples until 5 hours have elapsed. Results for insulin-producing tumor characteristically display a low or low normal FBS and the usual sharp rise after glucose (remaining within normal GTT values), then a slower fall to hypoglycemic levels that do not rapidly return to normal range. If the curve has not reached 50 mg/100 ml in 5 hours, the test is prolonged 1 additional hour. The curve for alimentary hypoglycemia shows normal FBS, marked rise after glucose with the peak greater than normal GTT values, then a rapid fall to hypoglycemia within 2–4 hours. Functional hypoglycemia typically has normal FBS, a rise after glucose but within normal GTT values, then a fall to hypoglycemia within 2–4 hours. Diabetics may sometimes produce a GTT curve in which the 2-hour value is elevated but which continues to decrease to mild hypoglycemic levels between 2 and 4 hours before returning to FBS (Fig 27–1).

Unfortunately, interpretation is not as simple as would appear from this description. A considerable minority of insulin-producing tumors are reported to demonstrate a "flat" curve, or sometimes even a diabetic-type curve, rather than what would be expected. In addition, it was found in at least one study that 23% of the presumably normal population sampled produced an asymptomatic blood glucose level below 50 mg/100 ml between 2 and 5 hours during the oral GTT, with a few as low as 35 mg/100 ml. Thus, the diagnosis of organic hypoglycemia from GTT curves must be made with caution.

The major utility of the 5-hour oral GTT in patients with hypoglycemia is to suggest etiologies other than islet cell tumor, specifically those just mentioned in which hypoglycemia is provoked by food intake rather than fasting.

PLASMA INSULIN-GLUCOSE RATIO.—The immunoreactive insulin-glucose (IRI/G) ratio should be less than 0.3 (the immunoreactive insulin measured in microunits per milliliter, the glucose in milligrams per 100 ml). The ratio is abnormal if greater than 0.3 in nonobese persons, and in

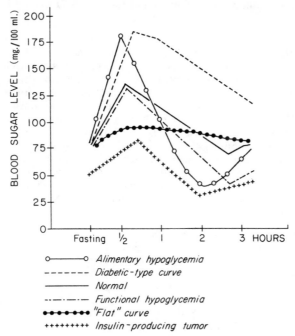

Fasting   ½   1   2   3 HOURS

○————○ *Alimentary hypoglycemia*
−−−−−− *Diabetic-type curve*
———— *Normal*
−··−··—··− *Functional hypoglycemia*
●●●●●●● *"Flat" curve*
+++++++++ *Insulin-producing tumor*

Fig 27–1.—Representative oral glucose tolerance curves.

obese persons, if greater than 0.3 with serum glucose below 60 mg/100 ml. Hyperinsulinism due to insulinoma results in serum insulin levels inappropriately high in relation to the low serum glucose values. In some instances the IRI/G ratio may be abnormal when the actual serum insulin value is within normal range. (Instead of IRI/G, some use G/IRI.)

TOLBUTAMIDE TOLERANCE TEST FOR INSULINOMA.—The test is performed in the same way as in the diagnosis of diabetes, but normal values are different. In patients with insulin-producing tumors the fall in blood sugar is greater than that of most normals—down to the 40–65% of FBS range compared to normals, who are usually over 50% of FBS.

Since there is occasional overlap, of greater significance is the fact that insulin tumor hypoglycemia persists for more than 3 hours, whereas in most normals the blood sugar level has returned to fasting values by 3 hours. In a few normals and in those with functional hypoglycemia, values return to at least 80% of FBS by 3 hours. Adrenal insufficiency also returns to at least 80% by 3 hours, although the initial decrease may be as great as that in insulin tumor. Some patients with severe liver disease give curves similar to those of insulin tumor. However, this is not frequent and usually is not a real diagnostic problem. The tolbutamide test is apparently more sensitive than the oral glucose tolerance test for the diagnosis of islet cell tumor, but has the disadvantage that the characteristic responses of functional or alimentary hypoglycemia to the oral GTT cannot be demonstrated.

PROINSULIN.—Insulin is derived from a precursor called proinsulin synthesized in the pancreas, which is metabolically inactive and larger in size ("big insulin"). Proinsulin consists of an alpha and a beta chain connected by an area called "connecting peptide" (C-peptide). Proinsulin is enzymatically cleaved within beta cells into equal quantities of insulin and C-peptide. Radioimmunoassay measurement of insulin includes both proinsulin and regular insulin. Normally, about 5–15% of so-called immunoreactive insulin (that which is measured by RIA) is proinsulin. In many (but not all) patients with insulinomas, the amount of circulating proinsulin is increased relative to total insulin. In diabetics with insulin deficiency being treated with insulin, proinsulin within that person's own immunoreactive insulin values may be increased. Measurement of proinsulin necessitates special procedures such as Sephadex column chromatography and is not widely available.

EFFECTIVENESS OF METHODS.—Since islet-cell insulinomas are not common, it is difficult to compile large series of patients in whom all detection methods were used. Thus far, the most accurate method is prolonged fasting with periodic insulin plus glucose measurement, or such measurement if symptoms develop. This may take up to 72 hours. After an overnight fast, approximately two thirds of tumors may be revealed by IRI/G ratio and about 50% with FBS alone. After a 48-hour fast, IRI/G uncovers approximately 85% of tumors, and after 72 hours, over 95%. Blood sugar alone detects about 70% of patients at 72 hours. Roughly 80% display abnormal proinsulin level (percent of total insulin) and tolbutamide test results.

Besides these procedures, leucine and glucagon tests have been used. However, these are somewhat less sensitive than IRI/G or tolbutamide.

The majority of islet cell tumors are located in the body or tail of the pancreas; about 90% are benign adenomas. Pancreatic artery angiography may be very helpful to pinpoint the exact location of the tumor. Most institutions, however, are able to detect less than 50% by arteriography.

SERUM C-PEPTIDE MEASUREMENT.—As noted previously, C-peptide is a by-product of insulin production. Although it is released in quantity equal to insulin, serum C-peptide levels do not exactly parallel those of insulin, due to differences in serum half-life and catabolic rate. Nevertheless, C-peptide values correlate well with insulin values in terms of the position of each in relation to its own normal range (i.e., if one is decreased, the other likewise is decreased). Therefore, C-peptide can be used as an indicator of insulin secretion.

Occasional patients produce hypoglycemia by self-administration of insulin. Since insulin assay cannot differentiate between exogenous insulin and that produced by insulinoma, measurement of C-peptide can be helpful. If self-administration of insulin is suspected, C-peptide assay should be performed on the same specimen that showed elevated insulin. In hyperinsulinism from islet cell tumor, C-peptide is elevated; in that due to exogenous insulin, C-peptide is low. Some of those who take insulin develop insulin antibodies; this offers an alternate method for detection.

OTHER ETIOLOGIES. — Five other etiologies of hypoglycemia should be mentioned. They are:

1. Certain nonpancreatic tumors, presumably either by glucose utilization or by production of an insulinlike substance. The great majority have been intra-abdominal neoplasms of large size, usually described as fibrosarcomas or spindle cell sarcomas. Hepatoma is next most frequent.

2. Leucine sensitivity of infancy and childhood. Symptoms are produced by ingestion of cow's milk, which contains the amino acid leucine. Diagnosis is made by a leucine tolerance test, similar to the oral GTT but using oral leucine.

3. Alcohol hypoglycemia may occur either in chronic alcoholics or occasional drinkers. Malnutrition, chronic or temporary, seems an important predisposing factor. Fasting for 12 – 24 hours precedes alcohol intake; symptoms may occur immediately, but most often follow 6 – 34 hours later.

4. Overdose of insulin in a diabetic. Since the patient may be found in coma without any history available, insulin overdose must be a major consideration in any emergency-room comatose patient.

5. Hypoglycemia of latent diabetes (usually mild; p. 319).

REFERENCES

Andres, R.: Aging and diabetes, Med. Clin. North Am. 55:835, 1971.

Baker, R. J.: Newer considerations in the diagnosis and management of fasting hypoglycemia, Surg. Clin. North Am. 49:191, 1969.

Blonde, L., and Riddick, F. A.: Hypoglycemia: The "undisease," South. Med. J. 69: 1261, 1976.

Cohen, B. D.: Abnormal carbohydrate metabolism in renal disease, Ann. Intern. Med. 57:204, 1962.

Conn, J. W.: Hypertension, the potassium ion, and impaired carbohydrate tolerance, N. Engl.J. Med. 273:1135, 1965.

Fajans, S.: What is diabetes? Definition, diagnosis, and course, Med. Clin. North Am. 55:793, 1971.

Frethem, A. A.: Clinics on endocrine and metabolic diseases. 10. Relation of fasting blood glucose level to oral glucose tolerance curve, Proc. Staff Meet. Mayo Clin. 38:110, 1963.

Fulop, M., and Hoberman, H. D.: Alcoholic ketosis, Diabetes 24:785, 1975.

Grunt, J. A., et al.: Blood sugar serum insulin and free fatty acid interrelationships during intravenous tolbutamide testing in normal young adults and in patients with insulinoma, Diabetes 19:122, 1970.

Hofeldt, F. D., et al.: Postprandial hypoglycemia; fact or fiction? J.A.M.A. 233:1309, 1975.

Horwitz, D. L., et al.: Circulatory serum C-peptide: A brief review of diagnostic implications, N. Engl. J. Med. 295:207, 1976.

Ibarra, J. D.: Hypoglycemia, Postgrad. Med. 51:88, 1972.

Jackson, W. P. U.: The cortisone-glucose tolerance test with special reference to the prediction of diabetes, Diabetes 10:33, 1961.

John, J.: Hyperthyroidism showing carbohydrate metabolism disturbances, J.A.M.A. 99:620, 1932.

Kaplan, N. M.: Tolbutamide tolerance test in carbohydrate metabolism disturbances, Arch. Intern. Med. 107:212, 1961.

Kraft, J. R.: Detection of diabetes mellitus in situ (occult diabetes), Lab. Med. 6:10, 1975.

Liechty, R. D., et al.: Islet cell hyperinsulinism in adults and children, J.A.M.A. 230: 1538, 1974.

McDonald, G. W.: Reproducibility of the oral glucose tolerance test, Diabetes 14: 473, 1965.

Mackay, N., et al.: Observer error in Dextrostix estimations of blood-sugar, Lancet 2: 269, 1965.

Madison, L. L.: Ethanol-Induced Hypoglycemia, in Levine, R., and Luft, R. (eds.): *Advances in Metabolic Disorders* (New York: Academic Press, Inc., 1968), vol. 3, p. 85.

Medford, F. E.: An evaluation of the glucose oxidase skin test in the diagnosis of diabetes mellitus, W. Va. Med. J. 60:255, 1964.

Merimee, T. J., and Tyson, J. E.: Stabilization of plasma glucose during fasting: Normal variations in two separate studies, N. Engl. J. Med. 291:1275, 1974.

Milstein, J. M.: Hypoglycemia in the neonate, Postgrad. Med. 50:91, 1971.

Munch-Peterson, C. J.: Glycosuria of cerebral origin, Brain 54:72, 1931.

Raskin, T. J., et al.: Oral glucose tolerance as a test of liver function, Gastroenterology 25:548, 1953.

Seltzer, H.: Insights about diabetes and hyperinsulinism gained from the insulin immunoassay, Postgrad. Med. 46:73, 1969.

Service, F. J., et al.: Insulinoma: Clinical and diagnostic features of 60 consecutive cases, Mayo Clin. Proc. 51:417, 1976.

Shatney, C. H., and Grage, T. B.: Diagnostic and surgical aspects of insulinoma, Am. J. Surg. 127:174, 1974.

Siperstein, M. D.: The glucose tolerance test: A pitfall in the diagnosis of diabetes mellitus, Adv. Intern. Med. 20:297, 1975.

Sowton, S.: Cardiac infarction and the glucose tolerance test, Br. Med. J. 1:84, 1962.

Spellacy, W. N.: A review of carbohydrate metabolism and the oral contraceptives, Am. J. Obstet. Gynecol. 104:448, 1969.

28 / Thyroid Function Tests

THYROID FUNCTION TESTS make up an important segment of laboratory medicine. Many patients have at least one sign or symptom that suggests thyroid disease. On the other hand, thyroid dysfunction produces a wide variety of effects without any single one being diagnostic. There has been a continual search for a laboratory test that will provide a clear-cut diagnosis. Enumeration of the classic signs and symptoms of thyroid disease is the best way to emphasize the necessity for such a test.

SIGNS AND SYMPTOMS OF THYROID DISEASE

Hyperthyroid.—Thyrotoxicosis may be produced by a diffusely hyperactive thyroid (Graves' disease) or a hyperfunctioning nodule (Plummer's disease). Many patients have eye signs such as exophthalmos, lid lag or stare. Other symptoms include tachycardia; warm, moist skin; heat intolerance; nervous hyperactive appearance; loss of weight; and tremor of fingers. Less frequent symptoms are diarrhea or congestive heart failure. Hemoglobin is usually normal; WBC count is normal or slightly decreased. There is sometimes an increase in lymphocytes. Patients may have various combinations of these clinical symptoms or have only minimal changes. It is in clinically borderline cases that thyroid function tests are of especially great help.

Hypothyroid.—Myxedema develops from thyroid hormone deficiency. Most common signs and symptoms include nonpitting edema of eyelids, face and extremities; loss of hair in the outer third of the eyebrows; large tongue; cold, dry skin with cold intolerance; lethargic appearance and mental activity. Cardiac shadow enlargement on chest x-ray is common, with normal or slow heart rate. Anorexia and constipation are frequent. Laboratory tests show anemia in over 50% of myxedema patients, with a macrocytic but nonmegaloblastic type in about 25%. The WBC count is usually normal. The cerebrospinal fluid usually has elevated protein level with normal cell counts, for unknown reasons. Again, the classic picture of myxedema is often completely missing or only partially developed; symptoms may be vague and misleading or may suggest some other disease.

Conditions that superficially resemble or simulate hypothyroidism in the infant (cretinism) include mongolism and Hurler's disease (because of mental defect, facial appearance and short stature); various types of dwarfism, including achondroplasia (because of short stature and retarded bone

333

TABLE 28-1.—THYROID FUNCTION TESTS

1. Thyroid uptake of iodine
   RAI
2. Thyroxine tests
   a) "Direct" measurement
      T_4 iodine
         PBI
         BEI
      T_4 by column
      T_4 by isotope
         Competitive protein binding (T_4D; Murphy-Pattee)
         RIA
         "Corrected" T_4
         Free thyroxine (dialysis method, Sterling)
   b) "Indirect" measurement
      T_3 uptake (resin uptake)
      Free thyroxine index (Clark and Horn)
3. Triiodothyronine tests
   T_3 RIA
4. Tissue utilization of thyroxine
   Basal metabolic rate
   Cholesterol
   Achilles tendon reflex
5. Pituitary and hypothalamic area tests
   TSH assay
   TRF test
6. Other
   Stimulation and suppression tests
   Thyroid scan
   LATS assay

age); and nephrosis (because of edema, high cholesterol and low T_4). Myxedema in older children and adults may be simulated by the nephrotic syndrome, mental deficiency (because of mental slowness) and sometimes simple obesity.

There is a comparatively large group of laboratory procedures that measure one or more aspects of thyroid function (Table 28–1). The multiplicity of these tests implies that none is infallible or invariably helpful. To get best results, one must have a thorough knowledge of each procedure, including what aspect of thyroid function is measured, reliability in diagnosis of thyroid conditions and false results caused by nonthyroid conditions. In certain cases, a brief outline of the technique involved when the test is actually performed helps clarify some of these points.

THYROID HORMONE PRODUCTION

Thyroid hormone production and utilization involves several steps (Fig 28–1). Thyroid gland activity is under the control of thyroid-stimulating hormone (TSH), produced by the anterior pituitary. In turn, the pituitary is controlled by thyrotropin-releasing factor (TRF) from the hypothalamus.

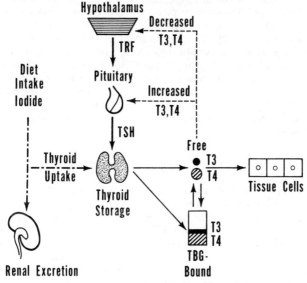

Fig 28–1.—Iodine and thyroxine metabolism.

The main raw material of thyroid hormone is inorganic iodide. Thyroid hormone synthesis begins when inorganic iodide is extracted from the blood by the thyroid. Within the thyroid, inorganic iodide is converted to organic iodine, and one iodine atom is incorporated into a tyrosine nucleus to form monoiodotyrosine. Monoiodotyrosine then incorporates a second iodine atom to form diiodotyrosine. Diidotyrosine may condense with itself to form thyroxine (T_4) or with monoiodotyrosine to form triiodothyronine (T_3). Thyroid hormone is stored in the thyroid acini as thyroglobulin, to be reconstituted and released when needed. In serum, T_4 comprises about 90% of thyroid hormone material, and T_3 about 3%. Weight for weight, T_3 is much more active than T_4, and many investigators feel that T_3 is the metabolically active form of thyroid hormone. Although some T_3 is secreted by the thyroid as part of thyroid hormone, most of it is probably derived from peripheral tissue deiodination of T_4. Due to the small amount of circulating T_3, the iodine of T_4 represents about 95% of total serum iodine. Almost 99% of both T_4 and T_3 are reversibly bound to serum proteins, predominantly to thyroid-binding globulin (TBG), an alpha$_1$ globulin, with a lesser amount carried by albumin and pre-albumin molecules. Hormone bound to TBG is metabolically inactive, as though it were in storage. The quantity of metabolically active nonbound ("free") T_4 or T_3 depends to some extent on the degree of saturation of TBG. Normally, TBG is about 15–30% saturated, but the actual proportion depends on the amount of T_4 produced by the thyroid plus the total quantity of TBG available to bind T_4. Since TBG-bound T_4 is not metabolically active, free thyroxine has a better correlation with thyroid hormone activity in certain situations than does total thyroxine.

There is a feedback control mechanism between serum levels of free T_4 and T_3 and the hypothalamus or pituitary. Decreased levels of free T_4 and T_3 stimulate TRF release, whereas increased serum T_4 and T_3 are thought to exert a direct inhibitory effect on pituitary secretion of TSH.

Certain drugs affect aspects of thyroid hormone production. Perchlorate and cyanate inhibit iodide trapping by the thyroid. The thiouracil compounds inhibit thyroid hormone synthesis within the gland from iodine and tyrosine. Iodine in large amounts tends to decrease thyroid vascularity and acinar hyperplasia and is thought to interfere briefly with thyroxine synthesis and to have some inhibitory effect on thyroid hormone release in Graves' disease.

THYROID UPTAKE OF IODINE

RADIOACTIVE IODINE UPTAKE. — The degree of thyroid hormone production normally determines how much iodine will be extracted from the bloodstream. A small dose of radioactive iodine is given, and the amount that enters the gland provides an indirect measure of thyroid activity. The test is said to have a clinical accuracy of 70–95%, gives definitely better results in hyperthyroidism than in the hypothyroid range, and is more accurate in Graves' disease than in thyrotoxicosis caused by hyperfunctioning ("toxic") nodule. In fact, 50–80% of patients with toxic nodular goiter are said to have normal RAI. Thyroid uptake is usually measured 24 hours after the test dose is administered. An occasional patient with thyrotoxicosis has unusually fast iodine turnover, so that maximal gland iodine concentration is reached before 12 hours and thus falls into normal range before 24 hours. In such cases, a 2-hour uptake is recommended, although some investigators prefer a 4-hour or a 6-hour determination.

Any condition that alters thyroid requirements for iodine will affect the RAI. Iodine deficiency goiter will elevate the RAI results, and excess organic or inorganic iodine will saturate the thyroid and produce low RAI values. In cirrhosis, 25–50% of patients are said to have abnormally high RAI due to dietary deficiency of iodine, although the deficiency is not severe enough to produce clinical symptoms. The RAI is affected by most of the same diseases that affect protein-bound iodine (PBI), but it differs in that some diseases, such as iodine-deficiency goiter, give abnormal RAI but not PBI, and hypoproteinemia gives abnormal PBI but not RAI. The RAI is affected by many, but not all, of the same drugs, medications and chemicals that interfere with the PBI (p. 488). The RAI may be elevated during the last trimester of pregnancy.

Normal values for the 24-hour uptake were formerly considered to be 15–40%; for the 2-hour uptake, 1.5–15%. Reports from several areas in the last few years have noted a significant drop in the normal 24-hour value (and presumably, in the early uptake level also); this has been attributed to iodine incorporated in food or contaminating the environment. This makes it difficult to interpret RAI results unless each laboratory periodically redetermines its own normal values — a procedure hardly ever done because of the nature of the test. Another drawback is that the patient receives a certain amount of radiation (especially if a scan is done); whereas thyroid hormone assays, even those using radioisotopes, do not involve irradiation of the patient.

THYROXINE TESTS

These procedures attempt to directly measure serum thyroxine and thus directly measure the actual hormonal activity of the thyroid. In actuality, many of these tests measure iodine, not thyroxine, but since more than 95% of serum iodine is normally part of thyroxine, iodine measurement approximates thyroxine measurement unless something markedly increases serum free iodine. The PBI was the first of these tests to be developed and is the best known and studied. The others were introduced subsequently in efforts to avoid some of the drawbacks of the PBI.

PROTEIN-BOUND IODINE. — As mentioned previously, thyroxine normally contains most of the serum iodine and is mainly bound to certain serum proteins. The PBI method precipitates serum proteins and measures the iodine present, thus providing a close but indirect estimation of thyroxine. There are various modifications of the PBI, but all are very similar and have the same three basic steps:

1. Protein-bound iodine is removed from the serum by chemical precipitation of serum proteins. The iodine of thyroxine is organic iodine, incorporated directly into the thyroxine molecule, rather than existing as inorganic ion (such as KI).

2. Protein is eliminated in order to isolate the iodine. This may be accomplished by chemical ("wet") digestion or by incineration in a special furnace ("dry ash"). During either process, organic iodine is converted to iodide ion.

3. Iodide is measured by a chemical reaction whose color change is proportional to the amount of iodide present.

If no interfering factors are present, the PBI is a reliable test for thyroid function, achieving a clinical accuracy of 90–95%. There is some overlap between normal and hypo- or hyperthyroid ranges, since the normal range is relatively wide (4–8 μg/100 ml). There are unfortunately several pitfalls for this otherwise extremely useful test, both clinically and in the laboratory. Since thyroxine is carried to some extent by albumin and pre-albumin proteins, any condition which leads to marked decrease of these proteins (such as the nephrotic syndrome or severe liver disease) will falsely decrease PBI. However, contamination by organic or inorganic iodine is the main drawback of the PBI. Inorganic iodine (iodide) is found predominantly in medicines. Organic iodine is located in many types of x-ray contrast media. Contamination is a major headache in the laboratory, whether from unclean glassware, impurities in water or specimens with high iodine values influencing other tests done at the same time or later with the same equipment. Values above 20μg/100 ml are suspicious for contamination, and above 25 μg/100 ml are almost invariably due to iodine contamination.

Changes in TBG levels, whether congenital or disease- or drug-induced, will also change PBI values. TBG may be altered by physiologic increase in pregnancy or with estrogen therapy (most commonly in the form of birth control pills), and treatment by thyroid hormone, antithyroid drugs, adrenocortical steroids, or various other medications (p. 488). The rule of thumb is that high estrogen elevates the PBI, while all other medications (excluding iodine or thyroid hormone) decrease the PBI. For example, if the amount of TBG is increased, then the amount of thyroxine bound to TBG must also increase to preserve the normal degree of TBG saturation, although serum free thyroxine remains normal and thyroid function is not affected. Some of the medications decrease thyroxine binding to TBG rather than change TBG level, but the test results are basically the same.

BUTANOL-EXTRACTABLE IODINE.—Extraction of T_4 by butanol in an alkaline medium is a way to remove contaminating inorganic iodide and also the T_4 precursors mono- and diiodotyrosine. After butanol separation, the T_4 extract is measured by a PBI technique. Although inorganic iodide is eliminated, butanol-extractable iodine (BEI) still is affected by organic iodine contamination and by thyroid-binding protein abnormalities, whether congenital or drug-induced.

THYROXINE BY COLUMN.—Because of technical difficulties with the BEI, a simplified column chromatography technique with ion exchange resin (instead of butanol) was used by some laboratories to eliminate inorganic iodide and T_4 precursors. In general, results were similar to those of the BEI. Interference by organic iodine and by thyroid-binding protein alterations continued to be a problem.

THYROXINE BY ISOTOPE.—There are two subgroups with considerable similarity: competitive protein binding (Murphy-Pattee, CPB, T_4D) and radioimmunoassay (RIA). Both groups are available in a wide variety of modifications and trade names. Isotope-labeled T_4 competes with patient (nonlabeled) T_4 from the patient's serum for a T_4-binding substance (anti-T_4 antibody in RIA or thyroid-binding protein in T_4D). The amount of labeled hormone attached to the binder will depend on the amount of patient (nonlabeled) hormone. Patient hormone thus displaces a certain amount of radioactive hormone from the binder, and the amount of radioactive hormone displaced can be counted in a radiation detector and used to calculate the quantity of patient hormone in the specimen. Radioactive hormone counting is the test end-point rather than measurement of iodine, so that neither inorganic iodide nor organic iodine will affect test results. Since both methods measure total serum T_4 (bound and free), thyroid-binding protein alterations (congenital or drug-induced) continue to influence results in both T_4D and RIA. Besides minor technological points, the major difference between the two techniques is that T_4D is more prone to be falsely increased by changes in serum fatty acids, which may occur when specimens stand at room temperature for more than a day or are sent through the mail. Otherwise, both methods provide the same information.

TRIIODOTHYRONINE UPTAKE TEST.—Besides the thyroxine test group, measurement of T_3 can be used to investigate thyroid function. The first T_3 testing procedure was the T_3 uptake (T_3U). Actually, the name is somewhat misleading—first, because the test is an estimate of T_4 more than of T_3 and second, because the result is an indirect estimation that depends on TBG binding capacity rather than direct hormone measurement. It is unfortunate that many speak of the T_3U as "the T_3 test," making it difficult to know whether T_3 uptake or T_3 RIA is meant. In the T_3U, radioactive T_3 is added to patient serum. Radioactive T_3 and patient T_3 compete for binding sites on TBG. The free (nonbound) radioactive T_3 is separated from the TBG-bound fraction by adding another hormone binder, usually a special resin. This system actually measures the number of TBG binding sites available to T_3 rather than actual quantity of patient T_3. The number of T_3 binding sites is determined primarily by the number of sites occupied by T_4 (since T_4 constitutes most of thyroid hormone molecules) and by the total amount of TBG present. Assuming normal quantity of TBG, the T_3U thus becomes an indirect estimate of patient T_4. The T_3U values parallel T_4 assay values in hyper- and hypothyroidism. For example, in hyperthyroidism the amount of T_4 bound to TBG is increased so that most of the added radioactive T_3 has no place to go except onto the resin. The result is that resin uptake rises above normal.

The T_3U is not affected by inorganic iodide or by organic iodine. Rather T_3U is affected by changes in thyroid-binding protein, whether congenital or disease- or drug-induced. In these cases, however, the T_3U values travel in the opposite direction from values of other T_4 assay procedures. For example, TBG is normally one-third saturated by T_4, and if TBG is increased by the estrogen content of birth control pills, the additional TBG also becomes one-third saturated by T_4. This increases total serum T_4 values. The unsaturated portion of the additional TBG allows additional T_3 binding, which leads to decreased resin uptake. A comparison of T_4 assay and T_3U results is useful to detect changes in thyroid-binding proteins and to prevent erroneous diagnosis from either test alone. Unrelated to thyroid-binding protein alterations, T_3U may be falsely increased by supraventricular arrhythmias such as atrial fibrillation, and by severe acidosis. One report indicates a tendency to decrease in uremia.

Several modifications of the basic procedure are sold by commercial companies, and each modification has different areas where faulty technique would cause trouble. One source of confusion is that a commercial T_3 test that counts serum uptake gives exactly opposite results from one that counts resin uptake. The T_3 has been the subject of a growing number of clinical evaluations. Although some published reports are highly favorable, most indicate that accuracy is poor in hypothyroidism and that there is still a significant amount of overlap with normal values in mild hyperthyroidism. The main advantages are simplicity of performance, the fact that iodine contamination problems are eliminated and the possibility of calculating the free thyroxine index (FTI) in combination with a T_4 procedure.

FREE THYROXINE INDEX. — The free T_4 level of serum is not affected by TBG abnormalities, since TBG acts mostly as a storage depot. Free thyroxine, however, is difficult to assay directly by present methods (p. 458). Clark and Horn popularized a mathematical estimate of free thyroxine status. The estimate is calculated by multiplying the T_3U and T_4 results together. This is based on the fact that whereas T_3U and T_4 results parallel each other in hypo- and hyperthyroidism, they go in opposite directions when TBG-related factors influence test results. Multiplying T_3U and T_4

results together thus tends to cancel out the effects of TBG-related factors without affecting results in thyroid disease. Most reports indicate an excellent correlation to clinical thyroid status. When isotope T_4 methods are used for the FTI, iodine contamination as well as TBG effects are eliminated. Actual calculation of the FTI usually is not necessary. If one knows the normal values for the T_4 assay and for the T_3U, one simply decides whether assay values for the two tests have equivalent positions in their separate normal ranges (i.e., both increased or both near the middle of the normal range) or whether the values are divergent (i.e., one near the upper limit and the other near the lower limit). If the values are considerably divergent, there is a question of possible thyroid-binding protein abnormality. Therefore, it is more helpful to have the T_4 and T_3 values than the index number alone, for these values are sometimes necessary to interpret the index or provide a clue to technical error. Other names for FTI are T7 and T12.

"CORRECTED" T_4 BY ISOTOPE. — This method is also called "normalized" T_4, ETR and other trade names. Methods have been found to correct T_4 test results for effects of TBG abnormality. Whereas the usual T_4 test system employs only TBG from normal serum, this new technique compensates for patient TBG variations by first reacting the patient's thyroxine with normal TBG and then with the patient's own TBG. The result is a thyroxine test that is not affected by inorganic iodine or by organic iodine and should also not be affected by diseases or medications that alter TBG.

The major drawbacks of the other T_4 methods are thereby eliminated, and most of the diseases and medications that affect the other T_4 tests should theoretically no longer be a problem. Several reports claim excellent correlation to thyroid clinical status. However, some information is available that suggests more overlap in borderline cases than is desirable if thyroid function is to be evaluated by only one test. Laboratories have been slow to try this method, and much more data must be obtained before final evaluation can be made. In general, the corrected T_4 test provides the same information as the FTI. However, the corrected T_4 results alone are not sufficient to permit a diagnosis of TBG abnormality (one would need the combination of a definitely normal corrected T_4 and a definitely abnormal test that is TBG-dependent, such as the T_4 assay or the T_3U).

BRIEF COMPARISON OF THYROXINE MEASUREMENT TESTS. — The iodine end-point tests (PBI, BEI, T_4 by column) are in one way or another affected by iodine contamination and by conditions altering TBG. The T_3U and T_4 by isotope are affected only by TBG alterations. The corrected T_4 and FTI are not affected by either iodine or TBG.

TRIIODOTHYRONINE TESTS

TRIIODOTHYRONINE BY RADIOIMMUNOASSAY. — The T_3U measures unsaturated thyroid hormone binding sites on TBG and therefore is an indirect estimate of thyroid hormone level (actually more influenced by T_4 than by T_3), whereas the T_3 RIA measures total serum T_3 directly, using antibody against T_3. Since total serum T_3 includes both protein-bound and free segments, T_3 RIA is affected by alterations in thyroid-binding proteins in the same manner as T_4 RIA. Other information available indicates that T_3 RIA may be decreased in the presence of clinical euthyroidism in some patients with cirrhosis, with chronic renal failure, after starvation, during treatment with T_4, during treatment with dexamethasone, following surgery and during severe acute or chronic illness. Persons over age 60 may have normal values that are significantly lower than those under age 50 (reports have varied, possibly because of the population tested or the method or kit used, but most find 10–30% decrease). Finally, although T_3 RIA test kits are as easy to use as T_4 RIA kits, there seems to be more variation in results between T_3 kits from different manufacturers than between T_4 kits.

The T_3 RIA helps to detect "T_3 thyrotoxicosis." Some investigators have even stated that T_3 RIA is the most sensitive test for the usual thyrotoxicosis associated with T_4 increase, occasionally showing elevation in an early stage before T_4 levels have risen above normal upper limits. Nevertheless, a few patients have been noted to have clinical hyperthyroidism with elevated T_4 values but upper normal T_3 RIA results. This has been called "T_4 toxicosis" and seems to be more common after administration of iodine. Whether this represents true selective increase of T_4 or is due to assay problems, normal range differences, decreased peripheral conversion of T_4 to T_3 or other causes is not clear. T_3 RIA is not reliable in hypothyroidism due to considerable overlap in the hypothyroid and low normal range. A few reports suggest that some persons may have mildly hypothyroid T_4 levels but may have enough T_3 to maintain a clinically euthyroid state.

In T_3 thyrotoxicosis, an entity found in association with Graves' disease or with toxic nodular goiter, standard thyroxine and T_3U tests are normal. The 24-hour RAI may be normal (even low normal) or increased. Usually, T_3 suppression tests are abnormal and indicative of hyperthyroidism. At present, the most conclusive proof is obtained by quantitative T_3 measurement using radioimmunoassay (a different procedure from the standard T_3U test). The T_3 RIA demonstrates elevated total T_3 levels in T_3 thyrotoxicosis. However, since TBG abnormalities affect T_3 RIA, confirmation is advisable with the T_3 suppression test, TRF test or TBG assay. Use of corrected or normalized T_4 procedures may be misleading when TBG is increased. The corrected T_4 result will be normal, but the T_3 RIA may be elevated, simulating T_3 thyrotoxicosis. The combination of T_4 assay and T_3U results (FTI, but with both test results reported separately rather than as a single index number) would reveal the true situation. Iodine deficiency may also simulate T_3 thyrotoxicosis (p. 344).

TISSUE UTILIZATION OF THYROXINE

Another group of tests estimates thyroid function by assessing the effects of thyroid hormone on body metabolism or reactions. These include the Achilles tendon reflex (a physical measurement), basal metabolic rate and serum cholesterol.

ACHILLES TENDON REFLEX. — Thyroid hormone status affects the speed of muscle reflex. Equipment is available to measure contraction or relaxation time. Although a few investigators claim good results, the usual accuracy is 50–75% in hypothyroidism and 20–50% in hyperthyroidism. Diabetes mellitus, pernicious anemia and other neurologic disorders, and thiourea drugs prolong reflex time; estrogens and corticosteroids shorten it.

BASAL METABOLIC RATE. — This supposedly measures body reaction as a whole to circulating thyroid hormone. Most methods are indirect, utilizing rate of oxygen uptake by means of breathing a measured amount of oxygen in a closed-circuit tank apparatus. If increased amounts of oxygen are breathed in, theoretically the patient has an abnormally high basal metabolic rate, and vice versa for decreased metabolism. Unfortunately, so many variables are involved that the test is most reliable only when the clinical situation is already so obvious that it is not really necessary. A truly basal state is difficult to achieve and maintain. Anxiety, obesity, adrenal dysfunction and equipment malfunction are some of the other major obstacles to accurate results. The BMR is rarely used today.

CHOLESTEROL. — Cholesterol level is an indirect measurement of metabolic rate; this reflects a not-well-understood effect of thyroid hormone on cholesterol synthesis. Cholesterol is often elevated in myxedema and much less frequently is decreased in hyperthyroidism (in classic cases). Serum cholesterol measurement is, however, a poor test of thyroid function for several reasons:

1. Many diseases influence cholesterol metabolism in various ways.

2. Changes from normal range tend to occur only in far-advanced thyroid disease; much more so in hypothyroidism than in hyperthyroidism.

3. Cholesterol determination is one of the least accurate tests in the clinical laboratory. Also, the normal range itself is so wide that many persons could be abnormal and still have values within the population normal.

OTHER PROCEDURES

Thus far, discussion has been limited to the basic tests for diagnosis of hypothyroidism and hyperthyroidism. There are several other procedures that are helpful in special situations.

THYROID SCAN. — Thyroid uptake of radioactive isotopes such as ^{131}I may be counted by a special device which produces a visual overall pattern of gland radioactivity. This allows visual localization of areas that may be hyperactive or hypoactive. The procedure is useful in two situations:

1. To show whether thyrotoxicosis is caused by diffuse hyperplasia or by a hyperfunctioning nodule ("hot nodule" or "toxic nodule").

2. To demonstrate hypofunction in a nodule, thus increasing suspicion of carcinoma ("cold nodule").

Most reports agree that a hyperfunctioning nodule is rarely malignant. Single nonfunctioning nodules have a 10–20% incidence of malignancy. Truly nonfunctioning nodules are much more likely to be malignant than nodules that retain some function. The difficulty is that normal tissue above or below a nonfunctioning area may contribute some degree of apparent function to the nonfunctioning region.

THYROID-STIMULATING HORMONE TEST. — In some patients with myxedema, the question arises as to whether the etiology is primary thyroid disease or malfunction secondary to pituitary deficiency. This problem may be investigated by performing the RAI before and after administration of an appropriate amount of TSH. In pituitary insufficiency, the thyroid usually will respond to TSH; if hypofunction is primary disease of the thyroid, RAI uptake will not be significantly improved.

The procedure may be very useful in patients who have been on long-term thyroid hormone treatment and who must be reevaluated as to whether the original diagnosis of hypothyroidism was correct. The TSH test can be done while thyroid hormone is still being administered, whereas it would take several weeks after cessation of long-term therapy for the pituitary-thyroid relationship to reach pretherapy equilibrium.

THYROID SUPPRESSION TEST.—This is frequently called "T_3 suppression," although thyroid hormone could be used instead of T_3. A standard dose of T_3 is given daily for 1 week. In normal persons, exogenous T_3 (added to the patient's own thyroxine) will suppress pituitary secretion of TSH, leading to decrease in patient thyroid hormone manufacture. Values of RAI or T_4 after T_3 administration drop to less than 50% of baseline level. In hyperthyroidism, the thyroid is autonomous and continues to manufacture hormone (with little change in RAI or T_4 level) in spite of exogenous T_3. The suppression test is thought to be reliable and may be very useful in confirming the diagnosis of borderline hyperthyroidism, even though availability of T_3 RIA has decreased the number of patients with borderline function test results. The same basic technique may be used in conjunction with the thyroid scan to demonstrate that a nodule seen on original scan is autonomous. This is very helpful, since reports indicate that 50–80% of toxic nodular goiter patients have normal RAI and many have normal thyroxine tests. The procedure must be used with caution in elderly persons, especially those with cardiac disease.

SERUM THYROTROPIN ASSAY.—Direct assay of TSH is now available. Serum TSH has a diurnal rhythm, with serum levels relatively low during the day and high at night. In myxedema due to primary thyroid disease, serum TSH is elevated. In most cases of secondary (pituitary or hypothalamic) myxedema, serum TSH is low. Other causes for increased TSH levels include iodine deficiency goiter, thyroiditis, euthyroid goiter with enzyme defect and ^{131}I therapy for thyroid disease. On the other hand, certain patients with secondary hypothyroidism have normal TSH values when one would expect low TSH levels. The pituitary of these patients is able to secrete a small amount of TSH—not enough to maintain normal T_4 levels but enough to leave TSH within normal range. T_3 RIA may be decreased, but in some instances it may be low normal, either because of preferential secretion of T_3 rather than T_4 by subnormal TSH stimulation or because of problems with kit sensitivity in low ranges. Another problem concerns anti-TSH antisera in most (not all) TSH RIA kits which cross-react with chorionic gonadotropin; these kits will indicate variable degrees of false TSH increase during pregnancy. Finally, some (not all) TSH kits have poor sensitivity in the low range and cannot reliably differentiate low from low normal values. Theoretically TSH should be low in hyperthyroidism or in secondary hypothyroidism, but kit sensitivity problems may produce results in the low normal range. Likewise, apparent low TSH levels may be seen in occasional euthyroid persons.

Notwithstanding these difficulties, TSH assay is the most reliable way to confirm a diagnosis of primary hypothyroidism (by far the most common type of myxedema) and to demonstrate the adequacy of replacement therapy.

THYROTROPIN RELEASING FACTOR TEST. — Thyrotropin releasing factor (TRF) preparations are now becoming available. Decreased blood levels of free thyroid hormone stimulate the hypothalamus to produce TRF, which in turn induces the pituitary to produce TSH. By measuring serum TSH before and after injection of TRF, one can differentiate between hypothalamic and pituitary insufficiency in a patient with hypothyroidism and low serum TSH values. In addition, the TRF test may be useful to help confirm equivocal thyrotoxicosis if a T_3 suppression test is not advisable, since elevated serum free thyroid hormone suppresses pituitary production of TSH and makes the pituitary relatively resistant to TRF stimulation. Response of TSH to TRF is decreased by steroid or aspirin therapy, and some information suggests that the degree of response in males decreases with age. Finally, some instances have been reported in which patients did not respond to TRF in the expected manner, but without explanation. More data are needed on factors that affect this test.

THYROID TESTS IN IODINE DEFICIENCY

Iodine deficiency goiter is rare in the United States but still might be encountered by a physician. Iodine deficiency leads to increase in RAI. In mild or moderate deficiency there is said to be a decrease in T_4 assay and T_3U, but values usually remain within normal range. Often T_3 RIA is increased. Assay levels of TSH are usually normal. In severe iodine deficiency, T_4 assay and T_3U values often decrease, and T_3 RIA increases. TSH may be elevated, but only to a mild or moderate degree. Thus, iodine deficiency may simulate thyrotoxicosis (goiter and RAI increase), T_3 toxicosis (goiter with normal or decreased T_4 and elevated T_3 RIA) or even hypothyroidism (decreased T_4).

THYROID TESTS IN DIPHENYLHYDANTOIN (DILANTIN) THERAPY

There are conflicting statements in the literature concerning the effect of Dilantin on certain thyroid tests. Dilantin is known to compete for binding sites on TBG but apparently can influence certain tests by other means. The majority of reports indicate that T_4D or T_4 RIA, free T_4 and T_3 RIA are somewhat decreased, while T_3U, TSH assay and the TRF test are not significantly affected. T_4 is apparently decreased more than T_3 RIA. The test value may be decreased from pretreatment levels even though it may remain within normal range.

SELECTION OF THYROID TESTS

Each procedure measures one facet of thyroid hormone production, transport or utilization, and each has advantages and disadvantages. Selection should simply involve choosing what information is needed in the particular situation. Theoretically, the best single test to screen for hyperthyroidism is T_3 RIA, and for primary hypothyroidism, serum TSH assay. For general screening of thyroid function status, at the present time the most accurate single procedures that are readily available are the FTI and the "corrected" T_4 by isotope. However, if the patient has obvious clinical hyperthyroidism, all of the iodine end-point or isotope T_4 tests are equally good. Since the question is not that of diagnosis but only of confirmation, one test probably is sufficient. In obvious myxedema, any of the T_4 tests are adequate; the T_3U, T_3 RIA and RAI are significantly less efficient. In a patient with hyperthyroid symptoms but normal T_4, a T_3 RIA or T_3 suppression test (or possibly a TRF test or thyroid scan) may be useful to rule out T_3 thyrotoxicosis, laboratory error or borderline disease. In a patient with possible hypothyroidism but normal T_4, a TSH level can be very helpful. Except in special cases (such as thyroiditis), there is nothing to be gained by ordering more than one thyroxine test (PBI, BEI, T_4 by column or isotope) *at the same time*. All give the same information. They differ only in the particular agents that interfere with results. There is hardly ever any need for BMR or serum cholesterol. The RAI is no longer needed for diagnosis of hyper- or hypothyroidism. Normal values are changing, the test requires two patient visits plus the administration of radioactivity, results are not reliable in mild hypothyroidism, technique is often poor, and various other factors alter test results. However, there are a few situations in which RAI may be useful. In "factitious" hyperthyroidism (due to deliberate ingestion of thyroid hormone or its incorporation into medication such as diet control pills), the RAI is low when thyroxine tests are elevated. In TSH stimulation or T_3 suppression tests, RAI is the standard procedure used, although a thyroxine test could probably be substituted.

In any case, good clinical judgment is even more important than laboratory results. If the clinical status of the patient does not agree with the laboratory values, the test results should be rechecked.

A considerable number of persons take thyroid hormone without having conclusive evidence of hypothyroidism. A frequent question concerns the minimum time span after hormone administration before thyroid function tests will be reliable. One study suggests that four full weeks are necessary, although some statements in medical literature indicate that as little as two weeks may be sufficient. The TSH stimulation test can be done without stopping therapy.

Monitoring of Replacement Therapy

Desiccated thyroid and presumably other T_4 and T_3 combinations result in T_3 RIA values that may become elevated for several hours after administration and then decrease to normal range. T_4 values remain within normal range if replacement is adequate. In the few instances when clinical evidence and T_4 results disagree, TSH assay is helpful.

L-Thyroxine (Synthroid) results in T_3 RIA values that, in athyrotic persons, are approximately two thirds of those expected at a comparable T_4 level when thyroid function is normal. This is due to peripheral tissue conversion of T_4 to T_3. Values of T_3 RIA are more labile than those of T_4 and will be affected more by residual thyroid function. In general, both T_4 assay and

T_3 RIA levels depend on the dose of L-thyroxine and the frequency of administration. The standard test when L-thyroxine is used has been the T_4 assay.

Triiodothyronine (Cytomel) replacement therapy can be monitored clinically by serum TSH assay or T_3 RIA. The T_4 assay and T_3U tests remain below normal. After Cytomel administration, T_3 RIA levels peak in 1–2 hours and then fall, requiring nearly 24 hours to reach a plateau. Divided dose therapy would be difficult to monitor by T_3 RIA; single-dose therapy samples are drawn just before the next day's dose.

HASHIMOTO'S DISEASE

Hashimoto's disease is a form of chronic thyroiditis characterized histologically by marked lymphocytic infiltration of the thyroid gland. Clinically, the disease is much more common in females, and the main symptom is the onset of thyroid enlargement. The general category of Hashimoto's disease has been divided into two subgroups: so-called lymphocytic thyroiditis and ordinary (adult) Hashimoto's. Lymphocytic thyroiditis is most frequent in children and young adults, and patients present with a diffusely and slowly enlarging thyroid gland, with or without other minor symptoms. Thyroid function tests include a PBI, which is usually either elevated or high normal; and a BEI, which remains normal. Many patients show a PBI-BEI discrepancy of more than 1 μg/100 ml, whereas the normal limit is less than 1 μg/100 ml. Other thyroid function tests are variable, although the RAI is often elevated early in the disease. In fact, an elevated RAI with normal T_4 values definitely raises the possibility of active (early) chronic thyroiditis. Adult Hashimoto's disease is more frequent than lymphocytic thyroiditis. Again, it is most common in females but has a predilection for adults age 30–50. The goiter produced is often of relatively rapid onset. It is diffuse, although sometimes irregular. There may be pressure symptoms in the neck from the enlarged gland. As the disease progresses, hypothyroidism is frequent. Thyroid function test results usually are normal, except when hypothyroidism develops. There may be a PBI-BEI discrepancy above 1 μg/100 ml although not as frequently as in childhood lymphocytic thyroiditis. Thyroid scan often shows multiple areas of decreased isotope uptake. Exact diagnosis of Hashimoto's disease is important for several reasons: to differentiate the condition from thyroid carcinoma; because a diffusely enlarged thyroid raises the question of possible thyrotoxicosis; and because treatment with thyroid hormone gives excellent results, especially in childhood lymphocytic thyroiditis. Incidentally, adenomatous goiter is said to have a PBI-BEI discrepancy of 1–2 μg/100 ml in 10% of cases, and one report raises the possibility of a similar finding in rare cases of thyroid carcinoma.

Both subgroups of Hashimoto's disease are now considered to be either due to, or associated with, an autoimmune disorder against thyroid tissue. Autoantibodies against one or another element of thyroid tissue have been detected in most cases. In addition, there is an increased incidence of serologically detectable thyroid autoantibodies in the rheumatoid-collagen disease group, conditions themselves associated with disturbances in the body autoimmune mechanisms. Various systems have been devised for detection of circulating thyroid autoantibodies for aid in the diagnosis of Hashimoto's disease. The most readily available procedure is a rapid latex-agglutination slide test, called the thyroid antibody test (TA test). This primarily detects antibodies to thyroglobulin, and is similar in principle to the rheumatoid factor latex test (p. 260). Crude extract of thyroglobulin antigen is attached to an indicator (latex particles). Antithyroglobulin antibody in the serum (in significant titers) attacks the antigen and thereby clumps the latex particles. The TA test has been reported to be reasonably sensitive and specific. However, as with most screening tests, false positives and false negatives occur and must be expected. A small but significant percentage of patients with thyrotoxicosis, thyroid carcinoma and rheumatoid-collagen diseases have positive test results. Although there is an increased incidence of chronic thyroiditis histologically resembling Hashimoto's disease in thyrotoxicosis and thyroid carcinoma, some false positive TA tests occur without associated histologic thyroiditis, so that differentiation of these conditions by means of an autoantibody test cannot be made blindly. The TA test may also be positive in some cases of myxedema that cannot be established as being due to Hashimoto's disease. On the other hand, false negative results in TA tests have been reported in up to 30% of patients with Hashimoto's disease.

Another procedure, called the tanned red cell (TRC) test, is more sensitive to thyroid autoimmune disease. Most investigators find over 85% positive results in Hashimoto's, with lesser percentages in other thyroid disorders. Titers in disease other than chronic thyroiditis tend to be low. The TRC technique is preferable to the TA test. Since both tests are nonspecific, a negative TRC result would be stronger evidence against chronic thyroiditis.

Thyroiditis usually is classified as acute, subacute and chronic. Except for Hashimoto's disease, the other varieties are not common and will be mentioned only briefly. Acute thyroiditis usually is infectious in nature, and physical findings usually are those of localized infection. Thyroid function tests usually are normal. Subacute thyroiditis (De Quervain's, giant-cell, or granulomatous thyroiditis) is of unknown etiology but possibly is viral or autoimmune in nature. The majority of patients have some degree of pain in the thyroid area, but some do not. Histologically, there are areas of thyroid acini degeneration surrounded by multinucleated giant cells. If the disease is localized, the only functional abnormality is possible focal hyperfunction on thyroid scan. If the disease is more widespread, RAI uptake is low, and T_4 or T_3 tests show elevated or high normal levels due to release of thyroglobulin from damaged acini. Occasionally, patients present with actual symptoms of thyrotoxicosis. There may be an increased PBI-BEI discrepancy. Thyroid autoantibodies occasionally may be detected but are not common.

Finally, Riedel's struma is another type of chronic thyroiditis, consisting of extensive thyroid parenchymal fibrosis. In most cases, function tests are normal. In a few, results are hypothyroid.

In acute and subacute thyroiditis, nonspecific parameters of inflammation, such as the erythrocyte sedimentation rate (ESR), usually are abnormal. In Hashimoto's disease, about 50% of patients have an elevated ESR, more commonly in the childhood type. However, adenomatous goiter may also sometimes produce an increased ESR.

REFERENCES

Achilles Reflex Time in the Diagnosis of Thyroid Dysfunction, Med. Letter Drugs & Therapeutics 9:43, 1967.

Anderson, J. R., et al.: Diagnostic tests for thyroid antibodies: A comparison of the precipitin and latex-fixation (Hyland TA) tests, J. Clin. Pathol. 15:462, 1962.

Bauer, R. E.: The present status of the diagnosis of hypothyroidism, Ann. Intern. Med. 44:207, 1956.

Blahd, W. H. (ed.): *Nuclear Medicine* (2d ed.; New York: Blakiston Company, 1972).

Burger, A.: Reduced active thyroid-hormone levels in acute illness, Lancet 2:97, 1976.

Caplan, R. H., and Kujack, R.: Thyroid uptake of radioiodine: A re-evaluation, J.A.M.A. 215:916, 1971.

Carlson, H. E., and Hershman, J. M.: The hypothalamic-pituitary axis, Med. Clin. North Am. 59:1045, 1975.

Davis, P. J.: Factors affecting the determination of the serum protein-bound iodine, Am. J. Med. 40:918, 1966.

Dowling, J. T., et al.: Abnormal iodoproteins in the blood of eumetabolic goitrous adults, J. Clin. Endocrinol. Metab. 21:1390, 1961.

Evered, D.: Diseases of the thyroid gland, Clin. Endocrinol. Metabol. 3:425, 1974.

Gharib, H., and Wahner, H. W.: Clinical experience with assays for triiodothyronine, Med. Clin. North Am. 56:861, 1972.

Hershman, J. M.: Clinical application of thyrotropin-releasing hormone, N. Engl. J. Med. 290:886, 1974.

Larsen, P. R.: Triiodothyronine: Review of recent studies of its physiology and pathophysiology in man, Metabolism 21:1073, 1972.

Leboeuf, G., and Bongiovanni, A. M.: Thyroiditis in Childhood, in Levine, S. Z. (ed.): *Advances in Pediatrics* (Chicago: Year Book Medical Publishers, Inc., 1964), vol. 13, p. 183.

Magliotti, M. F., et al.: The effect of disease and drugs on the twenty-four hour I^{131} thyroid uptake, Am. J. Roentgenol. Radium Ther. Nucl. Med. 81:54, 1959.

Marsden, P., and McKerron, C. G.: Serum triiodothyronine concentration in diagnosis of hyperthyroidism, Clin. Endocrinol. (Oxf.) 4:183, 1975.

Marsden, P., et al.: Serum triiodothyronine in solitary autonomous nodules of the thyroid, Clin. Endocrinol. (Oxf.) 4:327, 1975.

McConahey, W. M., et al.: Comparison of certain laboratory tests in the diagnosis of Hashimoto's thyroiditis, J. Clin. Endocrinol. Metab. 21:879, 1961.

Meachim, G., and Young, M. H.: DeQuervain's subacute granulomatous thyroiditis: Histological identification and incidence, J. Clin. Pathol. 16:189, 1963.

Murphy, B. E. P.: In vitro tests of thyroid function, Semin. Nucl. Med. 1:301, 1971.

Nelson, J. C., et al.: Serum TSH levels and the thyroidal response to TSH stimulation in patients with thyroid disease, Ann. Intern. Med. 76:47, 1972.

Papapetrou, P. D., and Jackson, I. M. D.: Thyrotoxicosis due to "silent" thyroiditis, Lancet 1:361, 1975.

Patel, Y. C., et al.: Serum triiodothyronine, thyroxine and thyroid-stimulating hormone in endemic goiter: A comparison of goitrous and nongoitrous subjects in New Guinea, J. Clin. Endocrinol. Metab. 37:783, 1973.

Robertson, J. S.: Thyroid radioiodine uptakes and scans in euthyroid patients, Mayo Clin. Proc. 50:79, 1975.

Rose, N. R., and Witebsky, E.: Thyroid Autoantibodies in Thyroid Disease, in Levine, R., and Luft, R. (eds.): *Advances in Metabolic Disorders* (New York: Academic Press, 1968), vol. 5, p. 231.

Saxena, K. M., and Crawford, J. D.: Juvenile lymphocytic thyroiditis, Pediatrics 30: 917, 1962.

Sisson, J. C.: Principles of, and pitfalls in, thyroid function tests, J. Nucl. Med. 6:853, 1965.

Sterling, K., et al.: T-3 thyrotoxicosis, J.A.M.A. 213:571, 1970.

Vagenakis, A. G., et al.: Recovery of pituitary thyrotropic function after withdrawal of prolonged thyroid-suppression therapy, N. Engl. J. Med. 293:681, 1975.

Vagenakis, A. G., et al.: Studies of serum triiodothyronine, thyroxine, and thyrotropin concentration in endemic goiter in Greece, J. Clin. Endocrinol. Metab. 37:485, 1973.

Wellby, M. L.: A comparison of effective thyroxine ratio and free thyroxine in serum, Clin. Chim. Acta 45:255, 1973.

Werner, S. C. (ed.): *The Thyroid* (3d ed.; New York: Hoeber Medical Division, Harper & Row, 1971).

29 / Adrenal Function Tests

THE ADRENAL GLANDS produce several important hormones. A summary of the principal adrenal cortex hormones, their actions and their metabolites is shown in Figure 29 – 1. Histologically, the adrenal cortex is divided into three areas. A narrow outer (subcapsular) region is known as the zona glomerulosa. It is thought to produce aldosterone. The cortex middle zone, called the zona fasciculata, mainly elaborates 17-hydroxycortisone, also known as hydrocortisone or cortisol. This is the principal agent of the cortisone group. A thin inner zone, called the zona reticularis, manufactures compounds with androgenic or estrogenic effects. Pathways of synthesis for adrenal cortex hormones are outlined in Figure 29–2. The adrenal medulla produces epinephrine and norepinephrine. Production of cortisol is controlled by pituitary secretion of adrenal cortex stimulating hormone (ACTH). The pituitary, in turn, is regulated by a feedback mechanism involving blood levels of cortisol. If more cortisol is produced than needed, the pituitary is inhibited and decreases ACTH production; if more cortisol is needed, the pituitary increases ACTH.

Excess or deficiency of adrenal cortex hormones leads to several well-recognized diseases, which are diagnosed by assay of the hormone or its metabolites. In diseases of cortisol production, four assay techniques form the backbone of laboratory diagnosis: 17-hydroxycorticosteroids (17-OHCS), 17-ketosteroids (17-KS) 17-ketogenic steroids and direct measurement of cortisol. Before discussing the use of these steroid tests in various syndromes, it might be useful to consider what actually is being measured.

17-Hydroxycorticosteroids

These are C_{21} compounds that possess a dihydroxyacetone group on carbon number 17 of the steroid nucleus (Fig 29 – 3). In the blood, the principal 17-OHCS is hydrocortisone. In urine, the predominating 17-OHCS are tetrahydro metabolites (breakdown products) of hydrocortisone and cortisone. Therefore, measurement of 17-OHCS can be used to estimate the level of cortisone and hydrocortisone production. Estrogen therapy (including oral contraceptives) will elevate plasma 17-OHCS values, although degradation of these compounds is delayed and urine 17-OHCS levels are decreased.

17-Ketosteroids

These are C_{19} compounds with a ketone group on carbon number 17 of the steroid nucleus (see Fig 29 – 3). They are measured in urine only. In males, about 25% of 17-KS are composed of metabolites of testosterone.

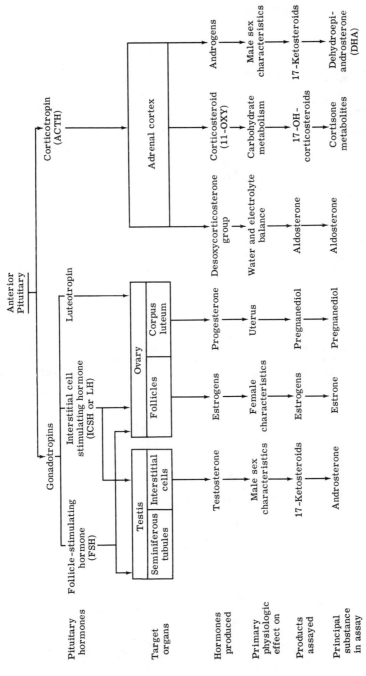

Fig 29 – 1.– Derivation of principal urinary steroids. (From *Handbook of Specialized Diagnostic Laboratory Tests* [7th ed.; Van Nuys, Calif.: BioScience Laboratories, 1966], p. 5.)

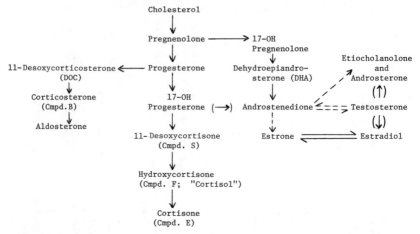

Fig 29–2.—Adrenal cortex steroid synthesis. Important classic alternate pathways are depicted in *parentheses,* and certain alternate pathways are omitted. *Dotted lines* indicate pathway which normally continues in another organ, although adrenal capability exists.

Fig 29–3.—Adrenal cortex steroid nomenclature. **A,** basic 17-OHCS nucleus with standard numerical nomenclature of the carbon atoms. **B,** configuration of hydrocortisone at the C-17 carbon atom. **C,** configuration of the 17-KS at the C-17 carbon atom.

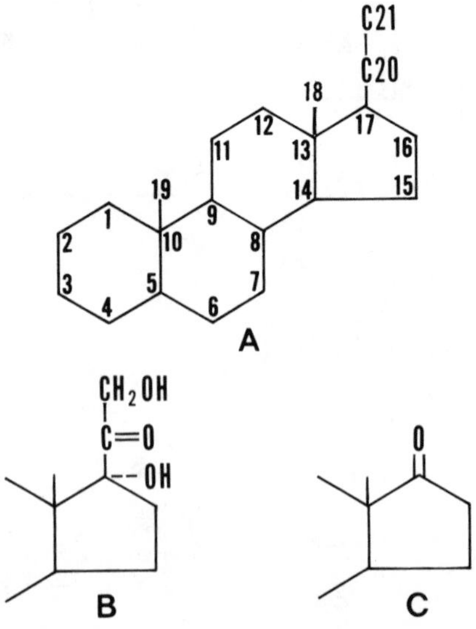

The remainder of 17-KS in males and nearly all 17-KS in females are derived from androgens other than testosterone, although lesser amounts come from early steroid precursors and a small percentage from hydrocortisone breakdown products. Testosterone itself is not a 17-KS. The principal urinary 17-KS is a compound known as dehydroisoandrosterone (dehydroepiandrosterone; DHA). This is formed in the adrenal and has a weak androgenic effect. It is not a metabolite of cortisone or hydrocortisone, and therefore 17-KS cannot be expected to mirror or predict levels of hydrocortisone production.

In adrenogenital or virilization syndromes, high levels of 17-KS usually mean congenital adrenal hyperplasia in babies and adrenal tumor in older children and adults. In both cases, steroid synthesis is abnormally shifted away from cortisone formation toward androgen production. High levels are occasionally found in testicular tumors, if the tumor produces androgens greatly in excess of normal testicular output. In Cushing's disease, 17-KS production is variable, but adrenal hyperplasia is often associated with mild- to moderate elevation, while adrenal carcinoma frequently produces moderate or marked urinary values. In adrenal tumor, most of the increase is due to DHA.

Low levels of 17-KS are not very important because of normal fluctuation and the degree of inaccuracy in assay. Low levels are usually due to a decrease in DHA. This may be caused by many factors, but the most important is stress of any type (such as trauma, burns, chronic disease, etc.). Therefore, normal 17-KS levels are indirectly a sign of health.

17-Ketogenic Steroids

These are C_{21} compounds that can be oxidized to 17-KS. The ketogenic steroids thus constitute the difference between 17-KS determinations done before and after oxidation. The 17-ketogenic compounds include the 17-OHCS group and also pregnanetriol. Pregnanetriol is a metabolite of 17-OH progesterone (a precursor of cortisone). Since pregnanetriol elevation occurs only in a very few conditions (such as the adrenogenital syndrome) in which 17-OHCS are not also elevated, in most situations a urinary 17-ketogenic steroid determination could be used (if desired) instead of urinary 17-OHCS. Whereas the metabolite of 17-OH-progesterone (pregnanetriol) is included in 17-ketogenic assays, the metabolite of progesterone (pregnanediol) is not a 17-ketogenic steroid.

A list of compounds that may interfere with 17-OHCS or 17-KS (and ketogenic) determinations is found on page 471.

Plasma Cortisol Measurement

Plasma cortisol exists in two forms, analogous to thyroxine; about 90% is bound to cortisol-binding protein (transcortin, an alpha$_1$ globulin) and physiologically inactive, and about 10% is unbound (free). Three basic assay techniques are used: Porter-Silber colorimetric, Mattingly fluorescent and radioassay. Porter-Silber is the most widely used of the older chemical methods. It measures cortisol, cortisone and compound S (see Fig 29–2) plus their metabolites. Ketosis and various drugs (p. 471) may interfere. The fluorescent procedure is based on fluorescence of certain compounds in acid media at ultraviolet wavelengths. It is more sensitive than Porter-Silber, faster, requires less blood and measures cortisol and compound B (but not compound S). Certain drugs (p. 471) that fluoresce may interfere. Radioassay has two subgroups, competitive protein binding (CPB) and radioimmunoassay (RIA). The CPB technique is the older of the two. It is based on competition between patient cortisol-like compounds and isotope-labeled cortisol for space on cortisol-binding protein. It measures cortisol, cortisone, compound S and compound B. Advantages are small specimen requirement and less interference by drugs. The RIA technique is based on competition between patient cortisol and isotope-labeled cortisol for anticortisol antibody. The method is nearly specific for cortisol, with less than 20% cross reaction with compound S. In certain clinical situations, such as congenital adrenal hyperplasia or the metyrapone test, it is important to know what "cortisol" procedure is being performed to interpret the results correctly. All techniques measure total blood cortisol, so that all will be falsely increased if increases in cortisol-binding protein levels occur due to estrogens in pregnancy or from birth control pills. Stress, obesity and severe hepatic or renal disease may falsely increase plasma levels. Androgens and dilantin may decrease cortisol-binding protein. In situations where cortisol-binding protein is increased, urine 17-OHCS or, better, urine free cortisol.(p. 356) may be helpful, since urine reflects blood levels of active rather than total hormone.

ADRENOGENITAL SYNDROME

This is a rare syndrome due to a congenital defect in one of several enzymes that take part in the chain of reactions whereby cortisone is manufactured from its precursors. Although formation of cortisone and hydrocortisone is blocked, the precursors of these steroids are still manufactured; the actual compound produced depends on where the defective enzyme has blocked the normal synthesis pathway. Most of the early precursors of cortisone are estrogenic compounds, which also are intermediates in the production of androgens by the adrenal cortex (see Fig 29–2). Normally, the quantitative production of adrenal androgen is small; however, if the steroid precursors pile up (due to block in normal formation of cortisone), some of this excess may be used to form more androgens.

Two things result from this situation. First, due to abnormally high production of androgen, secondary sexual characteristics are affected. If the condition is manifest in utero, pseudohermaphroditism (masculinization of external genitalia) results in females and macrogenitosomia praecox (accentuation of male genitalia) in males. If the condition does not become clinically manifest until after birth, virilism (masculinization) results in females and precocious puberty develops in males. Second, the adrenal glands themselves increase in size due to hyperplasia of the steroid-producing adrenal cortex. This results because normal pituitary production of ACTH is controlled by the amount of cortisone and hydrocortisone produced by the adrenal. In congenital adrenal hyperplasia, cortisone production is partially or completely blocked, the pituitary produces more and more ACTH in attempts to increase cortisone production and the adrenal cortex tissue becomes hyperplastic under continually increased ACTH stimulation.

This condition is diagnosed by the finding of increased 17-KS in the urine. 17-Ketosteroids are composed mainly of the metabolites or break-down products of androgens. In most cases, urinary pregnanetriol is also elevated.

VIRILIZATION SYNDROME

This rare syndrome occurs in older children and in adults. It is manifested by virilism in females and by excessive masculinization in males. It may be due to idiopathic adrenal cortex hyperplasia, adrenal cortex adenoma or cortex carcinoma. Tumor is more common than hyperplasia in these patients. Virilism in a female child or adult leads to hirsutism, clitoral enlargement, deepening of the voice, masculine contour and breast atrophy. The syndrome may be simulated in females by idiopathic hirsutism, arrhenoblastoma of the ovary and possibly by the Stein-Leventhal syndrome. Urinary 17-KS are elevated with normal or decreased 17-OHCS when the adrenal is involved. Ovarian arrhenoblastoma gives normal or only slightly elevated urine 17-KS, since androgen is produced in smaller quantities but is more potent, thus giving clinical symptoms without greatly increased quantities. In prepubertal males, the symptoms of virilism are those of precocious puberty; in adult males, excessive masculinization is difficult to recognize. A similar picture may be associated with certain testicular tumors.

CUSHING'S SYNDROME

About 50–60% of cases of Cushing's syndrome are due to simple hyperplasia of the adrenal cortex; most are idiopathic, but a few are secondary to pituitary basophil tumors. About 30–40% are caused by cortex adenomas, with cortex carcinomas accounting for 10% or less. Very uncommonly, the syndrome may be produced by nonadrenal tumors, mainly small cell undifferentiated ("oat cell") lung carcinoma. The highest incidence of the syndrome is found in adults, with females affected 4 times more often than males. Major symptoms and signs include body trunk obesity, "buffalo hump" fat deposit on the back of the neck, abdominal striae, osteoporosis and a tendency to diabetes, easy bruising and hypertension. Laboratory findings include hyperglycemia (either fasting or 2-hour postprandial) in about 50% of patients, hypokalemia with alkalosis in about 35% and lymphopenia with mild leukocytosis. Serum sodium may be elevated or normal. Total circulating eosinophils are decreased. Red blood cell counts and hemoglobin are often increased, sometimes to polycythemic levels.

Screening Procedures

SINGLE-SPECIMEN STEROID ASSAY.—Laboratory diagnosis of Cushing's syndrome requires proof of cortisol hypersecretion. For some time, assay of 17-OHCS by the Porter-Silber method in urine samples was the mainstay of diagnosis. Urine 17-KS were also used. 17-OHCS could be measured in plasma by the Porter-Silber technique, but this was technically more difficult. A single random 17-OHCS determination in either plasma or urine is not very reliable, although a definitely elevated value would increase suspicion of adrenal hypersecretion. Urine is said to be somewhat more helpful than plasma as a single test. About 15% of Cushing's syndrome patients are said to have consistently normal urine values, while some patients with obesity or with hyperthyroidism have consistently increased urine 17-OHCS. Elevated plasma 17-OHCS levels in random specimens may be produced by stress, obesity or increase in cortisol-binding protein due to estrogen increase (pregnancy or birth control pills), and patients with mild degrees of Cushing's syndrome may show normal values. Certain nonadrenal tumors (particularly lung "oat cell" carcinoma) may produce an ACTH-like material that leads to elevation of cortisol in both serum and urine. Plasma cortisol assay by fluorometric methods or by RIA is replacing plasma and urine 17-OHCS assays in many laboratories.

PLASMA CORTISOL DIURNAL VARIATION.—If plasma cortisol assay is available, a better screening test for Cushing's syndrome than a single determination consists of two plasma specimens, one at 8 A.M. and the other at 8 P.M. Normally there is a diurnal variation in plasma levels (not urine levels), with the highest values found between 6 and 10 A.M. and the lowest near midnight. The evening specimen ordinarily is less than 50% of the morning value. In Cushing's syndrome, diurnal variation is absent in nearly 90% of patients. Unfortunately, significant alteration of the diurnal pattern is not specific for Cushing's, being found in occasional patients with a wide variety of conditions. Stress, alteration of sleep patterns, ectopic ACTH syndrome, blindness, encephalitis, hypothalamic tumors, obesity, myxedema, psychosis, acute alcoholism and various drugs (morphine, prolonged steroid therapy, phenothiazines, reserpine and amphetamine) may alter or abolish normal drop in the evening cortisol level. A negative result (normal circadian rhythm) is probably more significant than an abnormal result.

URINE FREE CORTISOL.—About 1% of plasma cortisol is excreted by the kidney in the original "free" or unconjugated state; the remainder appears in urine as conjugated metabolites. Original Porter-Silber chromogenic techniques could not measure free cortisol selectively. Fluorescent methods or RIA can quantitate free cortisol, either alone or with compound S, depending on the method. The urine free cortisol measurement (24-hour collections) has been shown to give better separation of Cushing's syndrome patients from normal subjects than any urine test and better than a single plasma cortisol determination. Results seem to be as sensitive or possibly even better than those derived from determination of blood cortisol diurnal variation, with fewer false positives. Urine free cortisol will be influenced by some of the factors that affect blood cortisol, including stress and obesity. In cortisol-binding protein changes such as increase produced by estrogens, most reports indicate that urine free cortisol secretion is usually normal. Renal insufficiency may elevate plasma cortisol and decrease urine free cortisol. Hepatic disease may increase plasma cortisol but usually does not affect urine free cortisol significantly. The major difficulty with the test involves accurate collection of the 24-hour urine specimen.

SINGLE-DOSE DEXAMETHASONE TEST.—The most accurate simple screening procedure is said to be a rapid dexamethasone suppression test. Oral administration of 1 mg dexamethasone at 11 P.M. suppresses pituitary

ACTH production, so that the normal 8 A.M. peak of plasma cortisol fails to develop. Normal and obese persons produce 8 A.M. plasma cortisol values that are less than 50% of baseline levels (some require suppression to 5 μg/100 ml or less). The consensus is that over 95% of Cushing's syndrome patients exhibit abnormal test response (failure to suppress) with less than 5% false positive results (some have found more false positives in obese persons). Stress may negate the suppressive effects from small amounts of dexamethasone, so a barbiturate is usually given with the test dose. Estrogens or very serious illness may produce false positive tests (failure to suppress normally). Additional evidence to support abnormal screening test results may be obtained by using the standard dexamethasone suppression test.

The single-dose dexamethasone and diurnal variation tests may be combined. Plasma cortisol specimens are drawn at 8 A.M. and 8 P.M. Dexamethasone is administered at 11 P.M., followed by a plasma cortisol specimen at 8 A.M. next day.

Confirmatory Tests

Confirmation of the diagnosis depends mainly on tests that involve either stimulation or suppression of adrenal hormone production. It is often possible with the same tests to differentiate among the various etiologies of primary hyperadrenalism. Normally, increased pituitary ACTH production increases adrenal corticosteroid release. Increased plasma corticosteroid levels normally inhibit pituitary release of ACTH and therefore suppress further adrenal steroid production. Adrenal tumors, as a rule, produce their hormones without being much affected by suppression tests; on the other hand, they tend to give little response to stimulation, as though they behaved independently of the usual hormone control mechanism. Also, if urinary 17-KS are markedly increased (over twice normal), this strongly suggests carcinoma; adenoma is most often associated with normal or even low values, while hyperplasia produces mildly or moderately elevated levels. However, hyperplasia and carcinoma values overlap, and ketosteroid levels may be normal with either hyperplasia or carcinoma.

DEXAMETHASONE SUPPRESSION TEST. — The dexamethasone suppression test probably is the most widely used confirmatory procedure. Dexamethasone (Decadron) is a synthetic steroid with cortisone-type actions but is approximately 30 times more potent than cortisone, so that amounts too small for laboratory measurement may be given to suppress pituitary ACTH production. If low doses (2 mg/day) are used, patients with normal adrenals will show significantly decreased urine 17-OHCS values, while those with Cushing's syndrome from any etiology will not. If larger doses (8 mg/day) are used, those with cortical hyperplasia will usually show significantly depressed urine 17-OHCS, but those with hormone-producing adenomas or carcinoma will be relatively unaffected.

METYRAPONE TEST. — Metyrapone (Metopirone) blocks conversion of compound S to cortisol. This normally induces the pituitary to secrete more ACTH to increase cortisol production. Although production of cortisol is decreased, compound S is increased, as it accumulates proximal to the metyrapone block, and 17-OHCS or radioassay competitive binding methods for cortisol in either serum or urine will demonstrate sharply increased compound S in normal persons and those with cortex hyperplasia. Fluorescent or RIA measurements for cortisol do not include compound S, and therefore will be decreased. Adrenal tumors should not be significantly affected by metyrapone. Some authorities recommend measuring both cortisol and compound S. An increase in compound S verifies that lowering of plasma cortisol was accompanied by an increase in ACTH secretion. This maneuver also improves the ability of the test to indicate the status of pituitary reserve capacity, and the test is sometimes used for that purpose rather than investigation of Cushing's disease. To obtain both measurements, one would have to select a test method for cortisol that did not include compound S. Dilantin and estrogen administration will interfere with the metyrapone test. Compound S can be measured by a specific RIA method.

ACTH STIMULATION. — Injection of ACTH provides direct stimulation to the adrenal cortex. Patients with cortex hyperplasia and some adenomas display increased plasma cortisol and 17-OHCS levels. If urine collection is used, a 24-hour specimen taken the day of ACTH administration would demonstrate a considerable increase from preinfusion baseline values, which persists in a 24-hour specimen collected the day after ACTH. Normal persons should have increased hormone excretion the day ACTH was given but should return to normal in the next 24 hours.

SERUM ACTH. — Serum ACTH measurement by RIA is now available in many reference laboratories. At present, the assay techniques are too difficult for the average laboratory to perform in a reliable fashion.

There is a diurnal variation in serum ACTH levels corresponding to cortisol secretion, with highest values at 8–10 A.M. and lowest values near midnight. Stress and other factors that affect cortisol diurnal variation may blunt or eliminate the ACTH diurnal variation. In Cushing's syndrome due to adrenal tumor, the pituitary is suppressed by tumor-produced cortisol, so that serum ACTH is very low. In ectopic ACTH syndrome, serum ACTH is very high due to production of cross-reacting ACTH-like material by the tumor. In bilateral adrenal hyperplasia due to pituitary overactivity, serum ACTH can be either normal or elevated. It has been suggested that ACTH specimens obtained at 10–12 P.M. provide better separation of normal from pituitary hypersecretion than do specimens drawn in the morning.

PRIMARY ALDOSTERONISM

Aldosterone is the major electrolyte-regulating steroid of the adrenal cortex. Production is stimulated by ACTH, but is also influenced by serum sodium or potassium levels, and, in addition, aldosterone can be secreted under the influence of the renin-angiotensin system in quantities sufficient to maintain life even without ACTH. In plasma, some aldosterone is probably bound to alpha globulins. There is a circadian rhythm that corresponds to that of cortisol, peak levels occurring in the early morning and low levels (50% or less of A.M. values) in the afternoon. Ninety percent of breakdown and inactivation takes place in the liver. Aldosterone acts primarily on the distal convoluted tubules of the kidney, where it promotes sodium reabsorption with compensatory excretion of potassium and hydrogen ions.

Primary aldosteronism (Conn's syndrome) results from overproduction of aldosterone, usually by an adrenal cortex adenoma (carcinoma, nodular hyperplasia or glucocorticoid-suppressible aldosteronism are rare etiologies). Symptoms include hypertension, weakness and polyuria, but no edema. Hypokalemia is the most prominent laboratory finding; there usually is mild alkalosis and low urine specific gravity. Hypernatremia is found in classic cases, but a sizable minority of patients have high normal or normal serum sodium. Excretion of 17-OHCS and 17-KS is normal. Hemoglobin and WBC are also normal. Other diseases that may cause hypokalemia and hypertension include Cushing's syndrome, essential hypertension combined with mercurial or thiazide diuretic therapy and malignant hypertension.

Diagnosis of primary aldosteronism may be suggested by failure to raise serum potassium levels on regular diet plus 100 mEq potassium a day (in addition, urine potassium excretion should increase during potassium loading, assuming normal salt intake of 5–8 gm/day).

Besides primary aldosteronism, aldosterone may be increased in certain nonadrenal conditions ("secondary aldosteronism"):

1. Hyponatremia or low salt intake
2. Potassium loading
3. Generalized edema (cirrhosis, nephrotic syndrome, congestive heart failure)
4. Malignant hypertension
5. Renal ischemia of any etiology (including renal artery stenosis)
6. Pregnancy or estrogen-containing medications

Current explanations for the effects of these conditions on aldosterone point toward decreased effective renal blood flow (Fig 29-4). This triggers certain pressure-sensitive glomerular afferent arteriole cells called the juxtaglomerular apparatus into compensatory release of the enzyme renin. Renin acts on an alpha$_2$ globulin from the liver called renin substrate to produce a decapeptide, angiotensin I, which in turn is converted to an octapeptide, angiotensin II, by conversion enzymes in lung and kidney. Angiotensin II is a potent vasoconstrictor with a very short half-life (less than 1 minute), which also is able to stimulate the adrenal cortex to release aldosterone. There are several feedback mechanisms, one of which is mediated by retention of salt (and accompanying water) by increased aldosterone leading to increase in plasma volume, which in turn induces the juxtaglomerular apparatus of the kidney to decrease renin secretion. In addition, it is thought that angiotensin II can suppress renin secretion directly. The autonomic nervous system also affects renin output. Normally, renin production follows a circadian rhythm that roughly (not exactly) parallels that of cortisol and aldosterone (highest values in early morning). There are reports that renin normal values diminish somewhat with age. Upright posture is a strong stimulus to renin secretion.

The typical laboratory pattern for primary aldosteronism is that of increased aldosterone and decreased renin. Some other conditions have symptoms or laboratory findings that might suggest primary aldosteronism, but these can be differentiated by the combination of aldosterone and re-

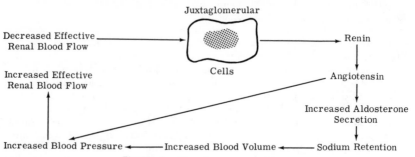

Fig 29—4. — Renal pressor system.

nin (Table 29–1). Some patients with Conn's syndrome have aldosterone values in the upper normal area rather than definitely elevated values. At times, either the renin or the aldosterone assay will have to be repeated to obtain a correct diagnosis.

Aldosterone Assays

Aldosterone can be assayed in 24-hour urine specimens or in plasma. Although RIA methods are now being applied, these are still much too difficult for the average laboratory. Even reference laboratories are not always dependable, especially for plasma aldosterone. Urine has the advantage that short-term fluctuations are eliminated and less overlap between normal and abnormal seems evident. Accurate collection of the 24-hour specimen is the major drawback. Plasma is much more convenient to obtain, but is more liable to be affected by short-term influences and other factors. Among these are diurnal variation and upright position, which both

TABLE 29–1. — TYPICAL RENIN-ALDOSTERONE PATTERNS IN
VARIOUS CONDITIONS

	PLASMA RENIN	ALDOSTERONE
Primary aldosteronism	Low	High
"Low-renin" essential hypertension	Low	Normal
Cushing's syndrome	Low	Low/normal
Licorice ingestion syndrome	Low	Low
High salt diet	Low	Low
Oral contraceptives	High	Normal
Cirrhosis	High	High
Malignant hypertension	High	High
Unilateral renal disease	High	High
"High-renin" essential hypertension	High	High
Pregnancy	High	High
Diuretic overuse	High	High
Juxtaglomerular tumor (Bartter syndrome)	High	High
Low salt diet	High	High
Addison's disease	High	Low
Hypokalemia	High	Low

greatly increase plasma aldosterone, whereas a 24-hour urine dampens these changes and instead reflects integrated secretion rate. Both plasma and urine aldosterone will be increased by low-sodium diets or lowered body sodium and decreased in the presence of high sodium intake. Potassium has an opposite effect; high potassium levels stimulate aldosterone secretion, while hypokalemia inhibits it. Since hypertensive patients are frequently treated by sodium restriction or diuretics, which increase sodium excretion, and since the body may be sodium depleted while still maintaining serum sodium within normal range, it is advisable to give patients a high-sodium diet or salt supplements for several days before collecting specimens for aldosterone (p. 490; renin assay is invalidated by salt loading and would have to be collected at some other time). Salt loading should not affect aldosterone values in primary aldosteronism, since the hormone is secreted autonomously and therefore production is not significantly affected by normal feedback mechanisms. As a further check, the 24-hour specimen (if urine is assayed) or a random urine specimen (if plasma is used) should be assayed for sodium. A finding of urine values less than 30 mEq/L suggests decreased sodium secretion, implying a sodium deficit and therefore a falsely increased aldosterone level. Some data indicate that aldosterone normal values, like those of renin, decrease somewhat with age. Certain drugs may change aldosterone secretion; most of these are agents that increase plasma renin (hydralazine [Apresoline], diazoxide [Hyperstat], nitroprusside and various diuretics such as furosemide [Lasix]). Glucose ingestion temporarily lowers plasma aldosterone levels.

Plasma Renin Assay

Plasma renin assay is complicated by the fact that renin cannot be measured directly, even by RIA. Instead, angiotensin I generation is estimated. This situation is standard in laboratory measurement of enzymes; usually the action of the enzyme on a suitable substrate is measured, rather than direct reaction of a chemical or antibody with the enzyme. Two related techniques are used: plasma renin activity (PRA) and plasma renin concentration (PRC). The PRA reflects the rate of angiotensin I formation per unit time. However, renin substrate (upon which renin acts) is normally not present in sufficient quantities for maximal renin effect. In PRC, excess renin substrate is added to demonstrate maximal renin effect; the result is compared to standard renin preparations to calculate the patient's renin concentration. In most cases PRA is adequate for clinical purposes and is technically a little more easy. Estrogens increase renin substrate, so PRC would be more accurate in that circumstance.

Plasma renin is a RIA technique of moderate or moderately great degree of difficulty; accurate results are highly dependent on the manner in which a laboratory performs the test. In addition, optimum conditions under which the assay should be performed are not yet standardized; and, although several kits are now commercially available, these kits demonstrate considerable variation in results when compared on the same plasma samples. In short, the majority of laboratories cannot be depended upon to produce accurate results, and even reference laboratories may at times have problems, especially with some of the kits. Renin is a very unstable enzyme, and for usable results must be drawn into a cold tube, the tube being kept cold while it is centrifuged and the plasma frozen immediately. Heparin cannot be used. The tourniquet should be removed before drawing the blood sample, since stasis may lower renin considerably. Certain factors influence renin secretion. Sodium depletion, hypokalemia, upright posture, various diuretics, estrogens and vasodilating antihypertensive drugs (hydralazine, diazoxide and nitroprusside) increase plasma renin. Methyldopa (Aldomet), guanethidine, L-dopa and propranolol decrease renin levels. Changes in body sodium have parallel effects on renin and aldosterone (e.g., low sodium stimulates production of both), whereas changes in potassium have opposite effects (low potassium stimulates renin but depresses aldosterone).

Although Conn's syndrome is typically associated with low plasma renin, other conditions (Table 29–1) may produce similar decreased values. In addition, nearly 25% of hypertensive patients display decreased plasma renin without having Conn's syndrome. Low salt diet plus 2 hours of upright posture are a combination of stimuli that, although renin values may increase, will not elevate renin in Conn's syndrome to normal range, while temporarily decreased renin from other etiologies will be stimulated enough to rise above the lower limits of normal. It has been advised not to use diuretics in addition to low salt plus upright posture, since the additional stimulation of renin production may overcome renin suppression in some patients with Conn's syndrome. Four hours' continual upright posture was originally thought to be necessary; subsequent data indicated that 2 hours was sufficient.

Several screening tests for renin abnormality have been suggested (p. 460). The furosemide test seems to be the one most widely used.

Unilateral renal disease is another etiology of hypertension that is potentially curable. It is estimated that 5% (or even more) of hypertensive persons have this condition, which makes it much more common than primary aldosteronism. Plasma renin is frequently elevated. Since renin assay may already be considered in a hypertensive patient to rule out Conn's syndrome, it could also serve as a screening test for unilateral renal disease. However, about half the patients (literature range 4–80%) who have curable hypertension due to unilateral renal disease have normal peripheral vein plasma renin. Other procedures (p. 137) yield better results in the detection of unilateral renal disease.

Renin measurement obtained from bilateral renal vein catheterization is being used in some medical centers as an index for potential curability as well as to indicate which kidney is the probable cause of the disease. Likewise, adrenal veins may be catheterized for adrenal phlebography and adrenal aldosterone in patients with Conn's syndrome for tumor localization. Adrenal radionuclide scanning using radioisotope-tagged agents such as cholesterol has produced encouraging results, both in Cushing's disease and Conn's syndrome, in those few centers that have access to the necessary radiopharmaceuticals.

ADDISON'S DISEASE

This condition is adrenocortical insufficiency from any cause. Tuberculosis used to be the most frequent etiology, but now is second to idiopathic atrophy. Steroid therapy, if long-term, causes cortex atrophy from disuse, and if steroids are abruptly withdrawn, symptoms will develop rapidly. Other etiologies are infection, idiopathic hemorrhage or replacement by metastatic carcinoma. The most frequent metastatic tumor is from the lung, and it is interesting that there often can be nearly complete replacement without any symptoms.

Weakness and fatigability are early manifestations of Addison's disease, often brought on by infection or stress. Other signs and symptoms of the classic syndrome are weight loss, hypotension of varying degree, a small heart, pigmentation of the skin and sometimes mild hypoglycemia. Laboratory studies show low serum sodium and chloride with elevated potassium. There may be a normocytic normochromic mild anemia and relative lymphocytosis with decreased neutrophils. The diagnosis may be suspected on clinical grounds and the finding of increased sodium and chloride in the urine despite low serum levels. Total circulating eosinophils usually are close to normal, although not always so.

ACTH Stimulation Test

A definitive diagnosis is possible using ACTH stimulation. The classic procedure is the 8-hour infusion test. If biologic rather than synthetic ACTH is used, many recommend 0.5 mg dexamethasone orally before starting the test to prevent allergic reactions. A 24-hour urine specimen is taken the day before the test. Twenty-five units of ACTH in 500 ml saline is given intravenously during an 8-hour period while another 24-hour urine specimen is obtained. In normal persons, there will be at least a two- to fourfold increase in cortisol or 17-OHCS levels. In Addison's disease, practically no response is found. If pituitary deficiency is suspected, the test should be repeated the next day, in which case there will be a gradual, although relatively small, response. If exogenous steroids have been given over long periods, especially in large doses, the test period may have to be prolonged up to 7 days. One group has circumvented this by using a continuous 24–48-hour infusion. If maintenance steroids are necessary during the test period, small doses of dexamethasone should be used to avoid measuring the treatment steroid along with endogenous production.

Most investigators now prefer a rapid ACTH stimulation test. After a baseline specimen is obtained, 25 units of ACTH or 0.25 mg cosyntropin (Cortrosyn or Synacthen), a synthetic ACTH preparation, is injected. There is variation in technique among descriptions in the literature. Some measure plasma cortisol and a few assay urinary 17-OHCS; some inject intramuscularly and others intravenously; some obtain a plasma cortisol specimen at 30 minutes after giving ACTH while others prefer 60 or 120 minutes, and some obtain samples at two intervals instead of one. A reasonable compromise seems to be intravenous injection (after a baseline blood specimen) and measurement of plasma cortisol at 30 and at either 90 or 120 minutes. Theoretically, patients with primary adrenal insufficiency should demonstrate little response, while patients with pituitary insufficiency or normal persons should have increased cortisol levels over twice baseline values. Since some persons with pituitary insufficiency may have a subnormal response, it has been suggested that aldosterone should be measured as well as cortisol. Aldosterone levels should increase in pituitary hypofunction but should not rise significantly in primary adrenal failure.

If steroid measurements are not available, the Thorn test is a reasonably satisfactory substitute, although not as accurate. First, a count of total circulating eosinophils is done. Then the patient is given 25 units of ACTH, either intravenously in the same way as the ACTH test just described or intramuscularly in the form of long-acting ACTH gel. Eight hours after ACTH is started, another total circulating eosinophil count is made. Normally, cortisone causes depression of eosinophil production. Therefore, a normal response to the test ACTH stimulation would be a drop of total circulating eosinophils to less than 50% of baseline values. A drop of less than 50% is considered suspicious for adrenal insufficiency. False positive responses (less than a 50% drop) may occur in any condition that itself produces eosinophilia (such as acute episodes of allergy).

A single "random" plasma cortisol specimen has been used as a screening procedure, since theoretically the value should be very low in Addison's disease and normal in other conditions, but most agree this is not reliable.

Plasma ACTH measurement also has been suggested, both to help confirm a diagnosis and to differentiate primary from secondary adrenal failure. In primary adrenal failure, ACTH should be high and cortisol should be low; in hypothalamic or pituitary insufficiency, ACTH and cortisol both should be low. A specimen for plasma ACTH can be drawn at the same time as baseline cortisol prior to stimulation tests, and can be frozen to be available if needed.

Some patients may produce equivocal rapid test results, and others may have been treated with substantial doses of steroids for considerable periods of time before definitive tests for etiology of Addison's disease are attempted. Under long-term steroid suppression, a normal adrenal cortex may be unable to respond immediately to stimulation. To perform definitive tests, the classic approach is to repeat the 8-hour ACTH infusion procedure daily for 5–7 days. Patients with primary Addison's disease should display little daily increment in cortisol values; those with secondary Addison's disease should eventually produce a stepwise increase in cortisol values. Some have used depot intramuscular synthetic ACTH preparations once daily instead of intravenous infusion.

ADRENAL MEDULLA DYSFUNCTION

The only syndrome in this category is produced by pheochromocytomas. Pheochromocytoma is a tumor of the adrenal medulla that often secretes epinephrine or norepinephrine. This causes hypertension, which may be continuous or intermittent. Although rare, pheochromocytoma is one of the few curable causes of hypertension, and thus should be tested for in any patient with hypertension of either sudden or recent onset. This is especially true for young or middle-aged persons. The original tests for pheochromocytomas were pharmacologic, based on the fact that epinephrine effects could be neutralized by adrenergic-blocking drugs such as Regitine. After basal blood pressure has been established, 5 mg Regitine are given intravenously and the blood pressure is checked every 30 seconds. The result is positive if systolic blood pressure decreases more than 35 mm Hg or diastolic levels decrease 25 mm Hg or more and remain decreased

3–4 minutes. Laboratory tests have proved much more reliable than the pharmacologic procedures, which have an appreciable percentage of false positives and negatives. The catecholamines epinephrine and norepinephrine are excreted by the kidney, about 3–6% free (unchanged) and the remainder as various metabolites (Fig 29–5). Of these metabolic products, the major portion is vanilmandelic acid (VMA), and the remainder (about 20–40%) are compounds known as metanephrines. Therefore, one can measure urinary catecholamines, metanephrines or VMA. Of these, metanephrine assay is considered by many to be the most sensitive and reliable single test. There are also fewer drugs that interfere. One report indicates that metanephrine excretion is relatively uniform and that a random specimen reported in terms of creatinine excretion can be substituted for the usual 24-hour collection in screening for pheochromocytoma. Although metanephrines are slowly gaining preference, VMA and catecholamine assay are still widely used. All three methods have detection rates within 5–10% of one another. A small but significant percentage of pheochromocytomas are missed by any of the three tests (fewer by metanephrines), especially if the tumor secretes intermittently. The VMA test has one definite advantage in that certain "screening" methods are technically more simple than catecholamine or metanephrine assay and therefore are more readily available in smaller laboratories. The VMA screening methods are apt to produce more false positive results, however, so that abnormal values (or normal results in patients with strong suspicion for pheochromocytoma) should be confirmed by some other procedure.

Catecholamine production may be increased after severe exercise (although mild or moderate exercise has no appreciable effect) and uncommonly by emotional stress. Uremia interferes with assay methods based on fluorescence. Other diseases that may increase catecholamine production (and thereby the excretion of either free catecholamines or their metabolites) are thyrotoxicosis, Cushing's disease, myocardial infarction, hemolytic anemia and occasionally lymphoma and severe renal disease. In addition, coffee and various other foods as well as some drugs may give falsely elevated VMA levels using some of the standard ("screening") techniques. An abnormal result with the "screening" VMA techniques should be confirmed by some other VMA method. Although other VMA methods or methods of metanephrines and catecholamine assay are more reliable, they too may be affected by certain substances, so that it is best to check with individual laboratories for details on substances that affect their particular

Fig 29–5. — Catecholamine metabolism.

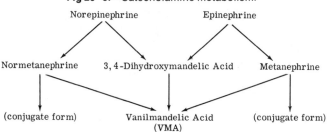

test method. Fasting blood sugar is elevated in about 50% of pheochromocytoma patients.

Cushing's disease, primary aldosteronism, unilateral renal disease (rarely bilateral renal artery stenosis) and pheochromocytoma, all discussed elsewhere, often produce hypertension. Hypertension due to these diseases is classifed as secondary hypertension, in contrast to primary idiopathic (essential) hypertension. Although patients with these particular diseases that cause secondary hypertension form a relatively small minority of hypertension patients, the diseases are important because they are surgically curable. The patient usually is protected against the bad effects of hypertension by early diagnosis and cure. Those patients who must be especially investigated are those who are young (under age 50), whose symptoms develop over a short period or who have a sudden worsening of the hypertension after previous mild stable blood pressure elevation.

REFERENCES

Amery, A., and Conway, J.: A critical review of diagnostic tests for pheochromocytoma, Am. Heart J. 73:129, 1967.

Bath, N. M., et al.: Plasma renin activity in renovascular hypertension, Am. J. Med. 45:381, 1968.

Beckerhoff, R., et al.: Problems associated with plasma renin activity measurements by angiotension I radioimmunoassay, Horm. Metab. Res. 7:342, 1975.

Boughton, A.: Application of adrenocorticotropic assays in a routine clinical laboratory, Am. J. Clin. Pathol. 64:618, 1975.

Brunner, H. R., and Gavras, H.: Clinical implications of renin in the hypertensive patient, J.A.M.A. 233:1091, 1975.

Conn, J. W.: Aldosteronism in hypertensive disease, Med. Times 98:116, 1970.

Conn, J. W., et al.: Preoperative diagnosis of primary aldosteronism, Arch. Intern. Med. 123:113, 1969.

Conn, J. W., et al.: Primary reninism: Hypertension, hyperreninemia, and secondary aldosteronism due to renin-producing juxtaglomerular cell tumors, Arch. Intern. Med. 130:682, 1972.

Dhuhy, R. G., et al.: Rapid ACTH test with plasma aldosterone levels: Improved diagnostic discrimination, Ann. Intern. Med. 80:693, 1974.

Eddy, R. L., et al.: Cushing's syndrome: A prospective study of diagnostic methods, Am. J. Med. 55:621, 1973.

Flint, L. D., and Jacobs, E. C.: Belated recognition of adrenocorticotropic hormone-producing tumors in post-adrenalectomized Cushing's syndrome, J. Urol. 112:688, 1974.

Foster, J. H., and Oates, J. A.: Recognition and management of renovascular hypertension, Hosp. Practice 10:61, 1975.

Kaplan, N. M.: The prognostic implications of plasma renin in essential hypertension, J.A.M.A. 231:167, 1975.

Kaplan, N. M., et al.: Single-voided urine metanephrine assays in screening for pheochromocytoma, Arch. Intern. Med. 137:190, 1977.

Katz, F.H., and Beck, P.: Plasma renin activity, renin substrate, and aldosterone during treatment with various oral contraceptives, J. Clin. Endocrinol. Metab. 39: 1001, 1974.

Katz, F. H., et al.: Diurnal variation of plasma aldosterone, cortisol, and renin activity in supine man, J. Clin. Endocrinol. Metab. 40:125, 1975.

Laragh, J. H.: An approach to the classification of hypertensive states, Hosp. Practice 9:61, 1974.

Lauler, D. P.: When to hospitalize for adrenal insufficiency, Hosp. Practice 3:35, 1968.

Lauler, D. P.: When to hospitalize for primary aldosteronism, Hosp. Practice 4:48, 1969.

Liddle, G. W., and Shute, A. M. : Cushing's Syndrome as a Clinical Entity, in Stollerman, G. H. (ed.): *Advances in Internal Medicine* (Chicago: Year Book Medical Publishers, Inc., 1969), Vol. 15, p. 155.

Liddle, G. W., et al.: Nonpituitary neoplasms and Cushing's syndrome, Arch. Intern. Med. 111:471, 1963.

Mills, I. H.: Primary aldosteronism, Clin. Endocrinol. Metab. 3:593, 1974.

Modlinger, R. S., and Gutkin, M.: Normal plasma renin in low renin hypertension, J. Clin. Endocrinol. Metab. 40:380, 1975.

Nelson, D. H.: Determining plasma and urinary corticosteroids, Postgrad. Med. 46:135, 1969.

Nichols, T., et al.: Steroid laboratory tests in the diagnosis of Cushing's syndrome, Am. J. Med. 45:116, 1968.

Oparil, S., and Haberk, E.: The renin-angiotensin system, N. Engl. J. Med. 291:389, 446, 1974.

Pertsemlidis, D., et al.: Pheochromocytoma: 1. Specificity of laboratory diagnostic tests. 2. Safeguards during operative removal, Ann. Surg. 169:376, 1969.

Ramirez, G., and Bates, H. M.: Measurement of urine sodium/potassium ratio, Lab. Management 13:18, 1975.

Ravasini, R. G., et al.: Adrenal scanning: Its use in medical and surgical routine, J. Nucl. Med. 15:526, 1974.

Rose, L. I., et al.: The 48-hour adrenocorticotropin infusion test for adrenocortical insufficiency, Ann. Intern. Med. 73:49, 1970.

Sambhi, M. P., et al.: Essential hypertension: New concepts about mechanisms, Ann. Intern. Med. 79:411, 1973.

Sawin, C. T.: Measurement of plasma cortisol in diagnosis of Cushing's syndrome, Ann. Intern. Med. 68:624, 1968.

Seabold, J. E., et al.: Iodocholesterol adrenal imaging in aldosteronism: Operative findings in 30 consecutive cases, J. Nucl. Med. 15:531, 1974.

Sealey, J. E., and Laragh, J. H.: Searching out low renin patients: Limitations of some commonly used methods, Am. J. Med. 55:303, 1973.

Sealey, J. E., et al.: Plasma prorenin: Cryoactivation and relationship to renin substrate in normal subjects, Am. J. Med. 61:731, 1976.

Spark, R. F.: Simplified assessment of pituitary-adrenal reserve, Ann. Intern. Med. 75:717, 1971.

Steinbeck, A. W., and Thiele, H. M.: The adrenal cortex (excluding aldosteronism), Clin. Endocrinol. Metab. 3:557, 1974.

Wallach, L., et al.: Stimulated renin: A screening test for hypertension, Ann. Intern. Med. 82:27, 1975.

Wolf, R. L.: Pheochromocytoma, Clin. Endocrinol. Metab. 3:609, 1974.

Zimmerman, B.: Pituitary and adrenal function in relation to surgery, Surg. Clin. North Am. 45:299, 1965.

30 / Pituitary, Parathyroid and Gonadal Function Tests; Tests in Obstetrics

TESTS OF PITUITARY FUNCTION

THE MOST COMMON AREAS of pituitary dysfunction are pituitary insufficiency in adults, growth hormone (GH) deficiency of childhood and acromegaly in adults.

Pituitary Insufficiency

Pituitary insufficiency in adults is most commonly due to postpartum hemorrhage (Sheehan's syndrome). Pituitary tumor must also be considered. Gonadal failure is usually the first deficiency to appear. It is followed some time later by myxedema. Diagnosis can be made, using indirect methods, by proving normal adrenal 17-ketosteroid (17-KS) response to ACTH stimulation or normal thyroid hormone response to TSH. The metyrapone (Metopirone) test (p. 357) can also be used. Growth hormone secretion can now be measured directly via radioimmunoassay (RIA). Values are elevated by sleep, exercise of any type and various foods. Therefore, basal levels should be drawn in the morning after awakening but before arising, subsequent to an overnight fast. Because basal normal range overlaps values found in hypopituitarism, only a clearly normal result is significant. In most cases, a stimulation test will be needed for diagnosis or confirmation. The two most frequently used procedures are insulin-induced hypoglycemia and arginine infusion. Pituitary insufficiency cannot be documented on the basis of either test alone, since about 20% of normal persons may fail to respond satisfactorily to insulin or to arginine. Estrogen administration tends to increase GH secretion, and some investigators obtained better results from arginine infusion after administration of estrogens.

Stimulation tests with other substances have been proposed, including glucagon, tolbutamide and L-dopa. Of these, L-dopa seems to have best results; some feel that it has accuracy equal to or better than insulin or arginine, and in addition is easier and safer to perform. One investigator found a greater number of unreliable results in older persons and in depressed patients. It has been suggested that propranolol improves GH response to glucagon.

Besides tests involving GH production, other procedures that have been used to evaluate various aspects of pituitary function are the metyra-pone (Metopirone) test (p. 357), based on the adrenal cortex hormone feed-back mechanism of ACTH and cortisol, but depending on hypothalamic as well as pituitary function; thyrotropin releasing factor (TRF) test (p. 344), involving ability of TRF to stimulate the pituitary directly to release TSH; tests involving pituitary gonadotropin (luteinizing hormone; LH) such as clomiphene (hypothalamic-pituitary axis) stimulation or LH releasing factor administration (direct pituitary action); and tests involving pituitary release of prolactin by direct pituitary stimulation (TRF), by blocking of hy-pothalamic inhibition (chlorpromazine) or by enhancement of hypothalam-ic inhibition (L-dopa).

Prolactin is a pituitary hormone. It stimulates lactation (galactorrhea) in females, but its function in males is less certain. The hypothalamus exerts an inhibitory effect, with one known pathway being under control of dopa-mine. There is a secretion pattern much like that of GH, with highest lev-els during sleep. Prolactin can be measured by RIA, and has been useful in evaluating inappropriate lactation in females. It is usually normal in gyne-comastia or hypogonadism in males, but occasionally may be elevated. Thyrotropin-releasing factor stimulates release of prolactin as well as TSH. Dopamine antagonists such as chlorpromazine or reserpine block the hy-pothalamic release inhibition pathway, leading to increased prolactin lev-els. Since TRF acts on the pituitary and chlorpromazine on the hypothala-mus, these agents can be useful as another way to assess hypothalamic and pituitary function. The greatest interest in prolactin stems from the discov-ery that most secreting pituitary tumors and 30% of so-called chromophobe (nonsecreting) adenomas induce elevated prolactin levels. According to available reports, chlorpromazine fails to induce normal degrees of prolac-tin elevation in most patients with pituitary tumors, whereas L-dopa will suppress prolactin values in normal fashion. Elevated prolactin levels that fail to increase significantly with chlorpromazine are thus highly suspi-cious for pituitary tumor. Besides pituitary tumor, prolactin elevation has been reported in the "empty sella" syndrome (enlarged sella turcica with-out tumor). Elevations usually, but not always, are relatively small.

Other conditions may produce elevated serum prolactin: renal failure (20% of patients), pregnancy, stress, anesthesia, hypoglycemia, primary hypothyroidism, acromegaly and certain medications (estrogens, pheno-thiazines, reserpine, methyldopa, Haldol).

Growth Hormone Deficiency

Growth hormone deficiency in childhood or infancy usually becomes part of the differential diagnosis of dwarfism. Among other etiologies of dwarfism are hypothyroidism, achondroplasia (and other chondrodys-trophies), so-called "primordial" (idiopathic) dwarfism and temporarily retarded growth. Diagnosis of hypothyroidism and the chondrodystrophies is discussed elsewhere. Diagnosis of GH deficiency consists of serum GH assay. Growth hormone values well within normal limits separate pituitary dwarfism from dwarfism having other etiologies. In equivocal cases, or to document a diagnosis further, GH stimulation tests can be used. Measure-ment of other pituitary hormones such as TSH and LH assists in differen-tiating isolated GH defect from hypopituitarism.

Acromegaly

Acromegaly is produced in adults by increase of GH, usually from an eosinophilic adenoma of the pituitary. About two thirds of these patients are females. Signs and symptoms include bitemporal headaches, disturbances of the visual field, optic atrophy, hand and face physical changes and decreased carbohydrate tolerance. About 65–75% of patients display sella turcica enlargement on skull x-rays. Growth hormone assay usually reveals levels above the upper limit of 5 ng/ml. The standard method of confirming the diagnosis is a suppression test using glucose. Normal persons nearly always respond with a decrease in GH levels to less than 50% of baseline levels, while acromegalic patients in theory have autonomous tumors and should show little if any effect of hyperglycemia. One recent study, however, noted relatively normal suppression in a significant percentage of acromegalics. Assay of serum prolactin with stimulation by chlorpromazine, as previously described, is now being used.

One report indicates that elevated cerebrospinal fluid (CSF) levels of various pituitary hormones such as prolactin, GH and TSH may occur in a large percentage of patients with pituitary tumors when suprasellar extension takes place.

TESTS OF GONADAL FUNCTION

The most common conditions in which gonadal function tests are used include hypogonadism in males and menstrual disorders, fertility problems and hirsutism or virilization in females. The hormones currently available for assistance include LH, FSH, testosterone and human chorionic gonadotropin (hCG).

Originally FSH and LH were measured together using bioassay methods, and so-called "FSH" measurements included LH. RIA techniques are able to separate the two hormones. LH cross-reacts with hCG in most RIA systems. Although this ordinarily does not create a problem, there is difficulty in pregnancy and in patients with certain neoplasms that secrete hCG. Several of the pituitary and placental glycopeptides (TSH, FSH, hCG, LH) are composed of at least two immunologic units, alpha and beta. All have the same immunologic response to the alpha fraction but a different response to the beta subunit. Antisera against the beta subunit of hCG eliminate interference by LH; and some investigators have reported success in producing antisera against the beta subunit of LH, which does not detect hCG. There is some cross reaction between FSH and TSH, but as yet this has not seemed important enough clinically in TSH assay to necessitate substitution of TSH beta subunit antiserum for antisera already available. Assay of FSH in serum is thought to be more reliable than in urine due to characteristics of the antibody preparations available.

Male Hypogonadism

Testicular function is mediated by LH (in males sometimes called interstitial cell stimulating hormone), which induces testosterone secretion by the Leydig cells of the testis. Follicle-stimulating hormone is also necessary for testicular function to stimulate seminiferous tubule (Sertoli cell) development. Testosterone has a feedback mechanism with pituitary LH via the hypothalamus. The adrenals also produce androgens, but normally this is not a significant factor in males. Testosterone in males has a diurnal variation of mild degree, with highest values in the morning. In primary hypogonadism (e.g., Klinefelter's syndrome or idiopathic gonadal failure), plasma testosterone is low and LH or FSH is high. Some investigators feel that FSH is more likely to be consistently elevated than LH. Patients with cirrhosis frequently have depressed testosterone levels. In secondary (pituitary or hypothalamic) hypogonadism, both testosterone and LH should be low. Stimulation tests are available for equivocal cases. The testis is directly stimulated by hCG, increasing testosterone secretion to at least twice baseline values. Clomiphene stimulates the hypothalamus, producing increase in both LH and testosterone. Gonadotropin-releasing hormone (LRH) is now available but not yet approved for general use.

Female Amenorrhea

In females, FSH and LH have a more complicated interrelationship than in males because of the menstrual cycle as well as menarche. While FSH rises to a peak early in the cycle with a second peak at the time of ovulation, LH has a single peak at ovulation; LH (and possibly FSH) is frequently released in short episodes followed by periods of relatively low secretion. Estrogen administration produces a rise in LH but not in FSH. Anovulation may occur in normal persons, and disorders of menstruation and fertility are a much more complicated group of disorders than sex hormone abnormalities in males. Hypogonadism may be suspected by the finding of decreased urinary estrogens or plasma estradiol. If primary hypogonadism (e.g., Turner's syndrome) exists, serum FSH should be high (LH may be normal or high); if pituitary or hypothalamic hypogonadism is present, FSH (and LH) should be low (sometimes low normal). Clomiphene stimulation may be used to confirm the diagnosis. Measurements of LH are sometimes used to establish exact time of ovulation with the menstrual cycle. Estrogens such as estradiol-17-beta can be measured in serum by RIA, and are helpful in confirming a diagnosis of female hypogonadism.

Female Hirsutism

This is a relatively common problem in which the overriding concern of the physician is to rule out an ovarian or adrenal tumor. Adrenal etiology leading to masculinization is more common in small children (adrenogenital syndrome, p. 354), while ovarian abnormality is more common in older children or adults. Adrenal virilization syndrome is discussed on page 355. Plasma testosterone is helpful in workup of patients with hirsutism. Urine determinations are less useful. In females, testosterone is derived from ovarian and adrenal androgens, the most important being androstenedione, mainly through conversion in peripheral tissues. The Stein-Leventhal (polycystic ovary) syndrome is usually associated with elevated plasma testosterone when virilization is present. Idiopathic hirsutism patients may have elevated testosterone values, but at least 40% are normal. Arrhenoblastomas frequently secrete testosterone. Virilization due to adrenal cortex etiology (adrenogenital syndrome) is usually accompanied by increased urine 17-KS, but reports differ on how frequently plasma testosterone is elevated. Estrogen administration may falsely increase plasma testosterone values, due to increase in testosterone-binding protein.

TESTS IN OBSTETRICS

Pregnancy

Pregnancy tests are based on the fact that the placenta secretes hCG, a hormone that has a luteinizing action on ovarian follicles but whose actual function is not definitely established. It reaches a level of about 500 international units (IU) of gonadotropic activity/L between the 28th and 32d days after the beginning of the last menstrual period. A peak is reached about the 63rd day, but ranging between the 50th and 80th days, with values reaching 200,000 IU, then slowly falling to levels between 2,000 and 10,000 IU. This level is maintained for the remainder of pregnancy, except for a brief rise and fall in the 3d trimester.

The first practical biologic test for pregnancy was the Ascheim-Zondek test, published in 1928. Urine was injected into immature female mice, and a positive result was indicated by corpus luteum development in the ovaries. This took 4–5 days to perform. Clinical accuracy is reported as up to 98%. A few false positives and negatives occur. The next widely used procedure was the Friedman test, which was similar except that female rabbits were used and the test took 3 days. Other variations on these procedures were used, but it was not until the frog tests were described that a significant advance occurred. Male frogs are used; urine or serum is injected and the frog is catheterized 1–2 hours later. The presence of spermatozoa is a positive result. The frog test has approximately a 95% reliability, although some report even better. False negative and false positive results do occur, although they are uncommon. Phenothiazine drugs (e.g., Thorazine) give a considerable number of false positives. The result is almost always positive at the 40th day of pregnancy, although sometimes sooner. All these biologic tests share the problems that go with using animals. In the past few years, it was discovered that antibodies to hCG could be produced by injecting the gonadotropin into animals. This raised the possibility of developing an immunologic pregnancy test using antigen-antibody reactions.

Both tube tests and slide tests are now available. In general, the tube tests require 2 hours to perform, but tend to be a little more accurate. The slide tests take 2–3 minutes. A few procedures based on chemical techniques are being marketed. There is significant variation in accuracy and sensitivity among all these tests (p. 492). In general, most immunologic tests are over 95% accurate and have a sensitivity between 1,000 and 3,000 IU/L. Each becomes positive between the 35th and 40th days (counting from the 1st day of the last menstrual period), sometimes sooner, and is almost always positive by the 41st day. Proteinuria (over 25 mg/100 ml) causes false positive results (p. 492) in many of the commercial slide tests; certain psychiatric drugs (such as Thorazine) give false positives in a few of the commercial procedures. In the 3d trimester, and occasionally even in the 2d, false negative results with any of the immunologic tests may be obtained in some patients, due to the much lower gonadotropin levels at this time. Occasional false positive results from some of the pregnancy tests have been reported in postmenopausal women and in hyperthyroidism; presumably this is due to increased LH, which cross-reacts with current antibody preparations to hCG.

Pregnancy tests are useful in certain situations other than early diagnosis of normal pregnancy. In possible abortion, a dying trophoblast is usually associated with low levels of hCG; this predicts present or inevitable abortion. However, normal levels are found in some instances where the embryo dies but the trophoblast continues to function. In ectopic pregnancy, the tests are positive only about half the time (using standard slide or tube procedures), so that a negative result definitely does not rule out this diagnosis. The RIA of hCG is much more sensitive than standard pregnancy tests (capable of detecting approximately 5 IU/L as compared to 700 IU/L for the most sensitive tube immunologic test) and therefore is more accurate in diagnosis of ectopic pregnancy. However, ectopic pregnancy is usually an emergency situation in which it is often not possible to wait until hCG assay by RIA can be obtained. Pregnancy tests have also been used for diagnosis of hydatidiform mole and chorionepithelioma, but hCG assay by RIA is preferred. Luteinizing hormone cross-reacts with hCG whether by standard pregnancy test or by RIA. This limits the sensitivity of the test to a level that will not detect usual amounts of LH. A new RIA procedure has been developed to measure the beta subunit of hCG; it avoids interference by LH and therefore is capable of increased accuracy with sensitivity to less than 5 IU/L.

Gestational Neoplasms

Neoplasms arising from chorionic villi, the fetal part of the placenta, include hydatidiform mole (the counterpart in tumor classification of benign adenoma) and choriocarcinoma (chorionepithelioma; the equivalent of carcinoma). Hydatidiform mole also has a subdivision, chorioadenoma destruens, in which the neoplasm invades the placenta but there is no other evidence of malignancy. The major importance of hydatidiform mole is a very high (10% or greater) incidence of progression to choriocarcinoma.

Several hormone assays have been proposed as aids in diagnosis. By far the most important is hCG, which is produced by the trophoblast cell component of fetal placental tissue. As just noted, hCG forms the basis for most pregnancy tests. Luteinizing hormone has a close biochemical and immunologic similarity to hCG (through its alpha subunit, p. 370), so that standard immunologic pregnancy tests could not be made more sensitive than 700–1,000 IU/L to avoid too many false positive results from cross-reaction with LH. Unfortunately, 25–30% of trophoblastic tumors produce hCG in amounts less than 1,000 IU/L. Antibodies to the specific beta subunit of hCG are now available, and RIA procedures using these antibodies can detect 5 IU/L or less without interference by LH, allowing detection of nearly all gestational tumors. Since normal placental tissue secretes hCG, the problem then is to differentiate normal pregnancy from neoplasm. Suspicion is raised by clinical signs and also by finding hCG levels that are increased more than expected by the duration of pregnancy or persist after removal of the placenta. Twin or other multiple pregnancies can also produce hCG above expected levels. Once neoplasm is diagnosed and treated, hCG measurement is a guideline for success of therapy and follow-up of the patient for possible recurrence.

Fetal and placental tissue produces other hormones that may be useful. Progesterone (or its metabolite pregnanediol) and estradiol are secreted by the placenta in slowly increasing quantity throughout most of pregnancy. It has been reported that up to 20 weeks of gestation, serum estradiol-17-beta is increased from values expected in normal pregnancy, with good separation of normal from molar pregnancy. Serum progesterone was increased in about 75% of nonaborted moles up to the 20th week. Urinary pregnanediol, on the other hand, is frequently decreased. Since hCG reaches its normal peak between the 50th and 80th days subsequent to the last menstrual period, finding increased serum progesterone and estradiol-17-beta during this time accompanied by decreased urine pregnanediol would suggest a hydatidiform mole or possibly a choriocarcinoma. Serum placental lactogen (hPL) is another placental hormone that rises during the 1st and 2d trimesters and then reaches a plateau during the last 2–3 months. The association of decreased levels of hPL in the 1st and 2d trimesters with increased hCG suggests neoplasm. There is, however, a small degree of overlap of hPL level in patients with mole and the normal range for pregnancy. One report suggests a possible inverse ratio between hPL values and degree of malignancy (the greater the degree of malignancy, the less serum hPL produced).

Production of hCG has been reported to occur in nearly two thirds of testicular embryonal cell carcinomas and about one third of testicular seminomas. Instances have been reported of hCG secretion by adenocarcinomas from other organs and rarely from certain other tumors (p. 494).

Fetal or Placental Function

Several hormone assays are available to help estimate whether placental function is normal or to predict impending fetal death. The two tests most widely used are urine estriol (or total estrogens) and serum placental lactogen. Estriol (E_3) is an estrogenic compound produced entirely by the placenta, using precursors derived from fetal liver and adrenal cortex. Thus, urine E_3 indicates function of the entire fetoplacental unit. After the 2d month of pregnancy, it is produced in steadily increasing amounts. The usual procedure is to obtain weekly or biweekly serial determinations after 30 weeks' gestation in high-risk patients, or as an immediate test if fetal distress occurs; 24-hour urine collections are preferred, since excretion fluctuates during the day. A marked decline from previous values, especially if sustained, is considered significant evidence of placental malfunction. Coupled with clinical evidence of fetal distress, or in a high-risk patient, cesarean section may be indicated. Those patients considered at high risk are diabetics, hypertensives and those with a history of stillbirths. The test is not valid in liver damage, such as occurs with Rh erythroblastosis or eclampsia. Bed rest tends to increase E_3 excretion. Urinary tract infection and certain drugs (p. 473) affect test results.

Since E_3 comprises about 95% of urinary estrogens in pregnancy, total estrogens (much easier technically) could be substituted for it. Results using total estrogens are a little more variable than E_3 patterns. Urine urobilinogen may falsely increase total estrogens.

Human placental lactogen (hPL; somatomammotropin) is a hormone produced only by the placenta, with metabolic activity similar in some degree to that of prolactin and GH. Values correlate roughly with the weight of the placenta and rise steadily in maternal serum during the 1st and 2d trimesters before entering a relative plateau in the 3d. Serum levels of hPL are higher than those attained by any other peptide hormone. Serum half-life is about 30 minutes. Although hPL cross-reacts with GH in most RIA systems, the high level of hPL relative to GH at the time of pregnancy when hPL is measured avoids clinical problems with GH interference. Serum hPL has been evaluated by many investigators as a test of placental function in the 3d trimester. Its short half-life is thought to make it a more sensitive indicator of placental failure than measurements of other hormones, especially urine measurements. Since hPL can fluctuate somewhat normally, serial measurements are more accurate than a single determination. Estriol, which reflects combined fetal and placental function, still seems to be used more than hPL.

Placenta Localization

Vaginal bleeding in the 3d trimester of pregnancy is most frequently caused by placenta previa. In this condition the placenta is located near the cervical opening instead of in its usual position near the upper end of the uterus. Placenta previa is therefore a hazard to normal delivery and might necessitate cesarean section. Radioisotope scanning and ultrasound B-mode scanning are now being used for placental localization. Placental scanning is over 90% accurate, and the fetal radiation dose using present-day isotopes is very small; much smaller than the fetus would receive from ordinary x-ray pelvimetry studies. Ultrasound B-scan, however, is clearly the procedure of choice, with over 95% accuracy and no radiation administered.

Fetal Maturity Tests.

Tests are also available for monitoring fetal maturity via amniocentesis. Bilirubin levels in erythroblastosis are discussed in Chapter 10 (p. 97). Amniotic creatinine, cell stain with Nile blue sulfate, fat droplet evaluation, osmolality and shake testing, alone or in combination, have been tried with satisfactory but not outstanding results. There is general although not unanimous agreement that the lecithin-sphingomyelin (L/S) ratio is the most accurate procedure currently available. Lecithin is a phospholipid and a major component of alveolar surfactant. Surfactant is a substance that lowers the surface tension of the alveolar lining, stabilizes the alveoli in expiration and helps prevent atelectasis. Surfactant deficiency causes neonatal respiratory distress syndrome (hyaline membrane disease). In amniotic fluid, sphingomyelin normally exceeds lecithin before the 26th week; thereafter, lecithin concentration is slightly predominant until approximately the 35th week, when lecithin swiftly rises to more than twice sphingomyelin levels. After lecithin level becomes twice that of sphingomyelin, there is no longer any danger of hyaline membrane disease. The L/S ratio thus becomes a test for fetal maturity. Certain precautions must be taken. Contamination by maternal vaginal secretions or bleeding into the amniotic fluid may cause a false increase in lecithin. The amniotic fluid specimen must be cooled immediately and kept frozen if not tested promptly, to avoid destruction of lecithin by certain enzymes in amniotic fluid.

Occasionally, amniotic puncture may enter the maternal bladder instead of the amniotic sac. Some have advocated glucose and protein determination, which is high in amniotic fluid and low in normal urine. To avoid confusion in diabetics with glucosuria, it has been suggested that urea and potassium be measured instead; these are relatively high in urine and low in amniotic fluid. Another potential danger area is the use of spectrophotometric measurement of amniotic fluid pigment as an estimate of amniotic fluid bilirubin content. Before 25 weeks' gestation, normal pigment levels may be greater than those usually associated with abnormality.

Congenital Anomalies

Besides giving information on fetal well-being, amniocentesis makes it possible to test for various congenital anomalies via biochemical analysis of amniotic fluid and tissue culture chromosome studies of fetal cells (p. 495). For example, amniotic fluid alpha fetoprotein (p. 215) is elevated in 90% or more of open neural tube defects such as spina bifida or anencephaly. Normal values depend on gestational age; moderate elevation normally occurs in the 1st trimester and declines during the 2d until very little remains by the 3d. Amniotic fluid fetoprotein may also become elevated due to placental injury, impending or actual fetal death, omphalocele and congenital nephrosis. One report indicates some degree of increase in diabetes and toxemia of pregnancy. If these conditions are ruled out, incidence of false positive results is reported to be less than 1%. Most of the false positive results are attributable to admixture of fetal blood with the amniotic fluid at the time of amniotic puncture, so that amniotic fluid with elevated fetoprotein values should be tested for fetal hemoglobin. Alpha fetoprotein is said to be elevated in maternal serum in about half the cases of fetal open neural tube defects. Levels in maternal serum are not helpful before 13–15 weeks' gestation (2d trimester). Even after this time, unless values are very high or clearly normal, interpretation may be difficult. Besides the various conditions which may elevate amniotic fluid fetoprotein and, therefore, maternal serum fetoprotein, twin (multiple) pregnancy may elevate maternal serum values but not amniotic fluid. Maternal blood specimens should be drawn before amniocentesis to avoid effects of possible fetomaternal hemorrhage. Since reagents from different sources may vary, each laboratory must determine its own normal values.

TESTS OF PARATHYROID FUNCTION

Hyperparathyroidism

Hyperparathyroidism is an uncommon disease, but nevertheless an important one, especially from the surgical standpoint. By far the most common manifestation is renal stones, but metabolic bone disease often is present, and peptic ulcer may be associated. The disease always enters into the differential diagnosis of hypercalcemia, because this is one of its most prominent laboratory signs. Typically, in addition to hypercalcemia, there is low serum phosphorus, elevated alkaline phosphatase and increased urine calcium (the Sulkowitch test is a commonly used semiquantitative urine method) due to the action of excessive parathyroid hormone (PTH). In the blood there tends to be a reciprocal relationship between serum calcium and phosphorus, with low serum phosphorus associated with high serum calcium and vice versa. Parathyroid hormone prevents renal tubular reabsorption of phosphorus, thus allowing serum phosphate to drain out into the urine, producing depressed blood levels. This is balanced by drawing calcium out of bone to raise serum calcium. Although the classic picture of primary hyperparathyroidism has just been described, in some cases one or more components may be lacking. Some patients have borderline or normal serum calcium, some have normal phosphorus and a considerable number have normal alkaline phosphatase. In these patients other tests are needed for preoperative diagnosis.

Hypercalcemia is considered by all authorities the most important laboratory clue to primary hyperparathyroidism. Unfortunately, other conditions besides parathyroid tumor may elevate serum calcium. The more common causes of hypercalcemia and metabolic bone disease, with their classic laboratory findings, are shown in Table 30–1. Here again, there may be variations in some of the values in patients. The clinical history, physical examination and other laboratory tests usually can separate out these other diseases. For example, in secondary hyperparathyroidism caused by chronic renal disease, there usually is anemia with an elevated blood urea nitrogen (BUN); these symptoms are absent in classic primary hyperparathyroidism. However, even in the primary disease, after long periods the kidney may be so damaged by calculi with superimposed infection or by renal tissue calcification that it is difficult to tell primary from secondary.

Bone scans and roentgenograms often will reveal metastatic carcinoma lesions (p. 402). Breast and lung carcinoma are the most frequent tumors associated with hypercalcemia. Myeloma also belongs in this group; the

TABLE 30–1.–DIAGNOSIS OF CALCIUM-
PHOSPHORUS DISEASES*

	SERUM CAL.	SERUM PHOS.	ALK. PHOS.	ACIDOSIS	URINE CAL.
Primary hyperparathyroidism	H	L	H/N‡		H
Vitamin D excess	H	N/L	N/H		H
Sarcoidosis	H	N	H		H
Secondary hyperparathyroidism	L/N	H	H	+	H
Renal acidosis	L/N	N/L	H	+	H
Sprue	L/N	N/L	H		L
Osteomalacia	L/N	L/N	H		L
Paget's disease	N	N	H		N/H
Metastatic neoplasm to bone†	N/H	N	N/H		N/H
Hypoparathyroidism	L	H	N		L
Osteoporosis	N	N	N		N/H
Hyperthyroidism	N/H	N/H	N/H		N/H

*H, N and L = High, Normal and Low; second letter, if present, means less common finding.

†Depends on primary tumor and type of bone lesion produced. Metastatic carcinoma to bone is one of the commonest etiologies of hypercalcemia, perhaps the most common.

‡Alkaline phosphatase is high in "textbook cases" of primary hyperparathyroidism.

bone scan, however, is less frequently abnormal than in carcinomas. Occasional tumors (especially lung carcinomas) secrete a PTH-like hormone ("ectopic PTH"), producing clinical hyperparathyroidism without necessarily having extensive bone metastases. Thiazide diuretics occasionally induce mild hypercalcemia. Laboratory error may produce apparent hypercalcemia, so that initial serum calcium elevation should be rechecked before extensive workups are begun. Conversely, hypercalcemia may not always be striking or continuous, and laboratory error can depress calcium as well as elevate it, so that a normal serum level does not rule out parathyroid tumor. False hypercalcemia may result from stasis when a tourniquet is left in place too long before venipuncture. Calcium carbonate antacids in large amounts may also be troublesome. Food may produce small increases in serum calcium, so that specimens should be drawn in the morning after overnight fasting. Since about half of total calcium is bound to serum protein (80% of the bound fraction is carried by albumin), decrease in albumin may decrease total calcium (about 0.8 gm/100 ml change for each 1.0 gm albumin change).

TOTAL VERSUS IONIZED CALCIUM. — Total calcium is composed of two roughly equal parts; an active fraction, ionized calcium, and an inactive fraction, protein-bound calcium. Since most laboratories only measure total calcium, and since protein-bound calcium (and therefore total calcium) is affected by changes in calcium-binding proteins (predominantly serum albumin), measurement of the relatively stable ionized fraction has been proposed as a better indication of calcium metabolism. Although ionized calcium is said to be almost always increased in primary hyperparathyroidism, myeloma, metastatic carcinoma to bone and possibly other conditions such as renal failure also may increase the ionized calcium level. Ionized calcium values are affected by pH of serum (decrease of 0.1 pH unit increases ionization by 1.5–2.5%). If serum is exposed to air and stands too long, pH slowly increases.

MEASUREMENT OF PARATHYROID HORMONE. — Serum PTH can now be measured directly by RIA. The parathyroids secrete intact hormone, which is metabolized to a smaller, metabolically inactive portion plus several even smaller fragments. Most of the RIA antisera that are available react either with a terminal carboxyl group (anti-C) or a terminal amine group (anti-N). Some antisera may react to other molecular groups. In general, anti-N reacts with intact hormone and a few of the smaller fragments that exist in measurable form for very short periods (half-life of intact PTH is about 20 minutes), whereas anti-C reacts with intact hormone plus several larger fragments that exist for longer periods (hours or days). Therefore, anti-N measures short-duration hormone, which is indicative of acute changes in PTH secretion. Anti-C measures primarily long-duration hormone, which is more influenced by long-term or chronic hormone changes. Anti-N is more useful in measuring hormone from catheterization of neck veins; anti-C is more useful for peripheral vein blood. Both antisera may show PTH elevation in patients with renal failure, although more show elevation with anti-C than anti-N.

Theoretically, PTH assay should differentiate parathyroid tumor from various other etiologies of hypercalcemia, since hypercalcemia with all other etiologies should show decreased PTH secretion. Unfortunately, when tested with presently available antisera, some patients with parathyroid adenoma display elevated serum calcium but have PTH levels within normal range; while some persons without parathyroid adenoma may have mildly elevated PTH with normal serum calcium. Diagnosis of parathyroid adenoma can be assisted by correlating PTH assay with serum calcium levels, based on the fact that PTH normally decreases as serum calcium increases. A parathyroid adenoma may produce a PTH level that is within population normal range but is higher than expected in relation to the degree of calcium elevation. Nomograms have been devised for various antisera to assist this differentiation.

Certain tumors (especially lung carcinoma) may secrete a PTH-like hormone ("ectopic PTH") that cross-reacts with present-day PTH antisera.

There are additional problems in PTH assay interpretation. The hormone has a diurnal variation, with lower values in the morning. Specimens should be drawn when patients are fasting in the morning without anticoagulants, and should be processed at cold temperatures, frozen immediately and transported in dry ice. Assay of PTH at present is very difficult; reliable antisera are not yet readily available from commercial sources, and homemade antisera in some reference laboratories seem to differ in reactivity.

Tubular reabsorption of phosphate (TRP; phosphate reabsorption index).—This procedure is an indirect measure of PTH by estimating PTH action on renal phosphate reabsorption. The patient should be on a normal phosphate diet; low phosphate (less than 500 mg/day) raises TRP normal values, while high phosphorus (3,000 mg/day) lowers normal limits.

The patient drinks several glasses of water and then voids completely. One hour after voiding, a blood sample is obtained for phosphorus and creatinine. Exactly 2 hours after beginning the test, the patient again voids completely, and the urine volume and urine concentration of creatinine and phosphate are obtained. It is then possible to calculate the creatinine clearance and find the amount of phosphorus filtered per minute by the glomeruli. Comparing this with the actual amount of phosphate excreted per minute gives the amount reabsorbed by the tubules per minute or the tubular reabsorption of phosphate (TRP). A rough approximation is afforded by the formula:

$$\% \text{ TRP} = 1 - \left[\frac{\text{Urine PO}_4 \text{ conc.} \times \text{serum creatinine conc.}}{\text{Urine creatinine conc.} \times \text{serum PO}_4 \text{ conc.}} \right] \times 100$$

A low index value of less than 80% means diminished TRP and thus suggests primary hyperparathyroidism. This test becomes increasingly unreliable when the creatinine clearance is low due to severe renal disease, and is definitely not reliable in the presence of renal insufficiency. About 5% of patients with renal stones but without parathyroid tumor have TRP of 70–80%, while about 20% of patients with parathyroid tumors have normal TRP values. Therefore, a TRP reduction is more significant than a normal result. Hypercalcemia due to malignancy usually displays decreased TRP. In addition, some patients with other conditions such as sarcoidosis and myeloma have been reported to have reduced TRP. In spite of all the exceptions, TRP seems to be one of the better simple diagnostic procedures for primary hyperparathyroidism.

STEROID SUPPRESSION. — Large doses of adrenocortical steroids given for 1 week do not affect the calcium level in most (but not all) patients with parathyroid tumor, whereas the steroids will suppress elevated calcium levels due to most other etiologies. Again, exceptions occur, especially with metastatic carcinoma to bone.

CALCIUM INFUSION TESTS. — Hypercalcemia from calcium infusion inhibits secretion of PTH; this in turn decreases renal tubule phosphate reabsorption, producing loss of phosphorus into the urine. Parathyroid tumors theoretically should not be influenced by serum calcium levels, and patients therefore would not display significant change in urinary excretion of phosphate, whereas calcium infusion should suppress the action of nonautonomous parathyroid glands and result in a decrease in urine phosphate. The original Ellsworth-Howard test has not proved to be sufficiently reliable, nor have rapid infusions and other test modifications. Newer suggestions based on measuring urine phosphate in the second 12-hour period after 4-hour calcium infusion or measuring serum PTH instead of urine phosphorus have not yet been sufficiently evaluated.

X-RAY FINDINGS. — Bone changes diagnostic of hyperparathyroid disease may be found radiologically in a significant minority of patients with primary hyperparathyroidism (one report quotes 20–25%, although this probably is higher than average experience). These are found most often in the phalanges, so that x-rays of the hands are often worthwhile. Patients with secondary hyperparathyroidism (chronic renal disease; malabsorption diseases) also may show these abnormalities. Other radiologic bone changes may be present (up to 45% of patients) but are not diagnostic.

Hypoparathyroidism

This is an uncommon condition. It used to occur when the parathyroids were inadvertently removed during thyroidectomy. Chemical hypocalcemia is rather frequent in hospitalized patients but usually not symptomatic. Decrease of serum albumin by 1 gm/100 ml produces decrease in serum calcium of approximately 0.8 mg/100 ml. Uremia is frequently associated with chemical hypocalcemia.

REFERENCES

Arnaud, C. D., et al.: Influence of immunoheterogeneity of circulating parathyroid hormone on results of radioimmunoassays of serum in man, Am. J. Med. 56:785, 1974.
Baker, H. W. G., and Hudson, B.: Male gonadal dysfunction, Clin. Endocrinol. Metab. 3:507, 1974.
Becker, R. L.: Gestational trophoblastic disease, Arch. Intern. Med. 137:221, 1977.
Behrman, S. J.: The complete fertility workup, Hosp. Practice 1:50, 1966.
Berk, H., and Sussman, L.: Spectrophotometric analysis of amniotic fluid during early pregnancy, Obstet. Gynecol. 35:170, 1970.

Brock, D. J. H., et al.: Effect of gestational age on screening for neural-tube defects by maternal plasma—AFP measurement, Lancet 2:195, 1975.

Buckman, M. T., and Peake, G. T.: Prolactin in clinical practice, J.A.M.A. 236:871, 1976.

Buffe, D., et al.: Alpha fetoprotein in amniotic fluid and maternal serum, N. Engl. J. Med. 295:51, 1976.

Cowett, R. M., et al.: Foam-stability test on gastric aspirate and the diagnosis of respiratory distress syndrome, N. Engl. J. Med. 293:413, 1975.

David, N. J., et al.: The diagnostic spectrum of hypercalcemia, Am. J. Med. 33:88, 1962.

Dawood, M. Y., et al.: Progesterone concentrations in the sera of patients with intact and aborted hydatidiform moles, Am. J. Obstet. Gynecol. 129:911, 1974.

Dawood, M. Y., et al.: Serum estradiol-17-B and serum HCG in patients with hydatidiform mole, Am. J. Obstet. Gynecol. 119:904, 1974.

Doe, R. P., and Gold, E. M.: The metyrapone test for pituitary function, Postgrad. Med. 46:157, 1969.

Eddy, R. L., et al.: Human growth hormone release, Am. J. Med. 56:179, 1974.

Edwards, C. R., and Besser, G. M.: Diseases of the hypothalamus and pituitary gland, Clin. Endocrinol. Metab. 3:475, 1974.

Eisenberg, H., et al.: Selective arteriography, venography, and venous hormone assay in diagnosis and localization of parathyroid lesions, Am. J. Med. 56:810, 1974.

Epstein, C. J.: Prenatal diagnosis of genetic disorders, Adv. Intern. Med. 20:325, 1975.

Franchimont, P., et al.: Female gonadal dysfunction, Clin. Endocrinol. Metab. 3:533, 1974.

Friedman, S.: Clinical uses of serum FSH and LH measurements, Obstet. Gynecol. 39:811, 1972.

Gluck, L., et al.: The interpretation and significance of the lecithin/sphingomyelin ratio in amniotic fluid, Am. J. Obstet. Gynecol. 120:142, 1974.

Goldstein, D. P.: Serum placental lactogen activity in patients with molar pregnancy and trophoblastic tumors: A reliable index of malignancy, Am. J. Obstet. Gynecol. 110:583, 1971.

Greenblatt, R. B.: Diagnosis and treatment of hirsutism, Hosp. Practice 8:91, 1973.

Hammond, C. B., and Parker, R. T.: Diagnosis and treatment of trophoblastic disease, Obstet. Gynecol. 35:132, 1970.

Hershman, J. M.: Clinical application of thyrotropin-releasing hormone, N. Engl. J. Med. 290:886, 1974.

Hobson, B. M.: Pregnancy diagnosis, J. Reprod. Fertil. 12:33, 1966.

Hsu, T.-H., et al.: Hyperprolactinemia associated with empty sella syndrome, J.A.M.A. 235:2002, 1976.

Johnson, P. M., and King, D. L.: The placenta: Evaluation by radionuclides and ultrasound, Semin. Nucl. Med. 4:75, 1974.

Jordan, R. M., et al.: Cerebrospinal fluid hormone concentration in the evaluation of pituitary tumor, Ann. Intern. Med. 85:49, 1976.

Jubiz, W., et al.: Single-dose metyrapone test, Arch. Intern. Med. 125:472, 1970.

Kahn, C. B., et al.: Laboratory assessment of diabetic pregnancy: A brief review, Diabetes 21:31, 1972.

Knochel, J. P.: The pathophysiology and clinical characteristics of severe hypophosphatemia, Arch. Intern. Med. 137:203, 1977.

Kolodny, H. D., and Sherman, L.: Laboratory aids in the diagnosis of pituitary tumors, Ann. Clin. Lab. Sci. 4:67, 1974.

Ladenson, J. H., and Bowers, G. N., Jr: Free calcium in serum. II. Rigor of homeostatic control, correlations with total serum calcium, and review of data on patients with disturbed calcium metabolism, Clin. Chem. 19:575, 1973.

Lamb, E.: Immunologic pregnancy tests, Obstet. Gynecol. 39:665, 1972.

Lawrence, A. M.: Glucagon in medicine: New ideas from an old hormone, Med. Clin. North Am. 54:183, 1970.

Lawrence, A. M., et al.: Growth hormone dynamics in acromegaly, J. Clin. Endocrinol. 31:239, 1970.

Lin, T., and Tucci, J. R.: Provocative tests of growth-hormone release: A comparison of results with seven stimuli, Ann. Intern. Med. 80:464, 1974.

Lipsett, M. B., et al.: Physiologic basis of disorders of androgen metabolism. Ann. Intern. Med. 68:1327, 1968.

Macri, J. N., et al.: Prenatal diagnosis of neural tube defects, J.A.M.A. 236:1251, 1976.

Malarkey, W. B.: Recently discovered hypothalamic-pituitary hormones, Clin. Chem. 22:5, 1976.

Malarkey, W. B., and Johnson, J. C.: Pituitary tumors and hyperprolactinemia, Arch. Intern. Med. 136:40, 1976.

Milunsky, A., and Alpert, E.: Antenatal diagnosis, alpha fetoprotein, and the FDA, N. Engl. J. Med. 295:168, 1976.

Milunsky, A., and Kimball, M. E.: Alpha-fetoprotein assays in all amniocentesis samples, Lancet 2:209, 1976.

Mitchell, M. L., et al.: Detection of growth-hormone deficiency: The glucagon stimulation test, N. Engl. J. Med. 282:539, 1970.

Murphy, B. E. P., et al.: Cortisol in amniotic fluid during human gestation, J. Clin. Endocrinol. 40:164, 1975.

Nelson, J. C.: Growth hormone secretion in pituitary disease, Arch. Intern. Med. 133:459, 1974.

O'Leary, J. A., and Bezjian, A. A.: Amniotic fluid fetal maturity score, Obstet. Gynecol. 38:375, 1971.

Ontjes, D. A.: Tests of anterior pituitary function, Metabolism 21:159, 1972.

Pak, C. Y. C., et al.: A simple and reliable test for the diagnosis of hyperparathyroidism, Arch. Intern. Med. 129:48, 1972.

Parfitt, A. M.: Investigation of disorders of the parathyroid glands, Clin. Endocrinol. Metab. 3:451, 1974.

Parks, J. S., et al.: Growth hormone responses to propranolol-glucagon stimulation: A comparison with other tests of growth hormone reserve, J. Clin. Endocrinol. 37:85, 1973.

Porter, B. A., et al.: The levodopa test of growth hormone reserve in children, Am. J. Dis. Child. 126:589, 1973.

Pottgen, P., and Davis, E. R.: Why measure total serum Ca? Clin. Chem. 22:1752, 1976.

Reiss, E.: Hyperparathyroidism: Current Perspectives, in Stollerman, G. H. (ed.): *Advances in Internal Medicine* (Chicago: Year Book Medical Publishers, Inc., 1974), Vol. 19, p. 287.

Rimoin, D. L.: Genetic defects of growth hormone, Hosp. Practice 6:113, 1971.

Rosenthal, A. F., et al.: Comparison of four indexes to fetal pulmonary maturity, Clin. Chem. 20:486, 1974.

Sarkozi, L., et al.: The origin of elevated amniotic fluid CPK levels and experimental verification of the time factor in intrauterine death, Clin. Chem. 19:658, 1973.

Schneider, A. B., and Sherwood, L. M.: Pathogenesis and management of hypoparathyroidism and other hypocalcemia disorders, Metabolism 24:871, 1975.

Scholz, D. A., et al.: Diagnostic considerations in hypercalcemic syndromes, Med. Clin. North Am. 56:941, 1972.

Shephard, B., et al.: Critical analysis of the amniotic fluid shake test, Obstet. Gynecol. 43:558, 1974.

Spellacy, W. N., et al.: Human growth hormone levels in normal subjects receiving an oral contraceptive, J.A.M.A. 202:451, 1967.

Strott, C. A., and Nugent, C. A.: Laboratory tests in the diagnosis of hyperparathyroidism in hypercalcemic patients, Ann. Intern. Med. 68:188, 1968.

Suh, H. K., and Frantz, A. G.: Size heterogeneity of human prolactin in plasma and pituitary extracts, J. Clin. Endocrinol. 39:928, 1974.

Vaitukaitis, J. L., and Ross, G. T.: Recent advances and evaluation of gonadotrophic hormones, Ann. Rev. Med. 24:295, 1973.

Weingold, A. B.: Monitoring the fetal environment, Postgrad. Med. 48:232; 201, 1970.

Woodhouse, N. J. Y.: Hypocalcemia and hypoparathyroidism, Clin. Endocrinol. Metab. 3:323, 1974.

31 / Tests for Syphilis

CLINICAL SYPHILIS usually is subdivided into primary, secondary, latent and tertiary stages. The primary stage begins after an average 3–6 weeks' incubation and is manifested by the development of a primary-stage lesion, or chancre, near the site of infection. The time of appearance is variable; the lesion often is inconspicuous and overlooked, especially in the female. The chancre usually heals and, in classic cases, skin and sometimes mucous membrane lesions develop about 4–6 weeks after appearance of a chancre, marking the secondary stage. After a few days or weeks, the secondary-stage lesions disappear, and the patient enters the latent stage. This lasts, on the average, 3–5 years. During this time, about half the untreated patients apparently become spontaneously cured or, at least, do not develop further evidence of the infection. About 25% remain in a latent ("late latent") status; the remaining 25% develop tertiary-stage sequelae such as neurologic, cardiovascular or ocular syphilis.

Diagnostic procedures in syphilis include dark-field examination, immunologic tests and cerebrospinal fluid examination, depending on the clinical situation.

Dark-Field Examination

Dark-field examination should be performed on all patients with primary and any suitable secondary lesions. Dark-field may be the only way to make an early diagnosis, since immunologic test antibodies often do not appear until late in the primary stage. The technique of obtaining the specimen without contamination by blood or surface bacteria is very important. The lesion should be cleansed thoroughly with water or normal saline and a sterile gauze pad. No soap or antiseptics are used. Care must be taken not to produce bleeding, since RBC will obscure the organisms. After having been blotted dry, the lesion will accumulate a clear serous exudate in a few minutes. If it does not, it may be abraded gently with gauze, but not enough to cause bleeding. The serous fluid exudate is taken off in a pipette or capillary tube for examination with a dark-field microscope. The causative organism, *Treponema pallidum,* has a characteristic morphology and motility under dark field, but experience is necessary for interpretation, since nonpathogenic varieties of spirochetes may be found normally in the genital areas.

Immunologic Tests

Immunologic tests for syphilis depend on the fact that diseases caused by infectious organisms are characterized by development of antibodies toward that organism. These antibodies can be specific or nonspecific

TABLE 31-1.—TYPES OF
IMMUNOLOGIC SYPHILIS TESTS

SPECIFIC	CROSS-REACTING	FORTUITOUS
TPI FTA	RPCF	STS

(Table 31-1), the nonspecific group either of cross-reacting type (sharing a common antigen with another organism) or fortuitous type (provoked by some nonspecific portion of the organism).

The first practical serologic test for syphilis (STS) was a complement-fixation technique invented by Wassermann. He used extract from a syphilitic liver. Subsequently, it was found that the main ingredient of the substance he used actually had nothing to do with syphilitic infection and was present in other tissues besides liver. It is a phospholipid that is now commercially prepared from beef heart and therefore called cardiolipin. The present-day STS reagent is a mixture of purified lipoproteins including cardiolipin, cholesterol and lecithin. Apparently, an antibody called reagin is produced in syphilis that will react with this cardiolipin-lipoprotein complex. Why reagin is produced is not entirely understood; it is not a specific antibody to *T. pallidum*. There is a lipoidal substance in spirochetes, and it is possible that this substance is similar enough to the cardiolipin-lipoprotein complex that antibodies produced against spirochetal lipoidal antigen may also fortuitously react with cardiolipin.

There are two basic types of STS procedures to detect reagin:

COMPLEMENT-FIXATION (CF) REACTION.—This was the procedure used by Wassermann. The original technique has been superseded by the Kolmar modification. There are several defects in this system. The patient's serum may be anticomplementary (contain substances that bind, and thus inactivate, complement). The CF test is a two-stage procedure, and the second stage of the reaction has to incubate overnight. Complement and sheep RBC are among the reagents needed, and these may be of poor quality. Contamination of glassware may give anticomplementary results.

FLOCCULATION REACTION.—In this system, the patient's serum is heated; for unknown reasons, heating seems to enhance the reaction. Then a suspension of cardiolipin antigen particles is added to the serum and mixed. If positive (reactive), the serum reagin antibody present will combine with the antigen, producing a microscopic clumping or flocculation of the antigen particles. The reaction is graded according to degree of clumping. It was found that the preliminary heating step could be eliminated if certain chemicals were added to the antigen, and this modification is called the rapid plasma reagin (RPR) test.

Not all serums from known syphilitics gave positive reactions to these tests. It was discovered that the number of positives could be increased by altering the ratio of antigen ingredients. However, usually when the percentage of positive results increased significantly, more false positives

TABLE 31-2.—STS PROCEDURES

CF TESTS	FLOCCULATION TESTS	
Kolmer (modified Wassermann)	VDRL	
	RPR	Most widely used
	Kahn	
	Hinton	
	Kline	
	Mazzini	

were reported. The various modifications in common use are listed in Table 31-2.

A peculiarity of the STS exists when antibiotic treatment is given. If the patient is treated early in the disease, the STS will revert to negative. However, the longer the disease has been present before treatment, the longer the STS takes to become negative; in many cases, it will never become negative even with adequate treatment (this is called "Wassermann fastness").

BIOLOGIC FALSE POSITIVE REACTION.—Another problem developed when some patients were found to give definitely positive STS but just as definitely did not have syphilis or any exposure to it. These are called biologic false positive reactions (BFP). The main known causes for BFP can be classified under three headings:

1. Acute BFP, due to many viral or bacterial infections and to many febrile reactions such as hypersensitivity or vaccination. These usually give low-grade or moderate (1-2+) STS reactions and return to normal within a few weeks.

2. Chronic BFP, due to chronic systemic illness such as the rheumatoid-collagen disease group, malaria or chronic tuberculosis.

3. Nonsyphilitic treponemal diseases such as yaws or pinta.

To add further to the confusion, some of these patients may have syphilis in addition to one of the diseases known to give BFP reactions. Because of this, everyone hoped for a way to use *T. pallidum* organisms themselves as antigen rather than depend on the nonspecific reagin system.

TPI TEST.—Syphilitic spirochetes can be cultured in rabbits. Eventually, a test was devised by Nelson called the *Treponema pallidum* immobilization, or TPI, test. This basically consists of incubating live syphilitic spirochetes with the patient's serum. If specific antisyphilitic antibody is present, it will attack the spirochetes and immobilize them, causing them to stop moving when viewed under the microscope. This involves an antibody that is different from reagin and that is specific against pathogenic *Treponema* spirochetes. Besides syphilis, other *Treponema* spirochetal diseases such as yaws may thus give positive reactions. The main disadvantages of this test are that it means working with live spirochetes, necessitates an animal colony, is difficult to perform accurately and is expensive. Antibiotics in serum kill the test spirochetes. Routine laboratories cannot do it using present techniques. The TPI behaves toward treatment like the

STS. If the patient is treated early, the TPI will revert to negative; if treated late, it may remain permanently reactive.

RPCF TEST. — The TPI is done using the Nichol strain of pathogenic spirochetes. It has been discovered that a certain nonpathogenic *Treponema* spirochete called the Reiter strain can be cultured more easily and cheaply on artificial media. Antigen prepared from this organism was adapted to a complement-fixation technique, and the result was the Reiter protein complement fixation (RPCF).

The Reiter antibody is different from the *Treponema*-immobilizing antibody of the TPI. Apparently, the nonpathologic Reiter and the pathologic Nichol spirochete share a common protein antigen, and it is this protein that is used in the RPCF. In addition, the Nichol organism has a specific antigen that results in the immobilizing antibody response of the TPI. Several investigators have found the RPCF to be almost as sensitive and specific as the TPI, although others have been definitely less enthusiastic about sensitivity in late syphilis. The Reiter antibody also appears at a different time from the TPI antibody. The main disadvantages of the RPCF are those inherent in all CF tests. The RPCF is practically never used in the United States.

FLUORESCENT TECHNIQUES. — Fluorescent techniques have been a relatively recent addition to laboratory methods. A procedure has been adapted for the detection of syphilis, using the Nichol spirochetes. Instead of living organisms, the spirochetes used are dead. The patient's serum is incubated on a slide with the organisms; afterward a preparation of antibodies produced by animals against human globulins is added. These animal anti-human-globulin antibodies were previously tagged with a fluorescein dye. Since human antibodies against syphilis are gamma globulins, the fluorescein-tagged animal antibodies against human globulin will combine with any antibodies against syphilis present in the patient's serum. If the patient's antibody has combined previously with the spirochetes, the fluorescent antiglobulin material will attach to the patient's antibody on the spirochetes, and the spirochetes will be fluorescent when viewed with an ultraviolet microscope (fluorescent treponemal antibody test; FTA).

Unfortunately, fluorescent work is not as simple as this description or the recent literature would imply. Many technical problems remain. These tests at present are not suitable for mass screening, although they are less time-consuming than the RPCF and easier than the TPI. Many substances will give varying degrees of natural fluorescence, and it is sometimes difficult to decide whether a preparation is actually positive or not. There may be nonspecific antigen-antibody binding of cross-reaction type, as well as specific reaction. When the animal anti-human-globulin antibody is conjugated with fluorescein, not all the fluorescein binds to it, and the free fluorescein remaining may stain various proteins, including the spirochetes, nonspecifically when the tagged mixture is added to the patient's serum.

The FTA underwent modification to become the FTA absorption test (FTA-ABS). Here the nonspecific cross-reacting antibodies are absorbed out of the patient's serum onto Reiter *Treponema* antigen. Antibody to T.

pallidum is not absorbed out by this technique, so the absorbed serum can then be run through the regular FTA procedure.

MHA TEST.—A microhemagglutination (MHA) test is now available, based on formalin-treated red cells sensitized with Nichol strain *T. pallidum* material. Patient serum is preabsorbed with Reiter *Treponema* reagent, as in the FTA-ABS technique. Antibody to *T. pallidum* prevents normal red cell agglutination when the test is performed. About 1–2% of sera contain nonspecific Forssman-type antibodies, so that reactive sera must be retested with nonsensitized control red cells.

Sensitivity and Specificity of Tests

The sensitivity and specificity of these tests should be discussed next. *Sensitivity* may be defined as the ability to detect syphilis, or the percentage of positive (reactive) test results in patients with syphilis. *Specificity* refers to the ability of the test to be reactive only in syphilis, or the percentage of positive results in persons who do not have syphilis ("false positive" reactions). Studies have been done in which duplicate samples from known syphilitic patients in various stages of their disease and also from normal persons were sent to various laboratories. Besides this, many reports have appeared from laboratories all over the world comparing one test with another in various clinical stages of syphilis, in nonsyphilitic diseases and in apparently normal persons. These are summarized in Table 31–3.

Note the considerable variation in results. Several factors must be involved besides the inherent sensitivity and specificity of the individual tests themselves.

1. Antibiotic treatment may cause some previously reactive syphilitic patients to become nonreactive.

2. Some persons may have unsuspected subclinical syphilis.

3. True BFP reactions, either acute or chronic, must be taken into account.

4. Most important, there is obvious variation in laboratory technique and ability. Some laboratories introduce their own modifications into standard techniques.

The time of appearance differs for the various antibodies. In general, the FTA-ABS test becomes positive in significant numbers of patients in the middle or end of the primary stage, followed by the MHA and RPCF, then the STS and finally the TPI. All these procedures usually give positive results in the secondary stage, and also probably in the early latent stage.

In tertiary (late) syphilis, there is a well-documented tendency for the STS to revert spontaneously to negative, even if the patient is untreated. This is reported to occur in a substantial minority of patients. The RPCF may do likewise, but only in a smaller minority of patients. The TPI in untreated tertiary syphilis is said to be usually positive (assuming good technique, etc.), but false negatives do occur—at least 5% and more likely 10%. The FTA-ABS and MHA are reported to be even more sensitive than the TPI in tertiary syphilis, although occasional false negatives may occur even with the FTA-ABS and MHA.

At this point it might be useful to summarize those tests for syphilis that have been described.

TABLE 31–3.—COMPARISON OF SEROLOGIC
TESTS FOR SYPHILIS
(APPROXIMATE PERCENTAGE REPORTED REACTIVE)

	STS	TPI	MHA	FTA-ABS
Primary	50–70 (48–96)°	35–65 (26–68)	75–85 (50–95)	85–86 (80–91)
Secondary	98–100	80–95 (67–99)	99 (96–100)	99–100
Latent	75–100	90–95 (84–100)	–	95–96
Tertiary	60–75 (55–95)	90–91 (78–100)	96 (90–99)	97 (95–100)
Congenital	70 (66–95)	82–93	–	99–100
Normal	1.0 (0.5–10.0)	2.0 (0.0–3.0)	0.9 (0.0–3.0)	0.8 (0.0–1.0)
Nonsyphilitic disease†	5.0 (5–45)	6.0 (2.8–8.0)	–	1.5 (0.6–14)‡
Biologic false positive diseases§	20–45	2.5	1.5 (0–11)	1.5 (0–16)‡

°Numbers in parentheses indicate range from the literature.
†Miscellaneous nonspirochetal diseases; patients had no history or clinical evidence of syphilis.
‡FTA-ABS reactive, TPI nonreactive (see text, p. 390).
§Nonspirochetal diseases known to produce a high incidence of BFP reactions in the STS.

STS.—The STS is cheap, easy to do and suitable for mass testing. Its sensitivity and specificity are adequate, and positivity develops reasonably early in the disease. Reagents are well standardized and reproducibility is good. Disadvantages are the problem of BPF reactions, relatively poor sensitivity in primary syphilis and the tendency in late syphilis for spontaneous reversion to negative.

TPI.—The TPI has been replaced by the FTA-ABS. At present, it is extremely difficult to find a laboratory that does the test.

FTA.—At present, the FTA-ABS seems well established. It has relatively good sensitivity in primary syphilis (except in very early disease) and has even better sensitivity in late syphilis than the TPI. It is said to be at least as specific as the TPI, possibly even more so. Nevertheless, there are some difficulties; for example, weak reactions are still a problem. Official recommendations are that equivocal or 1+ reactive specimens should be repeated, and the 1+ reclassified as "borderline" if the repeat test is nonreactive. However, if the serum that was 1+ reactive remains 1+ reactive when the test is repeated, it is considered to be "reactive" as though it had measured more than 1+. Therefore, a physician who receives a report that the FTA-ABS was "reactive" cannot tell whether the degree of reactivity was weak

(1+) or strong. This may be important, because there is some evidence that results on weakly reactive specimens sent to different laboratories may vary between nonreactive and reactive in a significant number of instances. In addition, several reports list a disturbingly high incidence of positive FTA-ABS reactions in patients who were STS positive but TPI negative. Some of these were eventually diagnosed as having syphilis; most of the remainder had 1+ reactions. Therefore, there are some data to suggest that 1+ reactions in the FTA-ABS may not be as reliable as those of stronger degree, and the physician has no way of knowing from the report which reactions are weak.

No laboratory test is free from the possibility of error, and the FTA-ABS is no exception. Surveys report up to 5–10% variation among laboratories. Occasional false positive FTA-ABS results have been reported in persons with hyperglobulinemia due to macroglobulins and in patients with antinuclear antibodies. In addition, atypical fluorescent patterns ("beaded") that could be misinterpreted as reactive have occurred in some patients with systemic lupus.

MHA.—The MHA is not as sensitive in primary syphilis as the FTA-ABS, although reactive in more than 50% of patients. It seems equally sensitive in secondary and possibly in late syphilis. Compared to FTA-ABS results, various studies have shown 90–98% overall correlation. Our laboratory has performed a comparison of this type, and found that nearly 85% of the disagreements represented either nonreactive MHA and 1+ reactive FTA-ABS, or 1+ reactive MHA and nonreactive FTA-ABS. Therefore, most disagreements seem to occur at low reactivity levels in which the accuracy of either test is open to some question. This being the case, there is reason to conclude that the MHA could be substituted for the FTA-ABS, except possibly in primary syphilis (in which case an FTA-ABS could be obtained if the MHA were nonreactive). The MHA is much easier to perform than the FTA-ABS and is less expensive.

Selection of Tests

The best selection of tests for syphilis depends on the clinical situation.

1. If the patient has possible primary syphilis, a dark-field examination should be performed. If this is negative or if a dark-field cannot be obtained, an FTA-ABS should be done. If the FTA-ABS is nonreactive, and if clinical suspicion is strong, the physician for practical purposes has the option of treating the patient without a conclusive diagnosis or of repeating the FTA-ABS in 2–3 weeks.

2. If the patient has confirmed early syphilis, an STS should nevertheless be obtained. If the STS is reactive, the degree of reactivity should be titered, since a falling titer after treatment provides evidence that treatment was effective.

3. If the patient has possible, equivocal or late syphilis, an FTA-ABS (or MHA) and STS should be done. If the FTA-ABS (or MHA) is reactive (2+ or more), the diagnosis is probable syphilis. If the FTA-ABS (or MHA) is weakly reactive (borderline or 1+ reactive), the test should be repeated in 1 month. If still weakly reactive, the diagnosis would be possible or probable syphilis, depending on the clinical picture. The STS results are useful mainly as additional evidence in equivocal cases.

4. If a routine screening STS is found to be positive in a person with no history or clinical evidence of syphilis, a confirmatory test should be done. *If the confirmatory test is negative,* the patient should be screened for diseases known to cause a high incidence of BFP reactions. In this respect, a weakly positive STS may be due only to an acute BFP etiology, and the STS should be negative in 2–3 months. *If the confirmatory test is positive,* past or present syphilis is a strong probability. Nevertheless, since false positive (and also false negative) reactions may occur occasionally even in the "confirmatory" tests, in certain patients it may be necessary to repeat the confirmatory test.

CONGENITAL AND CENTRAL NERVOUS SYSTEM SYPHILIS

CONGENITAL SYPHILIS. — This often gives a confusing serologic picture. Syphilitic infants usually have a positive STS. Sometimes, however, these infants have negative serologies at birth, and these may remain negative up to 3 months before the titer begins rising. On the other hand, if the mother has a positive STS, even though she was adequately treated, many infants will have a positive STS due to passive transfer of maternal antibodies through the placenta. The same is true for the TPI or FTA. If the mother has been adequately treated, the infant's positive serology will decline to negative by approximately 3–4 months and no treatment is necessary. The TPI may be positive for as long as 7 months. A modification of the FTA-ABS that is specific for IgM antibodies is reported to detect most cases of congenital syphilis in the newborn. Some investigators have experienced difficulty due to antibody transfer from the mother, although theoretically IgM should not cross the placenta.

CENTRAL NERVOUS SYSTEM *(CNS).* — This may also require serologic tests for diagnosis. The standard serologic tests for syphilis such as the Venereal Disease Research Laboratories (VDRL) usually, but not always, give positive results in the blood when they are positive in the cerebrospinal fluid (CSF). A lack of relationship is most often found in the tertiary stage, when the blood VDRL sometimes reverts to normal. Conversely, the CSF is very often negative when the peripheral blood VDRL is positive; since CNS syphilis usually is a tertiary form developing symptoms only after years of infection, in many patients with syphilis the CNS is not clinically involved at all. Despite lack of clinical CNS symptoms, actual CNS involvement is apparently fairly common and often begins as early as the secondary stage, although the clinical symptoms, if they develop, do not show up until the tertiary stage years later. The best criteria of disease activity are elevated cell count and CSF protein. The serology indicates disease that has been present for a certain length of time, without necessarily being currently active. The CSF serology (STS) usually is negative in those patients with so-called biologic false positive blood STS reactions.

The three most important forms of CNS lues are general paresis, tabes dorsalis and vascular neurosyphilis. In general paresis, the CSF serology almost always is positive in untreated patients. In tabes dorsalis, the CSF serology is said to be usually positive in early untreated disease, but up to 50% of late or so-called "burnt-out cases" may be negative. In vascular neurosyphilis, approximately 50% are positive. Sometimes the blood or CSF may have a negative STS but a positive FTA-ABS, since once the FTA-ABS is positive it usually remains reactive indefinitely unless the disease is treated early. If the CSF has a reactive FTA-ABS, the blood FTA-ABS is almost always reactive. The FTA-ABS is usually not done on CSF, since there is no problem of BFP reactions in the spinal fluid STS, and the blood FTA-ABS is reactive in most cases of CNS syphilis. The FTA-ABS has been shown to be more frequently reactive in the CSF of patients with syphilis than the VDRL. However, at present there does not seem to be a widespread feeling that this necessarily represents active CNS syphilis. Thus, the clinical importance of a reactive spinal fluid FTA-ABS is uncertain when the cell count, protein and spinal fluid VDRL are normal.

REFERENCES

Atwood, W. G., et al.: The TPI and FTA-ABS tests in treated late syphilis, J.A.M.A. 203:549, 1968.

Berner, J. E., et al.: Evaluation of the Reiter protein complement-fixation (RPCF) test for syphilis, Cleve. Clin. Q. 27:162, 1960.

Bradford, L. L., et al.: Fluorescent treponemal absorption and Treponema pallidum immobilization tests in syphilitic patients and biologic false positive reactors. Am. J. Clin. Pathol. 47:525, 1967.

Burns, R. E.: Spontaneous reversion of FTA-ABS test reactions, J.A.M.A. 234:617, 1975.

Carr, R. D., et al.: The biological false positive phenomenon in elderly men, Arch. Dermatol. 93:393, 1966.

Duncan, W. P., et al.: Fluorescent treponemal antibody-cerebrospinal fluid (FTA-CSF) test: A provisional technique, Br. J. Vener. Dis. 48:97, 1972.

Eng, J., and Wereide, K.: The TPI test in untreated syphilis, Br. J. Vener. Dis. 38: 223, 1962.

Goldman, J. N., and Lantz, M. A.: FTA-ABS and VDRL slide test reactivity in a population of nuns, J.A.M.A. 217:53, 1971.

Harner, R. E., et al.: The FTA-ABS test in late syphilis, J.A.M.A. 203:545, 1968.

Jaffe, H. W.: The laboratory diagnosis of syphilis: New concepts, Ann. Intern. Med. 83:846, 1975.

Kampmeier, R. H.: The late manifestations of syphilis: Skeletal, visceral, and cardiovascular, Med. Clin. North Am. 48:667, 1964.

Kolmer, J. A.: Clinical Diagnosis by Laboratory Examinations (3d ed.; New York: Appleton-Century-Crofts, Inc., 1961), p. 434.

McKenna, C. H., et al.: The fluorescent treponemal antibody absorbed (FTA-ABS) test beading phenomenon in connective tissue diseases, Mayo Clin. Proc. 48:545, 1973.

Mackey, D. M., et al.: Specificity of the FTA-ABS test for syphilis, J.A.M.A. 207: 1683, 1969.

Miller, J. N.: Value and limitations of nontreponemal and treponemal tests in the laboratory diagnosis of syphilis, Clin. Obstet. Gynecol. 18:191, 1975.

Monson, R. A. M.: Biologic false-positive FTA-ABS test in drug-induced lupus erythematosus, J.A.M.A. 224:1028, 1973.

Moore, M. B., and Knox, J. M.: Sensitivity and specificity in syphilis serology: Clinical implications, South. Med. J. 58:963, 1965.

Nicholas, L., and Beerman, H.: Present day serodiagnosis of syphilis: Review of some of the literature, Am. J. Med. Sci. 249:466, 1965.

Ravel, R.: Hemagglutination test for syphilis (MHA) as alternative to the FTA-ABS, Lab. Med. 7:22, 1976.

Shore, R. N., and Faricelli, J. A.: Borderline and reactive FTA-ABS results in lupus erythematosus, Arch. Dermatol. 113:37, 1977.

Sparling, P. F.: Diagnosis and treatment of syphilis, N. Engl. J. Med. 284:642, 1971.

Syphilis and Other Venereal Diseases (Symposium), Med. Clin. North Am., vol. 48 no. 3, May, 1964.

UNFORTUNATELY, there is no laboratory test to detect all cancer. There are, however, certain circumstances in which the laboratory may be of assistance.

Kidney

Renal carcinoma often causes microscopic hematuria, as does bladder carcinoma; this may be the only clue to the diagnosis. In addition, hypernephroma, on occasion, is a well-recognized cause of fever of unknown origin. The reported incidence of fever in renal cell carcinoma varies from 11 to 33%. It has rarely but repeatedly been associated with secondary polycythemia (about 3% of patients), although a large minority have anemia and the majority do not show hemoglobin abnormality.

In renal cell carcinoma (hypernephroma), symptoms and urinary findings vary according to the location, size and aggressiveness of the tumor. Hematuria is the most frequent finding, either gross or microscopic, being detected at some time in 75–80% of patients. Flank pain is much less commonly present, and a palpable abdominal mass usually suggests relatively large size. Proteinuria may sometimes be found. The intravenous pyelogram is the most useful screening test for renal cell carcinoma, and, if carefully done, will also detect many cases of carcinoma in the renal pelvis and ureters. Other procedures, such as kidney scanning or computerized axial tomography (CAT) are also useful.

Once a space-occupying lesion is identified in the kidney, the question arises as to its nature. B-mode ultrasound, CAT and drip infusion tomography seem to be excellent methods of distinguishing a solid renal tumor from a renal cyst. Selective renal angiography is equally effective, and could be performed if tomography were inconclusive. No technique is infallible, however, since, uncommonly, a tumor may become exceptionally cystic due to internal necrosis. Urine cytology has relatively little value at present in the diagnosis of renal cell carcinoma. Metastatic carcinoma or malignant lymphoma in the kidney usually does not produce significant clinical or urinary findings.

Prostate

Prostatic carcinoma often may be detected chemically because normal prostatic tissue is rich in the enzyme acid phosphatase, and adenocarcinomas arising from this area often retain the ability to produce this enzyme. Generally speaking, the presence of elevated serum acid phosphatase means that a prostatic carcinoma has metastasized. However, 10–15% of patients give elevated values without demonstrable metastasis. About 25% of patients with metastases but no skeletal invasion show abnormal values, and between 50 and 80% with bone involvement. Most prostatic skeletal metastases are osteoblastic in nature, and therefore alkaline phosphatase shows elevation in 70–90% of patients with bone metastases, depending on extent of involvement. One difficulty results from the fact that various widely used chemical methods vary in their specificity for prostatic acid phosphatase. Platelets are rich in nonprostatic acid phosphatase, and certain conditions might conceivably result in elevated serum levels if a relatively nonspecific method is used. Fortunately, in situations where prostatic acid phosphatase is needed, the likelihood of coexistent sources of nonprostatic acid phosphatase is small. Since L-tartrate will inhibit prostatic phosphatases, when there is doubt about the origin of elevated acid phosphatase, the test may be repeated with tartrate inhibition. After tartrate, elevated values suggest nonprostatic origin. There is dispute concerning the accuracy of this technique. Elevated values of prostatic phosphatase may be produced by prostatic infarcts as well as carcinoma. Acid phosphatase from bone marrow aspirate may be more sensitive and specific for bone metastasis than serum assay.

Another difficulty that sometimes arises comes from the fact that acid and alkaline phosphatase are very similar enzymes, differing mainly in their optimum pH. Therefore, when alkaline phosphatase is very high for any reason, some of the enzymes may react at a lower pH than usual, giving so-called spillage into the acid phosphatase range.

Prostatic acid phosphatase is heat and pH sensitive. Serum left at room temperature after exposure to air may exhibit significantly decreased activity after as little time lapse as 1 hour.

Certain acid phosphatase procedures have recently been marketed with claims of specificity for prostatic phosphatase. Unfortunately, these may also produce false high values when alkaline phosphatase is markedly elevated.

Gastrointestinal Tract

Tumors of the lower GI tract were discussed in Chapter 26. Screening tests include rectal examination and examination of the stool for occult blood. Tumor anywhere in the GI tract, benign or malignant, frequently results in blood found in the stool, sometimes gross, although much more often occult. The most frequent malignancies are from colon and rectum, stomach and the head of the pancreas. Many people advocate sigmoidoscopy as a routine screening test for rectal and sigmoid colon carcinoma in all people over age 40.

In carcinoma of the stomach, under the best conditions, x-ray examination is said to be about 90% accurate. Unfortunately, this still leaves open the question as to the nature of the lesion demonstrated. Gastroscopy is currently the best procedure for diagnosis, since instruments are available that allow visualization of most areas in the stomach and also permit biopsy. If gastroscopy is not available, gastric analysis for acid (after stimulation) may be helpful; achlorhydria would considerably increase suspicion of carcinoma. Cytology of gastric washings is useful. However, gastric cytology is not as successful as results from specimens of uterine or even of pulmonary neoplasia, since small gastric tumors may not shed many neoplastic cells, and interpretation of gastric Papanicolaou ("Pap") smears in general is more difficult. Gastric aspiration specimens for cytology should be placed in ice immediately to preserve the cells.

CARCINOIDS.—These are relatively uncommon tumors found mainly in the GI tract, although a minority are located in the lungs. The appendix is the most frequent site of origin; these are almost always benign. Carcinoids are next most frequent in the terminal ileum or rectum. Tumor in these locations frequently is malignant. When metastases are extensive, a characteristic syndrome is often produced. This is due to the production of the vasoconstrictor serotonin by liver metastases. The diagnosis can be made by testing for abnormal levels of the chief metabolic breakdown product of serotonin, 5-hydroxyindoleacetic acid (5-HIAA), in the urine. Although levels are usually elevated, sometimes they fluctuate, and repeat determinations may be needed if a normal result is obtained in the presence of characteristic symptoms. Surprisingly, malignant rectal carcinoids rarely produce this syndrome. Certain foods may elevate urinary 5-HIAA (p. 471).

Breast

Until 1960 diagnosis of mammary carcinoma depended on discovery of a breast mass by physical examination, followed by a biopsy of the lesion. It has been said that, with experience, carcinoma as small as 1 cm may be regularly detected by palpation. More recently, x-ray study of the breast (mammography) has begun to receive considerable attention. Several favorable reports have been published, and several mass screening surveys have been attempted. To date, available information on the status of mammography includes the following:

1. Breast carcinoma can be seen by mammography in some cases in which it is not palpable.

2. Screening surveys utilizing mammography are reporting detection of 2–3 times the normally expected rate of breast carcinoma.

3. Proper technique is of the utmost importance; this calls for special training and conscientious technicians.

4. Mammography is definitely not infallible. The average good radiologist will probably miss a malignant diagnosis in about 20% of cases, and call a benign lesion malignant in about 10%. *Biopsy is still essential for all breast lesions.*

5. Mammography is best in the postmenopausal or large breast where fatty tissue predominates. In these circumstances, probably 80–90% of malignant tumors can be diagnosed correctly, whereas the figure decreases to 55% for women under age 45.

6. Mammography is useful to indicate the site for biopsy when several breast masses are present, and has shown that the incidence of a carcinoma in the opposite breast from previous malignancy is 6–8% (incidence in pathology studies ranges 1–12%), while the prospect of simultaneous bilateral breast carcinoma is 2–3% (incidence in pathology studies ranges from 10–47% for lobular carcinoma in situ to 0.5–16% for infiltrating carcinomas. The majority of references indicate 1–2% for infiltrating carcinoma).

7. At present, mammography is not an ideal screening procedure, be-

cause only a rather limited number of satisfactory studies can be performed daily under present conditions in the average radiologic office.

When the diagnosis of breast cancer is first made or suspected, the question may arise as to which tests provide useful information that might influence type or extent of treatment. Bone scan detects lesions in 10–40% of patients on initial workup. The small amount of information available on results of initial-visit brain scanning suggests that fewer than 5% will be abnormal if there are no neurologic signs or symptoms. Surprisingly little data are available on the contribution of liver scan to initial (pretherapy) workup, but one study found that liver scan yielded only 1% true positive results.

Another possible aid in selection of therapy is estrogen receptor assay. It has been shown that approximately 30–40% of postmenopausal breast cancer patients respond to ovariectomy, adrenalectomy, hypophysectomy or estrogen therapy. Premenopausal patients respond less frequently. Certain tissues, such as premenopausal endometrium, have been shown to possess estrogen receptors within their cells. Normal breast tissue has low estrogen receptor activity. Estrogen receptor assay techniques involve tissue slices or cytoplasm (cytosol) extracts from the tumor to be evaluated. Radioactive estradiol and another estrogen-binding substance are added, and the tumor estrogen receptors compete with the estrogen binder for the labeled estradiol. The amount of labeled estradiol bound by the tumor estrogen receptors can then be determined. According to information available to date, about 50–60% of postmenopausal breast carcinoma patients have tumors that bind sufficient estrogen per unit of tissue to be considered estrogen receptive or "positive." About 60–70% of women whose tumors exhibit a positive estrogen receptor response are reported to respond to endocrine therapy (either estrogen or endocrine ablation); only 5–10% of those with negative estrogen receptor assay test seem to respond. There are several techniques for preparing tissue for the receptor assay, and some of the techniques differ significantly in the number of patient tumors that demonstrate apparently increased receptors. At present, it is necessary to secure at least 1 gm of tumor after eliminating all fat and normal breast tissue. The tumor must be fresh and must be frozen by dry ice within a short time (preferably within 15 minutes) after excision.

As the description of the test indicates, with present-day techniques the procedure is partially a bioassay, and therefore would be available only in larger institutions or reference laboratories.

Uterus

The mainstay of screening for uterine carcinoma is the Papanicolaou ("Pap") smear. For Pap examination of the cervix, material is best obtained directly from the cervix by some type of scraping technique. Reports indicate that obtaining two successive specimens at the same examination instead of one increases diagnostic yield significantly (as much as 86%). A single smear has a false negative rate of approximately 10–20%. Vaginal irrigation smears are reported to be 50–75% as accurate as the cervical scrape for detection of cervical carcinoma. For endometrial carcinoma screening, endometrial aspiration currently provides optimum results (average accuracy 90%; literature range 78–100%); next best is sampling of vaginal secretions in the posterior fornix, and least effective are routine cervical or vaginal smears or scrape slides (about 50% accurate; literature range 14–76%). Aspiration can be done by cannula suction or with an instrument called the Gravlee jet washer; averaging of results from evaluations to date indicate that accuracy is approximately the same.

Suspicious or definitely positive Pap smears should be followed up with a biopsy of the site indicated to confirm the diagnosis and determine the extent and character of the neoplasm. For the cervix, a conization procedure, or at least a 4-quadrant biopsy, is the method of choice. For the endometrium, dilatation and curettage (D & C) should be done.

Lung

Chest x-ray has been the usual means of detecting lung cancer. Unfortunately, best results are obtained from the less common peripheral lesions rather than the more usual bronchogenic carcinomas arising from major bronchi. In general, chest x-rays are not an efficient means of early diagnosis, and this is especially true for the miniature films used in mass survey-type work. If a patient over age 40 has symptoms such as chronic cough, hemoptysis or recurrent pneumonia, sputum samples should be collected for cytology. These should be obtained once daily (before breakfast and after rinsing the mouth with water) for 3 days. The material should be from a "deep cough"; saliva is not adequate. If adequate sputum cannot be obtained, aerosol induction may be helpful. If the specimen cannot be taken to the lab immediately, it should be collected in a fixative such as 70% alcohol. Twenty-four-hour collections are not advised, due to cell disintegration. A good specimen is the key to success in pulmonary cytology, because interpretation is more difficult than with uterine material.

When the diagnosis of lung cancer is first made, the question frequently arises as to which tests might help delineate extent of disease and thus establish operability. Bone scan is reported to detect lesions in approximately 35–45% of patients, the frequency correlating roughly with clinical stage of the disease. Brain scan data available suggest that fewer than 5% will be abnormal if there are no neurologic signs or symptoms. There is surprisingly little data on initial-workup liver scan, but one small study suggests less than 5% of patients have detectable lesions.

Pancreas

Zollinger-Ellison syndrome is caused by a gastrin-producing non-beta islet cell ("delta cell") tumor of the pancreas (gastrinoma). There frequently is more than one tumor. About 60% are malignant. Occasionally the tumor may occur in the wall of the duodenum, and rarely in the stomach. The three major components of the syndrome are intractable peptic ulcer, severe chronic diarrhea (30% of patients [literature range: 16–75%], with potassium loss especially prominent) and multiple peptic ulcers (12%) or ulcer in unusual locations (usually the jejunum; jejunal ulcer comprises 25% of cases). Steatorrhea may be present. About 20–25% (literature range 10–48%) are associated with abnormality in other endocrine organs, most commonly parathyroid adenoma. About 50% have a single duodenal ulcer. Diagnosis is based on demonstration of elevated serum gastrin and basal gastric hypersecretion and hyperacidity; some consider these an integral part of the syndrome. Basal (1-hour) acid secretion greater than 10 mEq HC1/hour and a ratio of basal acid secretion to maximal acid output (MAO) of 0.4 or greater should have serum gastrin assay; 15 mEq HCl/hour and a basal acid secretion to MAO ratio of 0.6 or greater is very suspicious (although not pathognomonic, p. 304). Serum gastrin assay is the method of choice for diagnosis. The majority of gastrinomas produce basal gastrin levels over 10 times the normal upper limit. Some feel that gastric analysis can therefore be eliminated. However, occasional gastrinoma patients have basal gastrin levels that are only mildly or moderately elevated. Somewhat increased basal serum gastrin can be found in conditions associated with achlorhydria, such as atrophic gastritis and pernicious anemia (if the antrum is not severely affected); after vagotomy; in patients with retained antrum following gastrojejunostomy, and in uremia. In addition, some patients with peptic ulcer have mild or moderate serum gastrin elevation and overlap with those occasional gastrinoma patients who have values that are not markedly elevated. Since overlap may occur, stimulation tests have been devised to assist differentiation. The standard procedure is calcium infusion. Patients with gastrinomas more than double baseline values, while ulcer patients fail to do so. Patients with pernicious anemia, however, frequently respond to calcium. Secretin is another stimulating agent for gastrinomas, whereas it is reported that achlorhydric patients do not respond.

Liver

Tumor in the liver is most often metastatic. The liver is more frequently subject to mestastases than any other organ; 25–50% of all (metastasizing) cancers reach the liver. The GI tract (including the pancreas), breast, kidney, lung, melanomas and sarcomas are especially apt to produce hepatic metastases.

Tests for detection include alkaline phosphatase, liver scan and liver biopsy (Chapter 19). Primary liver cell carcinoma (hepatoma) is more common in cirrhosis. On liver scan, it typically appears as a large, dominant, space-occupying lesion. The fetoprotein test (p. 215) is often positive. Liver biopsy is essential to verify a diagnosis of cancer in the liver, since nonneoplastic diseases may produce abnormalities identical to those of neoplasia in any of the tests.

Sympathetic Nervous System

Neuroblastoma is one of the most frequent tumors of childhood, during which it comprises the most frequent abdominal neoplasm except for Wilms' tumor of infancy. It usually presents as an abdominal mass, and frequently the only method of diagnosis is abdominal exploration with biopsy. Treatment by combined radiation and chemotherapy is beginning to produce worthwhile results, so that diagnosis has become of more than academic interest. Urine vanilmandelic acid (VMA) has been found elevated in over 90% of patients, although some elevations were not present initially. Homovanillic acid (HVA), a metabolic product of the catecholamine precursor dopamine, is reported to be abnormal in about 80% of patients. Combined VMA and HVA positive results include nearly 100% of patients. Bone marrow aspiration has been reported positive in up to 50% of patients. Therefore, bone marrow aspiration should be done in all patients, since the finding of marrow metastases rules out surgery alone as a curative procedure.

Pheochromocytoma has been discussed in Chapter 29.

Testes

Alpha fetoprotein (AFP) and beta-subunit chorionic gonadotropin (hCG) by radioimmunoassay (RIA) methods are elevated in certain gonadal tumors. In general, "pure" seminomas fail to produce AFP; hCG production in seminoma ranges from 0 to 37%. In embryonal cell carcinoma and malignant teratoma, 70% or more of patients display elevated AFP and 40–60% or more have elevated hCG; 85% or more produce either one or both. Elevation of AFP by RIA occurs in hepatoma (75–85%, p. 215) and has also been reported in significant numbers of patients with gastric and pancreatic carcinoma and occasional patients with lung carcinoma or other tumors, mostly in low titer. Elevated hCG is found in choriocarcinoma or hydatidiform mole (p. 373); and has also been reported in various other neoplasms, notably gastric, hepatic, pancreatic and breast carcinoma; melanoma and myeloma (again, usually in low titer).

Thyroid

Thyroid carcinoma seems to have generated a considerable number of misconceptions. About 20% of these tumors are "pure" papillary, about 10% "pure" follicular, about 50% mixed papillary and follicular and about 10% are called medullary. However, the "pure" papillary carcinoma usually has a few follicular elements if enough histologic sections are made, and the reverse is sometimes true in follicular tumors. In addition, some pathologists classify the tumors according to the predominant element unless the proportion of each is very close to the other. If this were done, about 65% would be called papillary and about 20% would be considered follicular. There is enough diversity in classification methods to create difficulty in relating pathology reports to statistics in the literature. Papillary and the majority of mixed papillary-follicular carcinomas metastasize primarily to regional lymph nodes. Prognosis is excellent in young adults but less so in older persons. Follicular carcinoma tends to produce hematogenous metastases, most often to lungs and bone.

The major screening test is the thyroid scan. The characteristic appearance of thyroid carcinoma is a single nonfunctioning nodule. A gland that is multinodular on scan has less chance of containing carcinoma than one with a solitary nodule. A nodule that demonstrates some degree of function has only a relatively small likelihood of being carcinoma, and a hyperfunctioning nodule is almost always benign. On occasion, a palpable nodule may represent metastatic carcinoma from another primary site in a lymph node close to the thyroid.

A significant number of patients are referred for thyroid scan while thyroid uptake of radionuclide is being suppressed by administration of thyroid hormone or by x-ray contrast media (p. 336). This frequently produces unsatisfactory or even misleading results. When thyroid cancer is discovered, either before or after initial therapy, patients may be referred for scanning to detect metastases. Unless all of the normal thyroid tissue is removed or is ablated by radioiodine therapy, enough of the scanning dose will be taken up by normal tissue to make such attempts useless in most cases. In addition, replacement thyroid hormone administration must cease for 2–4 weeks prior to scan. The dose of radioactive iodine for a metastatic tumor scan is 10 times the usual scan dose, and the optimum time to scan is 72 hours after dose administration.

Thermography and B-mode ultrasound have been used to help evaluate thyroid nodules for malignancy. Results of thermography to date have been rather disappointing. About 15–20% of thyroid nodules are cystic, and ultrasonography attempts to show whether a nodule is solid or cystic, since data suggest that thyroid nodules that are pure cysts are rarely malignant. Accuracy in several reports seems to be 80–95%, with ultrasonic impression that a nodule was solid being more reliable than evidence of a cyst.

MEDULLARY CARCINOMA OF THE THYROID. — This comprises 3–10% of thyroid carcinomas. It is derived from certain stromal cells known as "C" cells. The tumor has an intermediate degree of malignancy. It may occur sporadically or in a hereditary form. The familial variety is transmitted as an autosomal dominant, is usually present in both thyroid lobes and is frequently associated with other neoplasms (pheochromocytoma, mucosal neuromas) as part of the Sipple syndrome (multiple endocrine adenosis, type II). This also includes some degree of association with other endocrine abnormalities, such as parathyroid adenoma and Cushing's syndrome. The tumor may present in a variety of histologic patterns, but the classic form is solid nests of cells that are separated by a stroma containing amyloid. These tumors have aroused great interest, since most secrete abnormal amounts of the hormone calcitonin (thyrocalcitonin). Calcitonin has calcium-lowering action derived from inhibition of bone resorption; therefore, calcitonin acts as an antagonist to parathyroid hormone. Thyroid "C" cells produce calcitonin as a normal reaction to the stimulus of hypercalcemia. About 70–75% of medullary carcinomas produce elevated levels of serum calcitonin. In those that do not, elevated calcitonin can be induced by stimulation with calcium infusion or pentagastrin. Glucagon will also stimulate secretion, but not as effectively. A few medullary carcinomas are reported to secrete serotonin or prostaglandins. About 30% of patients experience diarrhea. Besides medullary thyroid carcinoma, calcitonin secretion has been reported in as many as 60% of bronchogenic carcinoma patients (oat cell and adenocarcinoma).

Metastatic Carcinoma to Bone

Any carcinoma, lymphoma or sarcoma may metastasize to bone, although those primary in certain organs do so much more frequently than others. Breast, prostate, lung, kidney and thyroid are the most common carcinomas. Once in bone they may cause local destruction that is manifested on x-ray by osteolytic lesions. In some cases there is osseous reaction with the formation of new bone or osteoid, and this appears on x-ray films as osteoblastic lesions. Prostate carcinoma is usually osteoblastic; breast and lung are more commonly osteolytic, but a significant number are osteoblastic. The others usually have an osteolytic appearance.

About half the carcinomas metastatic to bone replace or at least injure bone marrow to such an extent as to give hematologic symptoms. The degree of actual replacement often is relatively small in relation to the total amount of bone marrow, so that some sort of toxic influence of the cancer on the blood-forming elements has been postulated. Whatever the mechanism, about half the patients with metastatic carcinoma to bone have anemia when first seen (that is, a hemoglobin at least 2 gm/100 ml less than the lower limit of normal). When the hemoglobin is less than 8 gm/100 ml, nucleated red cells and immature white cells may appear in the peripheral blood, and thrombocytopenia may be present. By this time there is often extensive marrow replacement.

Because of bone destruction and local attempts at repair, the serum alkaline phosphatase is often elevated. Roughly one third of patients with metastatic carcinomas to bone from lung, kidney or thyroid have elevated alkaline phosphatase on first examination; for breast carcinoma this may be true in up to 50% of patients while for the prostate reports vary from 70 to 90%.

If an x-ray skeletal survey is taken, bone lesions will be seen in approximately 50% of patients with actual bone metastases. More are not detected on first examination because lesions must be over 1.5 cm to show on x-ray films, because parts of the bone are obscured by overlying structures and because the tumor spread may be concealed by new bone formation. Almost any bone may be affected, but the vertebral column is by far the most frequent.

Bone scanning for metastases is now available in most institutions, using radioactive isotopes of elements that take part in bone metabolism (see Chapter 22). Bone scanning will detect 10–40% more foci of metastatic carcinoma than will x-ray (p. 270) and is the method of choice in screening for bone metastases. Bone scan is considerably more sensitive than bone marrow examination in patients with metastatic carcinoma. However, tumors that seed in a more diffuse fashion, such as oat cell carcinoma of lung, neuroblastoma and possibly also malignant lymphoma, are exceptions to this rule and could benefit from marrow biopsy in addition to scan.

Bone marrow aspiration will show tumor cells in a certain number of patients with metastatic carcinoma to bone. Reports do not agree whether there is any difference in positive yield between the sternum and iliac crest. Between 7 and 40% of the patients with tumor in the bone have been said to have a positive bone marrow. This varies with the site of primary tumor, whether the marrow was tested early or late in the disease and whether random aspiration or aspiration from x-ray lesions was performed. The true incidence of positive marrows is probably about 15%. Prostatic carcinoma has the highest rate of yield, since this tumor metastasizes to bone the most frequently, mostly to the vertebral column and pelvic bones.

Several studies have shown that marrow aspiration clot sections detect more tumor than marrow smears and that needle biopsy locates tumor more often than clot section. Two needle biopsies are said to produce approximately 30% more positive results than only one.

The question often arises as to the value of bone marrow aspiration in suspected metastatic carcinoma to bone. In this regard, the following statements seem valid:

1. It usually is difficult or often impossible to determine either the exact tumor type or the origin (primary site) of tumor cells from marrow aspiration.

2. If localized bone lesions exist on x-ray and it is for some reason essential to determine their nature, a direct bone biopsy of these lesions using a

special needle is much better than random marrow aspiration or even aspiration of the lesion area. In this way, a histologic tissue pattern may be obtained.

3. If a patient has a normal alkaline phosphatase, no anemia and no bone lesions on bone scan (or skeletal x-ray survey if bone scan is not available), and in addition has a normal acid phosphatase level in cases of prostatic carcinoma, the chances of obtaining a positive bone marrow aspiration are less than 5% (exceptions are oat cell lung carcinoma and neuroblastoma).

4. If a patient has known carcinoma or definite evidence of carcinoma and has x-ray lesions of bone, there is usually no practical value in getting chemical studies or bone marrow aspiration apart from academic interest, except in certain special situations in which anemia or thrombocytopenia may be caused by a disease that the patient has in addition to the carcinoma.

Effusions and Tests for Cancer

In general, when an effusion occurs, the problem is differentiation among neoplastic, infectious and fluid leakage etiologies. Effusions due to neoplasms or infection are frequently termed "exudates," and those due to hydrostatic leakage from vessels are called "transudates." Several criteria have been proposed to separate transudates and exudates, and to differentiate among the three major diagnostic categories. Most work has been done on pleural fluids.

Protein content.—Protein levels over 3 mg/100 ml are characteristic of exudates. Transudates have protein content of less than 3 and usually less than 2 gm. Two studies found that 8% of exudates and 11–15% of transudates would be misdiagnosed if 3 gm were used as the dividing line. The majority of exudates that were misdiagnosed as transudates were neoplastic. A pleural fluid-to-serum protein ratio of 0.5 may be a slightly better dividing line; exudates usually have a ratio greater than 0.5. With this criterion, accuracy in identifying transudates improved, but 10% of the exudates, mostly of malignant origin, were incorrectly classified as transudates. Pulmonary infarct, rheumatoid-collagen diseases, acute pancreatitis and other conditions may produce effusions with protein content compatible with exudates.

Specific gravity.—Exudates typically have a specific gravity of 1.016 or more, and transudates less than 1.015. One study found about 25% error in misclassification of either transudates or exudates.

Glucose.—Pleural fluid glucose levels more than 10 mg/100 ml below lower limits of normal for serum, and especially when less than 20 mg/100 ml actual value, are reported to be suggestive of neoplasm or infection. Possibly 15–20% of malignant effusions have decreased glucose. Patient hypoglycemia, rheumatoid arthritis and infection are other etiologies.

Cell count and differential.—Many segmented granulocytes suggest infection (empyema); many mononuclear cells raise the question of lymphoid malignancy, carcinoma or tuberculosis. Several investigators state that sufficient exceptions occur to limit the usefulness of this information severely in diagnosis of individual patients.

Culture.—Culture is frequently performed for tuberculosis, fungus and ordinary bacteria. Pleural fluid culture for tuberculosis is said to be positive only in approximately 25% of known cases of tuberculosis effusion. Some feel that tuberculosis culture should be limited to those who are high-risk patients or have a positive skin test. Whereas tuberculosis is an important etiology of idiopathic pleural effusion, although less common at present in the United States, fungus is an uncommon cause of pulmonary infection except in patient groups with compromised immunologic defenses.

Cytology.—Cytology is reported to detect tumor cells in 30–67% of patients with malignant effusion. About 25–50% of all pleural effusions are associated with neoplasms. Interpretation is frequently difficult.

Effusion lactic dehydrogenase.—Pleural fluid-to-serum lactic dehydrogenase (LDH) ratio greater than 0.6 is reported to be typical of exudates. One study found that most transudates were correctly identified, but that nearly 30% of exudates were misclassified.

Combinations of criteria.—The more criteria that favor one category as opposed to the other, the more accurate the results become. One study found that the combination of pleural fluid-to-serum protein ratio and pleural fluid-to-serum LDH ratio correctly identified most transudates and exudates.

Miscellaneous Tests

Metastatic tumors to bone will produce hematologic symptoms if sufficient marrow replacement occurs. This must be distinguished from the anemia of neoplasia, which appears in a considerable number of patients without direct marrow involvement and whose mechanism may be hemolytic, toxic depression of marrow production or of completely unknown etiology. Generally speaking, one always suspicious sign of extensive marrow replacement is the presence of thrombocytopenia in a patient with known cancer. Another is the appearance of nucleated red cells in the peripheral blood, sometimes with slightly more immature white cells in addition. This does not occur in multiple myeloma, even though this disease often produces discrete bone lesions on x-ray and the malignant plasma cells may replace much of the bone marrow.

Serum lactic dehydrogenase (LDH) is sometimes elevated in extensive carcinomatosis, often without any obvious reason. This is especially true in lymphoma, where it has been reported abnormal in up to 50% of cases.

CARCINOEMBRYONIC ANTIGEN.—Gastrointestinal tract epithelium in early fetal life contains an antigen that has also been found in extracts from tumors in the adult GI tract. Immunologic tests have been based on antibodies against this antigen. The procedure was originally thought to be specific for colon adenocarcinoma; but as more experience was obtained and modifications of the original technique developed, it became evident that abnormal results could be obtained in malignancies of various organs, in certain benign diseases (usually involving tissue inflammation or destruction), in occasional benign tumors and in persons who smoke cigarettes. In colon carcinoma, different investigators have published widely divergent results, with percentage of tumor detected ranging from 59 to 97%. The smaller and earlier-stage tumors are less likely to give positive results.

Several basic RIA techniques have been published. The most frequently used is the Hansen procedure, using "Z-gel" as a radioactivity separation agent. At present an overnight incubation is required, so that 2 days are needed to perform the test. Normal values obtained by this procedure are 0–2.5 ng/ml. Among noncolonic tumors, 70–90% of lung, 85–100% of pancreatic and 45–60% of breast and gastric carcinomas are reported to produce abnormal results when tested by more than one investigator. Normal persons who smoke were CEA-reactive in nearly 20% of cases, and conditions associated with elevation in more than 10% of patients include pulmonary emphysema, benign rectal polyps, benign breast diseases, alcoholic cirrhosis and ulcerative colitis. Over 5 ng/ml (twice upper limits), abnormal results in colorectal, lung and pancreatic carcinoma decreased to 50–60%; breast and gastric, to 30%. Most other conditions were reduced to 5% abnormality or less, except for alcoholic cirrhosis (about 25%), acute ulcerative colitis (13%) and emphysema (20%). Over 10 ng/ml (4 times upper normal), abnormal results were found in 35% of colorectal, 25% lung, 35% pancreas and 15–20% gastric and breast carcinoma. All other benign conditions were less than 1% reactive except for emphysema (4%), acute ulcerative colitis (5%) and alcoholic cirrhosis (2%).

This data indicates that CEA results over 10 ng/ml are strongly suggestive of tumor; results in the 5–10 ng/ml range are moderately suspicious, and results less than 5 ng/ml are either equivocal or not helpful. The major recommended use for the test is to follow patients undergoing therapy; decrease of CEA from baseline suggests effective therapy, and increase suggests recurrence or additional tumor spread. There are, however, occasional exceptions to both these statements. Serial determinations are more reliable than single assays. In certain instances, such as patients with fever of unknown origin or vague abdominal complaints, CEA can be useful as a tumor screening test (results over 10 ng/ml would be highly suggestive of occult tumor and might indicate further studies).

TUMOR-SEEKING RADIOPHARMACEUTICALS. — Certain compounds have been found empirically to localize in neoplasms. These can be tagged with a radioisotope and used to detect tumor by scanning. Currently, gallium-67 citrate is the most widely used. Labeled bleomycin may be available in the near future. Both are not specific tumor markers; both may appear in certain organs or tissues (liver, spleen and bone, in the case of gallium) and in areas of localized infection (p. 164).

Gallium scan abnormality has been reported in approximately 90% of primary site lung carcinoma; 85% of Hodgkin's disease; 60–75% of non-Hodgkin's lymphoma (depending on cell type); 55% of acute leukemia lymph nodes; 75–85% of brain tumors; 75% of hypernephromas; 65% of breast carcinomas; 45% of melanomas, and about 30–35% of adenocarcinomas from GI tract, pancreas and ovary. Gallium is less sensitive than ordinary bone scan agents for detection of skeletal metastases. After 24 hours, gallium is excreted in the feces, so that colon activity may interfere unless adequate bowel cleansing is performed.

REFERENCES

Alexander, J. C.: Effect of age and cigarette smoking on carcinoembryonic antigen levels, J.A.M.A. 235:1975, 1976.

Bell, M.: Newer chemical diagnostic tests (neuroblastoma symposium), J.A.M.A. 205:105, 1968.

Blahd, W. H. (ed.): *Nuclear Medicine* (2d ed.; New York: McGraw-Hill Book Company, Inc., 1971).

Block, M. A.: Medullary thyroid carcinoma: A component of an interesting endocrine syndrome, CA 19:74, 1969.

Braunstein, G. D., et al.: Ectopic production of human chorionic gonadotropin by neoplasms. Ann. Intern. Med. 78:39, 1973.

Brennan, M. J.: Endocrinology in cancer of the breast, Am. J. Clin. Pathol. 64:797, 1975.

Brown, D. H.: The urinary excretion of vanilmandelic acid (VMA) and homovanillic acid (HVA) in children with retinoblastoma, Am. J. Ophthalmol. 62:239, 1966.

Cameron, A. J., and Hoffman, H. N.: Zollinger-Ellison syndrome, Mayo Clin. Proc. 49:44, 1974.

Clark, O. H., et al.: Evaluation of solitary cold thyroid nodules by echography and thermography, Am. J. Surg. 130:206, 1975.

Clark, R. C., et al.: Reproducibility of the technique of mammography (Egan) for cancer of the breast, Am. J. Surg. 109:127, 1965.

Cooley, R. N.: Diagnostic accuracy of radiologic studies of biliary tract, small intestine, and colon, Am. J. Med. Sci. 246:610, 1963.

Creutzfeldt, W., et al.: Pathomorphologic, biochemical, and diagnostic aspects of gastrinomas (Zollinger-Ellison syndrome), Hum. Pathol. 6:47, 1975.

Crowder, B. L., et al.: Gastrointestinal carcinoids and the carcinoid syndrome: Clinical characteristics and therapy, CA 18:213, 1968.

DeGroot, L. J.: Thyroid carcinoma, Med. Clin. North Am. 59:1233, 1975.

Delta, B. G., and Pinkel, D.: Bone marrow aspiration in children with malignant tumors, J. Pediatr. 64:542, 1964.

Dhar, P., et al.: Carcinoembryonic antigen (CEA) in colonic cancer, J.A.M.A. 221:31, 1972.

Egan, R. L.: Bilateral breast carcinomas: Role of mammography, Cancer 38:931, 1976.

Ellman, L.: Bone marrow biopsy in the evaluation of lymphoma, carcinoma, and granulomatous disorders, Am. J. Med. 60:1, 1976.

Gailani, S., et al.: Human chorionic gonadotrophins (hCG) in non-trophoblastic neoplasms, Cancer 38:1684, 1976.

Gershon-Cohen, Mammography, thermography, and xerography, CA 17:108, 1967.

Gilbertson, V. A.: X-ray examination of the chest — Unsatisfactory method of detection of early lung cancer in asymptomatic individuals, J.A.M.A. 188:1082, 1964.

Gomez-Uria, A., and Pazianos, A. G.: Syndromes resulting from ectopic hormone-producing tumors, Med. Clin. North Am. 59:431, 1975.

Gondos, R.: Recent developments in the cytologic diagnosis of vaginal, endometrial, and ovarian cancer, Ann. Clin. Lab. Sci. 4:420, 1974.

Goodwin, D. A., and Mears, C. F.: Radiolabeled antitumor agents, Semin. Nucl. Med. 6:389, 1976.

Grabstald, H.: Renal cell cancer (parts I, II and III), NY State J. Med. 64:2539, 2658, 2771, 1964.

Gyorkey, F., et al.: The usefulness of electron microscopy in its diagnosis of human tumors, Hum. Pathol. 6:421, 1975.

Haverback, B. J., Stubrin, M. I., and Majcher, S. J.: Serotonin and Related Substances, in Dowling, H. F. (ed.): *Disease-a-Month* (Chicago: Year Book Medical Publishers, Inc., April, 1966).

Hayes, T. P.: Brain and liver scans in the evaluation of lung cancer patients, Cancer 27:362, 1971.

Holyoke, E. D., et al.: CEA as a monitor of gastrointestinal malignancy, Cancer 35: 830, 1975.

Ivey, K. J., and Hansky, J.: Variability of serum gastrin levels in Zollinger-Ellison syndrome, Am. J. Dig. Dis. 20:513, 1975.

Kantor, S., et al.: Carcinoid tumors of the gastrointestinal tract, Am. Surg. 27:448, 1961.

Lange, P. H., et al.: Serum alpha fetoprotein and human chorionic gonadotropin in the diagnosis and management of non-seminomatous germ-cell testicular cancer, N. Engl. J. Med. 295:1237, 1976.

Lauby, V. W., et al.: Value and risk of biopsy of pulmonary lesions by needle aspiration, J. Thorac. Cardiovasc. Surg. 49:159, 1965.

Light, R. W., et al: Pleural effusions: The diagnostic separation of transudates and exudates, Ann. Intern. Med. 77:507, 1972.

Lilien, D. L., et al: A clinical evaluation of indium-111 bleomycin as a tumor-imaging agent, Cancer 35:1036, 1975.

Lipsett, M. B., et al.: Humoral syndromes associated with nonendocrine tumors, Ann. Intern. Med. 61:733, 1964.

Lipton, A., et al.: Urinary polyamine levels in patients with localized malignancy, Cancer 38:1344, 1976.

McCartney, W. H., and Hoffer, P. B.: The CEA assay as an adjunct to liver scanning in the detection of hepatic metastases. Scientific exhibit, Society of Nuclear Medicine, Philadelphia, June 16, 1975.

Meyer, J. S., and Steinberg, L. S.: Microscopically benign thyroid follicles in cervical lymph nodes, Cancer, 24:302, 1969.

Moore, T. L., et al.: Carcinoembryonic antigen assay in cancer of the colon and pancreas and other digestive tract disorders, Am. J. Dig. Dis. 16:1, 1971.

Myers, W. P. L., et al.: Endocrine syndromes associated with nonendocrine neoplasms, Med. Clin. North Am. 50:763, 1966.

Nathanson, L., and Fishman, W. II.: New observations on the Regan isoenzyme of alkaline phosphatase in cancer patients, Cancer 27:1388, 1971.

Newlands, E. S., et al.: Serum alpha-1-fetoprotein and H.C.G. in patients with testicular tumours, Lancet 2:744, 1976.

Ozgelen, F. N., et al.: Cytology in lung cancer, J. Thorac. Cardiovasc. Surg. 49:221, 1965.

Pearson, O. H.: Endocrine treatment of breast cancer, CA 26:165, 1976.

Pinsky, S. M., and Hankin, R. E.: Gallium-67 tumor scanning, Semin. Nucl. Med. 6: 397, 1976.

Ptak, T., and Kirsner, J. B.: The Zollinger-Ellison Syndrome, Polyendocrine Adenomatosis, and Other Endocrine Associations with Peptic Ulcer, in Stollerman, G. H., et al. (eds.): *Advances in Internal Medicine* (Chicago: Year Book Medical Publishers, Inc., 1970), vol. 16, p. 213.

Rao, N. V., et al.: Needle biopsy of parietal pleura in 124 cases, Arch. Intern. Med. 115:34, 1965.

Ratnaike, R. N., et al.: Comparative accuracy of methods used in diagnosis of gastric cancer, Med. J. Austr. 2:30, 1972.

Richman, S. D., et al.: Radionuclide studies in Hodgkin's disease and lymphomas, Semin. Nucl. Med. 5:103, 1975.

Sasaki, G. H., et al.: LevoDopa test and estrogen receptor assay in prognosticating responses of patients with advanced cancer of the breast to endocrine therapy, Ann. Surg. 183:392, 1976.

Schwartz, M. K.: Biochemical procedures in different forms of cancer, Med. Clin. North Am. 55:613, 1971.

Scott, W. G.: Mammography and the training program of the American College of Radiology, Am. J. Roentgenol. 99:1022, 1967.

Sears, H. R., et al.: Liver scan and carcinoma of the breast, Surg. Gynecol. Obstet. 140:409, 1975.

Sherlock, P., and Kim, Y. S.: Unusual gastrointestinal manifestations of cancer and newer techniques in the diagnosis of gastrointestinal cancer, Med. Clin. North Am. 50:747, 1966.

Shulman, J. J., et al.: The PAP smear: Take two, Am. J. Obstet. Gynecol. 121:1024, 1975.

Silberstein, E. B.: Cancer diagnosis: The role of tumor-imaging radiopharmaceuticals, Am. J. Med. 60:226, 1976.

So-Bosita, J. L., et al.: Endometrial jet washer, Obst. Gynecol. 36:287, 1970.

Stillman, A., and Zamcheck, N.: Recent advances in immunologic diagnosis of digestive tract cancer, Am. J. Dig. Dis. 15:1003, 1970.

Storey, D. D., et al.: Pleural effusion: A diagnostic dilemma, J.A.M.A. 236:2183, 1976.

Tickton, H. E., and Trujillo, N. P.: Enzymes in Neoplastic and Surgical Diseases, in Coodley, E. L. (ed.): *Diagnostic Enzymology* (Philadelphia: Lea & Febiger, 1970), p. 205.

Turnipseed, W. D., and Keith, L. M.: Altered serum gastrin levels in achlorhydric states, Am. J. Surg. 131:175, 1976.

Walsh, J. H., and Grossman, M. I.: Gastrin, N. Engl. J. Med. 292:1324, 1377, 1975.

33 / Congenital Diseases

CONGENITAL DISEASE will be considered as any clinical condition resulting from a genetically determined abnormality. Such a category provides a wide variety of unrelated disorders. Although a great many syndromes and diseases are known, only those for which adequate laboratory diagnostic tests are available will be included.

HEMATOLOGIC DISEASES

These include principally the hemoglobinopathies (p. 24), red cell glucose-6-phosphate dehydrogenase deficiency (p. 31) and the hemophilias (p. 62). These diseases were discussed in the appropriate sections on hematology. The Philadelphia chromosome abnormality found in chronic myelogenous leukemia was noted in reviewing that disease (p. 49).

DISEASES OF CARBOHYDRATE METABOLISM

RENAL GLUCOSURIA. — This is a disorder of the renal tubule glucose transport mechanism, mentioned on page 326.

LACTOSURIA. — A surprising number of infants, more commonly premature, show neonatal intolerance to lactose, clinically manifested by gastrointestinal upsets. Urinary lactose is increased and can be detected by one of the copper sulfate reducing sugar urine methods; glucose oxidase enzyme paper tests are negative. Specific chemical tests may then be done if desired to identify the substance positively as lactose. Benign lactosuria in adults is apparently not uncommon in the last trimester of pregnancy and the puerperium.

GALACTOSEMIA. — This is based on congenital inability to utilize galactose and thus differs from lactosuria, which represents a temporary inability to hydrolyze lactose, a major precursor of galactose. Normally, galactose is metabolized to galactose-1-phosphate and thence, through several intermediate steps, to glucose-1-phosphate. In galactosemia there is a deficiency of the enzyme galactose-1-phosphate uridyl transferase, which mediates the conversion of galactose-1-phosphate to the next step in the sequence toward glucose-1-phosphate. The defect is transmitted by a recessive gene, and the enzyme affected is located in red blood cells.

Galactosemia usually is not clinically evident at birth, but symptoms commence within a few days after beginning a milk diet. Vomiting, diar-

409

rhea and "failure to thrive" are common. Physiologic jaundice may seem to persist, or jaundice may develop later with hepatomegaly. Splenomegaly occurs in only about 10–30% of patients. Eye signs, consisting of lens cataracts, develop after several weeks in about 50%. Without treatment, mental retardation is a frequent sequel. The disease is treatable with a lactose-free diet if begun early enough.

There are multiple laboratory abnormalities. Urinalysis shows proteinuria and galactosuria. Galactose in the urine may be detected by a positive copper sulfate reducing test combined with a negative glucose oxidase method; urine chromatography or specific chemical tests are available for more precise identification. Currently, this is the way most of these patients have been detected. However, galactosuria depends on lactose ingestion, and may be absent if the infant refuses milk or persistently vomits. There is also abnormal amino acid urinary excretion, and this can be detected by urine paper chromatography, although little is added to the diagnosis by such information. Positive urine galactose results must be confirmed by some type of blood galactose determination, since occasional normal newborns have transient galactosuria. Serum chromatography for galactose is a valuable aid in confirmation of the diagnosis, and there are new screening tests available by which the galactose-1-phosphate uridyl transferase in RBC may be measured semiquantitatively. These enzymatic screening tests measure a red cell enzyme that is relatively unstable; therefore, it would be better to request serum chromatography if the specimen must be sent to a distant laboratory.

Hepatomegaly is a frequent finding, although the liver is not always palpable. Jaundice may or may not be present. Liver function tests should be interpreted with caution, since normal values in infants are different from those in adults; nevertheless, the SGOT is said to be often considerably elevated. Liver biopsy has been used in certain problem patients; the histologic changes are suggestive but not conclusive, and consist of early fatty metamorphosis, with a type of cirrhosis pattern often developing after about 3 months of age.

The galactose tolerance test was once the most widely used method for confirmation of galactosemia. However, there is considerable danger of hypoglycemia and hypokalemia during the test, and it has been replaced by chromatography and red cell enzyme assay.

DISACCHARIDE MALABSORPTION. — Occasionally this is a cause of chronic diarrhea or vomiting in newborns or infants. This probably is not common, especially compared to the frequency of diarrhea and vomiting in infants, but it is beginning to receive more attention. Certain enzymes present in small intestine mucosal cells aid absorption of various carbohydrates by preliminary hydrolyzation. Affected patients have varying degrees of specific enzyme deficiency, and thus cannot properly absorb the substance that depends on that enzyme. Clinically, the most common problems are with the disaccharides sucrose and lactose. Lactose is present in milk, while sucrose is a common source of carbohydrate supplement. A presumptive diagnosis can be made by careful substitution of foods, at least for lactose and sucrose. Of course, cessation of symptoms does not necessarily mean that intolerance was the real etiology. Of some help as a screening procedure is the fact that when excessive amounts of these carbohydrates reach the large intestine, bacterial fermentation often will turn the stool pH from normally neutral to strongly acid. In addition, a test (such as Clinitest) for reducing substances has also been advocated. Strongly acidic stool pH may be found in certain other conditions associated with diarrhea, expecially steatorrhea. To make a definitive diagnosis at present requires either specific carbohydrate tolerance tests or small intestine biopsy for enzyme assay.

One report indicates that the standard lactose tolerance test is not reliable in diabetics who are insulin-dependent. A lactose-alcohol tolerance test, in which the patient is premedicated with alcohol and blood galactose is measured after oral lactose rather than blood glucose, is said to be more reliable in such patients.

GLYCOGEN STORAGE DISEASE. — This abnormality contains a spectrum of syndromes resulting from defective synthesis or utilization of glycogen. Clinical manifestations depend on the organ or tissue primarily affected and the specific enzyme involved. The disease in one or another of its clinical syndromes may affect the liver, heart or skeletal muscle. The most common is von Gierke's disease, whose clinical manifestations primarily involve the liver.

Diagnosis in the various forms of glycogen storage disease involves biopsy of liver or muscle (depending on the particular disease variant) for glycogen and enzyme analysis (p. 494). In some cases, enzyme assay can be performed on other tissues. This is a very specialized area, and it is best to contact a pediatric research center rather than expose the patient to inappropriate or incomplete diagnostic procedures.

DISEASES OF LIPID STORAGE

HISTIOCYTOSIS-X. — This term was coined to include three closely related diseases of unknown etiology; all three are characterized by proliferation of histiocytic cells, but only one of the three is associated with lipid storage. Letterer-Siwe disease is a rapidly progressive fatal condition seen mostly in early childhood and infancy. There is widespread involvement of visceral and reticuloendothelial organs by atypical histiocytes, with accompanying anemia and thrombocytopenia. Bone marrow aspiration or, occasionally, lymph node biopsy is the usual diagnostic procedure. Eosinophilic granuloma is the benign member of the triad. It is seen most often in later childhood, and most commonly presents as isolated bone lesions. These usually are single but may be multiple. The lungs may occasionally be involved. The lesion is composed of histiocytes with many eosinophils and is diagnosed by direct biopsy. Hand-Schüller-Christian disease is somewhat intermediate between the other two in terms of chronicity and histology. Bone lesions, often multiple, are the major abnormalities. Soft tissue and reticuloendothelial organs sometimes may be affected. There may be very few systemic symptoms or there may be anemia, leukopenia and thrombocytopenia. The lesions are composed of histiocytes containing large amounts of cholesterol in the cytoplasm and accompanied by fibrous tissue and varying numbers of eosinophils. Diagnosis usually is by direct biopsy of a lesion.

GAUCHER'S DISEASE.—This is a disorder in which the glycolipid cerebroside compound kerasin is phagocytized by the reticuloendothelial system. There seem to be two subgroups of this disorder—a fatal disease of relatively short duration in infancy accompanied by mental retardation, and a more slowly progressive disease of older children and young adults without mental retardation. Splenomegaly is the most characteristic finding, but the liver and occasionally the lymph nodes also may become enlarged. The most characteristic x-ray findings are aseptic necrosis of the femoral heads and widening of the femoral marrow cavities; although typical, these findings may be absent. Anemia is frequent, and there may be leukopenia and thrombocytopenia due to hypersplenism. The serum acid phosphatase usually is elevated if the chemical methods used are not reasonably specific for prostatic acid phosphatase. There are several widely used chemical methods, and while none is absolutely specific for prostatic acid phosphatase, some are considerably more so than others. Definitive diagnosis is most easily made by bone marrow aspiration. Wright-stained bone marrow smears often show the characteristic Gaucher cells, which are large mononuclear phagocytes whose cytoplasm is filled with a peculiar linear or fibrillar material. Splenic puncture is even better than bone marrow aspiration, but is a more complicated procedure. Biopsy of the spleen, and sometimes the liver, can yield the diagnosis on histologic section with special stains—or, better, tissue analysis for lipids—but should be reserved for special problem patients.

NIEMANN-PICK DISEASE.—This is similar clinically and pathologically to the fatal early childhood form of Gaucher's disease, except that the abnormal lipid involved is a phospholipid sphingomyelin. Diagnosis is established by bone marrow aspiration, although the cells are not as characteristic as those of Gaucher's disease. Spleen or liver biopsy with histologic special stains or tissue lipid analysis are probably the most definitive studies.

DIAGNOSIS.—There are several diseases in the lipid storage category; a complete list is given on page 495. Definitive diagnosis can now be obtained by enzyme analysis of the patient's white blood cells or by tissue culture of fibroblasts obtained from the patient's skin. In addition, in most of these diseases it is possible to perform specific glycosphingolipid analysis from liver biopsy specimens. It is recommended that a university medical center specializing in such problems or the Neurological Diseases branch of the National Institutes of Health be contacted for details on how to proceed with any patient suspected of having a lipid storage disease. It is highly preferable that the patient be sent directly to the center for biopsy or required specimen collection, to avoid unnecessary and costly delays and to prevent damage to the specimen in transport.

DEFECTS IN AMINO ACID METABOLISM
(AMINOACIDOPATHIES)

Primary (Metabolic) Aminoacidopathies

PHENYLKETONURIA (PKU).—This condition is due to deficiency of a liver enzyme needed to convert the amino acid phenylalanine to tyrosine.

With its major utilization pathway blocked, phenylalanine accumulates in the blood and leads to early onset of progressive mental deficiency. This disease is one of the more common causes of hereditary mental deficiency, and one of the few whose bad effects can be prevented by early treatment of the infant. At birth the infant usually has normal serum levels of phenylalanine (less than 2 mg/100 ml) due to maternal enzyme activity, although some instances of mental damage in utero occur. After birth, and after beginning a diet containing phenylalanine (such as milk), serum levels begin to rise gradually. After they reach the 12–15-mg/100-ml level, utilization of phenylalanine by other metabolic pathways has reached such an extent that a characteristic substance known as phenylpyruvic acid begins to appear in the urine. This becomes detectable by urine screening tests (ferric chloride or Phenistix) at some time between 3 and 6 weeks of age. Since some degree of damage may have been done by that time, it is desirable to make an earlier diagnosis.

The most widely used screening test for elevated serum phenylalanine is the Guthrie test. This is a bacterial inhibition procedure. A certain substance that competes with phenylalanine in *Bacillus subtilis* metabolism is incorporated into culture media; this essentially provides a phenylalanine-deficient culture medium. *Bacillus subtilis* spores are seeded into this medium, but to produce significant bacterial growth, a quantity of phenylalanine equivalent to more than normal blood levels must be furnished. Next, a sample of the patient's blood is added, and the presence of abnormal quantities of serum phenylalanine is reflected by bacterial growth in the area where the specimen was applied. The Guthrie test, if properly done, is adequately sensitive and accurate, and will reliably detect definitely abnormal levels of serum phenylalanine (4 mg/100 ml or over). It also fulfills the requirements for an acceptable screening method. There are, however, two main drawbacks to the use of this procedure. First, the standard practice is to obtain a blood specimen from an infant before discharge from the hospital. Unfortunately, in the majority of patients, it takes 2 to 4 days on a high-protein (milk) diet before the serum phenylalanine reaches the definitely abnormal level of 4 mg/100 ml. Therefore, if the blood specimen is obtained before 4 full days on a milk diet are completed and definitely if obtained before 3 full days, a certain very significant percentage of PKU patients will be missed. Second, there are other possible causes of elevated neonatal serum phenylalanine such as liver disease, galactosemia or late development of certain enzyme systems. In fact, some reports state that the majority of initially positive Guthrie tests are not due to PKU. In some of these "false positive" patients, harm could be done by prolonged PKU treatment (low-phenylalanine diet). Therefore, an abnormal Guthrie test should be followed up by more detailed investigation, including, as a minimum, both the serum phenylalanine and tyrosine levels (the typical PKU patient has a serum phenylalanine level greater than 15 mg/100 ml with a serum tyrosine level less than 5 mg/100 ml. The tests may have to be repeated in 1–2 weeks if values have not reached these levels.)

ALKAPTONURIA (OCHRONOSIS).—The typical manifestations of this uncommon disease are the triad of arthritis, black pigmentation of cartilage (ochronosis) and excretion of homogentisic acid in the urine. Arthritis usually begins in middle age and typically involves the spine and the large joints. Black pigmentation of cartilage is most apparent in the ears, but may be noticed in cartilage elsewhere, or may even appear in tendons. The intervertebral disks often become heavily calcified and thus provide a characteristic x-ray picture. The disease is caused by abnormal accumulation of homogentisic acid, an intermediate metabolic product of tyrosine; this in turn is caused by a deficiency of the liver enzyme homogentisic acid oxidase, which mediates the further breakdown of the acid. Most of the homogentisic acid is excreted in the urine, but enough slowly accumulates in cartilage and surrounding tissues to cause the characteristic changes previously described. Diagnosis is accomplished by demonstration of homogentisic acid in the urine. Addition of 10% sodium hydroxide turns the urine black or gray-black. A false positive urine sugar test is produced by copper reduction methods such as Benedict's or Clinitest.

OTHER PRIMARY AMINOACIDOPATHIES. — These are numerous, varied and rare. They are mostly diagnosed through paper chromatography of urine (or serum), looking for abnormal quantities of the particular amino acid involved whose metabolic pathway has been blocked. The most widely known diseases (apart from phenylketonuria and alkaptonuria) are maple syrup disease and histidinemia. The most common is homocystinuria.

Secondary Aminoacidopathies

These are associated with a renal defect, usually of reabsorption, rather than a primary defect in the metabolic pathway of the amino acid in question. The serum levels are normal. The most common cause is a systemic disease such as Wilson's disease, lead poisoning or the Fanconi syndrome. In such cases, several amino acids usually are found in the urine. Aminoaciduria may occur normally in the first week of life, especially in premature infants. A much smaller number of patients have a more specific amino acid renal defect with one or more specific amino acids excreted; the most common of these diseases is cystinuria. Patients with cystinuria develop cystine renal calculi. Cystine crystals may be identified in acidified urine, providing the diagnosis. Otherwise, combined urine and serum paper chromatography are the diagnostic methods of choice.

DISORDERS OF CONNECTIVE TISSUE

HURLER'S SYNDROME (GARGOYLISM). — There actually are several subtypes of Hurler's, or Hurler-like syndromes, but the classic disease includes many of the following: short stature or dwarfism, moderate lumbar kyphosis, saddle nose, clouding of the ocular corneas, deafness, joint stiffness, hepatosplenomegaly and abnormalities of heart valves. There often are varying degrees of mental deficiency, but some patients have normal intelligence. The biochemical defect consists of abnormal tissue storage by connective tissue cells of certain mucopolysaccharides, chondroitin sulfate B and heparitin sulfate. There also is markedly increased urinary excretion of the substances, which are not detectable in normal persons except uncommonly during the first week of life. Rapid screening tests have been devised for demonstration of mucopolysaccharides or chondroitin sulfuric acid in the urine. However, these have been developed relatively recently, and probably are not widely available as yet.

OTHER. — There are other disorders involving primarily connective tissue; a complete list is presented on page 497. The most characteristic laboratory finding is elevated urine mucopolysaccharides. Differentiation can be made by chemical identification of the individual substance excreted, plus inheritance patterns and clinical signs. Tissue cell culture may prove to be the basic method of the future; fetal cells from amniocentesis have been used by one investigator. Some of these conditions display metachromatic granules in lymphocytes and occasionally in segmented neutrophils. Certain of these diseases are frequently included among the chondrodystrophies, since basic connective tissue defects frequently lead to cartilage abnormalities.

CHROMOSOMAL ABNORMALITIES

There are several conditions, some relatively common and some rare, that result either from abnormal numbers of chromosomes, defects in size or configuration of certain specific single chromosomes or abnormal composition of the chromosome group that determines sexual characteristics. Laboratory diagnosis, at present, takes two forms. First, chromosome charts may be prepared on any individual by culturing certain body cells, such as white blood cells from peripheral blood or bone marrow; introducing a chemical such as colchicine, which kills the cells at a specific stage in mitosis when the chromosomes become organized and separated, and then photographing and separating the individual chromosomes into specific groups according to similarity in size and configuration. The most widely used system is the Denver classification. The 46 human chromosomes are composed of 22 chromosome pairs and, in addition, 2 unpaired chromosomes, the sex chromosomes (XX in the female and XY in the male). In a Denver chromosome chart (karyotype) the 22 paired chromosomes are separated into 7 groups, each containing 2 or more individually identified and numbered chromosomes. For example, the 1st group contains chromosomes 1–3, the 7th group chromosomes 21–22. In addition, there is an 8th group for the 2 unpaired sex chromosomes. Chromosome culture takes a substantial amount of experience and care in preparation and interpretation.

The other, more widely used, technique provides certain useful information about the composition of the sex chromosome group. It was discovered by Barr that the nuclei of various body cells contains a certain stainable sex chromatin mass (Barr body) that appears for each X chromosome more than 1 that the cell possesses. Therefore, a normal male (XY) cell has no Barr body because there is only 1 X chromosome; a normal female (XX) has 1 Barr body, and a person with the abnormal configuration XXX would have 2 Barr bodies. The most convenient method for Barr body detection at present is called the buccal smear. It is obtained by scraping the oral mucosa, smearing the epithelial cells thus collected onto a glass slide in a monolayer and, after immediate chemical fixation, staining with certain special stains. Comparison of the results, together with the secondary sex characteristics and genitalia of the patient, allows presumptive diagnosis of certain sex chromosome abnormalities. The results may be confirmed, if necessary, by chromosome karyotyping.

Buccal smears should not be obtained during the 1st week of life or during adrenal corticosteroid or estrogen therapy, because these situations falsely lower the incidence of sex chromatin Barr bodies. Certain artifacts may be confused with the nuclear Barr bodies. Poor slide preparations may obscure the sex chromatin mass and lead to false negative appearances. Also, only about 40–60% of normal female cells contain an identifiable Barr body. The buccal smear is not capable by itself of demonstrating the true genetic sex; it is only an indication of the number of female (X) chromosomes present.

KLINEFELTER'S SYNDROME. — In this condition the patient looks outwardly like a male, but the sex chromosome makeup is XXY instead of XY. The external genitalia are usually normal, except for small testes. There is a tendency toward androgen deficiency and thus for gynecomastia and decreased body hair, but this may be slight or not evident. There also is a tendency toward mental deficiency, but many have perfectly normal intelligence. Patients with Klinefelter's syndrome are almost always sterile. Testicular biopsy used to be the main diagnostic method, with histologic specimens showing marked atrophy of the seminiferous tubules. At present, a buccal smear is the procedure of choice; it shows a "normal female" configuration with 1 Barr body (due to the 2 XX chromosomes). In the presence of unmistakably male genitalia, this usually is sufficient for clinical diagnosis. Chromosome karyotyping may be necessary to confirm the diagnosis in doubtful cases.

TURNER'S SYNDROME (OVARIAN AGENESIS). — This is the most frequent chromosomal sexual abnormality in females, as Klinefelter's is for males. In Turner's syndrome there is a deletion of 1 female (X) chromosome, so that the patient has only 45 chromosomes instead of 46, and only 1 female sex chromosome instead of 2. Typically, this leads to a female with relatively short stature but with normal body proportions. There is deficient development of secondary sex characteristics and small genitalia, although body hair usually is female in distribution. Some of these persons have associated anomalies such as webbing of the neck, coarctation of the aorta and short fingers. These patients do not menstruate, and actually lack ovaries. Diagnosis may be made in most cases by buccal smear; this should be "sex chromatin negative," since Barr bodies appear only when the female sex chromosomes number more than 1. If the buccal smear is "chromatin positive," a chromosome karyotype should be ordered, because some patients with Turner's syndrome have mixtures of normal cells and defective cells ("mosaicism").

MONGOLISM (DOWN'S SYNDROME). — This is a relatively frequent disorder associated with 2 different chromosome abnormalities. The majority of patients have an extra chromosome in the number 21–22 chromosome group (therefore producing 3 chromosomes in this group instead of 2, a situation known as "trisomy 21"). These patients have a total of 47 chromosomes. Their chromosome abnormality has nothing to do with the sex chromosomes, which are normal. This type of mongolism apparently is spontaneous, not inherited (that is, there is no family history of mongolism, and the parents have very little risk that they will have another similar child). Other patients with mongolism have an extra 21-type chromosome, but it is attached to one of the other chromosomes, most often in the 13–15 group (called the D group in some nomenclatures). This type of arrangement is called "translocation." It means that 1 of the parents had a normal total number of chromosomes, but 1 of the pair of number 21 chromosomes was attached to 1 of the number 15 chromosomes. The other number 21 and the other number 15 chromosome were normal. The cluster behaves in meiosis as though it were a number 15 chromosome. If the abnormal chromosome cluster is passed to the children, 2 situations could arise: a mongoloid child who received both the translocated 15–21 chromosome plus the normal number 21 chromosome, or a carrier who received the translocated 15–21 chromosome but did not receive the other (normal) number 21 chromosome.

Clinically, an infant or child with mongolism usually presents some combination of the following: prominent epicanthal folds at the medial aspect of the eyes, mental retardation or deficiency, broad hands and feet and a single long transverse crease on the palm instead of several shorter transverse creases. Other frequent but still less common associated abnormalities are umbilical hernia, webbing of the toes and certain types of congenital heart disease. There also is an increased incidence of acute leukemia.

Diagnosis usually can be made clinically, but chromosome karyotyping is a valuable means of confirmation and of diagnosis in equivocal cases. It probably is advisable to get chromosome karyotyping in most children with mongolism, because the type of chromosome pattern gives an indication of the prognosis for future children.

OTHER DISORDERS. — A wide variety of syndromes, usually composed of multiple congenital deformities and anomalies, are now found to be due to specific chromosomal abnormalities. The most common of these involve trisomy in the 13–15 (D) group and in the 16–18 (E) group. Some patients with habitual abortion have abnormal karyotypes. Various tumors have yielded abnormal chromosome patterns, but no one type of tumor had produced any consistent pattern (except for chronic myelogenous leukemia).

COMMONLY ACCEPTED INDICATIONS FOR BUCCAL SMEAR. — These include the following:
1. Ambiguous or abnormal genitalia
2. Male or female infertility without other known cause
3. Symptoms suggestive of Turner's syndrome or Klinefelter's syndrome, such as primary amenorrhea

INDICATIONS FOR CHROMOSOME KARYOTYPING. — These include selected patients in the groups just described for confirmation or initial diagnosis, and:
1. Mongoloid infants; also possible carriers
2. Mentally defective persons
3. Persons with multiple congenital anomalies

DISEASES OF SKELETAL MUSCLE

Several well-known disorders affecting skeletal muscle either are not congenital or do not as yet have any conspicuously useful laboratory test. Among these are myasthenia gravis, a disorder affecting muscle electrical impulse conduction at the neuromuscular junction, whose diagnosis is most often made by pharmacologic tests such as response to edrophonium chloride. A second group of disorders has the primary defect located in the central nervous system rather than in skeletal muscle itself. These comprise various neurologic diseases that secondarily result in symptoms of muscle weakness.

MUSCULAR DYSTROPHIES. — These comprise still another group, but one in which the clinical laboratory may be of assistance. The muscular dystrophies can be divided into several subgroups (p. 494). The most common is Duchenne's (pseudohypertrophic) dystrophy. This is usually transmitted as a sex-linked recessive disorder, although sporadic instances have been reported. The patient is clinically normal for the first few months of life; symptoms develop usually between age 1 and 6 years. The most frequent symptoms are lower extremity and pelvic muscle weakness. There is spotty but progressive muscle fiber dissolution, with excessive deposition or replacement by fat and fibrous tissue. The latter process leads to the most characteristic physical finding of the disease — pseudohypertrophy of the calf muscles. The usefulness of laboratory tests is based on the fact that certain enzymes are found in relatively high concentration in normal skeletal muscle. These include creatine phosphokinase, aldolase, SGOT and LDH, as well as others. Despite external pseudohypertrophy, the dystrophic muscles actually undergo individual fiber dissolution and loss of skeletal muscle substance; this is accompanied by release of these enzymes into the bloodstream. In many tissues SGOT, LDH and aldolase are found together. Pulmonary infarction, myocardial infarction and acute liver cell damage as well as other conditions cause elevated serum levels of these enzymes. Aldolase follows a pattern similar to SGOT in liver disease, and to LDH otherwise. Creatine phosphokinase (CPK) is found in significant concentration only in brain, heart muscle and skeletal muscle.

The two most helpful tests in Duchenne's muscular dystrophy are CPK and aldolase. They are elevated very early in the disease, well before clinical symptoms become manifest, and the elevations usually are over 10 times normal, at least for CPK. This marked elevation persists as symptoms develop. Eventually, after replacement of muscle substance has become chronic and extensive, the aldolase often becomes normal and the CPK may be either normal or only mildly elevated (less than 5 times normal). In the hereditary type of Duchenne's dystrophy, borderline or elevated CPK has been reported in variable numbers of carrier females; in one study, up to 80%. Aldolase is much less frequently abnormal; SGOT and LDH tend to parallel CPK and aldolase, but at a much lower level. Therefore, these enzymes frequently are normal in the later stages of the disease, when the more sensitive tests are still considerably abnormal, and are not of much use in detecting carriers.

The CPK isoenzyme pattern in Duchenne's dystrophy reveals increased MB isoenzyme as well as MM fraction (p. 227), especially in the earlier phases of the illness.

In fascioscapulohumeral dystrophy and limb-girdle dystrophy, conditions that resemble Duchenne's in many respects, CPK and aldolase are variable, but frequently are normal.

Other muscular disorders in which the serum enzymes may be elevated are trauma, dermatomyositis and polymyositis. The levels of elevation are said to be considerably below those seen in early cases of Duchenne's dystrophy. Neurologic disease does not show elevated levels, even when marked secondary muscular atrophy occurs.

Diagnosis in the muscular dystrophies may sometimes be made on the basis of the clinical picture and enzyme values. A more definitive diagnosis can be made by the addition of muscle biopsy. This becomes essential when the findings are not clearcut. The biceps or quadriceps muscles are the preferred biopsy location. The biopsy is best done in a pediatric or congenital disease research center where special studies (such as histochemical staining or electron microscopy) can be performed and the proper specimen secured for this purpose (these special studies provide additional information and are essential when biopsy results are atypical or present unexpected findings).

DISEASES OF MINERAL METABOLISM

WILSON'S DISEASE (HEPATOLENTICULAR DEGENERATION). — This most often becomes manifest between ages 7 and 15. Symptoms most often include dystonia (abnormal muscular rigidity) and tremor of the fingers, due to involvement of the basal ganglia (lentiform nuclei) of the brain. Dysarthria, mental disturbances and a flapping type of upper extremity intention tremor are frequent developments. Patients with Wilson's disease almost invariably have developed a postnecrotic type of liver cirrhosis by the time clinical symptoms are manifest; uncommonly, the initial symptoms are those of hepatic failure. Wilson's disease is characterized by inability of the liver to manufacture normal quantities of an $alpha_2$ globulin named ceruloplasmin, which is the plasma transport agent for copper. For reasons not entirely understood, excessive copper is deposited in various tissues, producing eventual damage. Damage to the basal ganglia of the brain and to the liver were mentioned earlier; the kidney is also affected, leading to aminoaciduria, and copper is deposited in the cornea, producing a discolored zone called the Kayser-Fleischer ring.

The triad of typical basal ganglia symptoms, Kayser-Fleischer ring and hepatic cirrhosis are diagnostic. However, the Kayser-Fleischer ring is seen in only about half the patients, and even in some of these slit lamp examination may be required for its identification.

Laboratory studies may be of value in diagnosis, especially in the preclinical or early stages. Plasma ceruloplasmin is always low (except in a few patients with late disease), is low from birth and is considered the best screening test for Wilson's disease. However, normal newborn infants apparently may have decreased ceruloplasmin levels, and the test is not considered reliable (except to rule out Wilson's disease if results are normal) until about 3 months of age. Elevation in ceruloplasmin, however, may occur in cirrhosis and with estrogen therapy. Certain other diseases may be associated with low plasma ceruloplasmin; these include the nephrotic syndrome, malabsorption syndromes such as sprue and infrequently a few other conditions. Another useful test, especially for confirmation, is liver biopsy. The characteristic findings are early or established postnecrotic-type cirrhosis plus demonstration of increased hepatic copper content by special stains (or tissue analysis, if available). For histologic staining of copper, fixation of the biopsy specimen in alcohol rather than the routine fixatives is recommended. Here again, it is advisable to wait 6–12 weeks after birth.

Other laboratory abnormalities that may be present are a characteristically low serum uric acid, rather frequent hypercalcemia and low serum phosphorus, aminoaciduria including many amino acids and sometimes glucosuria without hyperglycemia.

HEMOCHROMATOSIS. — This is an uncommon disease, predominantly affecting males, which is produced by excessive deposition of iron in various tissues, especially the liver. There is dispute as to whether hemochromatosis is due to an inborn error of metabolism or is a variant of nutritional cirrhosis in which iron deposition in body tissues is, for some reason, more pronounced. Most authors seem to favor the first hypothesis, so the disease is included in this chapter. At any rate, cirrhosis (usually Laennec's type) is always present when symptoms begin. Onset usually is between ages 40 and 60. Cirrhosis, diabetes mellitus and bronze skin pigmentation form the classic triad of hemochromatosis, although diabetes may not be manifest in 20–50% (at least, not clinically manifest when the patient is first seen), and skin pigmentation is absent in over 15%, depending on the stage of the disease. Hypogonadism and a history of alcoholism or poor nutrition are frequent.

Laboratory findings include those of diabetes mellitus, discussed in Chapter 27. Liver function tests are those expected in portal cirrhosis; in some cases there are minimal abnormalities. The body iron abnormality is expressed in a high serum iron level coupled with a decreased total iron-binding capacity (i.e., marked saturation of the TIBC). In addition, hemosiderin very often can be demonstrated in the urinary sediment by iron stains. Liver biopsy shows cirrhosis plus marked parenchymal deposition of iron.

Diagnosis is made more difficult because various other conditions may produce some of these laboratory changes. Hemosiderosis due to multiple blood transfusions over long periods can mimic idiopathic hemochromatosis closely, but a history of transfusions usually is available. A diabetic type of oral glucose tolerance test result is not uncommon in nonhemochromatotic cirrhosis, and there may be increased skin pigmentation. Hemolytic anemia may give similar serum iron and TIBC values, and is found occasionally in association with cirrhosis. Even liver biopsy may not always yield unequivocal results, because many patients with cirrhosis have increased hepatic iron deposition, and some of these may have enough to make a clearcut decision either difficult or impossible.

ABNORMALITIES OF GLANDULAR SECRETION

Cystic fibrosis (mucoviscidosis, or fibrocystic disease of the pancreas) is a hereditary condition that affects the exocrine glands of the body. It is best explained at present as due to a recessive gene whose full expression depends on a homozygous genetic status. The disease is rare in blacks. Both mucus-producing and nonmucus-producing exocrine glands are affected. The mucous glands produce abnormally viscid secretions that may inspissate, plug the glands and generate obstructive complications. In the lungs, this may lead to recurrent bronchopneumonia, the most frequent and most dangerous symptom of cystic fibrosis. Next most common is complete or partial destruction of the exocrine portions of the pancreas, leading to various degrees of malabsorption, steatorrhea, digestive disturbances and malnutrition. This manifestation varies in severity, and about 15% of patients have only a minimal disorder or even a normal pancreatic exocrine function. Less common findings are those of biliary cirrhosis, most often focal, due to obstruction of bile ductules and intestinal obstruction by inspissated meconium (meconium ileus), found in 10–15% of newborns with cystic fibrosis.

Nonmucus-producing exocrine glands such as the sweat glands do not ordinarily cause symptoms. However, they are also affected, because the sodium and chloride concentration in sweat is higher than normal in patients with cystic fibrosis, even though the volume of sweat is not abnormally increased. Therefore, unusually high quantities of sodium and chloride are lost in sweat, and this fact is utilized for diagnosis. Screening tests have been devised (silver nitrate or Schwachman test) that depend on the incorporation of silver nitrate into agar plates or special paper. The patient's hand is carefully washed and dried, since previously dried sweat will leave a concentrated chloride residue and give a false positive result. After an extended period, or after exercise to increase secretions, the palm or fingers are placed on the test surface. Excess chlorides will combine with the silver nitrate to form visible silver chloride. For definitive diagnosis, sweat is collected by means of a plastic bag arrangement or some other method such as iontophoresis, and the specimen is subjected to quantitative electrolyte analysis. A sweat chloride content greater than 60 mEq/L is considered definitely abnormal. For diagnostic sweat collection it is recommended that the hand not be used, because the concentration of electrolytes in the palm is significantly greater than elsewhere. Also, the quantity of sweat collected for analysis is important; volumes less than 50 mg are not considered reliable.

A further caution pertains to normal values in persons over age 15. In children 60 mEq/L of chloride or sodium is considered the upper limit of normal. However, one study demonstrated 5% of children with cystic fibrosis who revealed sweat sodium values below 60 mEq/L and 3% of controls with values of 60–70 mEq/L. In a group of normal adults, 34% were found to have sweat sodium concentration greater than 60 mEq/L and 4% over 90 mEq/L. The diagnosis is therefore more difficult in adults.

Besides ordinary sweat collection, iontophoresis using sweat stimulants such as pilocarpine is available. The apparatus consists of small electrodes that create a tiny electric current to transport the stimulating drug into the skin. The method is painless and reliable; it is preferred to sweat collection by bag if the equipment is available.

Clinically normal heterozygotes and relatives of patients with cystic fibrosis have been reported to give abnormal sweat electrolytes in 5–20% of instances, although some investigators dispute these findings.

ENZYME ABNORMALITIES

CONGENITAL CHOLINESTERASE DEFICIENCY.—Cholinesterase is an enzyme best known for its role in regulation of nerve impulse transmission via breakdown of acetylcholine at the nerve synapse and neuromuscular junction. Two categories of cholinesterase are distinguished: acetylcholinesterase ("true cholinesterase"), found in RBC and nerve tissue, and serum cholinesterase ("pseudocholinesterase"). Cholinesterase deficiency became important when it was noted that such patients were predisposed to develop prolonged periods of apnea after administration of succinylcholine, a competitor to acetylcholine. Serum cholinesterase is thought to have greatest effect in degradation of succinylcholine. Serum cholinesterase deficiency may be congenital or acquired; the congenital type is uncommon but is responsible for most of the cases of prolonged apnea. The patient with congenital deficiency seems to have an abnormal ("atypical") cholinesterase, of which several genetic variants have been reported. Serum cholinesterase assay is the best screening test for cholinesterase deficiency. If abnormally low values are found, it is necessary to perform inhibition procedures with dibucaine and fluoride to distinguish congenital deficiency ("atypical" cholinesterase) from acquired deficiency of the normal enzyme. Deficiency of normal enzyme may cause prolonged succinylcholine apnea, but not predictably and usually only in very severe deficiency. Acute or chronic liver disease is the most frequent etiology for acquired deficiency. Hypoalbuminemia is frequently associated in hepatic or nonhepatic etiologies. A considerable number of drugs lower serum cholinesterase levels (p. 474) and thus might potentiate the action of succinylcholine.

Cholinesterase is also decreased in organic phosphate poisoning (p. 432); this affects both red cell and plasma enzyme levels. Screening tests have been devised using "dip-and-read" paper strips. These are probably satisfactory to rule out phosphate insecticide poisoning, but are not accurate in diagnosis of potential for succinylcholine apnea.

ALPHA$_1$ ANTITRYPSIN DEFICIENCY.—This deficiency has been associated with two different diseases: pulmonary emphysema in adults (relatively common) and cirrhosis in children (rare). This type of emphysema is characteristically (although not invariably) more severe in the lower lobes. A substantial number of those with homozygous antitrypsin deficiency are affected; reports differ on whether heterozygotes have increased predisposition to emphysema or to pulmonary disease. The most useful screening test at present is serum protein electrophoresis; alpha$_1$ globulin peak is absent or nearly absent in homozygotes. More defintive diagnosis, as well as separation of severe from intermediate degrees of deficiency, may be accomplished by quantitation of alpha$_1$ antitrypsin using methods such as immunodiffusion. Estrogen therapy (birth control pills) may elevate alpha$_1$ antitrypsin levels. Since this protein is one of the "acute phase reactants" in the alpha$_1$ and alpha$_2$ electrophoretic group, it is frequently elevated in acute infections and tissue destruction, and sometimes in malignancy.

REFERENCES

Anderson, C. M., and Freeman, M.: Sweat test results in normal persons of different ages compared with families with fibrocystic disease of the pancreas, Arch. Dis. Child. 35:581, 1960.

August, G. P.: Diagnosis of disorders of sexual maturation, Pediatr. Clin. North Am. 18:313, 1971.

Bartholomew, C. G., and Dahlin, D. C.: Intestinal polyposis and mucocutaneous pigmentation (Peutz-Jeghers syndrome), Minn. Med. 41:949, 1958.

Basford, R. L., and Henry, J. B.: Lactose intolerance in the adult, Postgrad. Med. 41: A-70, 1967.

Bell, R. S.: The radiographic manifestations of alpha-1 antitrypsin deficiency, Radiology 95:19, 1970.

Bruns, W. T., et al.: Test strip meconium screening for cystic fibrosis, Am. J. Dis. Child. 131:71, 1977.

Burkhart, J. M., et al.: The chondrodystrophies, Mayo Clin. Proc. 40:481, 1965.

Carpenter, G. G., et al.: Phenylalaninemia, Pediatr. Clin. North Am. 15:313, 1968.

Carter, C. H., et al.: Classification of inborn errors of metabolism associated with mental retardation, J. Florida Med. Assoc. 54:1147, 1967.

Climie, A. R. W.: Muscle biopsy: Technique and interpretation, Am. J. Clin. Pathol. 60:753, 1973.

Crouch, W. H., Jr., and Evanhoe, C. M.: Inborn errors of metabolism, Pediatr. Clin. North Am. 14:269, 1967.

Denborough, M. A.: Serum creatine phosphokinase and malignant hyperpyrexia, Br. Med. J. 4:408, 1975.

Dmowski, W. P., and Greenblatt, R. B.: Abnormal sexual differentiation, Am. Fam. Physician 3:73, 1971.

Dubin, I. N.: Idiopathic hemochromatosis and transfusion siderosis: A review, Am. J. Clin. Pathol. 25:514, 1955.

Ellis, F. R., et al.: Serum creatine phosphokinase and malignant hyperpyrexia, Br. Med. J. 1:584, 1976.

Epstein, C. J.: Prenatal diagnosis of genetic disorders, Adv. Intern. Med. 20:325, 1975.

Ferguson-Smith, M. A.: Chromosomal abnormalities. II: Sex chromosome defects, Hosp. Practice 5:88, 1970.

Frias, J. L.: Developments in laboratory diagnosis of chromosomal abnormalities, Ann. Clin. Lab. Sci. 5:369, 1975.

Gatti, R. A., and Good, R. A.: The immunological deficiency diseases, Med. Clin. North Am. 54:281, 1970.

Gerbie, A. B., and Simpson, J. L.: Antenatal detection of genetic disorders, Postgrad. Med. 59:129, 1976.

Good, R. A.: Disorders of the immune system, Hosp. Practice 2:39, 1967.

Guthrie, R.: Guthrie test and repeated examinations (questions and answers), J.A.M.A. 197:303, 1966.

Heidelberger, K. P.: Alpha-1-antitrypsin deficiency: A review: 1963–1975, Ann. Clin. Lab. Sci. 6:110, 1976.

Hirschhorn, K.: Chromosomal abnormalities. I: Autosomal defects, Hosp. Practice 5: 39, 1970.

Lebenthal, E.: Small intestine disaccharide deficiencies, Pediatr. Clin. North Am. 20:757, 1975.

MacDonald, M. J., et al.: Use of the lactose-ethanol tolerance test in diabetes, Am. J. Med. Sci. 269:193, 1975.

MacDonald, R. A.: Hemochromatosis, Postgrad. Med. 41:56, 1967.

Malone, M. J.: The cerebral lipoidoses, Pediatr. Clin. North Am. 23:303, 1976.

Melicow, M. M., and Uson, A. C.: A periodic table of sexual anomalies, J. Urol. 91: 402, 1964.

Milhorat, A. T., and Goldstone, L.: The carrier state in muscular dystrophy of the Duchenne type, J.A.M.A. 194:110, 1965.

Milunsky, A.: Prenatal diagnosis of genetic disorders, N. Engl. J. Med. 295:377, 1976.

Mone, J. C., and Mathe, W. E.: Qualitative and quantitative defects of pseudocholinesterase activity, Anaesthesia 22:55, 1967.

Myers, K. R.: A summary review of the diagnosis and pathology of the primary familial periodic paralyses, Ann. Clin. Lab. Sci. 5:216, 1975.

Nyhan, W. L., and Tocci, P.: Aminoaciduria, in DeGraff, A. C., and Creger, W. P. (eds.): *Annual Review of Medicine* (Palo Alto, CA: Annual Reviews, Inc., 1966), vol. 17, p. 133.

O'Brien, W. M., et al. Biochemical, pathologic, and clinical aspects of alkaptonuria, ochronosis, and ochronotic arthropathy, Am. J. Med. 34:813, 1963.

Osoba, D.: Thymic function, immunologic deficiency, and autoimmunity, Med. Clin. North Am. 56:319, 1972.

Rennart, O. M.: Syndrome of the defective lysosome—the genetic mucopolysaccharidoses, Ann. Clin. Lab. Sci. 5:355, 1975.

Rifkind, B. M. (ed.): Disorders of lipid metabolism, Clin. Endocrinol. Metab. 2:3, 1973.

Sharp, H. L.: Alpha-1 antitrypsin deficiency, Hosp. Practice 6:83, 1971.

Shwachman, H.: The sweat test, Pediatrics 30:167, 1962.

Schwachman, H.: Changing concepts of cystic fibrosis, Hosp. Practice 9:143, 1974.

Schwachman, H.: Gastrointestinal manifestations of cystic fibrosis, Pediatr. Clin. North Am. 22:787, 1975.

Smith, D. W.: Dysmorphology (teratology), J. Pediatr. 69:1150, 1966.

Snyderman, S. E.: Diagnosis of metabolic disease, Pediatr. Clin. North Am. 18:199, 1971.

Stanbury, J. B., et al.: *The Metabolic Basis of Inherited Disease* (3d ed.; New York: McGraw-Hill Book Company, Inc., 1972).

Starfield, B., and Holtzman, N. A.: A comparison of effectiveness of screening for phenylketonuria in the United States, United Kingdom, and Ireland, N. Engl. J. Med. 293:118, 1975.

Viamonte, M., Jr., et al.: Angiographic findings in a patient with tuberous sclerosis, Am. J. Roentgenol. 98:723, 1966.

Waisman, H. A.: Some newer inborn errors of metabolism, Pediatr. Clin. North Am. 13:469, 1966.

Welsh, J. D.: Isolated lactose deficiency in humans: Report on 100 patients. Medicine 49:257, 1970.

Zundel, W. S., and Tyler, F. H.: The muscular dystrophies, N. Engl. J. Med. 273:537, 596, 1965.

34 / Laboratory Analysis of Therapeutic and Toxic Substances

THERAPEUTIC DRUG MONITORING

AMONG THE REASONS for obtaining drug levels in blood when prescribing certain medications are:

1. Estimation of therapeutic margin (index), to find (a) whether the administered dose attains recognized levels of therapeutic effectiveness; (b) how closely an effective dose approaches possible toxicity. If blood values are close to toxic levels, the physician may wish to ascertain whether a lower dose would still be effective.

2. Investigation of unexpected patient response to medication. A standard dose may be associated either with insufficient response or with toxicity. In either case, finding that drug blood levels are low, in the normal therapeutic range or increased permits a much more rational investigation. Some of the factors to be considered include: (a) patient compliance (Has the proper dose been taken, and if so, at the right time?); (b) patient biologic variation in drug absorption, utilization and excretion; (c) effects of drug interaction with other medications; (d) effects of organ disease (e.g., severe liver disease); and (e) which of several drugs given concurrently is responsible for toxicity (What changes are there from previous baselines?).

Drug monitoring is carried out in two basic situations: in an isolated attempt to find the reason for therapeutic failure (either toxic symptoms or nonresponse to therapy) and in obtaining a baseline value after sufficient time has elapsed for stabilization. Baseline values are needed to enable comparison with future values if trouble develops and to establish the relationship of a patient's drug blood level to accepted therapeutic range. Many authorities recommend baseline measurements when patients are placed on long-term therapy. They feel this information can be invaluable in future emergencies by saving time and eliminating guesswork.

To receive adequate service, the physician must provide the laboratory with certain information as well as the patient specimen. This includes the exact drug or drugs to be assayed, patient age, time elapsed from the last dose until the specimen was obtained, drug dose and route of administration. All of these factors affect normal values. It is also desirable to state the reason for the assay and provide a list of medications the patient is receiving.

425

Methods used in drug assay include gas-liquid chromography (technically difficult but especially useful when several drugs are being administered simultaneously, as frequently occurs in epileptics); thin-layer chromatography (more frequently used for the hypnotic drugs); radioimmunoassay (RIA); and enzyme-multiplied immunoassay (EMIT).

One of the major reasons that therapeutic drug monitoring has not achieved wider acceptance is that reliable results are frequently not available. Even when they are, the time needed to obtain a report may be several days rather than several hours. It is essential that the physician be certain that his reference laboratory, whether local or not, is providing reliable results. Reliability can be investigated in several ways: by splitting patient samples to be evaluated between the laboratory and a reference laboratory whose work is known to be good (but if isolated values are discrepant, a question may arise as to who is correct); by splitting samples and sending one portion one week and the remainder the next week; or by obtaining standards from commercial companies and submitting these as unknowns. Most good reference laboratories will do a reasonable amount of such testing without charge if requested to do so beforehand.

In some situations, assay results may be misleading without additional information. In certain drugs, e.g., diphenylhydantoin (Dilantin), digitoxin and quinidine, a high percentage is bound to serum albumin and only the nonbound fraction is metabolically active. This is similar to thyroid hormone protein binding, discussed in Chapter 28. The free (nonbound) fraction may be increased in hypoalbuminemia or in conditions that change protein binding, such as uremia or administration of drugs that block binding or compete for binding sites. Drug level assays measure total drug and do not reflect changes in protein binding. In addition, some drugs, diseases or metabolic states may potentiate or inhibit the action of certain therapeutic agents without altering blood levels or protein binding. An example is digoxin toxicity induced by hypokalemia.

Anticonvulsant Therapy

Most epileptics can be controlled with diphenylhydantoin (Dilantin), primidone (Mysoline), phenobarbital or other agents. Frequently, drug combinations are required. Therapy is usually a long-term project. When toxicity develops, many of these therapeutic agents produce symptoms that could be due to CNS disease, such as confusion, somnolence and various changes in mental behavior. Some of the drugs, such as primidone, must be carefully brought to therapeutic level by stages rather than in a single dose. Most antiepileptic drugs are administered to control seizures, but if seizures are infrequent, it is difficult to be certain that the medication is sufficient to prevent future episodes. When drug combinations are used, levels for all the agents should be obtained so that if only one drug is involved in toxicity or therapeutic failure, it can be identified.

When specimens are sent to the laboratory for drug assay, the physician should list all drugs being administered. Some are metabolized to substances which themselves have antiepileptic activity (e.g., primidone is partially metabolized to phenobarbital), and the laboratory would have to assay both the parent drug and its metabolite. Without a complete list of medications, there is a good chance that one or more drugs will be overlooked. Once drug blood levels have been obtained, the physician should remember that they are often not linear in relation to dose, so that a percentage change in dose may not result in the same percentage change in blood level. Repeated assays may be needed to guide dosage to produce desired blood levels. Finally, published therapeutic ranges may not predict the individual response of some patients to the drug. Clinical judgment as well as laboratory values must be used.

Some information on drug metabolism is necessary to interpret blood level information. Peak diphenylhydantoin levels are attained in 4–8 hours following oral intake and within 15 minutes after intravenous therapy. Serum half-life (time for half of the drug to disappear from serum) varies from 7–42 hours, with the average about 24 hours. Obtaining a steady state requires 5–10 days. Between 70 and 95% is bound to serum protein. Over two thirds is metabolized in the liver by hepatic cell microsomes. Certain drugs, such as disulfiram (Antabuse), isoniazid, Coumadin and chloramphenicol, increase diphenylhydantoin serum levels by interfering with its metabolism and thereby prolonging serum half-life. Decreased blood levels are said to occur in uremia. Administration of diphenylhydantoin by intramuscular injection rather than oral intake reduces blood levels about 50%. The therapeutic range for diphenylhydantoin is approximately 10–20 μg/ml (at least 3 hours after the last dose). For primidone, peak serum concentration occurs in 2–3 hours but may be prolonged in some patients. Half-life is 3–7 hours, but with long-term therapy it may be doubled or tripled. A steady state is reached in 4–7 days. About 50% is bound to serum protein. The therapeutic range is 7–15 μg/ml. Phenobarbital has an average half-life of 96 hours. Reaching a steady state takes 2–3 weeks. Therapeutic range is 15–40 μg/ml.

Lithium

Lithium carbonate is used for control of the manic phase of manic-depressive psychiatric states. Blood levels vary considerably during the day, so that some authorities recommend a lithium tolerance test (basal specimen, lithium dose and then specimens at 1, 3 and 6 hours after the dose) to ascertain the patient's handling of the medication. Specimens for conventional monitoring are usually obtained 12 hours after the last dose. The usual laboratory method is flame photometry; the usual therapeutic range is 0.5–2.0 mEq/L.

Procainamide

This agent is used to control certain cardiac ventricular arrythmias. Its serum half-life is approximately 3 hours. After administration, there is approximately 30% variation in serum levels during 3 hours and 50% during 6 hours. The usual therapeutic range is 4–8 mg/L. Toxicity begins in the 8–16 mg/L area and is common over 16 mg/L (3 hours after the last dose).

Quinidine

Quinidine is used to convert or suppress cardiac atrial and ventricular arrythmias. The therapeutic range is approximately 3–6 mg/L; the borderline between therapeutic range and toxicity is narrower than for procainamide. Oral dose half-life is 6–8 hours with serum peak at 2 hours.

Digoxin

This agent could be included in the section on toxicology, since the majority of serum assay requests are to investigate possible digoxin toxicity. However, since an increasing number of studies have demonstrated unsuspected overdosage or underdosage (30% toxicity and 11% underdigitalization in one study), requests for baseline levels are becoming more frequent. The volume of requests and the relative ease of performance (by RIA or EMIT) make this assay readily available, even in smaller laboratories. The widespread use of digoxin, the narrow borderline between therapeutic range and toxicity, and the nonspecific nature of mild or moderate toxic signs and symptoms that mimic a variety of common disorders (diarrhea, nausea, arrythmias and ECG changes) contribute to the need for serum assay.

Normal therapeutic range is 0.5–2.0 μg/100 ml. Serum half-life is approximately 32 hours. After an oral dose is given, serum levels rise to a peak in 30–90 minutes and then slowly decline until a plateau is reached about 6–8 hours after administration. Digoxin assay specimens must be drawn at least 6 hours after the last dose in either oral or intravenous administration, to avoid blood levels that are significantly higher than would be the case when tissue levels have equilibrated (the time span mentioned is minimum elapsed time; specimens may be drawn later; in many cases more information is obtained from a sample drawn shortly before the next scheduled dose).

Various metabolic disorders and medications may alter body concentration or serum levels of digoxin or may affect myocardial response to usual dosage. The kidney is the major route of excretion, and a decrease in renal function sufficient to raise serum creatinine will elevate serum digoxin levels. Hypothyroidism will also increase digoxin serum values. On the other hand, certain conditions affect patient response to digitalis without affecting blood levels. Myocardial sensitivity to digoxin, regardless of dose, is increased by acute myocardial damage, hypokalemia, hypercalcemia, hypermagnesemia, alkalosis, tissue anoxia and glucagon. Drugs that produce hypokalemia (including various diuretics, amphotericin B, corticosteroids or glucose infusion) thus predispose to toxicity. Other medications, such as phenylbutasone, diphenylhydantoin (Dilantin) and barbiturates (which enhance degradation), or Kaopectate, antacids, cholestyramine and oral aminoglycoside antibiotics (which interfere with absorption), tend to be antagonistic to the effect of digitalis.

In various studies, there is a certain amount of overlap in the area that statistically separates normally digitalized patients from those with toxicity. This overlap exists because it is difficult to recognize mild degrees of toxicity, because patient sensitivity to digitalis varies, and because the assay technique itself, no matter how well done, like all laboratory tests displays a certain amount of variation when repeated determinations are performed on the same specimen. Regardless of these problems, if the clinical picture does not agree with the level of toxicity predicted by digoxin assay values and laboratory quality control is adequate, the physician should not dismiss or ignore the assay results but should investigate the possibility of interference by improper specimen time interval, drug interaction or metabolic alterations. If necessary, the assay can be repeated.

Antibiotics

Methods of estimating antibiotic therapeutic effectiveness have been discussed elsewhere (pp. 163 and 165). Several antibiotics possess therapeutic ranges whose upper limits border on toxicity. Serum assays for several of these have been developed, most commonly using RIA. One example will be used to illustrate general principles. Gentamicin (Garamycin) is one of the aminoglycoside antibiotics that is active against gram-negative organisms including *Pseudomonas aeruginosa*. Unfortunately, side effects include ototoxicity and nephrotoxicity. Drug excretion is mainly through renal glomerular filtration. Serum peak levels and residual levels both provide valuable information. Residual levels are obtained just prior to the next dose. Specimens at this time correlate best with nephrotoxicity, especially when values are greater than 4 μg/ml. Peak levels are obtained approximately 30 minutes after the end of intravenous infusion and 1 hour after intramuscular injection. Peak levels correlate best with therapeutic effectiveness and possibly with ototoxicity. Normal values are usually considered 4–8 μg/ml. Values less than 4 μg/ml may be ineffective, while those over 10 μg/ml predispose to toxicity. Gentamicin assay is desirable because serum levels differ considerably between patients receiving the same dose, while serum gentamicin half-life is equally variable. Standard doses or use of nomograms based on serum creatinine fail to predict blood concentration accurately for peak or for residual levels in a substantial number of patients, even with adequate renal function. When renal function is impaired or when nephrotoxic antibiotics have previously been administered, serum assay becomes essential.

Morphine and Related Alkaloids

There has been considerable interest in assay methods for alkaloids in urine, to screen for possible drug abuse or to determine if known addicts remain free of illicit drugs while on treatment or afterward. Methods available include thin-layer chromatography, gas-liquid chromatography, fluorescent spectrophotometry, hemagglutination inhibition (HI) and RIA. Technically, HI and RIA are the simplest of these, have adequate sensitivity and are more likely than the others to yield reliable results in the average laboratory. Gas-liquid chromatography has the advantage that it can detect several drugs simultaneously.

Other Substances

A growing list of compounds can be assayed using various techniques, including salicylates, methotrexate, aminophylline (theophylline), various sedative and hypnotic drugs and various tranquilizers.

Overdose Therapy

Treatment of drug overdose by dialysis or other means can often be assisted with the objective information derived from serum drug levels. In some cases, drug screening may reveal additional drugs or substances, such as alcohol, which affect management or clinical response.

LABORATORY TOXICOLOGY

Toxicology includes a selected list of conditions that seem especially important in drug overdose and poisoning.

Lead

Lead exposure in adults is most often due to occupational hazard (as in exposure to gasoline additives and smelting) or to homemade "moonshine" whiskey distilled in lead-containing equipment. Children usually are affected when they eat lead-containing paint. The acute syndrome is uncommon. Symptoms may include "lead colic" (crampy abdominal pain, constipation, occasional bloody diarrhea), and in 50% of patients, hypertensive encephalopathy. Chronic poisoning is more common. Its varying symptoms may include lead colic, constipation with anorexia (85% of patients), peripheral neuritis (wrist drop) in adults and lead encephalopathy (headache, convulsions) in children. A "lead line" is frequently present just below the epiphyses (in approximately 70% of patients with clinical symptoms and 20–40% with abnormal exposure but no symptoms). Most patients develop slight to moderate anemia, usually hypochromic but sometimes normochromic. Basophilic stippled RBC are the most characteristic peripheral blood finding. Some authors claim stippling is invariably present; others report stippling absent in 70–80% of cases. Normal persons may have as many as 500 stippled cells per 1 million RBC. The reticulocyte count is usually greater than 4%.

Body intake of lead produces biochemical effects on heme synthesis (see Fig 20–2). Delta-aminolevulinic acid dehydrase (ALA-D), which converts ALA to porphobilinogen, is decreased as early as the 4th day after exposure begins. Once ALA-D is reduced, persistence of abnormality correlates with the amount of lead in body tissues (body burden), so that ALA-D remains reduced as long as significant quantities of lead remain. Therefore, after chronic lead exposure, low ALA-D values may persist for years even though exposure has ceased. The level of ALA-D is also a very sensitive indicator of lead toxicity and is usually reduced to 50% or less of normal activity when blood lead values are in the 30–50 μg/100 ml range. Unfortunately, ALA-D reaches a plateau when marked reduction takes place, so that it cannot be used to quantitate degree of exposure. In addition, this enzyme must be assayed within 24 hours after securing the blood specimen. Relatively few laboratories perform the test, although it is of only moderate technical difficulty.

Intake of lead ordinarily results in rapid urinary lead excretion. If excessive lead exposure continues, lead is stored in bone. If bone storage capacity is exceeded, lead accumulates in soft tissues. Blood lead levels depend on the relationship between intake, storage and excretion. Blood lead basically is a measurement of acute (current) exposure but is influenced by previous storage. Blood lead values of 10–20 μg/100 ml (whole blood) are considered normal. Values higher than 40 μg/100 ml are considered abnormal, and symptoms of lead poisoning are associated with levels higher than 80 μg/100 ml, although mild symptoms may occur at 50 μg/100 ml in children. Blood lead assay takes considerable experience and dedication to perform accurately. Contamination is a major headache – in drawing the specimen, in sample tubes, in laboratory glassware and in the assay procedure itself.

Another procedure frequently used is urine ALA. Blood and urine ALA increase when blood ALA-D is considerably reduced. Therefore, ALA also becomes an indicator of body lead burden, and urine ALA begins to increase when blood lead values are higher than 40 μg/100 ml. Disadvantages of urine ALA are difficulties in 24-hour urine collection or, if random specimens are used, the effects of urine concentration or dilution on apparent ALA concentration. In addition, at least one investigator found that urine ALA was normal in a significant number of cases when blood lead was in the 40–80 μg/100 ml (mildly to moderately abnormal) range. Light, room temperature, and alkaline pH all decrease ALA levels. If ALA determination is not done immediately, the specimen must be refrigerated and kept in the dark (collection bottle wrapped in paper or foil) with the specimen acidified, using glacial acetic or tartaric acid.

If a patient is subjected to continuous lead exposure of sufficient magnitude, blood lead, urine lead excretion, ALA-D and urine ALA all correlate well. If the exposure ceases before laboratory tests are made, blood lead (and sometimes even urine lead) may decrease relative to ALA-D or urine ALA. Assay of ALA-D is the most sensitive of these tests. In fact, certain patients whose urine ALA and blood lead are within normal limits may display mild to moderate decrease in ALA-D. It remains to be determined whether in all cases this reflects previous toxicity or simply means that ALA-D levels between 50 and 100% of normal are too easily produced to mean truly abnormal lead exposure.

Urine lead excretion has also been employed as an index of exposure, since blood lead values change more rapidly than urine lead excretion. However, excretion values depend on 24-hour urine specimens, with the usual difficulty in complete collection. A further problem is that excretion values may be normal in borderline or past exposure. Urine lead has been measured after administration of a chelating agent such as EDTA, which mobilizes body stores of lead. This is a more satisfactory technique than ordinary urine excretion for determining body burden (i.e., previous exposure). Abnormal exposure is suggested when 24-hour urine lead excretion is greater than 1 μg per milligram of Ca-EDTA administered. Disadvantages are those of incomplete urine collection, difficulty in accurate lead measurement and occasional cases of EDTA toxicity.

Erythrocyte protoporphyrin (zinc protoporphyrin) is still another indicator of lead exposure. Lead inhibits heme synthetase, an enzyme that incorporates iron into protoporphyrin to form heme. Decreased protoporphyrin conversion leads to increased RBC protoporphyrin. In normal persons, protoporphyrin is extracted and measured as a free base, so that the product has been called free erythrocyte protoporphyrin. In patients with lead poisoning, protoporphyrin is found complexed to zinc rather than iron, hence the term zinc protoporphyrin. Since protoporphyrin is fluorescent, most laboratory analytic techniques involve fluorescent methods. In fact, some have used visual RBC fluorescence (in a heparinized wet preparation using a microscope equipped with ultraviolet light) as a rapid screening test for clinical lead poisoning.

Urinary coproporphyrin III excretion is usually, although not invariably, increased in clinically evident lead poisoning. Since this compound fluoresces under Wood's light, simple screening tests have been devised based on fluorescence of coproporphyrin III in urine specimens under ultraviolet light.

Other Toxic Agents

HEAVY METALS. — Mercury, arsenic, bismuth and antimony are included. Urine is preferred over blood samples. Hair and nails are useful for arsenic examination.

ORGANIC PHOSPHATE. — Certain insecticides such as parathion and the less powerful malathion are inhibitors of the enzyme cholinesterase. This allows overproduction of acetylcholine at nerve-muscle junctions. Symptoms include muscle twitching, cramps and weakness; parasympathetic effects such as pinpoint pupils, nausea, sweating, diarrhea and salivation; and various central nervous system aberrations. Laboratory diagnosis is based on finding decreased cholinesterase in RBC or plasma. Levels in RBC reflect poisoning more accurately than do plasma values, which are reduced by many conditions and drugs. Screening tests are generally based on plasma measurement (p. 422). A normal result rules out anticholinesterase toxicity.

SALICYLATE. — Salicylate is discussed on p. 117. The Phenistix dipstick test on plasma and the ferric chloride test on urine are useful screening procedures.

BARBITURATES AND GLUTETHIMIDE (*Doriden*). — These are the most common vehicles of drug-overdose suicide. In testing, either anticoagulated (not heparinized) whole blood or urine can be used; blood is preferred. Thin-layer chromatography is used both for screening and to identify the individual substance involved. Chemical screening tests are also available. It is preferable to secure both blood and urine specimens plus gastric contents, if available.

PHENOTHIAZINE TRANQUILIZERS. — Urine is tested with Phenistix or ferric chloride procedure.

NARCOTIC ALKALOIDS. — Urine is most commonly used for screening purposes. A syndrome of pulmonary vasculitis in addicts caused by foreign-particle injection has been reported, with lung scan findings suggestive of embolization and multiple small chest x-ray infiltrates.

CARDIAC DRUGS. — The digitalis family, procainamide and quinidine may be toxic under certain conditions (p. 427). Radioisotope immunoassay techniques are available for digitalis family serum measurement. In general, patients with clear-cut evidence of digitalis toxicity and those who are clinically normal usually can be separated. In borderline or questionable situations, it is very difficult to rely on any theoretical upper limit of normal, since many factors (electrolyte concentrations, medications, acid-base, thyroid status and individual patient variation) may affect cardiac response to a given level of digitalis (p. 428).

ALCOHOL. — Most courts of law follow the recommendations of the National Safety Council on alcohol and drugs:

Blood alcohol

Below 0.05%: No influence by alcohol within the meaning of the law.

Between 0.05 and 0.10%: A liberal, wide zone in which alcohol influence usually is present, but courts of law are advised to consider the person's behavior and circumstances leading to the arrest in making their decision.

Above 0.10%: Definite evidence of being "under the influence," since most persons with this concentration will have lost, to a measurable extent, some of that clearness of intellect and self-control they would normally possess.

Alcohol has a considerable number of metabolic and toxic effects that may directly or indirectly involve the clinical laboratory. Liver manifestations include gamma glutamyl transpeptidase elevation (p. 211), fatty liver (p. 217), acute alcoholic hepatitis ("active cirrhosis," p. 217) or Laennec's cirrhosis; and may lead indirectly to bleeding from esophageal varices or to cytopenias from hypersplenism (p. 19) or through other mechanisms. Red cell macrocytosis is frequently associated with chronic alcoholism, and nutritional anemia such as that due to folic acid (p. 12) may be present. Other conditions include acute pancreatitis (p. 309), gastritis, alcoholic hypoglycemia (p. 331), various neurologic abnormalities, and subdural hematoma (p. 204). The chronic alcoholic is more susceptible to infection (p. 163). Finally, alcohol interacts with a variety of medications. It potentiates many of the CNS depressants, such as various sedatives, narcotics, hypnotics and tranquilizers (especially chlordiazepoxide (Librium) and diazepam (Valium). Alcohol is a factor in many cases of overdose, even when the patient has no history of alcohol intake or denies intake. The presence of alcohol should be suspected when toxicity symptoms from barbiturates or other medications are associated with blood levels that normally would be considered safe. Alcohol may antagonize the action of various other medications, such as Coumadin and diphenylhydantoin (Dilantin). When blood specimens are collected, a simple precaution, not always remembered, is to avoid alcohol wipes when cleansing the skin prior to venipuncture.

REFERENCES

Albahary, C.: Lead and hemopoiesis, Am. J. Med. 52:367, 1972.

Aldrich, F. D.: Cholinesterase assays: Their usefulness in diagnosis of anticholinesterase intoxication, Clin. Toxicol. 2:445, 1969.

Anderson, A. C., et al.: Determination of serum gentamicin sulfate levels, Arch. Intern. Med. 136:785, 1976.

Basalt, R. C., et al.: Therapeutic and toxic concentrations of more than 100 toxicologically significant drugs in blood, plasma, or serum: A tabulation, Clin. Chem. 21: 44, 1975.

Berman, P. H.: Management of seizure disorders with anticonvulsant drugs; current concepts. Pediatr. Clin. North Am. 23:443, 1976.

Butler, U. P., et al.: Steps to safer digitalization, Patient Care 8:105, 1974.

Chisolm, J. J.: Childhood lead intoxication, Med. Times 98:92, 1970.

Chisholm, J. J.: The continuing hazard of lead poisoning, Hosp. Practice 8:127, 1973.

Fried, F. E., and Malek-Ahmadi, P.: Bromism: Recent perspectives, South. Med. J. 68:220, 1976.

Garry, P. J.: Serum cholinesterase variants: Examination of several differential inhibitors, salts and buffers used to measure enzyme activity, Clin. Chem. 17:183, 1971.

Gibaldi, M., and Levy, G.: Pharmacokinetics in clinical practice. 2. Applications, J.A.M.A. 235:1987, 1976.

Green, M.: Immediate management of accidental poisoning in children, Hosp. Med. 3:114, 1967.

Hughes, J. M., and Merson, M. H.: Fish and shellfish poisoning, N. Engl. J. Med. 295:1117, 1976.

Kutt, H., and Penry, J. K.: Usefulness of blood levels of antiepileptic drugs, Arch. Neurol. 31:283, 1974.

Lamola, A. A., et al.: Zinc protoporphyrin (ZPP): A simple, sensitive, fluorometric screening test for lead poisoning, Clin. Chem. 21:93, 1975.

Lorny, P. P., and Vestal, R. E.: Drug prescribing for the elderly, Hosp. Practice 11:111, 1976.

Lum, G., et al.: Plasma levels and the antiarrhythmic effects of procainamide, Ann. Clin. Lab. Sci. 6:358, 1976.

Mason, M. F., et al.: Alcohol, traffic, and chemical testing in the United States: A résumé and some remaining problems, Clin. Chem. 20:162, 1974.

Morello, J. A.: Assays of antibiotic agents in serum, Lab. Med. 7:30, 1976.

Morgan, J. M., and Burch, H. B.: Comparative tests for diagnosis of lead poisoning, Arch. Intern. Med. 130:335, 1972.

Mulvihill, J. J., et al.: Fetal alcohol syndrome: Seven new cases, Am. J. Obstet. Gynecol. 125:937, 1976.

Nieburg, P. I., et al.: Red blood cell delta-aminolevulinic acid dehydrase activity: An index of body lead burden, Am. J. Dis. Child. 127:348, 1974.

Ravel, R., and Schall, R. F., Jr.: Pitfalls in iodine-125 digoxin measurement, Ann. Clin. Lab. Sci. 6:365, 1976.

Smith, T. W.: Measurement of serum digitalis glycosides: Clinical implications, Circulation 43:179, 1971.

Vincent, W. F., and Ullman, W. W.: Measurement of urinary delta-aminolevulinic acid in detection of childhood lead poisoning, Am. J. Clin. Pathol. 53:963, 1970.

Vincent, W. F., and Ullman, W. W.: The preservation of urine specimens for delta-aminolevulinic acid determinations, Clin. Chem. 16:612, 1970.

Wilder, B. J., and Perchalski, R. J.: How assay methods can guide drug therapy for epileptic patients, Mod. Med. 43(13):68, 1975.

Winek, C. L.: Laboratory criteria for the adequacy of treatment and significance of blood levels, Clin. Toxicol. 3:541, 1970.

Young, D. S., et al.: Effects of drugs on clinical laboratory tests, Clin. Chem. 21(5):1D, 1975.

Zarkowsky, H. S.: The Lead Problem in Children: Dictum and Polemic, in Gluck, L. (ed.): *Current Problems in Pediatrics* (Chicago: Year Book Medical Publishers, Inc., July, 1976).

35 / Special Category Tests

THIS CHAPTER includes tests that should be mentioned for special reasons but seem better left out of the main text for the sake of succinctness. Some are too new, and original reports need independent confirmation; some have generated highly favorable evaluations that have not been confirmed by the experience of others; some are older tests that are being replaced but occupy a prominent place in the older medical literature, and others are rarely used procedures that might be useful in very unusual circumstances. The tests are listed by the chapters in which they could have been placed.

Chapter 2. Factor Deficiency Anemia

FIGLU AND MMA.—*Formiminoglutamic acid* (FIGLU) is a compound that is derived from the amino acid histidine and requires active folic acid (tetrahydrofolic acid) for normal metabolism to glutamic acid. In significant folic acid deficiency, FIGLU cannot be properly utilized and is excreted into the urine in abnormal quantities. Vitamin B_{12} deficiency will also influence FIGLU metabolism to some extent, because B_{12} is necessary for the conversion of folic acid to metabolically active tetrahydrofolic acid. Urine assay for FIGLU has proved rather difficult, and several techniques are available. Some of these have poor sensitivity, others are not sufficiently specific and others are technically difficult. To circumvent some of the problems of sensitivity and specificity, a loading dose of oral histidine (15 gm, in 3 divided doses in 12 hours) with a 24-hour urine collection for FIGLU has proved helpful. Challenge with a loading dose of histidine augments FIGLU excretion in folic acid-deficient states. Excretion of FIGLU after histidine loading is reported to be a reasonably accurate parameter of folic acid deficiency. However, FIGLU measurement is not widely available. Histidine may produce a reticulocyte response in megaloblastic anemia. Collection of urine must be done using a container with acid as a preservative. Many diseases produce elevated FIGLU excretion, so false positive results will be common. Treatment of megaloblastic anemia returns FIGLU to normal.

Methylmalonic acid (MMA) excretion has been proposed as a specific test for B_{12} deficiency. However, the assay is difficult and not always reliable; patients with mild serum B_{12} decrease and mild megaloblastosis may still have normal MMA values, and some patients with folic acid deficiency anemia are reported to have elevated urine MMA levels because of coexisting B_{12} deficiency. Treatment of B_{12} deficiency restores MMA to normal.

With availability of serum B_{12} and folic acid assay, there seems little use for FIGLU or MMA determination.

THE "THERAPEUTIC TRIAL." — In deficiency diseases, treatment with the specific agent that is lacking will give a characteristic response in certain laboratory tests. This response may be used as a confirmation of the original diagnosis. Failure to obtain the expected response means that doubt is cast on the original diagnosis; that treatment has been inadequate in dosage, absorption, utilization or type of agent used, or that some other condition is present that is interfering with treatment or possibly is superimposed on the more obvious deficiency problem. The two usual deficiency diseases are chronic iron deficiency and vitamin B_{12} or folic acid deficiency. When a test agent such as iron is given in therapeutic dose, a reticulocyte response should be manifest in 3–7 days, with values at least twice normal (or significantly elevated over baseline values if the baseline is already elevated). Usually, the reticulocyte count is normal or only slightly elevated in uncomplicated hematologic deficiency diseases. If the baseline reticulocyte values are already significantly elevated over normal range in a suspected deficiency disease, this suggests either previous treatment (or, in some cases, a response to hospital diet), wrong diagnosis or some other superimposed factor (such as recent acute blood loss superimposed on chronic iron deficiency anemia). If the baseline values are already over twice normal, it may not be possible to document a response. Once the correct replacement substance is given in adequate dosage, hemoglobin values generally rise toward normal at a rate of approximately 1 gm/100 ml/week.

Two major cautions must be made regarding the "therapeutic trial": (1) it never takes the place of a careful, systematic search for the etiology of a suspected deficiency state, and (2) the patient may respond to one agent and at the same time have another factor deficiency or more serious underlying disease.

A "therapeutic trial" usually is initiated with therapeutic doses of the test agent. This standard procedure will not differentiate vitamin B_{12} from folic acid deficiency, since therapeutic doses of either will invoke a reticulocyte response in deficiency due to the other. If a therapeutic trial is desired in these circumstances, a small physiologic dose should be used — such as 1 μg/vitamin B_{12}/ day for 10 days, or 100 μg folic acid /day for 10 days. At least 10 days should elapse between completion of one trial agent and beginning of another. Also, the patient should be on a diet deficient in folic acid or B_{12}, and baseline reticulocyte studies should be performed for a week on this diet before initiation of the actual trial. Generally, in vitamin B_{12} deficiency, the Schilling test (without intrinsic factor) gives the same information, and can be repeated with the addition of intrinsic factor to pinpoint the etiology. In folic acid deficiency, a therapeutic trial may be helpful in establishing the diagnosis. The main drawback of the "therapeutic trial" in diagnosis is the time involved.

ASSAY FOR INTRINSIC FACTOR AND FOR ANTIBODY TO INTRINSIC FACTOR. — In vitro techniques have been described for assay of these substances. For intrinsic factor, aspiration of gastric juice is necessary. The specimens from routine gastric analysis are satisfactory. Antibody to intrinsic factor is said to occur in approximately two thirds of pernicious anemia patients. Presence of antibody is reported to be virtually diagnostic for pernicious anemia. Neither of these two assays seems at present to be widely used or readily available.

SERUM FERRITIN. — Ferritin is a major iron-storage protein located in reticuloendothelial cells. Radioimmunoassay can detect the small quantity normally present in serum. Reports indicate that serum ferritin is, in most cases, a reliable indicator of body iron stores. Information obtained is equivalent to that obtained from bone marrow iron examination. Normal mean values are about 3 times as high in adult males as in females; the sex difference is much less in children and the elderly. Values are decreased in chronic iron deficiency and increased in iron overload. Serum ferritin values are elevated in patients with acute or chronic liver disease, acute or chronic infection or inflammation, many patients with chronic illnesses which have an inflammatory component (such as rheumatoid arthritis), chronic hemolytic anemias, and some patients with leukemia or neoplasia. Bone marrow iron may be normal or increased in these patients; and serum ferritin levels may not always be above normal population range (although presumably increased over what would have been the expected value before illness). In chronic renal disease, ferritin is normal or slightly elevated. Transfusions tend to elevate ferritin levels.

Serum ferritin provides more information than serum iron alone, because serum iron may be decreased in both iron deficiency and certain chronic diseases while ferritin is decreased only in chronic iron deficiency. However, if chronic inflammation or neoplasia is superimposed on chronic iron deficiency, serum ferritin may be falsely elevated into normal range.

REFERENCES

Chanarin, I.: *The Megaloblastic Anaemias* (Oxford: Blackwell Scientific Publications, 1969).

Chanarin, I., et al.: Urinary excretion of histidine derivatives in megaloblastic anemia and other conditions and a comparison with the folic acid clearance test, J. Clin. Pathol. 15:269, 1962.

Drysdale, J. W. et al.: Human isoferritins in normal and disease states, Semin. Hematol. 14:71, 1977.

Herbert, V.: Detection of malabsorption of vitamin B_{12} due to gastric or intestinal dysfunction, Semin. Nucl. Med. 2:220, 1972.

Jacobs, A. and Worwood, M.: Ferritin in serum: Clinical and biochemical implications, N. Engl. J. Med. 292:951, 1975.

Lipschitz, D. A., et al.: A. clinical evaluation of serum ferritin as an index of iron stores, N. Engl. J. Med. 290:1213, 1974.

Chapter 4. Depletion Anemia

PAROXYSMAL COLD HEMOGLOBINURIA. — This is a rare but famous cause of hemolytic anemia. The most frequent etiology is syphilis. Cold temperatures trigger episodes of intravascular hemolysis, producing hemoglobinuria. The Donath-Landsteiner test detects cold-acting antibodies responsible for this hemolysis.

SICKLE HEMOGLOBIN SCREENING TESTS. — *Dithionate tests.* — These tests (Sickledex and other trade names) are becoming widely used. They seem to be based on deoxygenation of sickle hemoglobin, which then becomes insoluble and precipitates in certain media. The test is said to be reliable, with certain drawbacks that should be appreciated. False negative results may be obtained in patients whose hemoglobin is less than 10 gm/100 ml (or hematocrit 30%) unless hematocrit is adjusted by removing plasma. Reagents may deteriorate and inactivate. Dysglobulinemia (Waldenström's, myeloma, cryoglobulinemia) may interfere. Infants aged less than 6 months may react negatively, because fetal hemoglobin is not yet completely transferred to adult hemoglobin. Certain rare non-S sickling hemoglobins will be positive.

Murayama test. — Recently proposed as a specific screening test for Hgb S, this test is based on differential solubility of S. hemoglobin at different temperatures. The only other non-S hemoglobin thus far reported positive is C (Harlem), which is rare and which also sickles in other sickling tests, but migrates with Hgb C on electrophoresis. However, the Murayama test is too cumbersome in its present form to use in most laboratories.

REFERENCES

Nalbandian, R. M., et al.: Sickledex test for hemoglobin S: A critique, J.A.M.A. 218: 1679, 1971.
Nalbandian, R. M., et al.: Molecular basis for the specific test for hemoglobin S (Murayama test), Ann. Clin. Lab. Sci. 1:26, 1971.

Chapter 6. Leukemia, Lymphomas and Myeloproliferative Syndromes

SERUM MURAMIDASE (LYSOZYME) ASSAY. — Muramidase (formerly called lysozyme) is an enzyme that is present in many body secretions and in serum. The majority of serum activity is derived from monocytes and cells from the myelocytic series (except blasts). Most excretion occurs via kidney tubules, and serum levels therefore have a direct relationship to renal function as estimated by serum BUN or creatinine.

Serum muramidase has been used to help differentiate among different types of leukemia. More than 90% of patients with myelomonocytic and "pure" monocytic leukemia have elevated values. Patients with lymphocytic leukemia almost always have normal or low values. In chronic myelogenous leukemia that is positive for the Philadelphia chromosome, values are usually normal, and in the form negative for the Philadelphia chromosome, serum muramidase levels are elevated. In acute myelogenous leukemia, values are usually elevated, but may be normal or even reduced.

VITAMIN B_{12} AND B_{12} BINDING CAPACITY ASSAY. — In polycythemia vera, serum B_{12} levels have been reported increased in approximately 35% of patients and serum B_{12} binding capacity in approximately 70%, whereas these assays are usually normal in patients with secondary polycythemia. In patients with other types of hematologic disease, B_{12} binding capacity increases roughly in proportion to the size of the granulocyte mass. The greatest increases, therefore, tend to occur in chronic myelogenous leukemia.

CYTOCHEMICAL STAINS IN HEMATOPOIETIC MALIGNANCY. — The myelo-peroxidase reaction and Sudan black B stain are positive in blast cells of acute myelocytic leukemia but negative in acute lymphocytic leukemia. The naphthol AS or ASD-acetate (NASDA) esterase reaction is positive before and after exposure to fluoride in granulocytes, whereas in mono-cytes or monoblasts, the NASDA esterase is positive but is inhibited by fluoride.

SUBCLASSIFICATION OF ACUTE LEUKEMIA. — A French-American-British cooperative group has proposed that current subcategories of acute leuke-mia (lymphocytic and myelocytic) be further subclassified into subgroups on the basis of criteria derived from morphologic examination of peripheral blood and bone marrow using Wright's stain and cytochemical techniques.

CLASSIFICATION OF NON-HODGKIN'S LYMPHOMA. — Although the Rappa-port classification is currently the one most widely used, at least in the United States, several others have been proposed. Thus far, these include the classifications of Dorfman, Lukes, a British pathology group (Bennett and colleagues) and the so-called Kiel classification (Lennert, Gerard-Mar-chant and colleagues). Although certain categories in each format roughly correspond to categories in the Rappaport system, exact superimposition does not seem possible, and in some instances it is difficult to determine precisely what morphologic criteria are being used to classify groups and subgroups.

REFERENCES

Bennett, J. M.: Proposals for the classification of the acute leukemias: French-Amer-ican-British Cooperative group, Br. J. Haemat. 33:451, 1976.

Bennett, M. H., et al.: Classification of non-Hodgkin's lymphomas, Lancet 2:405, 1974.

Dorfman, R. F.: Classification of non-Hodgkin's lymphomas, Lancet 1:1295, 1974.

Gerard-Marchant, R., et al.: Classification of non-Hodgkin's lymphomas, Lancet 2: 406, 1974.

Gilbert, H. S., et al.: Serum vitamin B-12 content and unsaturated vitamin B-12 bind-ing capacity in myeloproliferative disease, Ann. Intern. Med. 71:719, 1969.

Herbert, V.: Diagnostic and prognostic values of measurement of serum vitamin B-12 binding proteins, Blood 32:305, 1968.

Lukes, R. J., and Collins, R. D.: Immunologic characterization of human malignant lymphomas, Cancer 34:1488, 1974.

Perillie, P. E., and Finch, S. C.: Lysozyme in leukemia, Med. Clin. North Am. 57: 395, 1973.

Seligman, B. R., et al.: Serum muramidase levels in acute leukemia, Am. J. Med. Sci. 264:69, 1972.

Chapter 7. Blood Coagulation

TESTS FOR FIBRINOLYSIN. — The following tests are in limited use and merit some attention:

Staphylococcal clumping. — Staphylococci contain a substance that un-der proper conditions will agglutinate the organisms in the presence of fibrinogen or fibrin split products. The test is not widely used; it is report-ed to have sensitivity slightly greater than the "Fi" test.

Ethanol gelation. — It is postulated that certain concentrations of ethyl alcohol allow breakup of abnormal complexes formed by fibrinogen and fibrin monomer, with subsequent gel formation by the fibrin monomer. With certain modifications, the procedure has been praised by some but reported to have inadequate sensitivity by others.

SCREENING TEST FOR FLETCHER FACTOR. — One report indicates that Fletcher factor deficiency will increase the APTT using kaolin (but not el-lagic acid) as the activator and 3 minutes as the duration of activation per-mitted, whereas the kaolin APTT became normal when duration of activa-tion was increased to 10 minutes. Some patients had mild rather than marked prolongation of the 3-minute APTT, and some of these were found to have partial Fletcher factor deficiency. Coumadin was found to produce abnormality similar to that of Fletcher factor deficiency. More data are needed.

TESTS FOR COAGULATION SCREENING. — *Activated Whole Blood Clot-ting Time.* — Whole blood is drawn into a vacuum tube containing a contact factor activator. The tube is incubated in a heat block at 37° C and tilted every 5 seconds. Normal upper limit is about 2 minutes. The test is claimed to be very reproducible. It can be used both for coagulation defect screen-ing and to monitor heparin therapy. It is said to have approximately the same sensitivity as the activated partial thromboplastin time (APTT) in coagulation defects, and in heparin assay is more linear than APTT at greater heparin effects. Disadvantages are the need for a portable heating unit and inability to automate the procedure (the fact that the test is done at the bedside is considered by its proponents to be an advantage). The test is not sensitive to platelet variations.

Activated Plasma Recalcification Time (APRT). — Citrate-anticoagulated blood is obtained. Platelet-rich plasma is prepared; material to activate the contact factor is added; incubation at room temperature is followed by warming to 37° C, and calcium is added to begin the clotting process. Up-per normal range is about 35 seconds. The test is said to have approximate-ly the same sensitivity as the APTT in coagulation factor defects. In addi-tion, platelets affect the test. Disadvantages include need for centrifugation and two incubation periods.

TESTS FOR HEPARIN THERAPY MONITORING. — *Whole Blood Recalcifica-tion Time (WBRT).* — Whole blood is drawn into a tube with citrate antico-agulant. Calcium chloride is added to an aliquot of the whole blood to begin the clotting process. Normal upper limit for clotting is about 2 minutes at 37° C or 5 minutes at room temperature. The test is said to be adequately reproducible. The WBRT is used primarily to monitor heparin therapy. Its advantage is that whole blood clotting may be a more truthful representa-tion of the varied effects of heparin than tests that circumvent part of the normal clotting process. Only one very cheap reagent is needed. The WBRT is sensitive to platelet variations and is more linear than the APTT at greater heparin effects. The major disadvantage is inability to automate. One report states that the test must be performed within 1 hour after veni-puncture.

Whole Blood Activated Recalcification Time (BART). — This is similar to the WBRT except that a contact factor activator has been added to the anticoagulant tube. Normal upper limit is about 90 seconds. The test is said to be linear at all heparin concentrations. Platelets will affect results. The test can be automated.

Whole Blood Activated Partial Thromboplastin Time. — Two milliliters of nonanticoagulated whole blood are added to an APTT reagent at the bedside. The tube is tilted every 15 seconds at room temperature until a clot begins. Normal upper limit is about 2½ minutes. The test is said to have a good correlation with the Lee-White clotting time in all ranges of heparin effect and to be more sensitive to heparin than the APTT.

Plasma Recalcification Time (PRT). — Anticoagulated blood is obtained, the specimen is centrifuged at low speed to obtain platelet-rich plasma and calcium is added to an aliquot of the plasma to begin the clotting process. Normal upper limit is approximately 130 seconds. The test is used to monitor heparin therapy and produces results similar to whole blood recalcification methods. Values are reasonably linear at higher concentrations of heparin. Platelets affect the results when platelet-rich plasma is used.

Thrombin Time. — One aliquot of diluted thrombin is added to 1 aliquot of patient plasma. Clotting time upper limit is approximately 20 seconds. The test is simple and said to be very sensitive to heparin effect. It is not affected by Coumadin. As originally performed, the method was nonlinear and greatly prolonged in higher degrees of heparin effect, like the APTT. Certain modifications may have partially corrected this problem. Reagent source and composition may affect results considerably.

Polybrene Neutralization Test. — Polybrene, like protamine, is a substance that will neutralize heparin. The test consists of adding thrombin to aliquots of patient platelet-rich plasma, then adding increasing concentrations of Polybrene. The Polybrene concentration that neutralizes heparin present (indicated by clot formation) can be related to heparin concentration by a standard curve. A major advantage is freedom from interference by Coumadin.

Antithrombin-III. — Antithrombin-III (AT-III) is a substance that acts with heparin to neutralize thrombin and the activated forms of factors IX, X and XI. Tests that assay functional levels of AT-III are said to be useful in monitoring heparin therapy. In addition, decreased AT-III levels have been found in disseminated intravascular coagulation and in various patients who exhibited a tendency to thrombosis.

TESTS FOR MONITORING COUMADIN THERAPY. — *Thrombotest (Owren).* — This uses a special thromboplastin reagent designed to measure factor IX in addition to those affecting the Quick 1-stage PT test (prothrombin, VII and X). However, there is controversy whether it responds adequately to severe factor IX deficiency, since it has been reported that factor IX must be reduced below 10% of normal to affect the test. In a significant minority of patients the results will be below the recommended therapeutic range of 25% of normal (corresponding to a PT of about 1½ times normal) when the PT is within therapeutic range.

P & P test (Ware and Stragnell modification). — The name relates to early experiments implying that the test measured only prothrombin and proconvertin (factor VII). Actually, the procedure is similar to the PT test except that a 1:10 dilution of patient plasma is made and extra factor V and fibrinogen are added. The main advantage is said to be increased sensitivity to changes in factor VII. However, increased sensitivity may lead to more fluctuation in test values, and the Coumadin dose may have to be adjusted more often.

REFERENCES

Baden, J. P.: The precise management of heparin therapy, Am. J. Surg. 124:777, 1972.

Belko, J. S., and Warren, R.: The recalcification time of blood, A.M.A. Arch. Surg. 76: 210, 1958.

Breen, F. A., and Tullis, J. L.: Ethanol gelation: A rapid screening test for intravascular coagulation, Ann. Intern. Med. 69:1197, 1968.

Coagulation test predicts thrombosis, Lab. World 27:40, 1976.

Galliani, G. L., et al.: Blood recalcification time: A simple and reliable test to monitor heparin therapy, Am. J. Clin. Pathol. 65:396, 1976.

Grann, V. R., et al.: Polybrene neutralization as a rapid means of monitoring blood heparin levels, Am. J. Clin. Pathol. 58:26, 1972.

Hattersley, P. G.: Progress report: The activated coagulation time of whole blood (ACT), Am. J. Clin. Pathol. 66:899, 1976.

Hattersley, P. G., and Hayse, D.: The effect of increased contact activation time on the activated partial thromboplastin time, Am. J. Clin. Pathol. 66:479, 1976.

Marder, V. J., et al.: Detection of serum fibrinogen and fibrin degradation products, Am. J. Med. 51:71, 1971.

Moore, C. B., and Beeler, M. B.: Thrombotest versus one-stage prothrombin time determinations, N. Engl. J. Med. 264:681, 1961.

Reno, W. J., et al.: Evaluation of the BART test (a modification of the whole-blood activated recalcification time test) as a means of monitoring heparin therapy, Am. J. Clin. Pathol. 61:78, 1974.

Rodman, T., et al.: A comparison of laboratory methods for the control of anticoagulant therapy with prothrombinopenic agents, Am. J. Med. 31:547, 1961.

Shanberge, J. N., et al.: The whole blood recalcification clotting time: A convenient method for monitoring heparin therapy, Lab. Med. 5:30, 1974.

Stewart, C.: The laboratory control of heparin therapy, Med. J. Aust. 1:1160, 1971.

Ts'ao, C-H., et al: Effects of source and concentration of thrombin, and divalent cations, on thrombin time of heparinized blood, Am. J. Clin. Pathol. 65:206, 1976.

Vura, R. C., and Speicher, C. E.: The activated plasma recalcification time: A measurement encompassing the activated partial thromboplastin time and platelet function, with improved detection of bleeders, Am. J. Clin. Pathol. 64:80, 1975.

Chapter 13. Renal Function Tests

PHENOLSULFONPHTHALEIN (PSP) EXCRETION TEST. — More than 85% of PSP is actively excreted by the renal proximal tubular epithelium; less than 5% is filtered at the glomerulus, and the remainder is excreted by the liver. Thus, PSP excretion is a measure of one tubular "function" and indirectly of tubular health. The 15-minute measurement is the most important in this respect, but a 2-hour specimen should also be done. It is most important to hydrate the patient beforehand and to have some urine in the bladder when dye is injected; this volume of urine is not a factor in the results, but helps to recover all the excreted dye. Also essential are accurately timed specimen collection and care taken to ensure complete bladder emptying at the collection periods even if catheterization is necessary (however, catheterization for this test alone is not justified clinically because of the risk of introducing infection). Normal values are 25% or greater excretion at 15 minutes; 40–60% at 1 hour, and 60–80% at 2 hours. The importance of the 15-minute specimen lies in the fact that relatively early or mild bilateral renal disease may decrease function enough to influence the early collection specimen, whereas the later specimens may still fall within the normal range, since they represent an additive or cumulative effect over the longer time intervals.

The PSP gives similar information to clearance procedures over much of the same area. It is not quite as dependent on renal blood flow, although this is a factor; also, it takes a total of 2 hours, during which most patients can hold their urine. Disadvantages are that the patient is not always able to void accurately for the 15-minute specimen, which is often the most important value, or even for the other specimens. A certain constant percentage of the PSP dye is excreted into the urine on each cycle of blood flow to the kidney. Therefore, the 15-minute value may be low, although over a prolonged period the total values for 2 hours when added together may be almost within normal range, as noted previously. However, when kidney function is moderately to considerably decreased, the 2-hour value also starts falling. Obviously, it is necessary to be sure that the urine collection is complete so that all the PSP dye is recovered. If the patient has significant residual urine, the results may be falsely low.

In the usual case of chronic diffuse bilateral renal disease, the first demonstrable abnormality is impairment of the concentration test. As the disease progresses, the creatinine clearance and 15-minute PSP start to become reduced. Then the specific gravity becomes fixed and the creatinine clearance, followed by the 2-hour PSP, both show considerable decrease.

Fig 35–1.—Comparison of renal function tests in chronic diffuse bilateral renal disease.

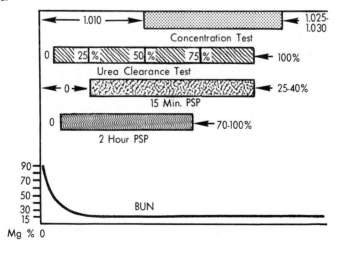

Finally, both these tests show a marked decrease and the BUN starts to rise, followed shortly by the blood creatinine (Fig 35–1).

BETA-2 MICROGLOBULIN (B_2M) ASSAY.—B_2M, a component of cell membranes, is excreted by glomerular filtration and nearly all resorbed and metabolized by renal tubule cells. Serum B_2M increases roughly in proportion to GFR decrease. Significant degrees of proximal tubule function loss produce increased urine B_2M excretion. B_2M has been used to estimate GFR, to detect patients with tubule damage and to differentiate primary glomerular from primary tubule disease. In chronic azotemia (serum creatinine over 4 mg/100 ml), urine B_2M no longer differentiates primary tubule disease.

FREE WATER CLEARANCE.—In acute tubular necrosis and end-stage chronic bilateral renal disease, urine sodium excretion is typically fixed at 40–100 mEq/L. However, this may not occur at the onset of renal failure. One study indicates that changes in renal concentrating ability, reflected in free water clearance, can indicate acute tubular necrosis in its early stage before the BUN or creatinine rise significantly, and help differentiate prerenal azotemia from renal failure due to intrinsic kidney damage. Free water clearance is calculated in two steps:

$$\text{Osmolar (osmolal) clearance} = \frac{\text{urine osmolality} \times \text{urine volume (ml/hr)}}{\text{plasma osmolality}}$$

$$\text{Free water clearance (ml/hr)} = \text{urine volume (ml/hr)} - \text{osmolar clearance}$$

Normally, osmolar clearance should be a negative number. Prerenal azotemia also displays a negative result (farther from 0 than −0.40). In early acute tubular necrosis, the result becomes close to 0 (closer to 0 than −0.15). When acute renal failure is well established, the result is very close to 0 (closer than −0.10) and may even be a positive number.

Verification of this data is needed. In the one or two cases we have investigated with this method, we had difficulty in obtaining accurate timed urine specimens.

FRACTION OF EXCRETED SODIUM (FE_{Na}).—One investigator reports that patients with prerenal azotemia tend to reabsorb more urine sodium after glomerular filtration than do patients with severe intrinsic renal damage such as acute tubular necrosis or chronic renal failure. The formula used is:

$$FE_{Na} = \frac{\text{urine Na} \times \text{serum creatinine}}{\text{serum Na} \times \text{urine creatinine}} \times 100$$

The normal or prerenal azotemia level is said to be less than 2.0. Diuretics may inhibit sodium reabsorption and produce a falsely elevated value. Confirmation by other investigators is needed.

REFERENCES

Baek, S. M. et al.: Free-water clearance patterns as predictors and therapeutic guides in acute renal failure, Surgery 77:632, 1975.

Espinal, C. H.: The FE_{Na} test: Use in the differential diagnosis of acute renal failure, J.A.M.A. 236:579, 1976.

Pullman, T. N.: Kidney function tests in clinical practice, Med. Clin. North Am. 43: 469, 1959.

Wibell, L., et al.: Serum B$_2$-microglobulin in renal disease, Nephron 10:320, 1973.

Chapter 14. Bacterial Infectious Diseases

HEMOLYTIC REACTIONS OF BACTERIA ON BLOOD AGAR. — These hemolytic reactions may be altered by the type of blood used. Alpha streptococci produce green alpha hemolysis on human blood or sheep blood agar, but not on rabbit blood. *Hemophilus* species will not grow well on sheep blood agar.

The type of agar base and other conditions of culture technique can also influence hemolysis in group A streptococci. Failure to incubate isolation plates under reduced oxygen tension (CO_2 atmosphere or stab technique) may result in failure to produce recognizable beta hemolysis.

COUNTERIMMUNOELECTROPHORESIS (CIE). — This technique has been applied to the diagnosis of infectious disease through detection of specific bacterial antigens. CIE places an antibody specific against a certain antigen into a small circular hole cut into agar and applies the substance to be tested (CSF, serum, urine, etc.) into a second hole nearby. The agar is then submitted to electrophoresis in such a way as to force the contents of the two wells toward each other. If specific antigen to the antibody is present, a visible precipitin line will result when antigen and antibody meet. The method is relatively easy to perform and takes less than 1 hour to complete. Thus far, the most widely used application is diagnosis of bacterial meningitis. Antibodies against the most common infectious agents *(H. influenzae*, meningococcus, pneumococcus and streptococcus B) are available. Detection rate is said to be 60–80%, with some investigators able to report even better results. Presently available antisera are more sensitive for *H. influenzae* and meningococcus than for pneumococcus. Other body fluids or even nonfluid material may be subjected to the same procedure, although results to date are less impressive than with CSF. The major technical difficulty has been variation in potency of commercial antisera.

This technique has also proved useful in diagnosis of systemic *Candida* infection, although there has been some overlap between patient groups who are colonized by *Candida* and those with actual infection.

NITROBLUE TETRAZOLIUM (NBT) TEST. — Neutrophils increase their phagocytic activity during acute bacterial infections. If neutrophils are incubated with NBT dye, activated neutrophils will phagocytize the reagent and reduce it to a colored formazan compound. After inspection of 100 neutrophils, the percent containing formazan granules is reported. Monocytes will also ingest NBT; they are not counted when performing the test. In general, acute bacterial infection increases the NBT count, while viral and tuberculous infections do not. The test is generally employed to indicate the presence of acute bacterial infection. Some conditions other than bacterial infection that may elevate the NBT score ("false positives") include age less than 2 months (normal infants), echovirus infection, malignant lymphomas (especially Hodgkin's disease), hemophilia, malaria, certain parasitic infestations, *Candida albicans* and *Nocardia* infections and possibly the taking of oral contraceptives. Certain conditions may (to varying degree) induce normal scores in the presence of bacterial infection ("false negatives"); these include antibiotic therapy, localized infection, systemic lupus, sickle cell anemia, diabetes mellitus, agam-maglobulinemia and certain medications (steroids, phenylbutazone). In chronic granulomatous disease, phagocytosis becomes markedly impaired; the NBT test score is 0, and the procedure serves as a screening method for this disorder.

Many evaluations of NBT have been published, and there is marked disagreement as to its value. The majority of reports are favorable. A substantial minority of authors found large numbers of false positive or negative results and concluded that the test is useless. Various modifications of the original method have been used, including variations in technique involving anticoagulant, incubation temperature control, smear thickness and method of calculating data, all of which may affect test results.

REFERENCES

Anderson, G. L., and Deinard, A. S.: The nitroblue tetrazolium (NBT) test: A review, Am. J. Med. Technol. 40:345, 1974.

Chitwood, L.: Isolation and identification of Group A streptococci with commercially available reagents, Lab. Med. 2:26, 1971.

Feigin, R. D., and Pickering, L. K.: Role of the nitroblue tetrazolium dye test in diagnosis of infections, South. Med. J. 68:237, 1975.

Kozinn, P. J., et al.: The precipitin test in systemic candidiasis, J.A.M.A. 235:628, 1976.

Lace, J. K., et al.: An appraisal of the nitroblue tetrazolium reduction test, Am. J. Med. 58:685, 1975.

Rytel, M. W.: Counterimmunoelectrophoresis in diagnosis of infectious disease, Hosp. Practice 10:75, 1975.

Sommers, H. M.: ASCP Microbiology Check Sample MB-37, 1968.

Chapter 16. Viral, Rickettsial and Miscellaneous Infectious Diseases

STREPTOCOCCUS MG. — This is a test for the mycoplasma-induced antibodies of primary atypical pneumonia. The test is based on the unusual reactivity of these antibodies for material from this strain of the streptococcal organism. The majority of investigators feel that the test is not as sensitive as cold agglutinins. The "strep MG" test gives positive results in less than 40% of cases, although reports range from 10 to 80%.

TICK HEMOLYMPH TEST FOR ROCKY MOUNTAIN SPOTTED FEVER (BERGDORFER PROCEDURE). — A live tick is needed. The tick should be picked off with tweezers, working gently without pulling to avoid breaking the mouth parts. The tick should not be crushed. When finally detached from the skin, the tick should be placed in a small bottle with a piece of moist tissue and sent either to the state health department (if the test can be done there) or to Dr. Willy Bergdorfer, Rickettsial Disease Section, Rocky Mountain Laboratory, Hamilton, MT 59840. The test consists of obtaining a drop of tick hemolymph and examining tick hemocytes with a special stain for the organisms.

REFERENCES

Fighting spotted fever, Med. Lab. 10(10):23, 1974.

Purcell, R. H., and Chanock, R. M.: Role of mycoplasmas in human respiratory disease, Med. Clin. North Am. 51:791, 1967.

Chapter 18. Cerebrospinal Fluid Examination

COLLOIDAL GOLD REACTION. — This is based on the fact that in certain pathologic CNS conditions, a suspension of colloidal gold in sodium chloride will be precipitated, giving characteristic color changes in standard dilutions. The color normally is wine red, but may change to a blue and even to a clear color, depending on the degree of precipitation. Each dilution tube is given a number 0 to 5, depending on the degree of color change. There are 10 tubes, each with a different dilution, so the results are reported as a series of 10 numbers.

A reading of 1 in all tubes is within normal limits. A reading of 2 is of doubtful significance and, to be significant, at least 1 of the 10 tubes must read 3 or over. According to classic theories, globulin tends to precipitate the gold particles in the solution, while albumin tends to "protect" the finely dispersed colloidal state. More recent work indicates that the gamma globulins have the strongest precipitating action, while most but not all of the protective function seems to be in the albumin and alpha globulins. When gamma globulin is increased without significant albumin or alpha globulin increase, color changes are mostly in the lower dilution tubes, producing a "first-zone" curve (for example, 5553211111). This is characteristically found in syphilitic general paresis and in multiple sclerosis, but not always in either. When both the albumin and the globulin are increased in the same general proportions, but only moderately, or when the gamma globulin is only very slightly increased, a "second-zone" curve is produced in which the middle dilution tubes show precipitation and thus have color change (for example, 1113321111). Theoretically, the albumin or alpha globulin was present in sufficient quantities to prevent precipitation in the first zone, but was diluted out after the first few tubes. Due to the relatively mild gamma globulin increase, this globulin also is supposed to be diluted out, but not until the last tubes. A second-zone curve is classically found in tabes dorsalis; again, many other conditions can occasionally produce a similar effect. In patients with high total protein levels, the precipitating action of the gamma globulin may not appear until the last dilution tubes, by which time the albumin and alpha globulin are diluted enough to unmask the gamma globulin effect. This is called a "third-zone" or "end-zone" curve and classically is found in acute bacterial meningitis. The colloidal gold curve, however, is not nearly as specific as one would gather from this simplified account, since, for example, acute bacterial meningitis can give any of the three types of curves as well as no curve at all, and many other diseases can occasionally give one or the other type of curve. Again, for example, although multiple sclerosis classically gives a first-zone curve, a considerable number show a midzone or no curve. The main clinical use of the colloidal gold curve is in the diagnosis of multiple sclerosis, general paresis and tabes dorsalis. It is not a routine test, and its use should be confined mainly to situations in which these three diseases are possibilities.

Cerebrospinal fluid electrophoresis can substitute for colloidal gold; chronic infections or diseases produce elevated gamma globulin levels.

REFERENCES

Bloomfield, N.: Behavior of isolated plasma proteins in the colloidal gold test, Am. J. Clin. Pathol. 41:15, 1964.

Merritt, H. H., and Fremont-Smith, F.: *The Cerebrospinal Fluid* (Philadelphia: W. B. Saunders Company, 1937).

Chapter 19. Liver and Biliary Tract Tests

CEPHALIN FLOCCULATION TEST. — In acute and chronic liver cell necrosis or inflammation, abnormal globulins are often produced. Depending on their nature, they may be precipitated by certain substances such as zinc sulfate or buffered thymol, or be detected by excessive attachment to certain surfaces such as colloidal gold or cephalin-cholesterol particles. Zinc sulfate turbidity tests have been demonstrated to be nearly specific for gamma globulin. The thymol turbidity test responds either to changes in gamma globulin or to lipoproteins migrating in the beta globulin area. The cephalin flocculation test (ceph. floc.) is more complex and responds to either of two stimuli. Gamma globulin will precipitate the cephalin emulsion, but is normally prevented from doing so by certain stabilizing factors, probably in the alpha$_1$ globulin area. In acute hepatic parenchymal cell injury, the stabilizing factors vanish from serum in 24–48 hours, allowing normal amounts of gamma globulin present to give a positive ceph. floc. reaction. On the other hand, excessively large amounts of gamma globulin may be sufficient to overcome normal amounts of stabilizing factor present and likewise give a positive result. However, the ceph. floc. does not seem to depend primarily on hypergammaglobulinemia, since certain types of globulins have a peculiar reactivity out of proportion to their actual quantity.

The technique of the ceph. floc. consists of incubating the patient's serum with a cephalin-cholesterol emulsion in the dark for 24 hours. Any resulting flocculation or precipitation is graded 1 to 4 plus. Normal serums are negative, but 1+ is regarded as within normal range and only 2+ or over is considered significant to rule out error in visually estimating very weak reactions. As noted earlier, results are usually positive in acute hepatocellular injury from any cause, except when very mild. The stabilizing factor remains absent until hepatocellular healing is well established, but following relatively mild or brief episodes, the ceph. floc. may be elevated only a few days. The test cannot show the degree of damage or the amount of tissue affected. Results are usually normal in certain diseases such as obstructive jaundice without superimposed infection, chronic passive congestion (as opposed to acute types), small to moderate degrees of metastatic carcinoma and solitary liver abscess. However, occasionally some of these conditions may give a positive result, especially with extensive metastasis and jaundice. Since there must be active cell necrosis to get a positive result (unless abnormal globulins are present), there usually are negative results in fatty liver, inactive cirrhosis, often in moderately active cirrhosis or in healing stages of acute diseases. Positive results may be found in a certain percentage of cases in primarily nonhepatic diseases, as mentioned earlier, although some of these may also have liver involvement. These include collagen diseases, infectious mononucleosis, SBE, viral pneumonia, malaria, pernicious anemia and a few others.

Both the SGOT and SGPT, if they show elevation, do so before the ceph. floc. becomes abnormal, but they all return to normal ranges considerably in advance of the ceph. floc. Therefore, the ceph. floc. sometimes will be abnormal in the presence of normal enzyme studies, due either to a minimal amount of hepatocellular damage or to obtaining the tests after the enzymes had returned to normal. In general, the ceph. floc. is less sensitive than the SGOT, but is elevated longer and is more specific for hepatic cell acute destruction. It may be helpful to assess activity of cirrhosis and as a parameter of therapy in hepatitis.

The ceph. floc. is probably of most use as a means to confirm acute liver cell damage in a patient when the SGOT is normal or only minimally elevated. There usually is little use in getting a ceph. floc. if the SGOT is elevated. With the advent of enzyme tests, such as SGPT, which are more specific for hepatocellular injury, the ceph. floc. is considered obsolete. The ceph. floc. is not reliable in the neonatal period, and before age 6 months may sometimes be normal even with extensive acute liver cell damage.

ZINC SULFATE TEST. — This demonstrates elevations of gamma globulin, but serum protein electrophoresis can do this more informatively.

THYMOL TURBIDITY TEST. — Results of this test roughly correlate with the results of the ceph. floc. This test seems less sensitive than the ceph. floc. and becomes positive later, but tends to remain positive longer.

ORNITHINE CARBAMYL TRANSFERASE (OCT). — This enzyme is found mainly in liver and, to a much lesser extent, within intestinal mucosa. Since it takes rather extensive intestinal infarction to provoke significant OCT elevation, this enzyme is nearly specific for liver cell disease. It is even more sensitive than SGOT to hepatocellular injury, and reportedly may be elevated in some cases without histologic cell changes.

ISOCITRIC DEHYDROGENASE (ICD). — This behaves like the SGOT in liver disease. Although ICD is found in cardiac muscle and several tissues besides liver, it is not elevated in myocardial infarction and usually is abnormal only in liver disease.

ALKALINE PHOSPHATASE ISOENZYMES. — Alkaline phosphatase can be separated into single enzymes that are relatively specific for bone, liver, placenta and intestine. The easiest method is heat fractionation; bone isoenzyme is heat inactivated, while liver is heat stable. Placenta has the greatest heat stability. More than 30% heat stable suggests liver origin; less than 30% heat stable suggests bone. Normals are 15–35% heat stable, creating overlap with bone. This method has not been reliable in my laboratory. Chemical fractionation is too cumbersome. Electrophoresis is just becoming available, and promises to be the best separation method. An interesting isoenzyme, called "Regan," migrates in the placenta area and is found in some patients with cancer.

5-NUCLEOTIDASE. — This is a member of the alkaline phosphatase group, but is thought to be more specific (and possibly more sensitive) than alkaline phosphatase for hepatobiliary tract disease. However, one study suggests elevation in some patients with bone lesions.

LEUCINE AMINO PEPTIDASE (LAP). — This is an enzyme produced exclusively by the liver. In general, it tends to parallel the alkaline phosphatase, although it is not as sensitive. Bone lesions do not affect this test. When originally reported, LAP was thought to indicate pancreatic carcinoma, but all agree now that this theory was wrong and that the only association occurs when pancreatic carcinoma causes biliary obstruction, just as alkaline phosphatase is elevated in the same situation.

OTHER ENZYMES. — *Guanase* is indicative of acute hepatocellular damage; sensitivity is somewhat greater than that of SGOT. Guanase is also located in brain, kidney and intestine.

Aldolase has tissue specificity and sensitivity similar to that of SGOT.

Alcohol dehydrogenase is said to be relatively (not completely) specific for acute hepatocellular damage, although elevation may occur in fatty liver and metastatic tumor. Infectious mononucleosis, uncomplicated early extrahepatic obstruction and inactive portal cirrhosis are said to have normal levels.

Sorbitol dehydrogenase is relatively specific for acute hepatocellular damage and is similar in this respect to SGPT. Occasional elevation is noted during infection.

IMMUNOGLOBULIN LEVELS. — Marked IgM increase has been reported in 80% of patients with biliary cirrhosis, but elevated levels may occur in extrahepatic obstruction and other diseases. Reports of increased IgA in alcoholic cirrhosis are even less specific and frequent. Immunoglobulins have not, therefore, been very helpful.

CELL COMPONENT ANTIBODIES. — Antibodies have been described that react against specific structures in cells, as demonstrated by immunofluorescent technique. Antimitochondrial antibodies are found in 80–100% of biliary cirrhosis patients and may aid in the diagnosis of this uncommon disease. False positive results have been reported in some patients with drug-induced cholestasis and chronic active hepatitis, as well as in a relatively small number of patients with extrahepatic obstruction, acute infectious hepatitis, rheumatoid arthritis and other conditions. Anti-smooth-muscle antibodies were reported in 45–70% of patients with chronic active ("lupoid") hepatitis and have been found in biliary cirrhosis and, less frequently, in other liver diseases (except alcoholic cirrhosis). An immunofluorescence expert is needed to set up and interpret these procedures. Liver biopsy is still needed.

CHOLESTEROL AND CHOLESTEROL ESTERS. — Cholesterol is synthesized in several tissues, but the liver is the chief organ in its manufacture, alteration and degradation. Normally about 70% is esterified and about 30% in the free form. Esterification is affected much more than total cholesterol by liver damage. In moderate degrees of acute or chronic liver damage, cholesterol esters may decrease to the 40–50% range. They usually do not fall below 20% without severe liver parenchymal destruction. The total cholesterol is reduced below normal ranges (150–250 mg/100 ml) only in severe damage, most often chronic. However, the usefulness of cholesterol as an index of liver function is severely handicapped by the technical difficulties of the test itself. Laboratories have considerable variation in accuracy even from day to day, so it is difficult to know if a slightly or moderately reduced value is genuine or not. Also, the normal range is so wide that a patient could have the usual normal value decreased by one-third or more and still be within population normal ranges. Furthermore, other diseases such as hyperthyroidism, severe infections and malnutrition will lower serum cholesterol. On the other hand, certain types of liver diseases are associated with increased cholesterol; these include biliary obstruction, especially biliary cirrhosis and many cases of cholangitis. Nonhepatic diseases that cause elevated values are hypothyroidism, nephrotic syndrome, idiopathic hypercholesterolemia and often diabetes.

BROMSULPHALEIN TEST (BSP). — The liver excretes bilirubin by conjugating it with glucuronide molecules and then releasing it into the bile. It has been found that certain synthetic substances such as BSP dye are handled by the liver in a similar manner. On injection into the blood stream, the dye is mostly bound to serum albumin. As it passes through the intrahepatic sinusoidal circulation, BSP is somehow absorbed into the hepatic cells. Once there, some of the dye is conjugated with glutathione molecules, and all the absorbed BSP, whether conjugated or still free, is excreted into the bile. About 1% is excreted in urine without liver involvement, and a small percentage seems to be removed by other tissues. The rate of hepatic uptake is proportional to the amount of BSP in the plasma, meaning that a fairly constant percentage is removed by the liver on each passage through it. Therefore, the great bulk of the dye is removed from plasma relatively early, with the remaining amount getting progressively less as time passes. The four variables concerned in the test may be summarized as follows: the amount of dye injected, the plasma volume in which it is diluted, the ability of the hepatic parenchymal cell mass to remove the BSP and the patency of the bile ducts through which the excreted final products must pass to the duodenum.

The standard dose of BSP has been empirically set at 5 mg/kg of body weight, after experimentation with other concentrations. The reason this particular value is used comes from studies that show the ability of the liver in normal persons to remove practically all of the dye in the test period of 45 minutes. While normal persons almost always have less than 5% remaining in the serum at 45 minutes and less than 2% serum retention at 60 minutes, a large majority of patients with damaged livers due to various causes show elevated serum values, allowing good separation of normal from abnormal. Furthermore, plasma volume is normally not a significant factor due to the extremely efficient ability of the liver to take up and excrete BSP. To report values as percentage of test dose retained, it is assumed that body weight is related to plasma volume in a proportion of 1 kg to 50 ml, meaning that 5 mg is injected for each 50 ml of plasma. This gives a theoretical initial concentration of 10 mg/100 ml plasma. The amount of BSP remaining in the plasma in mg/100 ml is measured at the end of the test period, and the percentage of the initial dose is then calculated.

Since normal liver removal and excretion of the dye depends on normal hepatic blood flow, normal liver cells and normal bile duct excretory channels, it follows that a variety of diseases affecting one or more of these components will lead to impaired BSP excretion. In posthepatic bile obstruction such as may be caused by common duct stone or carcinoma of the head of the pancreas, there will be BSP retention if the obstruction is complete, sometimes even if obstruction is incomplete. Gallbladder disease will not affect BSP values unless infection spreads to the biliary duct system or stones reach the common bile duct. Severe acute liver damage will cause BSP serum elevation due to lack of ability to extract the dye. Small degrees of acute damage may not show values above the normal range, even if there is an increase in serum retention over what the same patient would show with a normal liver. Therefore, in hepatitis, BSP results are variable; if jaundice is present, however, BSP is almost invariably elevated. The jaundice of acute viral hepatitis is an intrahepatic type due to cell edema and destruction with collapse of bile sinusoids and thus temporary obstruction. The BSP test is the best single test for detection of cirrhosis, and may be the only one with elevated values when the cirrhosis is inactive. The same is true for fatty liver. The reason for this behavior in cirrhosis is the presence of fibrosis and irregularly regenerating liver cell nodules, which cause distortion and rearrangement of intrahepatic blood flow as well as actual loss of liver cells by fibrous tissue replacement. Nevertheless, despite reasonably good sensitivity, BSP test results may occasionally be normal in moderate degrees of cirrhosis or in severe fatty liver. Passive congestion of the liver secondary to congestive heart failure may cause temporary BSP elevation due to intrahepatic blood stasis and hepatic cell anoxia. Shock or hypotension from various causes will cut down hepatic blood flow and give elevated values. Results are normal in hemolytic anemias unless some other cause of liver damage is present. Elevation of BSP is the most frequent abnormality in metastatic carcinoma to the liver, although the mechanism involved is often obscure. The same is true in granulomas and other space-occupying lesions. Transient degrees of BSP elevation have been reported in some cases of acute pancreatitis, high fever, recent abdominal surgery, severe stress situations such as trauma and acute severe upper gastrointestinal hemorrhage. In summary, BSP elevation by itself means that something abnormal is taking place in the liver, but more information from history, physical examination, laboratory studies or the clinical situation is needed to show the etiology.

Certain substances will interfere with the test. These include PSP, iodine, morphine and other opium derivatives and sometimes barbiturates. Some of the x-ray contrast media for gallbladder studies will produce false results, so that a BSP should wait until 3 days afterward if gallbladder x-rays have been done. Otherwise, the x-ray department should be asked whether the particular substance they use is one that will affect the BSP.

False negatives may result from incorrect estimation of the dose or losing some of the dye outside the vein when it is injected. The dose is estimated according to the formula: weight in pounds divided by 22 equals ml BSP to be used. Regarding dosage, the problem of obesity sometimes arises. The weight-volume correlation obviously does not hold true in a markedly obese patient, whose adipose tissue will cause a significant overdose of dye when calculated on the same basis as for a normally built person. There is no formula to correct for obesity. Since adipose tissue has about two thirds of the blood flow found in muscle, it may be possible to find the ideal weight for the patient from published tables and add two thirds of the weight he possesses over that value to calculate the BSP dose more accurately. However, this is just a rough approximation and is no guarantee that true compensation is achieved.

Another important question is the usefulness of the BSP test when jaundice is present. When jaundice is over 5 mg/100 ml bilirubin level, the BSP will almost always be elevated unless the elevated bilirubin is due to pure hemolysis. In milder degrees of jaundice, the test still may be worthwhile, since a normal or near normal result can be of considerable help, especially in differentiating cirrhosis from other causes of bilirubinemia or indicating only slight degrees of parenchymal liver damage. The test is most helpful in patients with normal or only minimally elevated bilirubin. As mentioned earlier, elevated values may be caused by upper GI bleeding, but normal values in such a case would be helpful in ruling out cirrhosis as a cause for the bleeding. The dye may be given by syringe injection or intravenous tubing. Care should be taken to avoid extravasation of dye out of the vein, since the dye is very irritating to tissue, and also the test results may be affected. A few patients get hypersensitivity reactions to BSP; these are usually mild and treatable with antihistamines. Rarely, they are severe and may be fatal.

Indocyanine green (Cardio-Green) is a dye that is metabolized by liver cells in a manner similar to BSP. Evaluations suggest results equivalent to BSP, although the dye is slightly less sensitive for inactive cirrhosis. Cardio-Green has one advantage: no tissue toxicity or hypersensitivity reactions have been reported. The dye is 5 times more expensive than BSP and has not had the same degree of clinical evaluation and publicity.

ROSE BENGAL EXCRETION (HEPATOGRAM).—Rose bengal is a dye that is extracted from blood by hepatic parenchymal cells and excreted into the bile. Isotope-tagged rose bengal has been used as a test of biliary tract patency; failure to detect isotope excretion into the intestine on repeated monitoring over a 24–48-hour time span suggests complete biliary obstruction. Contrary to the expectation of many physicians, rose bengal cannot reliably distinguish between intrahepatic and extrahepatic obstruction in most cases, although severe hepatocellular damage can be inferred if the liver fails to extract more than 10% of the dye in 20 minutes. The main usefulness of the test lies in documenting complete biliary tract obstruction in patients with moderately or markedly elevated serum bilirubin levels. Rose bengal also concentrates with bile in the gallbladder, so that gallbladder visualization helps rule out abnormality in that organ. Ultrasound or CAT scanning provide more information than rose bengal in most instances.

REFERENCES

Breen, K. J., and Schenker, S.: Liver function tests, CRC Crit. Rev. Clin. Lab. Sci. 2: 573, 1971.

Fitzgerald, M. X. M., et al.: Value of differential alkaline phosphatase thermostability in clinical diagnosis, Am. J. Clin. Pathol. 51:194, 1969.

Hanger, F. M.: The meaning of liver function tests, Am. J. Med. 16:565, 1954.

Sherlock, S.: Chronic active hepatitis, Postgrad. Med. 50:206, 1971.

Walker, G., and Doniach, D.: Antibodies and immunoglobulins in liver disease, Gut 9:266, 1968.

West, M., and Zimmerman, H. J.: Serum enzymes in hepatic disease, Med. Clin. North Am. 43:1, 1959.

Zimmerman, H. J., and West, M.: Serum enzymes in gastrointestinal diseases, Med. Clin. North Am. 48:189, 1964.

Chapter 20. Cardiac, Pulmonary and Miscellaneous Diagnostic Procedures

MYOGLOBIN IN DIAGNOSIS OF MYOCARDIAL INFARCT. Myoglobin is found in cardiac and skeletal muscle. The few studies so far available indicate that the mean time for the peak value of serum myoglobin after myocardial infarct is reached in approximately 8-12 hours. During this time, serum myoglobin is abnormal in approximately 90% of patients. By 12 hours after admission, serum levels in a few patients may already have returned to normal range. By 12-24 hours after admission, probably fewer than 50% remain elevated. Another investigator found that myoglobin appeared intermittently, and that serial determinations within the first 6-18 hours increased the chances of detecting abnormality.

Myoglobin is excreted by renal glomerular filtration. There is evidence that myoglobinuria may appear as early as 3 hours after onset of infarct symptoms. In several patients, values returned to upper normal limits by 30 hours, but remained elevated longer in most cases. Another study recorded 90% sensitivity 24 and 48 hours after hospital admission, diminishing to 76% by 72 hours.

Besides cardiac muscle injury skeletal muscle injury due to trauma, ischemia or inflammation may release myoglobin. Nondestructive conditions affecting muscle such as delirium tremens and severe exertion also may produce myoglobinuria, and it has also been reported in some patients with diabetic acidosis, hypokalemia, systemic infection with fever, barbiturate poisoning and certain more uncommon etiologies. Since myoglobin is excreted through the kidneys, renal function might also influence results.

RATIO OF TOTAL LDH TO FAST-MOVING (LDH-1) ISOENZYME.—This has been proposed as a test for myocardial infarct, to improve specificity of total LDH and to demonstrate increase in LDH-1 that is significant but does not exceed normal population range. There have been conflicting reports on the usefulness of this technique.

ARTERIAL OXYGEN SATURATION.—Proposed as an ancillary test for pulmonary embolization, arterial oxygen saturation gives support to the diagnosis if the arterial oxygen pressure is below 80 mm Hg. However, exceptions occur, and it is not yet clear whether the number of exceptions is great enough to impair the usefulness of the test seriously.

PROTAMINE SULFATE TEST.—This test (p. 70) may be positive in embolization. Sensitivity depends on which test modification is used; thus far, results have been variable with all techniques. My personal experience disclosed many false positives and negatives in embolization.

RADIOISOTOPE PULMONARY FUNCTION TESTS.—Radioactive xenon is a gas that can be either inhaled or injected intravenously. Inhalation fills the alveoli for a few moments before the gas is exhaled. If injected intravenously, xenon quickly diffuses into the alveoli and then is exhaled. In either case a stationary rapid imaging device such as the Anger scintillation camera can photograph alveolar distribution of the gas. Conditions that alter ventilatory distribution, such as emphysema or space-occupying lesions, produce various abnormalities in the distribution of xenon. In pulmonary embolization the xenon scan is typically normal in the presence of defects on perfusion scans with isotope-labeled particles that outline pulmonary blood distribution. However, if emphysema is present, both the ventilation and the perfusion scan will be abnormal, and this provides a way to differentiate embolization from emphysema. Unfortunately, emboli sometimes occur in areas with preexisting severe emphysema. Xenon tests are available at present only in large hospitals. The gas is very expensive and necessitates special apparatus to avoid contamination of the room.

Isotope-labeled particles can be inhaled via aerosol; this allows visualization of the pattern of the major bronchi. It is claimed that this method can distinguish pure emphysema from that secondary to bronchitis. The technique is still experimental.

C-REACTIVE PROTEIN.—This is produced during conditions that cause acute tissue destruction or inflammation. The protein gets its name from its ability to precipitate with pneumococcus somatic C-polysaccharide. The test is performed with antiserum against C-protein and is reported in a semiquantitative 0 to 4+ fashion. This technique has roughly the same usefulness as the ESR, but has never attained the same degree of popularity.

REFERENCES

Blahd, W. H. (ed.): *Nuclear Medicine* (2d ed.; New York: McGraw-Hill Book Company, Inc., 1971).

Dalen, J. E., et al.: Pulmonary angiography in acute pulmonary embolism: Indications, techniques, and results in 367 patients, Am. Heart J. 81:175, 1971.

Kagan, L., et al.: Serum myoglobin in myocardial infarction: The "staccato phenomenon," Am. J. Med. 62:86, 1977.

Levine, R. S., et al.: Myoglobinuria in myocardial infarction, Am. J. Med. Sci. 262: 179, 1971.

Mills, J., and Drew, D.: Pulmonary embolism without arterial hypoxemia, Ann. Intern. Med. 75:972, 1971.

Nutter, D. O.: The isoenzymes of lactic dehydrogenase. I. Myocardial infarction and coronary insufficiency, Am. Heart J. 72:315, 1966.

Saranchak, H. J., and Bernstein, S. H.: A new diagnostic test for acute myocardial infarction: The detection of myoglobinuria by radioimmunodiffusion assay, J.A.M.A. 228:1251, 1974.

Chapter 21. Serum Proteins

Several screening tests have been devised for the detection of hyperlipoproteinemia. Two (K-agar and TEKIT precipitest) are based on precipitation by a sulfated polysaccharide, the other (Beta-L) involves precipitation of beta lipoprotein by specific antiserum. Very little has been published regarding sensitivity and accuracy of these procedures; however, each seems about 85–90% sensitive in detecting hyperlipoproteinemia. More independent evaluation is needed.

REFERENCES:

Boyle, E., Jr., et al.: Evaluation of rapid screening methods for the detection of abnormal lipid states related to atherosclerosis, Ann. Clin. Lab. Sci. 2:393, 1972.

Searcy, R., et al.: A screening procedure for detecting and characterizing hyperlipoproteinemia, Clin. Chim. Acta 38:291, 1972.

Chapter 22. Bone and Joint Disorders

ANTINUCLEAR ANTIBODIES (ANA) TEST MORPHOLOGY. — A peripheral (nuclear border) antinuclear staining reaction (in contrast to a solid or a "speckled" nuclear staining pattern) is said to be fairly specific for systemic lupus. Most of these patients have active disease; the incidence is much less in treated or inactive disease. Treated or inactive lupus is more apt to show solid or speckled (broken) nuclear fluorescent patterns, and these may also be found in significant numbers of persons with other collagen diseases or in some persons with rheumatoid arthritis.

REFERENCE:

Rothfield, N. F.: Serologic tests in rheumatic diseases, Postgrad. Med. 45:116, 1969.

Chapter 24. Serum Electrolytes

MAGNESIUM DEFICIENCY. — This may occasionally produce symptoms much like those of hypocalcemia, including tetany. The most common etiologies are steatorrhea, nasogastric suction accompanied by large quantities of magnesium-free intravenous fluids, diabetes and alcoholism or alcoholic cirrhosis. Diagnosis is made by serum assay for magnesium; this generally requires atomic absorption equipment. Since this is relatively expensive and is not applicable to many other laboratory tests, most small hospitals do not have this equipment and therefore do not have magnesium determination readily available.

SERUM WATER. — This can be estimated by a refractometer (total solids meter), which measures the effects of serum proteins on the refractive index. Serum proteins constitute the major determinant of serum colloid osmotic pressure, which regulates plasma and extracellular water equilibrium. Therefore, serum water estimates intravascular colloid osmotic pressure in contrast to serum osmolality, which measures intravascular osmotic pressure, an entity responding to electrolyte changes but not influenced significantly by colloid (protein). Serum water is influenced by changes in either protein or water. Elevated serum water suggests excess water; decreased serum water indicates water deficit. Unfortunately, decreased serum protein also leads to increased water values, and since decreased albumin is common in seriously ill patients, this fact plus the rather high cost of the instrument has limited the use of the test. Nevertheless, even protein abnormality does not totally destroy the usefulness of serum water determination, because a relative dilution caused by hypoproteinemia may be treated by administration of albumin. Normal serum water values are 93–94 gm/100 ml.

REFERENCES:

Agarwal, B. N., and Agarwal, P.: Magnesium deficiency in clinical medicine: A review, J. Am. Med. Wom. Assoc. 31:72, 1976.

Mansberger, A. R., et al.: Refractometry and osmometry in clinical surgery, Ann. Surg. 169:672, 1969.

Wacker, W. E. C., and Paresi, A. F.: Magnesium metabolism, N. Engl. J. Med. 278: 658, 712, 772, 1968.

Chapter 27. Tests for Diabetes and Hypoglycemia

SKIN TEST FOR HYPERGLYCEMIA. — A simple skin test utilizing glucose oxidase test paper has been proposed for the detection of diabetes mellitus. Evaluation has disclosed such erratic results that, in its present form, this procedure seems to have little value.

TOLBUTAMIDE TOLERANCE TEST. — Tolbutamide (Orinase) is a sulfonyl-urea drug that apparently has the ability to stimulate insulin production from pancreatic beta cells. This drug has been used for treatment of mild diabetics who produce insulin, but of insufficient quantity. In 1956 tolbuta-mide was first proposed as a test for diabetes. A special water-soluble form of tolbutamide is given intravenously. There is normally a prompt and con-siderable fall in blood glucose levels with a maximum at 30–45 minutes, followed by a return to normal values between 1 ½ and 3 hours. The coun-teracting forces responsible are thought to be primarily liver production of glucose from glycogen induced by epinephrine release in answer to the hypoglycemia. In diabetics, there is both diminished and delayed re-sponse to intravenous tolbutamide. There is little correlation between the degree of test abnormality and the likelihood that a patient would respond to actual tolbutamide therapy. The test must be preceded by adequate car-bohydrate diet, as described for the GTT.

The tolbutamide test is regarded by some as the most specific laboratory test for diabetes now available. However, this does not mean that it is ac-tually specific for diabetes. Some investigators did find significant numbers of false positives, although reduced in frequency, when patients with ab-normal GTTs from a variety of nonpancreatic etiologies were retested with tolbutamide. Nevertheless, nonpancreatic causes of abnormal GTT (oral or IV), mentioned in Chapter 27, may give a normal tolbutamide curve. When they do produce abnormality, levels may remain below those diag-nostic for diabetes. The sensitivity of the tolbutamide test is apparently somewhat less than that of the oral GTT and definitely less than the C-GTT. Many mild diabetics have abnormal response to tolbutamide, but there is a definite overlap of results in the borderline area. A considerable number of the very mild diabetics have close to normal results. The overall sensitivity of the tolbutamide test seems to be about that of the intra-venous GTT.

The tolbutamide test is not used in the last trimester of pregnancy, due to a combination of increased insulin requirement and increased adrenal ste-roid levels. The tolbutamide test has been used with the same schedule of steroid pretreatment as the C-GTT. Results are too meager as yet, but there seems to be somewhat increased sensitivity at the expense of decreased specificity (some abnormal responses found in obesity and old age). The tolbutamide test at present has not been widely accepted in clinical medi-cine for the diagnosis of diabetes, although it has been proved one of the most reliable tests for insulin-producing tumors. It is agreed that further evaluation is needed.

HYPEROSMOLAR NONKETOTIC COMA. — This is uncommon but is being reported with increased frequency. The criterion for diagnosis is very high blood sugar (usually well over 500 mg/100 ml) without ketones in either plasma or urine. The patients usually become severely dehydrated. Plasma osmolality is high due to dehydration and hyperglycemia. Most patients are maturity-onset mild diabetics, but nondiabetics may be affected. Associated precipitating factors include infections, severe burns, high-dose corticosteroid therapy and renal dialysis. Occasional cases have been reported due to Dilantin and to glucose administration during hypothermia.

LACTIC ACIDOSIS SYNDROME. — This syndrome is rare and may have several etiologies. It is most frequently reported with phenformin (DBI) therapy of diabetes or as a nonketotic form of diabetic acidosis. The most common cause of elevated blood lactate is tissue hypoxia from shock. Arterial blood is said to be more reliable than venous for lactic acid determination. Tourniquet blood stagnation must be avoided, and the specimen must be kept in ice until analyzed.

REFERENCES:

Danowski, T. S.: Non-ketotic coma and diabetes mellitus, Med. Clin. North Am. 55: 913, 1971.
Gordon, E. E., and Kabadi, U. M.: The hyperglycemic hyperosmolar syndrome, Am. J. Med. Sci. 271:253, 1976.
Lubowitz, H., et al.: Lactic acidosis, Ann. Intern. Med. 134:148, 1974.
McCurdy, D. K.: Hyperosmolar hyperglycemic nonketotic diabetic coma, Med. Clin. North Am. 54:683, 1970.
Oliva, P. B.: Lactic acidosis, Am. J. Med. 48:209, 1970.
Unger, R. H., and Madison, L. L.: A new diagnostic procedure for mild diabetes mellitus, Diabetes 7:455, 1958.

Chapter 28. Thyroid Function Tests

TBG QUANTITATIVE ASSAY. — Methods are now available for measuring actual TBG levels by means of electrophoresis-isotope combination techniques. This was useful when thyroid test abnormalities due to TBG alterations were suspected. With use of the "corrected" T_4 by isotope or free thyroxine index, TBG assay should rarely be needed.

FREE THYROXINE ASSAY. — Theoretically, free thyroxine levels should closely reflect thyroid function and not be affected by agents that alter TBG. Free thyroxine can be measured by performing a T_4 by isotope procedure, isolating the radioactive hormone that fails to bind to TBG (usually done by dialysis) and then calculating what percentage of radioactivity this fraction represents. This fraction has the same relationship to the radioactivity binding to TBG as free thyroxine has to thyroxine bound to TBG. If one then quantitates serum thyroxine via the PBI or some other method, the free thyroxine radioactive fraction multiplied by total thyroxine quantity yields the quantity of free thyroxine. The main drawback of this procedure is technical difficulty plus the unexpected finding that serum free thyroxine levels may be elevated in persons seriously ill from a variety of diseases (interestingly, these seriously ill patients may also display decreased T_3 RIA and free T_3 results and slightly reduced T_4 values). Presence of heparin may elevate free thyroxine. With use of the free thyroxine index or "corrected" T_4, free thyroxine assay should rarely be needed.

LONG-ACTING THYROID STIMULATOR ASSAY.—Long-acting thyroid stimulator (LATS) is an IgG-type antibody whose origin is still debated but which is associated with stimulation of thyroid hormone production. There is especially good correlation with exophthalmos and pretibial myxedema. This antibody is found only in Graves' disease, not in toxic nodular goiter. Elevated values have been reported in a small percentage of other thyroid diseases, but usually in low titer. At present, an average of 40–60% of patients with Graves' disease have significantly elevated LATS levels, although possibly current bioassay methods are not sensitive enough. Current methods are difficult and expensive, and the T_3 suppression test gives similar information in borderline Graves' disease, so the necessity for LATS assay is rare. Nevertheless, there are reports of a few patients with exophthalmos, normal thyroid function test results, normal T_3 suppression and positive LATS assay results. Since the classic test procedure is a mouse thyroid bioassay, and since LATS infusion into humans has not been proved to simulate the human thyroid, LATS is now being referred to as "mouse thyroid stimulator" (MTS).

More recently, another immunoglobulin was found that prevented adsorption of LATS onto human thyroid tissue and was therefore called "LATS-protector." This has subsequently been shown to stimulate production of cyclic AMP and thyroid hormone by the thyroid and is now being called "human thyroid stimulator" (HTS). Assay for HTS at present involves a rather complicated tissue radioreceptor technique. One report indicates that HTS is present in all instances of Graves' disease. More data are needed.

REVERSE T_3.—Peripheral tissue deiodination of T_4 yields 2 forms of T_3: 1 form that is metabolically active, containing 2 iodine atoms on the phenol ring and a single atom of the tyrosyl ring, and 1 form that is relatively inactive, containing 1 iodine atom on the phenol ring and 2 atoms on the tyrosyl ring ("reverse T_3"). These 2 forms of T_3 are immunologically different. Radioimmunoassay techniques have been developed to measure reverse T_3. There is usually a reciprocal relationship between active T_3 and reverse T_3, suggesting that conditions lowering formation of active T_3 shift deiodination toward reverse T_3. Serum reverse T_3 is increased (with corresponding active T_3 decrease) in starvation, anorexia nervosa, severe illness of various types, following surgery and in amniotic fluid or cord blood. Reverse T_3 itself does not seem to influence TSH secretion or TRF response significantly.

"DYNAMIC" THYROID BLOOD FLOW STUDY (CAROTID-THYROID TRANSIT TIME).—A technique has been described whereby a radioisotope compound is injected intravenously and the number of seconds difference between the time when isotope appears in the common carotids and when it appears in the thyroid is measured. This test is said to be more accurate than the RAI, especially in hypothyroidism. It also has the advantage that less radiation is given to the patient. Both the study and a thyroid scan can be completed together in 1 day rather than the 2 days needed for the RAI. Disadvantages include the necessity for a stationary rapid imaging device such as the Anger camera and the fact that most conditions affecting the RAI likewise affect the "dynamic" flow study.

REFERENCES:

Anderson, B. G.: Free thyroxine in serum in relation to thyroid function, J.A.M.A. 203:577, 1968.

Ashkar, F. S., and Smith, E. M.: The dynamic thyroid study—A rapid evaluation of thyroid function and anatomy using 99m-Tc as pertechnetate, J.A.M.A. 217:441, 1971.

Burger, A., et al.: Reverse T3 in screening for neonatal hypothyroidism, Lancet 2:39, 1976.

Carter, J. N., et al.: Effect of severe, chronic illness on thyroid function, Lancet 2: 971, 1974.

Clague, R., et al.: Thyroid-stimulating immunoglobulins and the control of thyroid function, J. Clin. Endocrinol. Metab. 43:550, 1976.

Gharib, H., and Mayberry, W. E.: Diagnosis of Graves' ophthalmopathy without hyperthyroidism: Long-acting thyroid stimulator (LATS) determination as laboratory adjunct, Mayo Clin. Proc. 45:444, 1970.

Green, W. L.: Humoral and genetic factors in thyrotoxic Graves' disease and neonatal thyrotoxicosis, J.A.M.A. 235:1449, 1976.

Hall, R., et al.: Thyroid stimulators in health and disease, Clin. Endocrinol. (Tokyo) 4:213, 1975.

Hershman, J. M., et al.: Reciprocal changes in serum thyrotropin and free thyroxine produced by heparin, J. Clin. Endocrinol. Metab. 34:574, 1972.

Kodding, R., et al.: Reverse triodothyronine in liver disease, Lancet 2:314, 1976.

Kriss, J. P.: The Long-Acting Stimulator and Thyroid Disease, in Stollerman, G. H., et al. (eds.): Advances in Internal Medicine (Chicago: Year Book Medical Publishers, Inc., 1970), vol. 16, p. 135.

Nicod, P., et al.: The failure of physiologic doses of reverse T3 to affect thyroid-pituitary function in man, J. Clin. Endocrinol. Metab. 43:478, 1976.

Chapter 29. Adrenal Function Tests

TESTS IN PRIMARY ALDOSTERONISM.—The technical difficulty of aldosterone and renin determinations has led to various screening tests for Conn's syndrome and, in some instances, to procedures that might replace renin for diagnosis. Now that more reliable renin determination is becoming available through RIA and while simplification of aldosterone technique continues, the need for alternatives to aldosterone and renin determinations has greatly decreased. However, original good results from most of the screening procedures have not yet been sufficiently evaluated by others. The new procedures include the following:

Deoxycorticosterone (DOCA) Suppression Test.—Deoxycorticosterone is reported to suppress aldosterone secretion in secondary aldosteronism but not in Conn's syndrome. It is a precursor of aldosterone.

Alpha-fluorohydrocortisone (fludrocortisone) Suppression Test.—This is similar to DOCA suppression. Fludrocortisone is a hydrocortisone analogue with marked salt-retaining action.

Spironolactone Test.—Potassium clearance is measured before and after 3 days of oral spironolactone (with the patient on a high-salt diet). More than 50% reduction in clearance suggests aldosteronism (either primary or secondary).

Furosemide (Lasix) Test. — The patient remains upright for 4 hours following an oral dose of the diuretic furosemide. Plasma renin is then drawn. The original report states 80% agreement with low-salt diet renin response in hypertensive patients, with the 20% disagreement containing both false positives and false negatives.

Saline Infusion. — Large quantities of saline given intravenously over a 2-day period are said to suppress aldosterone to less than 50% of baseline values in conditions other than primary aldosteronism.

Twenty-four-hour Urine Potassium. — Patients with hypokalemia who have primary aldosteronism usually have normal potassium excretion (over 40 mEq/day), while most others have low excretion as the body attempts to conserve potassium.

Plasma Aldosterone with Saline Infusion. — Plasma aldosterone is reported to be suppressed to less than 50% of baseline (recumbent for 8 hours) values by infusion of 2 L saline over a 2-hour period, whereas levels in primary aldosteronism remain greater than 50%. Saline infusion causes more marked suppression than does a high-salt diet.

17-KETOSTEROIDS. — These can be fractionated into alpha (androsterone and etiocholanolone) and beta (dehydroepiandrosterone). Increase of 17-KS in adrenal carcinoma is most often due to beta fraction increase. The normal ratio of beta to alpha is less than 0.2. Alternatively, the "Allen Blue" test is a reasonable estimate of DHA. Not all carcinomas are positive with either of these procedures, and neither is indicated if urine 17-KS are normal; therefore the use of these tests is decreasing.

SARALASIN TEST. — This is a test for renin-mediated hypertension. Saralasin (an angiotensin II analogue) is a competitive inhibitor of angiotensin II and therefore acts as an angiotensin blocking agent. An intravenous bolus of saralasin is reported to produce significant decrease in blood pressure in patients with renin-produced hypertension but not in normal persons or those with other etiologies for hypertension. These are primarily patients with unilateral renal disease. Some data suggest that such patients may respond to saralasin even if peripheral blood renin assay is within normal range. Premedication by salt depletion is said to be necessary in some cases. More evaluation is needed, but evidence is accumulating that saralasin may become the test of choice in screening for high-renin hypertension.

REFERENCES

Biglieri, E. G., et al.: A preliminary evaluation for primary aldosteronism, Arch. Intern. Med. 126:1004, 1970.
Birchall, R., and Batson, H. M., Jr.: Test for pathologic secretion of aldosterone, J.A.M.A. 206:2114, 1968.
Espiner, E. A., et al.: Effect of saline infusions on aldosterone secretions and electrolyte excretion in primary aldosteronism. N. Engl. J. Med. 277:1, 1967.

Frawley, T. F.: Cushing's Syndrome, in *Clinician* (Chicago: G. D. Searle & Co., 1971), vol. 1, p. 37.

Kem, D. C., et al.: Saline suppression of plasma aldosterone in hypertension, Arch. Intern. Med. 128:380, 1971.

Kopin, I. J., et al.: Dopamine-beta-hydroxylase: Basic and clinical studies, Ann. Intern. Med. 85:211, 1976.

Leutscher, J. A., et al.: Effects of sodium loading, sodium depletion and posture on plasma aldosterone concentration and renin activity in hypertensive patients, J. Clin. Endocrinol. Metab. 29:1310, 1969.

MacDonald, W. G., and Todoroff, T. G.: Negative results: The urinary sodium-ACTH test for adrenal competence, Am. J. Med. Sci. 252:446, 1966.

Marks, L. S., et al.: Saralasin bolus test: Rapid screening procedure for renin-mediated hypertension, Lancet 2:784, 1975.

Ramirez, G., and Bates, H. M.: Measurement of plasma dopamine beta-hydroxylase activity, Lab. Management 12:15, 1974.

Smilo, R. P., and Forsham, P. H.: Diagnostic approach to hypofunction and hyperfunction of the adrenal cortex, Postgrad. Med. 46:146, 1969.

Wallach, L., et al.: Stimulated renin: Screening test for hypertension, Ann. Intern. Med. 82:27, 1975.

Chapter 30. Pituitary, Parathyroid, Gonadal Function Tests; Tests in Obstetrics

PARATHYROID FUNCTION.—*Neck Vein Catheterization.*—In general, parathyroid hormone (PTH) increase from veins in only one side of the neck suggests parathyroid tumor, while increase in both sides suggests secondary hyperparathyroidism or ectopic PTH. Even this procedure does not always disclose PTH elevation in parathyroid tumor or always differentiate primary from secondary hyperparathyroidism with absolute accuracy. Results vary according to whether large or small vessels are catheterized and in what areas, and success thus depends on the skill and experience of the operator. Such procedures are therefore best carried out in an institution that has someone with an interest and extensive experience in this technique.

Chloride-Phosphate Ratio (C/P).—One group of investigators found that serum chloride (in mEq/L) divided by serum phosphorus (phosphate, in mg/100 ml) was above 33 in nearly 95% of patients with primary hyperparathyroidism and below 33 in about the same percentage of patients with hypercalcemia from other etiologies. The test is not useful if the serum calcium is normal or if a significant degree of renal failure is present. Ectopic PTH syndrome would also give false results. Some reports indicate too much overlap between primary hyperparathyroidism and other diseases to rely on the C/P ratio. More evaluation is needed.

Urine Cyclic AMP (cAMP) Excretion.—One of the effects of PTH is production of cAMP in the kidney, which mediates tubular reabsorption of phosphate. In primary hyperparathyroidism, cAMP excretion is increased; in hypercalcemia from other causes or in secondary hyperparathyroidism, cAMP is decreased. Cyclic AMP can also be used to differentiate primary hypoparathyroidism from pseudohypoparathyroidism (normal parathyroids but kidneys refractory to PTH). Injection of PTH will not increase cAMP in patients with pseudohypoparathyroidism. Cyclic AMP is reported to follow a diurnal rhythm in most persons (peak either between 9 A.M. and 3 P.M. or between 3 A.M. and 9 P.M.), so that a 24-hour urine collection is preferred. Decreased renal function may decrease cAMP excretion. More evaluation is needed as to its diagnostic accuracy or usefulness in possible hyperparathyroidism.

Selenomethionine Isotope Scanning.—Used to localize hyperactive parathyroid glands, results have been rather disappointing for a majority of those who have tried this technique.

Modified Calcium Infusion Procedure.—This has been recently reported to improve specificity of the old Ellsworth-Howard infusion test. Independent evaluation is needed.

Radioreceptor Test for Pregnancy.—Now available as an RIA kit (Biocept-G, Wampole Laboratories), this is based on the principle of competitive binding (p. 338) in which radioactive human chorionic gonadotropin (hCG) competes with patient hCG for tissue receptor sites on a preparation of bovine corpus luteum material. The procedure takes about 1 hour to perform. It is said to detect as little as 0.2 IU/ml of hCG, and may be reactive as early as 6–8 days after ovulation if fertilization occurs (compared to 25 days after ovulation for most standard immunologic pregnancy tests). Luteinizing hormone crossreacts; this may be a problem in menopausal or postmenopausal women. There is also an LH rise at midcycle, although supposedly below the detection level of the test. This may necessitate serial studies. More clinical evaluation is needed. Assay for beta-hCG by RIA might accomplish most of the same results.

REFERENCES

Aro, A., et al.: Hypercalcemia: Serum chloride and phosphate, Ann. Int. Med. 86:664, 1977.
Drezner, M. K., et al.: Renal cyclic adenosine monophosphate: An accurate index of parathyroid function, Metabolism 25:1103, 1976.
Eisenberg, H., et al.: Selective arteriography, venography, and venous hormone assay in diagnosis and localization of parathyroid lesions, Am. J. Med. 56:810, 1974.
Landsman, R., and Saxena, B. B.: Radioreceptorassay of human chorionic gonadotropin as an aid in miniabortion, Fertil. Steril. 25:1022, 1974.
Murad, F., and Pak, C. Y. C.: Urinary excretion of adenosine 3′, 5′-monophosphate, and guanosine 3′, 5′-monophosphate, N. Engl. J. Med. 286:1382, 1972.
Pak, C. Y. C., et al: Simple and reliable test for diagnosis of hyperparathyroidism, Arch. Intern. Med. 129:48, 1972.
Reeves, C. D., et al.: Differential diagnosis of hypercalcemia by the chloride/phosphate ratio. Am. J. Surg. 130:166, 1975.

Chapter 32. Laboratory Aspects of Cancer

URINE LACTIC DEHYDROGENASE (LDH).—This has been proposed as a screening test for urinary tract carcinoma. This procedure is not the same technique used for serum LDH, because urine contains an inhibitor that must be dialyzed out before assay is performed. Despite several enthusiastic reports, it has been found that other conditions such as urinary tract infection can also elevate urine LDH; to date, this test has not been widely used.

URINE HYDROXYPROLINE.—Hydroxyproline is a collagen component whose urinary excretion is increased in various disorders with increased osteoblastic activity as well as some diseases involving osteolysis and collagen metabolism. Significantly increased 24-hour excretion is reported in about half of patients with tumors having bone metastases, and normal results were obtained in most patients with tumors who did not have bone involvement. Some of those with skeletal metastases and elevated urine hydroxyproline had normal alkaline phosphatase levels. Some investigators use hydroxyproline/creatinine ratios. The test may be useful in some cancer patients by suggesting occult bone metastasis, although a bone scan is probably more sensitive.

EFFUSION CEA.—One report indicates that carcinoembryonic antigen (CEA) assay on effusion fluid can correctly identify malignant effusions in a high percentage of cases. Effusion CEA is said to indicate malignancy if greater than 10 ng/ml (Hansen method) or if double the plasma CEA level when effusion values are between 5 and 10 ng/ml. This work needs confirmation.

REFERENCES

Hosley, H. F., et al.: Hydroxyproline excretion in malignant neoplastic disease, Arch. Intern. Med. 118:565, 1966.
Nystrom, J. S., et al.: Carcinoembryonic antigen titers on effusion fluid, Arch. Int. Med. 137:875, 1977.
Schmidt, J. D.: Significance of total urinary lactic dehydrogenase activity in urinary tract disease, J. Urol. 96:950, 1966.

Chapter 33. Congenital Diseases

X-RAY IN LACTASE DEFICIENCY.—An upper GI series with small bowel follow-through may be helpful in suggesting lactase deficiency. Fifty grams of lactose is added to the barium suspension. Certain roentgenographic findings (such as barium-lactose dilution, intestinal dilatation and intestinal "hurry") point toward need for additional studies. Gastrectomy procedures may produce false positive results.

FAMILIAL DYSAUTONOMIA (RILEY-DAY SYNDROME).—This is a familial disorder characterized by a variety of signs and symptoms including defective lacrimation, relative indifference to pain, postural hypotension, excessive sweating, emotional lability and absence of the fungiform papilli on the anterior portion of the tongue. Most of those affected are Jewish. Helpful laboratory tests include increased urine homovanillic acid (HVA) and decreased serum dopamine-beta hydroxylase (DBH), an enzyme that helps convert dopamine to norepinephrine. Besides the Riley-Day syndrome, DBH may also be decreased in mongolism (Down's syndrome) and Parkinson's disease. It has been reported to be elevated in about 50% of patients with neuroblastoma, in stress and in certain congenital disorders that have not been adequately confirmed. There is disagreement as to values in patients with hypertension.

MALIGNANT HYPERPYREXIA (MALIGNANT HYPERTHERMIA).—This is a rare complication of anesthesia triggered by various conduction and inhalation agents, which results in sudden tachycardia, tachypnea, metabolic acidosis, hypercalcemia and markedly elevated temperature. A defect in muscle cell membrane transport has been postulated. The majority of cases have been familial. Creatine phosphokinase (CPK) elevation without known cause has been proposed as a screening test; there is marked difference of opinion among investigators as to the usefulness of the procedure, either in screening for surgery or in family studies. Likewise, disagreement exists as to the CPK isoenzyme associated with abnormality; BB has been reported by some, although the majority found MM to be responsible.

REFERENCES

Britt, B. A.: Malignant hyperthermia: A pharmacogenetic disease of skeletal and cardiac muscle, N. Engl. J. Med. 290:1140, 1974.

Kopin, I. J., et al.: Dopamine-beta-hydroxylase, Ann. Intern. Med. 85:211, 1976.

Laws, J. W., and Neale, G.: Radiological diagnosis of disaccharidase deficiency, Lancet 2:139, 1966.

Preger, L., and Amberg, J. R.: Sweet diarrhea: Roentgen diagnosis of disaccharidase deficiency, Am. J. Roentgenol 101:287, 1967.

Riley, C. M., and Moore, R. H.: Familial dysautonomia differentiated from related disorders: Case reports and discussion of current concepts, Pediatrics 37:435, 1966.

Rosenquist, C. J., et al.: Intestinal lactase deficiency: Diagnosis by routine upper gastrointestinal radiography, Radiology 102:275, 1972.

DIAGNOSTIC PROCEDURES THAT COMPLEMENT AND SUPPLEMENT LABORATORY TESTS

The clinical pathologist frequently meets situations in which laboratory tests alone are not sufficient to provide a diagnosis. If this happens, certain diagnostic procedures may be suggested to provide additional information. These procedures are noted together with the laboratory tests that they complement or supplement. Nevertheless, it seems useful to summarize some basic information about these techniques and some data that, for various reasons, are not included elsewhere.

Diagnostic Ultrasound

Ultrasound is based on the familiar principle of radar, differing primarily in the frequency of the sound waves. Very high frequency (1–10 MHz) sound emissions are directed toward an object, are reflected (echo production) by the target and return to the detector, with a time delay proportional to the distance traveled. Differences in tissue or material density result in a series of echoes produced by the surfaces of the various tissues or substances that lie in the path of the sound beam.

In "A-mode" (amplitude) readout, the echo signals are seen as spikes (similar to an ECG tracing format) with the height of the spike corresponding to intensity of the echo and the distance between spikes depending on the distance between the various interfaces (boundaries) of materials in the path of the sound beam. The A-mode technique is used mainly for the head, since the skull prevents adequate B-mode visualization by current techniques.

In "B-mode" (brightness-modulated; bistable) readout, the sonic generator (transducer) is moved in a line across an area while the echoes are depicted as tiny dots corresponding to the location (origin) of the echo. This produces a pattern of dots, which gives a visual image of the shape and degree of homogeneity of material in the path of the sound beam (the visual result is a tomographic slice or thin cross section of the target, with a dot pattern form somewhat analogous to that of a nuclear medicine scan).

"Gray-scale" is a refinement of B-mode scan readout in which changes in amplitude (intensity) of the sonic beam produced by differential absorption through different material in the path of the beam is transmuted into shades of gray in the dot pattern. This helps us to recognize smaller changes in tissue density (somewhat analogous to an x-ray).

The B-mode ultrasound technique is now the basic technique for most routine work. Limitations include problems with very dense materials, such as bone or x-ray barium, which act as a barrier both for signal and echo, and air, which is a poor transmitter of high-frequency sound (lungs; air in distended bowel or stomach, etc.).

In "M-mode" (motion) readout, the sonic generator and detector remain temporarily in one location, with each echo being depicted as a small dot relative to original echo location; this is similar to A-mode, but it uses a single dot instead of a spike. However, a moving recorder shows changes in the echo pattern that occur if any structures in the sonic beam path move; changes in location of the echo dot are seen in the areas that move but not in the areas that are stationary. The result is a series of parallel lines, each line corresponding to the continuous record of one echo dot, stationary dots producing straight lines and moving dots becoming a wavy or ECG-like line. In fact, the technique and readout is somewhat analogous to that of the ECG, if each area of the heart were to produce its own ECG tracing and all were displayed together as a series of parallel tracings. The M-mode technique is used primarily in studies of the heart (echocardiography), particularly aortic and mitral valve function.

USES OF DIAGNOSTIC ULTRASOUND.—With continuing improvements in equipment, capabilities of ultrasound are changing rapidly. A major advantage is that ultrasound is completely "noninvasive"; in addition, no radiation is administered and no acute or chronic ill effects have yet been substantiated in either tissues or genetic apparatus. Some of the major areas in which ultrasound may be helpful are:

Differentiation of Solid from Cystic Structures.—This is helpful in diagnosis of renal space-occupying lesions, nonfunctioning thyroid nodules, pancreatic pseudocyst, pelvic masses, and so on. When a structure is thought to be a cyst, accuracy should be 90–95%. Ultrasound is the best method for diagnosis of pancreatic pseudocyst.

Abscess Detection.—In the abdomen reported accuracy (in a few small series) varies between 60–90%, with 80% probably a reasonable present-day expectation. Abscess within organs such as the liver may be seen and differentiated from a cyst or solid tumor. Obvious factors affecting accuracy are size and location of the abscess as well as interference from air or barium in overlying bowel loops.

Differentiation of Intrahepatic from Extrahepatic Biliary Obstruction.—This is based on attempted visualization of dilated biliary tract ducts in extrahepatic obstruction. Present-day accuracy is probably about 80–90%.

Ultrasound may be useful in demonstrating a dilated gallbladder when cholecystography is not possible or suggests nonfunction. It may also be helpful in diagnosis of cholecystitis. Reports indicate about 90% accuracy in detection of gallbladder calculi.

Diagnosis of Pancreatic Carcinoma. – Although islet cell tumors are too small to be seen, acinar carcinoma can be detected in approximately 75–80% of instances. Pancreatic carcinoma cannot always be differentiated from pancreatitis.

Guidance of Biopsy Needles. – Ultrasound is helpful in biopsies.

Placental Localization; Visualization and Measurement of the Fetus; Diagnosis of Hydatidiform Mole. – Ultrasound is the method of choice in obstetrics to avoid irradiation of mother or fetus.

Detection and Delineation of Abdominal Aortic Aneurysms. – Ultrasound is the current method of choice for these aneurysms. Clot in the lumen, which causes problems for aortography, does not interfere with ultrasound. For dissecting abdominal aneurysms, however, ultrasound is much less reliable than aortography. Thoracic aneurysms are difficult to visualize by ultrasound with present techniques.

Detection of Periaortic and Retroperitoneal Masses of Enlarged Lymph Nodes. – Ultrasound current accuracy is probably 80–90%. There is at present very little reliable data that compare ultrasound to scanning with tumor-seeking radiopharmaceuticals (currently, radiogallium or bleomycin) or to computerized axial tomography.

Ocular Examination. – Although special equipment is needed, ultrasound has proved useful for detection of intraocular foreign bodies and tumors, as well as certain other conditions. This technique is especially helpful when opacity prevents adequate visual examination.

Cardiac Diagnosis. – Ultrasound using M-mode technique is the most sensitive and accurate method for detection of pericardial effusion, capable of detecting as little as 50 ml of fluid. A minor drawback is difficulty in finding loculated effusions. Mitral stenosis can be diagnosed accurately, and useful information can be obtained about other types of mitral dysfunction. Ultrasound can also provide information about aortic and tricuspid function, although not to the same degree. Entities such as hypertrophic subaortic stenosis and left atrial myxoma can frequently be identified. The thickness of the left ventricle can be estimated. Finally, vegetations of endocarditis may be detected on mitral, aortic or tricuspid valves in over half the patients.

REFERENCES

Dallow, R. L.: Ultrasonography of the eye and orbit, Appl. Radiol. 4:81, 1975.
Doust, B. D.: Role of ultrasound in obstetrics and gynecology, Hosp. Practice 8:143, 1973.
Freeman, L. A., (ed.): Diagnostic ultrasound issue, Semin. Nucl. Med. 5:287, 1975.
Hill, B. A., et al.: Diagnostic sonography in general surgery, Arch. Surg. 110:1089, 1975.

Maklad, N. F., et al.: Ultrasonic diagnosis of postoperative intra-abdominal abscess, Radiology 113:417, 1974.

Roundtable on diagnostic ultrasound, Patient Care 9:110 (Nov. 15), 1975; 9:20 (Dec. 1), 1975.

Computerized Axial Tomography (CAT Scan)

Computerized axial tomography scanning combines radiologic x-ray emission with nuclear medicine-type radiation detectors (rather than direct x-ray exposure of photographic film in the manner of ordinary radiology). The first CAT scanner (EMI) employed a pencil-like x-ray beam, detected on the opposite side of the object being scanned by a sodium iodide crystal similar to those used in nuclear medicine scanning. Tissue density of the various components of the object being scanned determined how much of the x-ray beam reached the detector, as in conventional radiology. However, the beam source traveled in a line across the object to be scanned, then stopped, turned its direction 1 degree, traveled in a line back across the object, rotated another degree and continued the process until it had moved 180° around the object being scanned (the beam source stayed at the same level relative to the top and bottom edge of the object but moved in an arc halfway around the object). This meant that the beam source had traversed the object 180 times from 180 different angles. A computer secured tissue density measurements from the detector as this was going on and eventually constructed a composite tissue density image similar in many aspects to those seen in ordinary x-rays. The image corresponds to a thin cross-section slice through the object (3–15 mm thick), i.e., a tissue cross-section slice viewed at a right angle (90°) to the direction of the x-ray beam.

To decrease the time required for a complete study, some manufacturers used multiple beams with multiple detectors and some used a fan-shaped (triangular) beam with multiple gas-filled tube detectors on the opposite side of the object to be scanned (corresponding to the base of the x-ray beam triangle). The beam source moved in a complete 360° circle around the object to be scanned without going back and forth across the object each time the direction of the beam was changed.

With the original EMI machine CAT scanning was limited to the head. Equipment capable of scanning any portion of the body is now available from an ever-increasing number of manufacturers. Evaluation of CAT results to date for the brain may be found on page 205. "Total body" CAT scanning has to date been limited to a relatively few institutions, and evaluation is in its early stages. Few data are available comparing CAT to ultrasound, nuclear medicine procedures and radiologic techniques in thoracic and abdominal diseases. Some information on biliary tract and pancreatic scanning is included in the sections that discuss laboratory tests for these areas.

REFERENCES

Alfidi, R. J., et al.: Computed tomography of the liver, Am. J. Roentgenol. 127:69, 1976.

Baker, H. L., et al.: Computer assisted tomography of the head: An early evaluation, Mayo Clin. Proc. 49:17, 1974.

Christie, J. H., et al.: Computed tomography and radionuclide studies in the diagnosis of intracranial disease, Am. J. Roentgenol. 127:171, 1976.

Davis, K. R., et al.: Cerebral infarction diagnosis by computerized tomography: Analysis and evaluation of findings, Am. J. Roentgenol. 124:643, 1975.

Payne, J. T., and McCullough, E. C.: Basic principles of computer-assisted tomography, Appl. Radiol. 5:53, 1976.

Stanley, R. J., et al.: Computed tomography of the body: Early trends in application and accuracy of the method, Am. J. Roentgenol. 127:53, 1976.

Wiggans, G., et al.: Computerized axial tomography for diagnosis of pancreatic cancer, Lancet 2:233, 1976.

Nuclear Medicine Scanning

Nuclear medicine organ scans involve certain compounds that selectively localize in the organs of interest when administered to the patient. The compound is first made radioactive by tagging with a radioactive element. (An exception is iodine used in thyroid diagnosis, which is already an element; in this case a radioactive isotope of iodine can be used. An isotope is a different form of the same element with the same chemical properties as the stable element form but physically unstable due to differences in the number of neutrons in the nucleus, this difference producing nuclear instability and leading to emission of radioactivity.) After the radioactive compound is administered and sufficient uptake by the organ of interest is achieved, the organ is "scanned" with a radiation detector. This is usually a sodium iodide crystal. Radioactivity is transmuted into tiny flashes of light within the crystal. The location of the light flashes corresponds to the locations within the organ from which radioactivity is being emitted; the intensity of a light flash is proportional to the quantity of radiation detected. The detection device surveys ("scans") the organ and produces an overall pattern of radioactivity (both the concentration and the distribution of activity), which it translates into a visual picture of light and dark areas.

Rectilinear scanners focus on one small area; the detector traverses the organ in a series of parallel lines to produce a complete (composite) picture. A "camera" device has a large-diameter crystal and remains stationary, with the field of view size dependent on the size of the crystal. The various organ scans are discussed in chapters that include biochemical function tests referable to the same organ.

The camera detectors are able to perform rapid sequence imaging not possible on a rectilinear apparatus, and this can be used for "dynamic flow" studies. A bolus of radioactive material can be injected into the bloodstream and followed through major vessels and organs by data storage equipment or rapid (1–3 second) serial photographs. Although the image does not have a degree of resolution comparable to that of contrast medium angiography, major abnormalities in major blood vessels can be identified, and the uptake and early distribution of blood supply in specific tissues or organs can be visualized.

Data on radionuclide procedures are included in areas of laboratory test discussion when this seems appropriate.

REFERENCE

Blahd, W. H. (ed.): Nuclear Medicine (2d ed.; New York: McGraw-Hill Book Company, Inc., 1971.

Appendix

A Compendium of Useful Data and Information

EFFECTS OF AGE ON LABORATORY TESTS

Apparent age-related increase in abnormal results has been reported in a wide variety of tests in patients over age 50.

1. Antinuclear antibodies; rheumatoid factor; VDRL; serum globulin (Br. J. Ven. Dis. 42:40, 1966; Ann. Rheum. Dis. 28:431, 1969)
2. Cholesterol; triglyceride (p. 253)
3. BUN (J. Lab. Clin. Med. 73:825, 1969)
4. Oral GTT values (p. 318)
5. ESR (p. 232)
6. Creatinine clearance (p. 131)
7. D-xylose test (p. 300)
8. Serum calcium (New England J. Med. 281:367, 1969 – however, most investigators do not find any significant difference)
9. Gastric acidity (p. 304)
10. T_3 RIA (p. 341)

SUBSTANCES THAT INTERFERE WITH CERTAIN LABORATORY TESTS

(Compiled from various sources; see especially Clin. Chem. 21 (5):1D, 1975)

I. Pheochromocytoma tests
  A. Catecholamines
    Poor preservation during collection
    Large doses of B complex vitamins
    Certain broad-spectrum antibiotics (ampicillin, Declomycin, Erythromycin, tetracyclines)
    Formaldehyde-forming drugs (Mandelamine, Uritone) in urine
    Ascorbic acid (vitamin C)
    Bananas
    Chlorpromazine (Thorazine)
    Hydralazine (Apresoline)
    Methyldopa (Aldomet)
    Isuprel or epinephrine-like drugs (inhalation)
    Quinine or quinidine

Salicylates
Uremia (fluorescent substances)
B. Vanillylmandelic acid (VMA)
  1. Screening tests (Gitlow method, etc.)
    Tea
    Coffee
    Citrus fruits
    Vanilla
    Bananas
    Chocolate
    Aspirin
    5-hydroxyindoleacetic acid (5-HIAA)
  2. Fluorescent techniques
    Same medications as catecholamines
    Glyceryl guaiacolate (cough medicines)
C. Metanephrines
  1. IVP x-ray media that contain methylglucamine (Renovist, Renografin), Pisano method
  2. Very few specific reports to date; presumably most compounds that increase catecholamines would increase metanephrines

II. 5-hydroxyindoleacetic acid (5-HIAA)
A. Substances that contain large amounts of serotonin (affects any method)
  Tomatoes
  Red plums
  Avocado
  Eggplant
  Bananas
B. Method of Udenfriend
  Methocarbamol (Robaxin)
  Mephenesin carbamate (several proprietary muscle-relaxant compounds)
  Glyceryl guaiacolate (many proprietary cough medicines)
  Phenothiazines (Thorazine, etc.)
  P-hydroxyacetanilide

III. 17-hydroxycorticosteroids (17-OHCS)
A. Increase

Acetone (in urine)	Monase
Ascorbic acid (vitamin C)	Oleandomycin
Atarax	Paraldehyde
Chloral hydrate	Quinine or quinidine
Colchicine	Reserpine
Doriden	Spironolactone
Estrogens or contraceptive drugs	Thorazine and similar phenothiazines
Fructose (in urine)	
Glucose (in urine)	Valmid
Librium	Vistaril
Mandelamine	
Meprobamate	

B. Decrease
   Apresoline
   Phenergan
   Reserpine
   Salicylate
IV. 17-ketosteroids (17-KS)

Acetone (in urine)
Amphetamine
Atarax (Vistaril)
Cephalothin
Diamox
Digitoxin
Diuril
Doriden
Librium
Meprobamate
Metabolites of progesterone (in urine)
Nalidixic acid (NegGram)

Oleandomycin
Penicillin
Pyridium
Quinine
Reserpine
Seconal
Spironolactone
Thorazine
Valmid

V. Anticoagulants
   A. Drugs that potentiate Coumadin (increase PT)

Aldomet (methyldopa)
Anabolic steroids
Analexin (phenyramidol)
Antabuse (disulfiram)
Atromid-S (clofibrate)
Benemid
Butazolidin and Tandearil
Chloral hydrate
Choloxin and cholestyramine
Clofibrate
Dextran
Diabinese
Diazoxide (Hyperstat)
Dilantin
Edecrin (ethacrynic acid)
Estrogens
Glucagon
Hepatotoxic agents
Indocin
Isoniazid (INH)
MAO inhibitors
Nalidixic acid (NegGram)

Orinase (tolbutamide)
PAS
Ponstel (mefenamic acid)
Quinidine and quinine
Reserpine
Ritalin (methylphenidate)
Salicylates (over 1 gm/day)
Sulfas
Tempra, Tylenol (acetaminophen)
Thiouracil drugs
Thyroid hormone
Vitamin B complex
Various antibiotics (Chloromy-
   cetin, Kantrex, tetracycline,
   penicillin)
Zyloprim

   B. Drugs that decrease response to Coumadin (decrease PT)

Antacids
Barbiturates
Digitalis
Diuretics (except Edecrin)
Doriden (glutethimide)
Estrogens
Griseofulvin

Haldol (haloperidol)
Meprobamate
Paraldehyde
Placidyl (ethchlorvynol)
Rimactane (rifampin)
Steroids

C. Drugs that antagonize action of heparin
   Antihistamine (large doses)   Phenothiazines (Thorazine, etc.)
   Digitalis   Polymyxin B (Coly-Mycin)
   Penicillin   Tetracycline

VI. Drugs that interfere with absorption
   Dilantin: blocks folic acid; decreases B_{12} and D-xylose
   Cholestyramine: decreases digoxin
   Colchicine: decreases B_{12}, carotene, D-xylose
   Kaopectate: decreases digoxin
   Neomycin: blocks folic acid; decreases B_{12} and D-xylose

VII. Effects of estrogens (birth control pills)
   Decrease albumin, glucose tolerance, T_3 uptake test, plasma cholin-
      esterase; may decrease folic acid
   Increase transferrin, TBG (thus alters various T_4 and T_3 RIA tests),
      triglycerides, total lipids, serum iron, iron-binding capacity, plas-
      ma cortisol, urine aldosterone, serum $alpha_2$ globulins, growth
      hormone, $alpha_1$-antitrypsin, neutrophil alkaline phosphatase,
      ceruloplasmin, RBC cholinesterase, serum vitamin A and caro-
      tene.
   Potentiate Coumadin (increases PT); invalidate metyrapone test

VIII. Technicon Autoanalyzer drug effects
   SGOT increased by diabetic acidosis, PAS, Vistaril, barbiturates
   Glucose oxidase-peroxidase interference by vitamin C., hydralazine,
      iproniazid (Marsilid), INH, tolazamide (Tolinase), acetaminophen
   Neocuproine glucose increased by reducing substances (15 mg/100
      ml creatinine plus 10 mg/100 ml uric acid raises glucose 20 mg/
      100 ml)
   Lipemia decreases cholesterol, bilirubin, albumin, LDH, alkaline
      phosphatase

IX. Miscellaneous
   Alkaline phosphatase: increased by many brands of human serum
      albumin (derived from placental tissue)
   SGOT: erythromycin increases colorimetric method, but not UV
      methods
   Heparin: antagonized by ascorbic acid; increases T_4 up to 60 min-
      utes after injection; increases free thyroxine; increases plasma
      insulin when used as specimen anticoagulant
   Plasma cortisol: spironolactone produces increase by fluorometric
      method
   Lithium therapy: frequent slight elevation of TSH and decrease in
      T_4; occasional clinical hypothyroidism
   Urine estriol: false increase from glucosuria, urinary tract infection,
      Mandelamine, hydrochlorothiazide, steroids; both serum and
      urine estriol affected by ampicillin and neomycin
   Porphobilinogen: false positive from phenothiazines
   Methyldopa (Aldomet): may increase bilirubin, reducing-substance
      methods for creatinine, uric acid and glucose, SMA 12/60 SGOT
      method, catecholamines or VMA; may produce lupus erythemato-
      sus (LE) syndrome

X. Digitalis

A. Conditions that increase risk of digitalis toxicity
Renal function decrease (especially when serum creatinine is increased)
Hypokalemia (diuretic or steroid therapy, cirrhosis, diabetic acidosis)
Hemodialysis
Hypothyroidism
Liver disease (hypokalemia and thiamine deficiency)

B. Drugs that potentiate digitalis effects
Adrenergic drugs (ephedrine, Isuprel, etc.)   Propranolol
Calcium intravenous therapy   Quinidine
Diuretics (except spironolactone)   Serpasil (reserpine)
Insulin   Thyroid hormone
Ismelin (guanethidine)
Intravenous glucose in water

C. Drugs that may decrease digitalis effect
Cholestyramine
Diphenylhydantoin (Dilantin)
Kaopectate
Oral aminoglycoside antibiotics
Phenobarbital
Phenylbutazone

XI. Drugs that affect kidney function
Amphotericin B
Aminoglycoside antibiotics (gentamicin, Kanamycin, Neomycin, Tobramycin)
Diuretics
Guanethidine (Ismeline)
Indomethacin (Indocin)
Methicillin
Methyldopa (Aldomet)
Polymyxin antibiotics (colistin, Coly-Mycin, polymyxin B)
Tetracyclines (intravenous)

XII. Serum cholinesterase (decrease)
Atropine
Barbiturates
Chloroquine
Epinephrine
Opiates
Phenothiazines
Prostigmin
Quinidine

XIII. Effects of ascorbic acid (vitamin C) in large doses
A. Increased
Tests that depend on reducing-substance reactions: creatinine, blood glucose (neocuproine, Folin-Wu, ferricyanide methods), uric acid, urine glucose by Benedict's or Clinitest methods
B. Decreased
Antagonist to heparin
Serum or urine glucose using glucose oxidase (Clinistix, etc.)

Serum vitamin B$_{12}$
Occult blood using orthotolidin (Hematest or Hemastix)
  C. Interferes with blood volume determination using RBC tagging
XIV. Drugs that may affect liver function
  A. Exclusively cholestatic (androgenic/anabolic steroids, estrogens)
    Dianabol (methandrostenolone)
    Enovid (norethynodrel)
    Halotestin (fluoxymesterone)
    Nilevar (norethandrolone)
    Norlutin (norethindrone)
  B. Cholestatic plus hepatocellular toxic component

Butazolidin	Nicotinic acid
Dilantin	Nilevar (norethandrolone)
Ilosone	Phenothiazines (Thorazine)
Librium	Tapazole (methimazole)
Marsilid (iproniazid)	Tetracycline (intravenous)
Meprobamate	

  C. Cytotoxic

Diabinese (chlorpropamide)	Nitrogen mustards
Dialose (laxative)	Novobiocin
Gold salts	Oxacillin
Halothane	Oxyphenisatin acetate (stool
Imuran (azathioprine)	softener ingredient)
Indocin	PAS
Isoniazid (INH))	Phenurone (phenacetylurea)
Methotrexate	Probenecid
Methyldopa	Zoxazolamine (Flexon)
Monamine oxidase inhibitor (Marsilid, Nardil)	

  D. Reported but not in detail

Allopurinol	Papaverine
Carbenicillin	Procainamide
Clofibrate	Rifampin
Florantyrone	Thiothixene
Lincomycin	Tolazamide
Metaxalone	Troleandomycin

XV. Drugs that increase renin activity
  Hydralazine (Apresoline)
  Diazoxide (Hyperstat)
  Minoxidil
  Sodium nitroprusside
  Spironolactone (Aldactone)
  Thiazide diuretics
XVI. Drugs other than hydralazine and procainamide reported to produce
    the LE syndrome (mostly case reports)
  Various anticonvulsants (Dilantin, Mesantoin, Mysoline, Tridione, Zarontin), sulfonamides, estrogens, PAS, tetracyclines, streptomycin, griseofulvin, propylthiouracil, phenothiazines, Sansert, reserpine, phenylbutazone, quinidine, clofibrate, gold salts

REFERENCES

Martin, E. W., et al.: *Hazards of Medication* (Philadelphia: J. B. Lippincott Co., 1971).

Sode, J., and Walsh, F. M.: CAP-ASCP annual meeting, October 1972.

Sunderman, F. W., Jr.: Drug interference in clinical biochemistry, CRC Crit. Rev. Clin. Lab. Sci. 1:427, 1970.

Weindling, H., and Henry, J. B.: Drug interaction and clinical laboratory data, Lab. Med. 6:24, 1975.

Young, D. S., et al.: Effects of drugs on clinical laboratory tests, Clin. Chem. 21 (5): 1D, 1975.

NORMAL (AVERAGE) BLOOD VALUES AT VARIOUS AGES*

	BIRTH	5 DAYS	2 WEEKS	3 MONTHS	6 MONTHS	2 YEARS	8 YEARS
Red blood cells (millions/cu mm)	5.5	5.5	5.0	4.1	4.5	4.8	5.0
Hemoglobin (gm/100 ml)	18.0	18.0	17.0	11.0	11.5	13.0	14.0
White blood cells (thousands/cu mm)	16.0	20.0	12.0	10.0	9.5	9.0	8.0
Platelets (thousands/cu mm)	350.0	400.0	300.0	260.0	250.0	250.0	250.0
Differential on peripheral blood							
%Neutrophils	45	55	35	35	40	40	60
%Lymphocytes	25	20	55	55	53	50	30
Nucleated RBC (per 100 WBC)	5	3	0	0	0	0	0

*Compiled from various sources.

LABORATORY DIFFERENCES IN PROTHROMBIN TIME (PT) DUE TO REAGENTS FROM DIFFERENT MANUFACTURERS*

THROMBOPLASTIN	SUGGESTED THERAPEUTIC RANGE (SECONDS)†
1. Thrombotime (Pfizer)	23 – 29.5
2. Manchester (Poller)	25 – 41.0
3. Dried (Hyland)	20 – 27.0
4. Fibroplastin (BioQuest)	19 – 28.0
5. Simplastin (Warner-Lambert)	20 – 29.0
6. Brain (Ortho)	18 – 24.5
7. Dried (Dade)	16.5 – 21.5
8. Activated (Dade)	13.5 – 18.0
9. Simplastin-A (Warner-Lambert)	20.0 – 29.0

*From Miale, J. B., and Kent, J. W.: Standardization of the therapeutic range for oral anticoagulants based on standard reference plasmas, Am. J. Clin. Pathol. 57:80, 1972, Table 8.

†Each is equivalent to a range of 10 to 20% reduction in the coagulation factors affected by oral anticoagulants.

SIMPLIFIED GUIDE TO ANEMIA DIAGNOSIS USING A MINIMUM OF TESTS
—AIMED AT MOST IMPORTANT DISEASE CATEGORIES

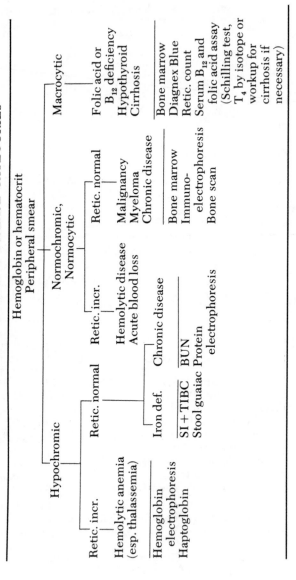

Hemoglobin or hematocrit
Peripheral smear

Hypochromic

Retic. incr.
Hemolytic anemia
(esp. thalassemia)

Hemoglobin
electrophoresis
Haptoglobin

Retic. normal

Iron def.

$\overline{SI + TIBC}$
Stool guaiac

Chronic disease

$\overline{BUN}$
Protein
electrophoresis

Normochromic,
Normocytic

Retic. incr.

Hemolytic disease
Acute blood loss

Retic. normal

Malignancy
Myeloma
Chronic disease

Bone marrow
Immuno-
electrophoresis
Bone scan

Macrocytic

Folic acid or
B_{12} deficiency
Hypothyroid
Cirrhosis

Bone marrow
Diagnex Blue
Retic. count
Serum B_{12} and
folic acid assay
(Schilling test,
T_4 by isotope or
workup for
cirrhosis if
necessary)

SERUM IRON (SI) AND TOTAL IRON-BINDING CAPACITY (TIBC)

SI decreased; TIBC decreased	Chronic diseases (including chronic infections, cirrhosis, rheumatoid-collagen, nonbleeding cancer)
	Uremia
SI decreased; TIBC increased	Iron deficiency anemia Pregnancy in third trimester
SI increased; TIBC decreased	Hemachromatosis (a minority say that the TIBC is increased) Iron therapy overload (TIBC may be normal) Hemolysis (if severe) °Hemolysis (mild); thalassemia; lead poisoning; sideroachrestic anemia
SI increased; TIBC increased	Estrogen medication Acute hepatitis (some report TIBC low normal)

Notes:

1. There is considerable (rather inexplicable) difference of opinion in the literature, sometimes quite contradictory, on findings in a variety of conditions.

2. SI has diurnal variation, highest values in A.M.; some report considerable day-to-day variation.

3. Combination of disease may exist; e.g., chronic blood loss anemia (which increases TIBC) superimposed on some other chronic disease (which depresses TIBC).

°SI may be normal or (more often) increased; TIBC may be normal or increased.

NEPHRITOGENIC STRAINS OF LANCEFIELD GROUP A STREPTOCOCCI

4	25
12 (most frequent)	Red Lake
18	

ENTEROPATHOGENIC STRAINS OF *E. COLI*
(Serotypes reported to cause infant diarrhea)

O26:B6°	O119:B17
O55:B5	O125:B15
O86:B7	O126:B16
O111:B4	O127:B8
O119:B11	O127:B12

°O refers to somatic antigen, B to one of the "capsule" antigens.

PRIMARY GLOMERULAR DISEASE (SIMPLIFIED)*

	LIGHT MICROSCOPE	ELECTRON MICROSCOPE	CLINICAL
I. Lipoid nephrosis			
A. Minimal change (Nil disease)	Normal	Endothelial footplate fusion	NS
B. Focal sclerosis	Focal mesangial sclerosis	Footplate fusion + subepithelial deposits	NS
II. Membranous GN	Wire-loop BM thickening; spike and dome pattern in silver stains	1. Extramembranous: diffuse BM subepithelial deposits; EM spikes into deposits	Microscopic hematuria
		2. Membranous: diffuse BM thickening without subepithelial deposits or spikes	NS
III. Proliferative GN			
A. Postinfectious GN (acute poststreptococcal; mesangial GN)	Mesangial cell proliferation	Subepithelial humps	Hematuria; C3 low initially
B. Latent GN	Mild focal and segmental mesangial cell proliferation	Mesangial deposits	Mild hematuria
C. Rapidly progressive GN (subacute; crescentic)	Poststreptococcal lesions + epithelial crescents	1. Subepithelial humps	Hematuria and proteinuria, or NS; C3 low initially

D. Membranoproliferative GN (mesangiocapillary; hypocomplementary)	Mesangial proliferation + capillary wall thickening	2. Fibrin deposition	Hematuria and proteinuria, or NS; C3 normal
		1. Mesangial proliferation + either subepithelial deposits or BM double-contour appearance	Many have persistently low C3; most have hematuria; majority have NS
		2. Lobular GN; same as (1), but with mesangial thickening	
		3. Dense deposits within BM (dense deposit disease)	
E. Focal proliferative GN (IgA disease)	Focal cellular proliferation at edge of glomerulus	Focal mesangial hypercellularity	Hematuria
IV. Chronic GN	Widespread glomerular sclerosis; varying degrees of change in remaining glomeruli	Mesangial sclerosis and proliferation	Slowly progressive to renal failure; may have episodes of hematuria or NS

*Glomerulonephritis = GN; nephrotic syndrome = NS; basement membrane = BM.

WIDAL'S TEST – SEROLOGIC GROUPS
(O ANTIGENS) OF THE
PATHOGENIC SALMONELLAE

GROUP	ORGANISM
A	*paratyphi A*
B	*paratyphi B*
	typhimurium
C	*paratyphi C*
	choleraesuis
	Newport
D	*typhi (typhosa)*
	enteritidis
	sendai
E	*anatum*

CLASSIFICATION OF ENTEROBACTERIACEAE

TRIBE	GENERA
Escherichieae	*Escherichia* (incl. *E. coli* and *alkalescens-dispar*
	Shigella
Edwardsielleae	*Edwardsiella*
Salmonelleae	*Salmonella*
	Arizona
	Citrobacter (incl. *E. freundii*)
Klebsielleae	*Klebsiella*
	Enterobacter (formerly *Aerobacter*)
	Serratia
Proteeae	*Proteus*
	Providencia (*Proteus inconstans*)

REFERENCE

Douglas, G. W., and Washington, J. A.: *Identification of Enterobacteriaceae in the Clinical Laboratory* (Atlanta: Microbiology Branch, National Communicable Disease Center, 1969).

CRITERIA FOR ABNORMAL ORAL GLUCOSE TOLERANCE TESTS*

| | U.S. PUBLIC HEALTH SERVICE | | | FAJANS & CONN | | UNIVERSITY GROUP DIABETES PROGRAM | |
	BLOOD	SERUM	POINTS†	BLOOD	SERUM		
Fasting	110	130	1	—	—		
1 hour	170	195	½	160	185		
1½ hour	—	—	—	140	160	Blood‡	Serum‡
2 hours	120	140	½	120	140	500 or more	600 or more
3 hours	110	130	1	—	—		

*Glucose values in mg/100 ml.
†Definite diabetes = 2 points; possible diabetes = 1 point
‡Sum of fasting, 1-, 2- and 3-hour values in mg/100 ml

REFERENCES

Standardization of the oral glucose tolerance test: Report of Committee on Statistics of the American Diabetes Association, Diabetes 18:299, 1968.
Fajans, S. S.: What is diabetes: Definition, diagnosis, and course, Med. Clin. North Am. 55:793, 1971.

COMPARISON OF TESTS FOR HEPATITIS B (HBAg)
Approximate sensitivity: CEP = 1

Counterimmunoelectrophoresis (CEP)	1
Complement fixation (CF)	10–20
Reversed passive latex agglutination (Antigex)	20
Reversed passive hemagglutination (Auscell)	150
Radioimmunoassay (Ausria I)	200
Radioimmunoassay (Ausria II)	1,500

DISTRIBUTION OF MONOCLONAL GAMMOPATHIES

DISEASE	% OF TOTAL
Multiple myeloma IgG = 60% IgA = 25% Bence-Jones only = 14–25%	65
Waldenström's	10
Franklin's disease (Heavy chain disease)	1
Lymphomas and leukemias	6
Cancer	8
Not associated with neoplasia	10

REFERENCES

Mattioli, C., and Tomasi, T. B., Jr.: Human Serum Immunoglobulins, in Dowling, H. F. (ed.): *Disease-a-Month* (Chicago: Year Book Medical Publishers, Inc., April, 1970).

Osserman, E., and Takatsuki, K.: Plasma cell myeloma: Gamma globulin synthesis and structure, Medicine 42:357, 1963.

RHEUMATOID FACTOR TESTS*

	ROSE-WAALER SENSITIZED SHEEP CELL	POLTZ-SINGER LATEX	HYLAND RA TEST	EOSIN SLIDE
Adult RA	64% (58–78)†	76% (53–94)	82% (78–98)	90% (88–92)
Normal	5.6 (0.3–13)	1.0 (0.2–3)	8 (0.7–15)	5 (0.2–8.6)
Collagen disease	15–39	17–20	14–67	10–50
Procedure	Tube	Tube	Slide	Slide

*Average % positive and reports from various publications.

†Numbers in parentheses refer to the range of values found in different reports.

TESTS FOR SYSTEMIC LUPUS ERYTHEMATOSUS (SLE)
(APPROXIMATE % POSITIVE)

	SLE	SCLERODERMA	OTHER COLLAGEN DISEASES	RHEUMATOID ARTHRITIS	OTHER
LE cell	60–80	0–20	<5	5–25	Lupoid hepatitis; drugs (hydralazine, procaina-mide)
Antinuclear antibody	95–100	75–80	10	10–50	Chronic liver disease Thyroid disease Acquired hemolytic anemia Old age
Serum complement (C′)	Low in 60% with active disease	Normal (rarely low)	Normal or high	Normal or high	Normal

USEFUL FLUID AND ELECTROLYTE INFORMATION*

Normal daily output
   Insensible loss (skin and lungs) 600–1,000 ml/day
                 Urine 500–1,500 ml/day

Average composition of certain body fluids (± 20%)

	Na	K	Cl (mEq/L)
Gastric	50	10	100
Bile	150	5	100
Small intestine	100	5	100
Perspiration (visible sweating)	30	0	30

Normal production of certain body fluids

Saliva	500–1,500 ml/day
Gastric	1,000–3,000 ml/day
Bile	300–1,000 ml/day
Pancreas	1,000–1,500 ml/day
Small intestine	1,000–2,000 ml/day
Visible sweating (at bed rest and/or high fever)	1,000–2,000 ml/day

Note: Normally, most GI secretions (fluid and electrolytes) are reabsorbed before they reach the rectum.

Daily nutritional requirements
A. Caloric requirements
   1st 10 kg body weight: 100 calories/kg
   10–20 kg body weight: 100 calories plus 50 calories for every kg over 10
   Over 20 kg body weight: 1500 calories plus 20 calories for every kg
     over 20
B. Fluid requirements
   1 ml fluid for every calorie needed
C. Electrolyte requirements
   Na: 3 mEq/100 cal
   K: 2 mEq/100 cal
   Cl: 2 mEq/100 cal

*Compiled from various sources.

DATA FOR DIABETES TOLERANCE TESTS

  I. Oral glucose tolerance test
     The ideal body weight dosage that may be used for adults is 1.75
     gm/kg. For infants and children, 2.5 gm/kg up to age 1 1/2, then 2.0
     gm/kg up to age 3 has been recommended.
 II. Intravenous glucose tolerance test
     Most investigators use a standard dose of glucose (in a 50% solution)
     amounting to 0.33 gm/kg of ideal body weight. Some use a standard
     dose of 25 gm, regardless of weight. For children, the recommended
     dose is 0.5 gm/kg.

III. Cortisone glucose tolerance test

After a standard 3-day carbohydrate diet, oral cortisone acetate is given at 8½ hours and again at 2 hours before the test glucose dose. A person over 160 lb gets 62.5 mg cortisone, and under 160 lb, 50 mg (at each time period). Afterward, the standard oral GTT is performed. Normal values are less than 160 mg/100 ml at 1 hour, 150 mg/100 ml at 1½ hours and less than 140 mg/100 ml at 2 hours (whole blood).

IV. Tolbutamide tolerance test

Inject 20 ml sterile Orinase Diagnostic (1 gm of water-soluble sodium tolbutamide) intravenously over 2–3 minutes' time. Blood samples are taken fasting and at 20 and 30 minutes after tolbutamide. At 20 minutes, normal values are less than 75% of FBS. Between 75 and 85% (of FBS) is considered borderline, between 85 and 89% highly suspicious (90% of patients in this group have diabetes) and over 89% is thought to show definite diabetes. At 30 minutes, over 76% of FBS is said to be virtually (99%) diagnostic. Either the 20- or 30-minute value is diagnostic when within the diabetic zone, even if the other is not.

Note: These are not the normal values to be used when investigating hypoglycemia.

BLOOD GLUCOSE METHODS

I. Folin-Wu

Technical: Copper reduction method. Manual only. Historically famous but little used today. Measures reducing substances such as creatinine, uric acid, glutathione and ergothionine in addition to most sugars.

Clinical: Performed on whole blood. Results 20–30 mg/100 ml higher than true glucose, but can fluctuate widely, as much as 10–70 mg/100 ml. Interference by metabolic reducing substances as noted and by vitamin C (large doses).

II. Neocuproine

Technical: Reducing-substance method. Automated only, using serum, on Technicon SMA 12/60.

Clinical: Results are 15% above manufacturer's stated 110 mg/100 ml fasting upper limit of normal for serum. Same basic interferences as Folin-Wu.

III. Somogyi-Nelson

Technical: Needs protein-free filtrate. Manual method only. Time consuming. Whole blood or serum.

Clinical: Although not entirely specific for glucose, results are fairly close to true glucose values.

IV. Ferricyanide

Technical: Widely used in Autoanalyser equipment. Serum only.

Clinical: Although a reducing method, results are within 5% of true glucose. Considerable increase in uric acid or vitamin C interferes.

V. Orthotoluidine

Technical: Need boiling apparatus. Manual or automated. Serum only. *(Continued on p. 490.)*

COMPOUNDS THAT INTERFERE WITH RESULTS OF THYROID TESTS

	PBI or T4		RAI UPTAKE		T3 UPTAKE EFFECT
	EFFECT	DURATION	EFFECT	DURATION	
Inorganic iodides	*PBI (Not T4)*				
Lugol's, KI, SSKI, etc.	Incr	1–4 wk	Decr	1–3 wk	None
Omade					
Organic iodine	*PBI (Not T4)*				
1. X-ray contrast media					
Teridax (gallbladder)	Incr	30 yr	None		None
Cholografin (gallbladder)	Incr	3–4 mo	Decr	3 mo	None
Telepaque (gallbladder)	Incr	6–12 wk	Decr	2 mo	None
Diodrast	Incr	2 wk	Decr	1–3 mo	None
Dionosil (bronchogram)	Incr	1–5 mo	Decr	2–5 mo	None
Lipiodol (bronchogram)	Incr	1–2 yr	Decr	1–3 yr	None
Pantopaque (myelogram)	Incr	3–12 mo	Decr	3–12 mo	None
Hypaque (IVP)	Incr	4–7 da	Decr	1–2 wk	None
Renografin (IVP)	Incr	1–4 wk (?)	Decr	1–2 wk	None
Salpix (uterosalpingogram)	Incr	2 wk	Decr	1 mo	None
2. Iodinated vaginal suppositories	Incr	4 wk	Decr	4 wk	None
Floraquin, Vioform, etc.					
Betadine					
Other medications	*PBI or T4*				
Thyroxine	Incr	2–4 wk	Decr	1–2 wk	Incr
Thyroid extract	Incr	4–6 wk	Decr	1–2 wk	Incr
Iodothiouracil	Incr	sev wk	Decr	2–8 da	Decr
Estrogens	Incr	2–4 wk	Occ incr		Decr
Triiodothyronine (T3)	Decr	2–4 wk	Decr	?	Decr
Propylthiouracil or Tapazole	Decr	5–7 da	Decr	2–8 da	Decr

Thiocyanate	Decr	2–3 wk	Decr	2–8 da	Decr
Dilantin	Decr	7–10 da	None		None
Androgens	Decr	3 wk	None	1 wk	Incr
Adrenal corticoids or ACTH	Decr	1–2 wk	Decr	?	Incr
Salicylates (large doses)	Decr	?	Decr	?	None
Phenylbutazone	Decr	2 wk	Decr	?	Incr
Perphenazine (Trilafon) after 6–10 weeks' treatment	Occ incr		?		Occ decr
Chlorpromazine (Thorazine)	None		Decr/Nl	?	None
Mercurial diuretics	None*		?	?	None
Thiazide diuretics	Decr†	?	None		None
Antihistamines (without iodine)	None		Decr	2–7 da	None
Orinase	None		Decr	2–7 da	None
Dicumarol	None		None		Incr
Sulfonamides	Decr (?)		Decr	1 wk	?
PAS or isoniazid (prolonged Rx)	Occ decr	?	Decr	1–2 wk	?
Pentothal	?		Decr	1 wk	?
Penicillin (large doses only)	None		None		Incr
Gold salts	Decr	Sev wk	None		None
Metrecal	Incr‡	?	None		?
Lithium carbonate	Nl§/Decr	?	Incr	?	Nl/Decr

*The wet ash PBI method is decreased 1–3 days.
†Not affected by 2–3 days' therapy.
‡BEI is also increased; T_4 is normal.
§Nl = normal.

Clinical: Measures glucose and other aldoses; results close to true glucose. Dextran produces false increase.

VI. Glucose oxidase

Technical: Manual or automated. Serum only. Enzymatic method.

Clinical: True glucose method. However, in the oxidase-peroxidase modification, interference by vitamin C (decrease) and by hydralazine, iproniazid (Marsilid), INH, acetaminophen, tolazamide (Tolinase).

VII. Hexokinase

Technical: Manual or automated. Serum only. Enzymatic method.

Clinical: True glucose. To date, few interferences reported.

PLASMA RENIN

Plasma renin determination may be very helpful in the diagnosis (or exclusion) of primary aldosteronism. However, to interpret results, it is necessary to keep in mind certain technical aspects of current methods. Renin is an enzyme. Most enzymes cannot be measured directly, but are estimated indirectly by observing their effect on a known quantity of substrate. In the case of renin, the situation is even more complex, since the substrate (which results in production of angiotensin) cannot be directly measured and must be estimated indirectly by observing its effect on an indicator system and comparing the results with a known amount of angiotensin. In addition, renin is a very unstable enzyme and must be kept at freezing temperature as much as possible to preserve its activity. Collection methods are very important; if the specimen is not collected and processed correctly, a false low value may result.

One possible collection protocol is outlined below. It incorporates a provocative test—low-sodium diet plus upright posture—to help differentiate primary from secondary aldosteronism. Urinary aldosterone determinations should not be collected during a low-salt diet because sodium deficiency stimulates aldosterone secretion. In fact, urine sodium should be obtained on all aldosterone specimens as a check on possible sodium deficiency. The protocol, therefore, incorporates a section with a high-salt diet to ensure proper collection of aldosterone. If desired, a plasma renin specimen may be obtained during this time to help rule out unilateral renal disease. If unilateral renal disease is not a possibility, step 2 may be omitted. If aldosterone collection is not desired, steps 1–3 may be omitted.

Protocol for Plasma Renin and Urine Aldosterone Determinations

1. Patient off medications, placed on 9 gm (180 mEq) high-sodium (normal potassium) diet for 4 days. (Note: can use normal diet plus 6 gm salt tablets extra per day.)

2. Fasting plasma renin specimen drawn the morning of the 4th day before patient stands or sits up (specimen 1). (Note: this can be omitted if unilateral renal disease screening is not desired.)

3. Twenty-four-hour urine for aldosterone and sodium collected during the 4th day. (Note: can also get metanephrine determination on the same specimen to rule out pheochromocytoma.)

4. Patient then placed on a 0.5 gm (10 mEq) low-sodium (normal potassium) diet for 3 days.

5. After awakening the morning of the 4th day, the fasting patient is placed upright (standing or leaning; not allowed to sit or lie down) for 2 hours. Lab notified when the 2-hour period will end; patient kept upright until lab draws blood specimen.

6. Plasma renin specimen drawn while patient is still upright (specimen 2); test ends.

Note: Heparinized collection tube is placed in ice water before the specimen is obtained and kept in ice bath as long as possible before the blood is actually drawn. The tourniquet should be released for a few seconds before blood is drawn, since it has been reported that venous stasis may decrease blood renin. The tube is returned to the ice bath immediately after the specimen is drawn and kept in ice water. It is centrifuged still packed in ice and the plasma is withdrawn, frozen immediately and sent to the reference laboratory packed in dry ice (do not send specimen on weekend).

A high-sodium diet decreases aldosterone secretion in normal persons. In patients with hypertension due to primary aldosteronism or unilateral renal disease, aldosterone is elevated. Plasma renin levels should be decreased in normal persons and those with primary aldosteronism, and increased in hypertension due to unilateral renal disease. A low-sodium diet should confirm results. Renin levels should be high in normal persons, whereas the previous elevated renin level seen in unilateral renal disease remains elevated and the decreased level seen in primary aldosteronism remains decreased. (Although some rise in plasma renin may occur, even in primary aldosteronism, values do not reach normal range.)

INTERPRETATION OF TRF TEST
(500 ug TRF intravenously)

	BASELINE SERUM TSH (uU/ML)	INCREASE IN SERUM TSH AT 30 MIN. (uU/ML)
EUTHYROID	10 or less (97%) [usually 6 or less; 20% less than 1.5]	2 or more (95%) [usually 6-30]
HYPERTHYROID	10 or less [usually 4 or less]	Less than 2
PRIMARY HYPOTHYROID	More than 10 (93%)	2 or more [usually 20 or more] Same as Euthyroid
SECONDARY HYPOTHYROID (Pituitary)	10 or less [usually 6 or less]	Less than 2 (60%) 2-50 (40%)
TERTIARY HYPOTHYROID (Hypothalamus)	10 or less [often less than 2]	2 or more (95%) Less than 2 (5%)

REFERENCES

Bath, N. M., et al.: Plasma renin activity in renovascular hypertension, Am. J. Med. 45:381, 1968.

Conn, J. W.: Aldosteronism in hypertensive disease, Med. Times 98:116, 1970.

Conn, J. W., et al.: Preoperative diagnosis of primary aldosteronism, Arch. Intern. Med. 123:113, 1969.

SURVEY OF PREGNANCY TESTS

TEST	TYPE	TIME	SENSITIVITY (% PREGNANT WOMEN DETECTED)		ACCURACY (% NEGATIVE IN NON-PREGNANT WOMEN)		SENSITIVITY (NONCONC.) URINE IU/L	PROTEIN	AFFECTED BY PHENOTHIAZINES	OTHER
			AVERAGE	RANGE	AVERAGE	RANGE				
Gravindex	Slide	2 min	92.5	70–99	98	92–100	3,000	Yes	No†	¶
Hyland HCG	Slide	2 min	83	50–94	94	93–100	2,000	Yes	Yes	
Natatel	Slide	2 min	—	95	—	100 (?)	?	No	No	
Pregslide	Slide	2 min	—	91–96	—	95.3–98.7	3,000	Yes	Yes	
DAP	Slide	2 min	—	97	—	97	2,000	No†	No†	
Prequest	Slide	2 min	—	96	—	96	5,000	?	?	
Pregnosis	Slide	2 min	96.5	96.2–97.1	99	98.9–100	2,000	No	No°	$
Planotest (Pregnosticon slide)	Slide	2 min	98.5	98–99	98.5	96.0–99.5	2,500	No	No	
Pregnosticon Dri-Dot	Slide	2 min	—	100	—	94	1,000–2,000	?	?	
Pregnosticon	Tube	2 hr	98.5	86–100	99	97–100	1,000	No	Occ.	
Pregnosticon-Accusphere	Tube	2 hr	—	98	—	90	750–1,000	No	?	
UCG	Tube	2 hr	93.5	69–97	96	90–100	2,000	No	No	
Prepurin	Tube	2 hr	98.5	96–99	97	94–100	4,000	?	No	
Twentisec	Chemical-color	20 sec	—	89.5	—	94	?	?	?	
LPT	Chemical-color	5 min	—	93°	—	93°	?	?	Yes	§‖
Aschheim-Zondek (A-Z)	Mouse	96 hr	98	83–100	98	90–100	600–700	?	?	
Friedman	Rabbit	48 hr	98	86–100	99	95–100	1,000–5,000	?	?	
Frog, male	Frog	2 hr	94–97	62–100	98	93–100	1,000–5,000†	?	Yes	
Frog, female	Toad	2 hr	90–97	80–99	99	78–100	1,000–5,000†	?	Yes	

No average % accuracy given if fewer than 3 evaluations.
°Manufacturer's data only available.
†Concentrated; 3–5 times less sensitive unconcentrated (Postgrad. Med. 42:A–48, 1967).
‡One report differs from others.
§False positive results with oral contraceptives.
‖False positive results in some persons with hepatitis or with salicylate or chloramphenicol therapy.
¶One report indicates high incidence of false positive reactions in postmenopausal women.

492

FREQUENCY OF METASTASES TO CERTAIN ORGANS (%)

PRIMARY SITE	LYMPH NODES	LIVER	LUNGS	BONE	BRAIN
Urinary bladder	30–40% (12–85)°	15–30 (9–43)	20–30 (15–40)	15–40 (2–55)	Rare
Prostate	65–85 (65–100)	20 (20–24)	40 (13–66)	70 (33–92)	Uncommon
Lung	70–80 (64–93)	30–40 (30–58)	–	20–40 (15–45)	15–20 (11–41)
Breast	70–75 (65–80)	40–60 (33–65)	55–60 (54–61)	(45–65) (44–78)	10–15 (6–29)
Colon	50 (12–58)	30–60 (24–83)	10–20 (5–38)	6 (3–11)	2 (1–4)
Uterus (corpus)	14	1–28	3–30	3	Rare
Uterus (cervix)	65 (46–77)	20–40 (9–42)	15–40 (4–52)	5–15 (1–20)	Uncommon
Melanoma	Frequent	39–68	7	2	5–39
Stomach	60–80 (50–89)	35–45 (33–68)	10–25	5–7 (3–10)	1–12
Kidney	40 (16–89)	35–45 (12–49)	50–60 (34–71)	30–40 (23–81)	7–10 (3–15)

°Parentheses enclose range found in the literature. Lack of parentheses indicates average expected frequency.

It is surprising how little well-documented information of this type is available in recent years. Most, but not all, of the data are derived from autopsy material, and therefore presumably represent the maximum chance for organ involvement. However, the data are not uniform in terms of patient clinical course (treatment or no treatment). In the case of bone, the statistics almost certainly underestimate true incidence, as autopsy usually includes only the spine. The purpose of this review is to provide some framework for preoperative workup in patients with cancer. If an organ has low metastatic potential as reflected in autopsy findings, presumably at an early stage the metastatic potential would be still lower, and scan of that organ would probably have a low cost-benefit ratio.

ECTOPIC TUMOR HORMONE PRODUCTION

Tumors may develop in certain organs that produce hormones and as a result are frequently associated with clinical syndromes. Tumors from other locations may also produce these hormones. It might be useful to list some of these syndromes, the associated tumor, the principal hormones secreted and the most commonly reported ectopic hormone-secreting neoplasms.

Plummer's disease: Hyperfunctioning thyroid adenoma; thyroid hormone (ovarian teratoma) or TSH (choriocarcinoma)

Thyroid medullary carcinoma: Calcitonin (lung carcinoma)

ACTH-induced Cushing's syndrome: Pituitary adenoma; ACTH (lung oat cell carcinoma, thymoma and various other tumors)

Hypoglycemia: Pancreatic islet beta cell tumor; insulin (hepatoma, fibrosarcoma).

Hypercalcemia: Parathyroid tumor; PTH (lung carcinoma, hypernephroma)

Inappropriate ADH syndrome: Hypothalamic disorder; ADH (lung carcinoma; a few other tumors reported)

Polycythemia: Erythopoietin (hepatoma, hypernephroma, cerebellar hemangioblastoma)

Gonadotropin: Choriocarcinoma; HCG (testicular tumors, lung carcinoma; the beta subunit of HCG is a common tumor marker, as noted on page 400)

Pheochromocytoma syndrome: Adrenal medulla pheochromocytoma; epinephrine (neuroblastoma)

Carcinoid syndrome: GI tract carcinoid; serotonin (oat cell lung carcinoma; pancreatic carcinoma)

GLYCOGEN STORAGE DISEASES (GLYCOGENOSES)

Type I.   Glucose-6-phosphatase deficiency (hepatorenal; von Gierke's)
Type II.   Acid maltase deficiency (Pompe's)
Type III. Debranching enzyme deficiency (limit dextranosis; Cori)
Type IV. Branching enzyme deficiency (amylopectinosis; Anderson)
Type V.   Myophosphorylase deficiency (McArdle)
Type VI. Liver phosphorylase deficiency (Hers)
Type VII. Phosphofructokinase deficiency
Type VIII. Hepatic phosphorylase kinase deficiency

Diagnosis: Liver in Type I, III, IV, VI and VIII; muscle in Type II, III, V and VII (glycogen content and enzyme analysis).

MUSCULAR DYSTROPHIES

Duchenne
Limb-girdle
Fascioscapulohumeral
Myotonic dystrophy/atrophy
Myotonia congenita
Ocular myopathies
Congenital muscular dystrophy

CONGENITAL MYOPATHIES

Central core disease
Nemaline (rod) myopathy
Myotubular (centronuclear) myopathy

LIPID STORAGE DISEASES

DISEASE	LIPID	WBC	DIAGNOSIS BY FIBROBLAST CULTURE	LIVER BIOPSY
A. Glycolipid storage diseases				
1. Ganglioside storage				
Tay-Sachs	GM_2	No	Yes	No
Tay-Sachs variant (hexosamidase A+B deficiency)	Globoside and GM_2	?	Yes	Yes
Metachromatic leukodystrophy	Sulfatide	Yes	?	Yes
Generalized ganglio-sidosis	GM_1	Yes	?	Yes
2. Ceramide storage				
Gaucher's	Glucosyl	Yes	Yes	Yes
Krabbe's (globoid leuko-dystrophy)	Galactosyl	Yes	?	Yes
Fabry's	Trihexoside	Yes	?	Yes
Lactosyl ceramidosis	Lactosyl	No	Yes	Yes
Niemann-Pick	Sphingomyelin	Yes	?	Yes
B. Other lipid storage diseases				
Wolman's*	Triglyceride (neutral lipid) and cholesterol esters	No	?	Yes
Refsum'st	Phytanic acid	No	Yes	Yes

*Calcification in adrenals on x-ray is typical.
†Plasma fatty acids can be analyzed for phytanic acid.

REFERENCES

Arey, J. B.: The lipidoses: Morphologic changes in the nervous system in Gaucher's disease, GM_2 gangliosidoses and Niemann-Pick disease, Ann. Clin. Lab. Sci. 5:475, 1975.

Brady, R. O.: The genetic mismanagement of complex lipid metabolism, Bull. NY Acad. Med. 47:173, 1971.

Danes, B. S.: The use of WBC cultures in the study of genetic metabolic disease, Hosp. Practice 5:52, 1970.

SELECTED SKIN TESTS

DISEASE	TEST	ANTIGEN	TIME	POSITIVE
Brucellosis	Brucellin	Brucellergen (killed bacteria)	24–48 hr	Over 5 mm reaction
Tularemia	Foshay	Killed bacteria	48 hr	Over 5 mm reaction
Lymphogranuloma venereum	Frei	Killed virus	48 hr	(p. 188)
Echinococcosis	Casoni	Fluid from hydatid cyst	15–30 min	"Immediate" reaction
Scarlet fever	Schultz-Charlton	Antitoxin	24 hr	Blanched area
Diphtheria susceptibility	Schick	Diphtheria toxin	3–6 da	Reaction over 10 mm
Scarlet fever susceptibility	Dick	Erythrogenic toxin	24 hr	Reaction over 10 mm
Sarcoidosis	Kveim	Sarcoid tissue	6 weeks	(p. 231)
Tuberculosis	Mantoux	PPD or OT	24–48 hr	(pp. 155–156)
Systemic fungal infection	Histoplasmin, etc.	Killed fungi	48 hr	(pp. 170–171)
Trichinosis	*Trichinella*	Killed larvae	15 min	(p. 195)

DISORDERS OF CONNECTIVE TISSUE (MUCOPOLYSACCHARIDOSES)

NAME	PHYSICAL ANOMALIES	MENTAL DEFICIENCY	URINARY MUCOPOLYSACCHARIDES
Hurler	Marked	Moderate	Dermatan sulfate (chondroitin sulfate B) Heparan (heparitin) sulfate (approx. 2:1)
Hunter	Moderate	Variable or none	Dermatan sulfate Heparan sulfate (approx. 1:1)
Sanfillipo A and B	Mild	Marked	Heparan sulfate
Morquio	Marked	None	Keratan sulfate
Scheie	Mild	None	Dermatan sulfate Heparan sulfate (approx. 2:1)
Maroteaux-Lamy	Moderate	None	Dermatan sulfate
"Atypical"	Moderate	None	?

Note: All are transmitted as autosomal recessive except for Hunter, which is sex-linked.

REFERENCES:

McKusick, V. A., et al.: The genetic mucopolysaccharidoses, Medicine 44:1, 1965.
Neufield, E. F.: Mucopolysaccharidoses: The biochemical approach, Hosp. Practice 7:107, 1972.

CURRENT AVAILABILITY OF SPECIAL LABORATORY PROCEDURES

It is difficult to obtain certain tests, either because of unusual technical complexity or because the test is currently new and not yet widely accepted. Therefore, it may be useful to have the names and addresses of several United States laboratories that advertise facilities to provide these tests.

The following points must be emphasized:

1. This listing is not an endorsement. The author does not guarantee results from any of these laboratories, and has not checked any of them for accuracy.

2. Laboratories other than the ones listed may provide identical services. These are only the ones presently known to the author.

Bio Science Laboratories
7600 Tyrone Avenue
Van Nuys, CA 91405

Interlab Associates, Inc.
Box 59-3585
AMF, Miami, FL 33159

Clin-Chem Laboratories
1106 Commonwealth Avenue
Boston, MA 02215

Laboratory Medicine Data
P. O. Box 22282
Houston, TX 77027

Biochemical Procedures
12020 Chandler Boulevard
North Hollywood, CA 91607

Reference Laboratory
12926 Saticoy
North Hollywood, CA 91609

Linden Laboratories, Inc.
731 West Peachtree Street N.E.
Atlanta, GA 30308

Leary Laboratory, Inc.
43 Bay State Road
Boston, MA 02215

Nichols Institute
1300 South Beacon Street
San Pedro, CA 90731

New England Nuclear Corp.
Biomedical Assay Laboratories Div.
15 Harvard Street
Worchester, MA 01608

Bioanalysis
1701 Berkeley Street
Santa Monica, CA 90404

Center for Laboratory Medicine
16 Pearl Street
Metuchen, NJ 08840

Bio-Assay Laboratory
P. O. Box 6113
Dallas, TX 75222

REFERENCE

Young, D. S., et al.: Directory of rare analyses, Clin. Chem. 23:323, 1977.

SPECIMEN COLLECTION

To a pathologist, nothing is quite as upsetting as listening to an outraged complaint about laboratory results and tracing the difficulty to improper specimen collection. Sometimes, too, the correct specimen may not be collected at the proper time or in the proper way. Even when these criteria are met, the specimen may appear in the laboratory with inadequate identification or instructions, or be delayed in transit enough to cause damage. Finally, at times the test or specimen ordered is not what would be best in the particular situation. It is surprising, although understandable, how one can order the most complicated series of diagnostic manipulations and not realize that the specimens on which all results depend are being collected by personnel who may not have the slightest idea how to perform their task. Even when collection routine is optimum, the patient may be confused, incontinent or otherwise fail to provide the specimen in its entirety without close supervision. This is especially important for 24-hour collections. In some cases, such as PSP, BSP or clearance tests, exact timing to the minute is essential to calculate results.

For 24-hour urine specimens the collection period begins when the patient has voided. At the end of the time period, the patient voids again, and this specimen is added to the others collected during the time period. Most 24-hour urine specimens should be refrigerated or kept in an ice water bath during the collection to control bacterial growth. In some cases, a preservative may be added instead.

It is usually advisable to have a creatinine excretion determination done to provide an additional check on completeness of collection. A 24-hour creatinine value below normal range suggests incomplete collection. Although there is moderate fluctuation in daily excretion, 24-hour creatinine values should vary less than 10–15% from day to day.

Fresh specimens are needed in some cases, such as culture, cytology or enzyme tests.

A partial list of special collection situations discussed in the book are noted below.

ALA, p. 431.
Aldosterone (urine), p. 490.
Bacterial culture, routine, p. 157.
Bacterial meningitis, p. 201.
Blood culture, pp. 158; 162–163.
Blood sugar, pp. 317–318.
Cryptococcus, p. 169.
Cytomegalic inclusion disease, p. 182.
Entamoeba histolytica, p. 192.
Fungus culture, p. 172.
Gastric contents for cytology, p. 395.
Growth hormone, p. 368.
Hemolysis effects on blood specimens (on LDH, p. 224).
Lactic acid, p. 458.
Lipoproteins, p. 257.
Renin, p. 490.
Sputum for cytology, p. 398.
Trichomonas, p. 195.
Tuberculosis culture (urine, p. 123; sputum and gastric, p. 155).
Urine culture, p. 158–159.
Urine urobilinogen, p. 116.
Venous blood pH specimens, p. 277.
Virus culture, pp. 177–178.

TABLE OF REPRESENTATIVE NORMAL VALUES

There actually is little justification to provide a table of normal values for clinical chemistry procedures. There are usually several methods for assaying any substance, and with exceptions such as electrolytes, BUN and a few others, each method gives different normal values. For example, enzyme procedures have different results depending on temperature, pH and other conditions of assay. In addition, modifications of every basic technique inevitably appear (sometimes modifications of modifications), each with its own normal range. In addition, there may be local population factors that alter normal range data provided by kit manufacturers. Therefore, each laboratory must provide its own normal range for the particular techniques that it uses and the population it serves. Attempts to apply the same normal range blindly to a test that is performed in different laboratories will frequently be misleading. In spite of these comments, however, sufficient demand for a normal-value table has been generated so that one has been provided here. The figures listed represent "classic" procedures. The values are in some cases rounded off to be representative, rather than exact transcription of a single method. In some cases the reader is referred to passages in the text.

A new system of units of chemical and physical measurement (Système International d'Unités, or SI) has been proposed. It is based on the metric system, and it is designed to create uniformity in the type of reporting system used in clinical chemistry assays. To date, very few laboratories in the United States have adopted the SI system, so that SI units are not included in this normal-value table. The SI system, while useful to chemists, does little if anything to assist the physician, who still must contend with a multiplicity of normal ranges from different assays and from different methods for the same assay. In fact, while the transition from currently employed units to SI units is taking place, there will be yet another set of values to contend with. What is needed is a system such as the Centrinormal, in which ranges of most clinical chemistry assays (especially those whose critical values involve elevation from normal) are reported with the upper normal range set at 100. This eliminates memorization of normal ranges, bypasses the confusion that results when a different method with different normal range is substituted for a current test or a new test is introduced and allows physicians who have patients with laboratory results from different hospitals to obtain comparable data. In addition, one can readily note the degree of abnormality in terms of multiples of the upper limit of normal.

A. Blood
   1. Chemistry

A/G ratio	1.5–2.5
Albumin	4.0–5.5 gm/100 ml (Biuret)
	3.5–5.0 gm/100 ml (electrophoresis)
Ammonia	30–70 μg./100 ml
Bilirubin: total	0.2–1.5 mg/100 ml
direct	0.1–0.5 mg/100 ml
BSP (45 min)	0–5%
BUN	10–20 mg/100 ml
Calcium	8.5–10.5 mg/100 ml
Ceph. floc. (24 hr)	0–1+
Chloride	96–106 mEq/L
Cholesterol: total	150–300 mg/100 ml (p. 253)
esters	65–75%
CO_2 (comb. power)	20–30 mEq/L
Cortisol, plasma	5–20 μg/100 ml
Creatinine, serum	0.8–2.0 mg/100 ml
Folic acid (serum)	3–15 ng/ml
Gamma glutamyl transferase:	
males	0–30 mU/ml at 25° C
females	0–20 mU/ml at 25° C
Globulin	1.2–3.0 gm/100 ml
Glucose tolerance test, oral	(p. 483)
Iron, serum	60–150 mg/100 ml
Iron-binding capacity	250–350 mg/100 ml

Lipids: total   400 – 1,000 mg/100 ml
       phospholipids   200 – 300 mg/100 ml
       triglycerides   30 – 190 mg/100 ml (p. 253)
Magnesium   1.5 – 2.5 mEq/L
Osmolality, serum   285 – 300 mOsm/L
Phosphorus (inorg.)   2.5 – 4.5 mg/100 ml
Potassium   4.1 – 5.6 mEq/L
Sodium (serum)   136 – 145 mEq/L
Sugar (fasting)   70 – 110 mg/100 ml (p. 316)
Sugar (2-hr postprandial)   Less than 140 mg/100 ml
                               (p. 319)
Thymol turbidity   0 – 5.5 SH units
Total protein   6 – 8 gm/100 ml
Triglyceride   190 mg/100 ml (p. 253)
Uric acid   2.5 – 8 mg/100 ml
Vitamin B_{12} 200 – 1,000 pg/ml

2. Thyroid tests
   BEI or T_4 by column   3 – 7 μg/100 ml
   PBI   4 – 8 μg/100 ml
   RAI uptake   10 – 35%
   T_3 uptake   Below 0.87, hyper;
                               above 1.13, hypo (Res-O-Mat)
                               25 – 35% (Triosorb)
                               39 – 64% (Trilute)
                               90 – 110% (Thyopac)
   T_3 RIA   100 – 200 ng/100 ml
   T_4 by isotope   4 – 11 μg/100 ml (Murphy-Pattee)
                               5.5 – 14.5 μg/100 ml (Tetrasorb)
                               5.3 – 12.2 μg/100 ml (Tetralute and
                                 Res-O-Mat)

3. Serologies
   Antistreptolysin-O   0 – 200 units
   Febrile agglutinins   0 – 1:40
     (Weil-Felix)   (p. 186)

4. Enzymes
   Amylase   60 – 180 units/100 ml (Somogyi)
   Acid phosphatase   0.5 – 2 units/100 ml (Bodansky)
                               0.1 – 5 units/100 ml (King-
                                 Armstrong)
                               0.1 – 0.8 units/100 ml (Bessey-
                               Lowry)
                               0.1 – 2 IU/L (Babson)
                               0.1 – 2 units/100 ml (Gutman)
   Alkaline phosphatase   1 – 4 units/100 ml (Bodansky)
                               4 – 13 units/100 ml (King-
                               Armstrong)
                               0.8 – 2.5 units/100 ml (Bessey-
                               Lowry)
                               30 – 110 mU/ml (SMA 12/60)

CPK	1 – 12 IU/L (Okinaka-activated)
males	5 – 50 mU/ml (Oliver-Rosalki)
females	5 – 30 mU/ml (Oliver-Rosalki)
	0 – 12 units (Sigma)
	0 – 1.5 IU/L (Tanzer-Gilvarg – nonactivated)
	1 – 12 IU/L (Tanzer-Gilvarg – activated)
males	5 – 70 IU/L (Hughes – activated)
females	5 – 45 IU/L (Hughes – activated)
	25 – 145 mU/ml SMA 12/60
HBD: males	150 – 300 units/100 ml (Rosalki-Wilkerson)
females	95 – 210 mU/ml (Rosalki-Wilkerson)
	55 – 125 units (Sigma)
LAP: males	75 – 230 units (Goldberg-Rutenberg)
females	80 – 210 units (Goldberg-Rutenberg)
	70 – 200 units (Sigma)
LDH, total	200 – 500 units/ml (Wroblewski-LaDue)
	200 – 600 OD units (Teller)
	25 – 80 IU/L (Babson)
	5 – 50 IU/L (Wacker UV)
	30 – 110 mU/ml (Wacker UV)
	100 – 225 mU/ml (SMA 12/60)
LDH, heat stable	20 – 40% of total
Lipase	0 – 1.0 Sigma units
SGOT	8 – 40 units/100 ml (Reitman-Frankel)
	1 – 12 IU/L (Reitman-Frankel)
	15 – 36 units/ml (Henry)
	9 – 36 IU/L (Babson)
	5 – 40 units/100 ml (Karmen UV)
	5 – 20 mU/ml (Karmen UV)
	10 – 40 mU/ml (SMA 12/60)
SGPT	5 – 35 units/ml (Reitman-Frankel)
	1 – 12 IU/L (Reitman-Frankel)
	12 – 55 units/ml (Henry)
	5 – 25 mU/ml (Wroblewski)

5. Blood gases (arterial)

pH	7.38 – 7.42
P_{CO_2}	35 – 45 mm Hg
P_{O_2}	80 – 90 mm Hg (under age 65)
	75 – 85 mm Hg (over age 65)
O_2 sat.	96 – 97% (room air)
BE	0 ± 2

6. Clearances
    Urea: standard   40–65 ml/min
          maximum   60–100 ml/min
    Creatinine   90–120 ml/min
    Phosphate reabsorption   Over 80%
      (TRP, PRI)
7. Hematology and coagulation
    Hgb: males   14–18 gm/100 ml (p. 1)
          females   12–16 gm/100 ml
    Hematocrit: males   40–54%
                females   37–47%
    RBC: males   4.5–6.0 million
          females   4.0–5.5 million
    MCH   26–34 (p. 2)
    MCHC   31–37% (p. 3)
    MCV   80–100 cu μ (p. 2)
    Platelets   150–300,000
    WBC   4,500–11,000/cu mm
    Dif: lymphs   20–40%
       seg   50–70%
       bands   0–7
       eos   0–5%
       monos   0–7%
    Sed rate: males   0–15 mm/hr
            females   0–20 mm/hr
    Fibrinogen (quant)   200–400 mg/100 ml
    Coagulation time (Lee-   5–15 min
      White)
    PT   Control ± 2 sec (p. 477)
    PTT   40–100 sec (nonactivated)
    PRT   90–130 sec
8. Protein electrophoresis (cellulose acetate)
    Albumin   3.5–5.0 gm (50–65%)
    Alpha$_1$ 0.2–0.4 gm (2.5–5.5%)
    Alpha$_2$ 0.6–1.0 gm (7–12%)
    Beta   0.6–1.0 gm (7–15%)
    Gamma   0.7–1.3 gm (11–21%)
B. Spinal fluid (CSF)
    Sugar   40–70 mg/100 ml
    Protein   20–40 mg/100 ml
    WBC   0–5 mononuclears
    RBC   0
    Colloidal gold   No number more than 1
    Chloride   20 mEq/L higher than serum
C. Urine
    1. Adrenal chemistry
      Aldosterone   2–26 μg/24 hr (Kliman and
                        Peterson)
      Catecholamines   5–150 μg/24 hr
                        5–100 μg/25 hr (Lund)

Metanephrines	0.3–0.9 mg/24 hr (Pisano)
VMA	0.5–12 mg/24 hr
	0.5–7 mg/24 hr (Pisano)
17-KS male	10–25 mg/24 hr
female under 50	5–15 mg/24 hr
female over 50	4–8 mg/24 hr
17–OHCS: male	3–12 mg/24 hr
female	3–10 mg/24 hr
17–KG: male	8–25 mg/24 hr
female	5–18 mg/24 hr

2. Miscellaneous chemistry

Amylase	Up to 300 units/hr (p. 310)
Amylase clearance/creatinine clearance ratio	1–4% (p. 310)
Calcium	Less than 250 mg/24 hr (reg. diet)
Creatinine	1.0–1.8 gm/24 hr
Glucose	0–0.3 gm/24 hr
Potassium	26–123 mEq/24 hr
Protein	0–0.1 gm/24 hr
Sodium	30–90 mEq/L/24 hr (p. 141)
Uric acid	250–750 mg/24 hr
5-HIAA	1–7 mg/24 hr (Goldenberg)

3. Urinalysis

Protein	0–30 mg/100 (random)
	0–0.1 gm/24 hr
WBC	0–5/HPF
RBC	0–1/HPF
Urobilinogen	0–1 Ehrlich unit
	0–1:20
Sugar	Neg
Acetone	Neg

Index